Tilapia Culture

AF789932

Tilapia Culture

Second Edition

Abdel-Fattah M. El-Sayed
Oceanography Department
Faculty of Science
Alexandria University
Alexandria, Egypt

ELSEVIER

ACADEMIC PRESS
An imprint of Elsevier

Academic Press is an imprint of Elsevier
125 London Wall, London EC2Y 5AS, United Kingdom
525 B Street, Suite 1650, San Diego, CA 92101, United States
50 Hampshire Street, 5th Floor, Cambridge, MA 02139, United States
The Boulevard, Langford Lane, Kidlington, Oxford OX5 1GB, United Kingdom

Copyright © 2020 Elsevier Inc. All rights reserved.

No part of this publication may be reproduced or transmitted in any form or by any means, electronic or mechanical, including photocopying, recording, or any information storage and retrieval system, without permission in writing from the publisher. Details on how to seek permission, further information about the Publisher's permissions policies and our arrangements with organizations such as the Copyright Clearance Center and the Copyright Licensing Agency, can be found at our website: www.elsevier.com/permissions.

This book and the individual contributions contained in it are protected under copyright by the Publisher (other than as may be noted herein).

Notices
Knowledge and best practice in this field are constantly changing. As new research and experience broaden our understanding, changes in research methods, professional practices, or medical treatment may become necessary.

Practitioners and researchers must always rely on their own experience and knowledge in evaluating and using any information, methods, compounds, or experiments described herein. In using such information or methods they should be mindful of their own safety and the safety of others, including parties for whom they have a professional responsibility.

To the fullest extent of the law, neither the Publisher nor the authors, contributors, or editors, assume any liability for any injury and/or damage to persons or property as a matter of products liability, negligence or otherwise, or from any use or operation of any methods, products, instructions, or ideas contained in the material herein.

Library of Congress Cataloging-in-Publication Data
A catalog record for this book is available from the Library of Congress

British Library Cataloguing-in-Publication Data
A catalogue record for this book is available from the British Library

ISBN: 978-0-12-816509-6

For information on all Academic Press publications visit our website at
https://www.elsevier.com/books-and-journals

Publisher: Charlotte Cockle
Acquisition Editor: Patricia Osborn
Editorial Project Manager: Devlin Person
Production Project Manager: James Selvam
Cover Designer: Alan Studholme

Typeset by TNQ Technologies

Working together
to grow libraries in
developing countries
www.elsevier.com • www.bookaid.org

Contents

Preface to the Second Edition

Almost fourteen years have passed since the first edition of this book appeared in 2006, during which tilapia culture industry has witnessed an outstanding growth rate and faced a lot of challenges as well. Tilapia production by 2017 had increased by almost threefold over the production reported in the first edition of this book. This has been possible because of the impressive innovations and technical and extension developments in tilapia aquaculture, in addition to the governmental will and supports in many countries worldwide.

I was really delighted that the first edition of this book was well received by the scientific community all over the globe. The positive response and feedback of many researchers, students and tilapia practitioners encouraged me to think of a second edition, to update the relatively old information of the book, in order to keep abreast of rapid developments in tilapia culture research and technology. With a quick navigation in the different publishing media, I was able to find over 3000 documents, published after 2006, on tilapia culture and related disciplines. With such a huge amount of new information in hand, updating the book was certainly timely. However, it was impossible to include all these documents in this second edition, together with the almost 1000 references contained in the first edition. Therefore, publications that were directly related to the practices and enhancement of tilapia culture were selected.

It also took me a long while to decide whether to keep the old references of the first edition or to reduce them and replace them with the new references I intend to include. I finally decided to keep the old information, as far as it is relevant and useful, and just build on it. I believe this would be more helpful for the readers, especially young researchers and tilapia farming beginners, since they will find a comprehensive knowledge on the topic they are reading, covering a long time span. It is no surprise, therefore, that this new edition of *Tilapia Culture* includes over 1600 references. Managing and handling this huge number of references was a real headache.

The old chapters of the first edition remained unchanged; just reviewed, updated and the relevant new information published after 2006 was added. Also, several sections of these chapters have been rearranged and/or expanded. Two new chapters were added: one on tilapia distribution, transfers and introductions and their ecological impacts (Chapter 3) and the other on tilapia trade and marketing (Chapter 11). In addition, the new second edition delivers new contents in the existing chapters on taxonomic position of tilapias, the use of probiotics and other additives in tilapia culture, new technological innovations, sustainability approaches and practices, such as best management practices, and value chain analysis of tilapia farming.

I sincerely hope the readers will find this second edition useful, and they would appreciate the effort paid in bringing all this new information to them in a single volume. I hope also that the objectives for which this edition was issued have been achieved. Finally, I would very much welcome any feedback from my colleagues and fellow readers.

Professor Abdel-Fattah M. El-Sayed
Alexandria, Egypt

Chapter 1

Current state and future potential

Chapter outline

1.1 Historical review*

Aquaculture is the farming of aquatic organisms, including fish, molluscs, crustaceans and aquatic plants in freshwater, brackish water and seawater environments. Capture fisheries, on the other hand, is the exploitation of aquatic organisms by the public, as a common property resource, with or without appropriate licences. Aquaculture's contribution toward total global fisheries landings was very low during 1950—70, ranging from only 638,577 t (3.2%) in 1950 to 5.2% in 1970. Global aquaculture production continued to grow to 9.6% in 1980 and 16.3% in 1990. The average annual compounded growth rate of aquaculture production was 9% per year during 1970—2000, compared with only 1.3% for capture fisheries (Tacon, 2003). From 2000 to 2017, global aquaculture grew at a steady rate of 6.3% to reach 111.95 million metric tons (mmt) in 2017 (Fig. 1.1). About half of total global aquaculture production in 2017 was finfish (53.40 mmt, 47.7%), 83% of them came from freshwater environments.

Tilapia are freshwater fishes belong to family Cichlidae. They are native to Africa but have been introduced into many tropical, subtropical and temperate regions of the world during the second half of the 20th century (Pillay, 1990). The introduction of tilapia into those areas was for (1) farming as food fish, (2) recreational fishing, (3) aquatic weed control and (4) research purposes. Tilapia have many attributes that make them an ideal candidate for aquaculture, especially in developing countries. These include their:

1. Fast growth.
2. Tolerance to a wide range of environmental conditions (such as temperature, salinity and low dissolved oxygen).
3. Resistance to stress and disease.
4. Ability to reproduce in captivity and having short generation time.
5. Feeding on low trophic levels and acceptance of artificial feeds immediately after yolk-sac absorption.

Tilapia culture is believed to have originated some 4000 year ago, about 1000 years before carp culture was introduced into China (Balarin and Hatton, 1979). However, other than biblical references and illustrations from ancient Egyptians tombs, very little information is available

* It should be first mentioned that unless otherwise indicated, all data presented in this chapter were derived from FAO, 2019a (http://www.fao.org/fishery/statistics/global-aquaculture-production/query/en) and 2019b (http://www.fao.org/fishery/statistics/global-fisheries-production/query/en).

Tilapia Culture. https://doi.org/10.1016/B978-0-12-816541-6.00001-5
Copyright © 2020 Elsevier Inc. All rights reserved.

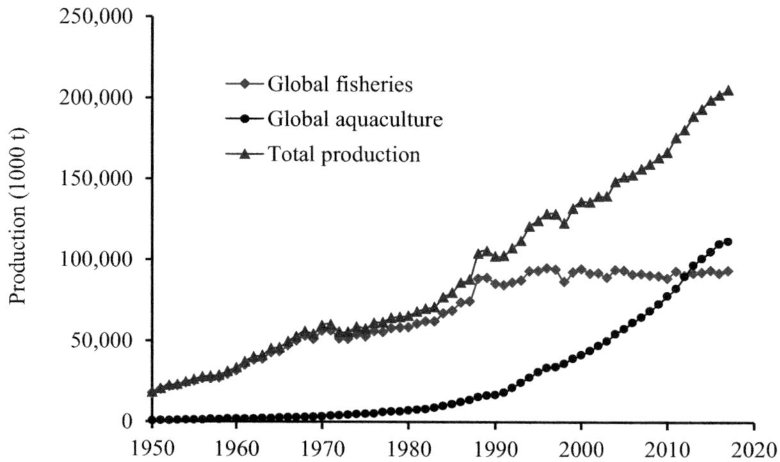

FIGURE 1.1 Global fisheries and aquaculture production during 1950–2017. *From FAO Fisheries and Aquaculture Statistics (http://www.fao.org/fishery/statistics/en) 2019a,b.*

on their culture during those early times. Current FAO aquaculture production statistics indicates that about 125 countries practice tilapia culture, since these countries reported tilapia production from aquaculture in 2017 (FAO, 2019a). The global development of tilapia culture has passed through three distinctive phases (Fig. 1.2).

1.1.1 Before 1970

The contribution of tilapia production to total global aquaculture production before 1970 was very minor, representing less than 1% of total production. For example, tilapia production in 1969 was only 24,633 t, representing 0.76% of total aquaculture production (3,238,079 t). Very few countries practiced tilapia culture during that period. Only seven countries reported tilapia production in 1950, increased to 12 countries in 1969. Taiwan, China, Egypt, Nigeria, Israel and Thailand were the major tilapia producers. The insignificant contribution of tilapia production during that period was mainly because aquaculture in general, and tilapia culture in particular, was not known as a food production system in most of the world countries.

1.1.2 From 1970 to 2000

Tilapia culture was gradually expanding worldwide during the period from 1970 to 2000. The number of countries practicing tilapia culture increased significantly to reach 88 countries in 2000, compared to only 12 countries in 1969. However, tilapia production in many of those countries was very limited. According to FAO aquaculture production statistics, out of those 88 countries, 45 countries produced less than 200 t yr^{-1} each. The production of farmed tilapia gradually increased to reach 1,189,926 t by 2000, representing 2.82% of total aquaculture production (5.7% of total fish production) in 2000. During that period, the

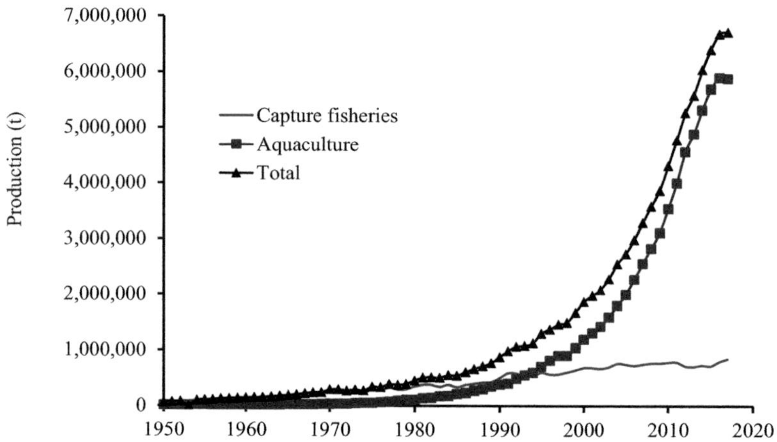

FIGURE 1.2 Global production of tilapia from aquaculture and capture fisheries during 1950–2017. *From FAO Fisheries and Aquaculture Statistics (http://www.fao.org/fishery/statistics/en) 2019a,b.*

annual growth of tilapia production fluctuated between <6% and >28%, with an average of 14.0%.

1.1.3 From 2001–now

Tilapia culture has witnessed a huge expansion during the past two decades. As a result, the number of countries practicing tilapia culture has reached 125 countries, as mentioned earlier. The production of farmed tilapia has also increased more than 350% to jump from 383,654 t in 2000 representing 2.82% of total aquaculture production reaching 5,714,901 t in 2017, representing 5.1% of total aquaculture production and 10.14% of total farmed fish production. The average annual growth of tilapia production during that period approached 10.6%.

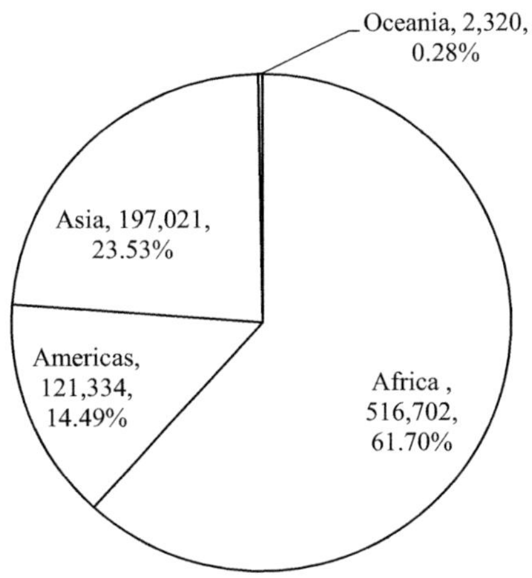

FIGURE 1.4 Tilapia production from capture fisheries (t, %) by region in 2017. *From FAO Fisheries and Aquaculture Statistics (http://www.fao.org/fishery/statistics/en) 2019b.*

1.2 Global tilapia production

1.2.1 Capture fisheries

Global landing of tilapia from capture fisheries has increased progressively during the 1950s through 1980s. Since then, the landings were almost stable, fluctuating around 500,000–837,447 t yr^{-1} (Fig. 1.2). Africa is, by far, the most important tilapia producer from capture fisheries, where it contributed about 61.7% of global landing in 2017, followed by Asia (23%) and the Americas (14.5%) (Figs. 1.3 and 1.4). Therefore, it is no surprise that among the world's top 10 tilapia producers from capture fisheries, six are African countries (Fig. 1.5). The top 10 producers included three Asian countries (Indonesia, Philippines and Sri Lanka) and one North American country (Mexico).

Among all tilapia species, Nile tilapia (*Oreochromis niloticus*) is the most important identified species in capture fisheries. In 2017, the production of that species amounted 278,720 t, representing 33.3% of total production. Other identified species include Mozambique tilapia (*Oreochromis mossambicus*), blue tilapia (*Oreochromis aureus*), jaguar guapote (*Parachromis managuensis*) and mango (Galilee) tilapia (*Sarotherodon galilaeus*). However, most of tilapia catches are not identified. For example, 54.7% of the catch in 2017 was reported under 'unidentified' cichlids, 'mouthbrooding' cichlids and 'unidentified' tilapias.

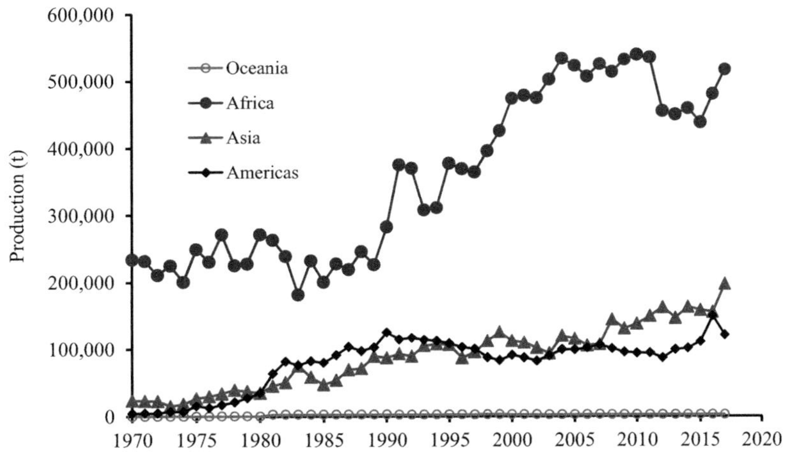

FIGURE 1.3 Tilapia capture by region during 1950–2017. *From FAO Fisheries and Aquaculture Statistics (http://www.fao.org/fishery/statistics/en) 2019b.*

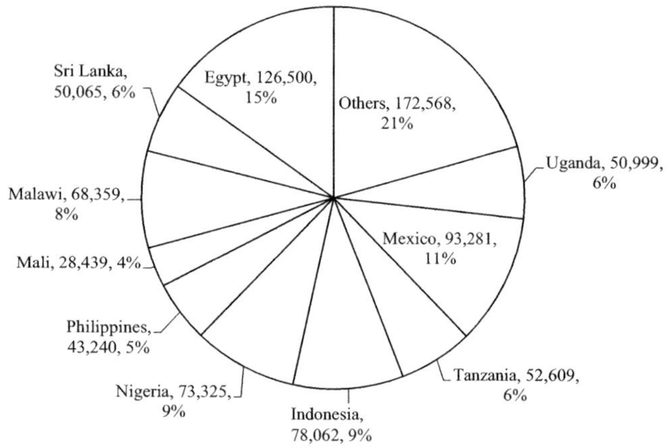

FIGURE 1.5 Top 10 producers of tilapia from capture fisheries (t, %) in 2017. *From FAO Fisheries and Aquaculture Statistics (http://www.fao.org/fishery/statistics/en) 2019b.*

1.2.2 Aquaculture

As pointed out earlier, the production of farmed tilapia has increased from 28,260 t in 1970 to 5,880,586 t in 2017. However, these values may be much less than the actual amounts produced. The under-reported tilapia production can be attributed to the following:

1. The reproductive characteristics of tilapia. The simple, frequent and asynchronous reproduction of tilapia makes the estimate of total production of these fishes almost impossible.
2. The poor management of evaluating and utilizing tilapia. The large amounts consumed by tilapia farmers' families and the amounts which are locally marketed informally may make production statistics incorrect and unreliable. For example, it has been reported that about 20% of aquaculture production in rural China is consumed by farmers' families. The global production of farmed tilapia may, therefore, be higher than the officially reported quantities.

The global production trends of farmed tilapia can be divided into two distinctive phases:

- During the 1950s through 1970s, tilapia culture grew at a relatively slow rate, where farmed tilapia production was much lower than that of capture fisheries (Fig. 1.2).
- In the 1980s through 1990s, tilapia culture has expanded at a much wider and more rapid rate, where the gap between tilapia landings from capture fisheries and aquaculture continued to narrow, until the production of farmed tilapia exceeded the landings from capture fisheries in 1993 (Fig. 1.2). Since then, tilapia culture has been growing at a very high rate, while tilapia landings from capture fisheries are about stable.

Since tilapia can tolerate a wide range of water salinity, they are currently farmed in freshwater, brackish water and even seawater environments; but freshwater tilapia aquaculture is dominating. The production of tilapia from freshwater systems reached 4,858,927 t in 2017, representing 82.6% of the total farmed tilapia production. The value of farmed tilapia has also witnessed a great increase during the past two decades. This value increased from about $US 239 million in 1986 to $US 11,031.1 million in 2017. As expected, the value of Nile tilapia represented between 65 and 70% of the total market value of farmed tilapia during the past decades (Fig. 1.6).

1.2.3 Major producers

Despite the fact that more than 125 countries practiced tilapia farming in 2017, only 5 countries (China, Indonesia,

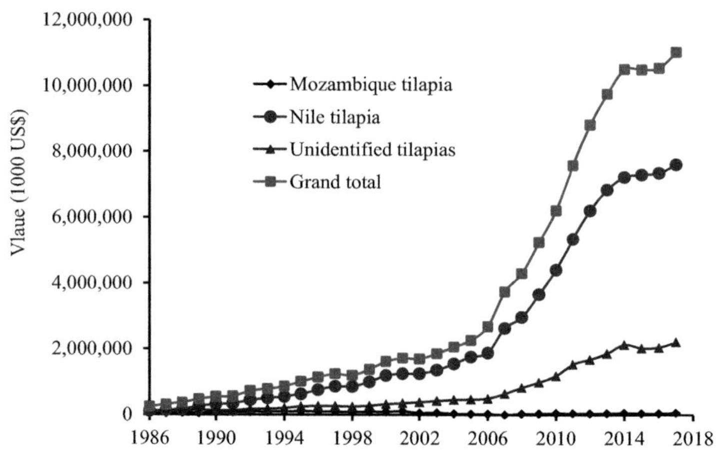

FIGURE 1.6 The value of important farmed tilapia during 1986–2017. *From FAO Fisheries and Aquaculture Statistics (http://www.fao.org/fishery/statistics/en) 2019a.*

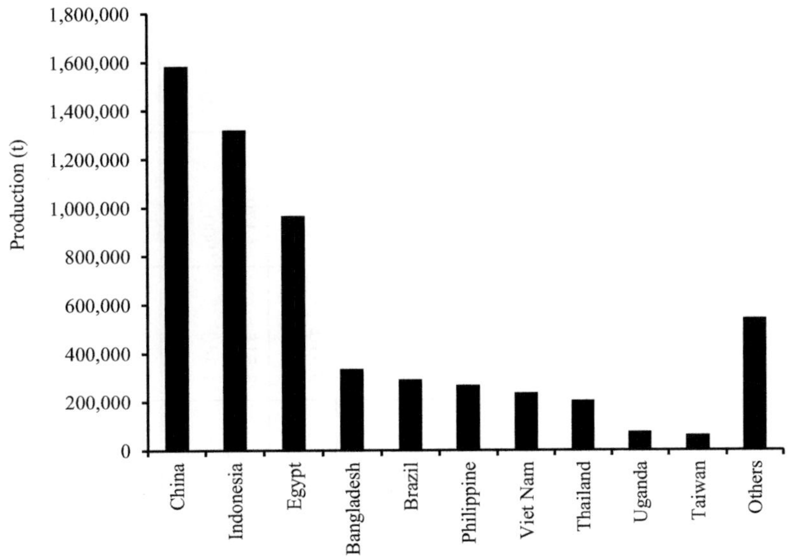

FIGURE 1.7 Top 10 producers of farmed tilapia (t) in 2017. *From FAO Fisheries and Aquaculture Statistics (http://www.fao.org/fishery/statistics/en) 2019a.*

Egypt, Bangladesh and Brazil) dominated the world production. Those countries yielded 76.5% of global tilapia production in 2017. China alone produced 1,584,680 t in 2017, representing 26.9% of total production, followed by Indonesia (22.4%), Egypt (16.5%), Bangladesh (5.7%) and Brazil (4.9%) (Fig. 1.7). However, the value of farmed tilapia in China in 2017 was $US 4308.7 million, representing only 2.9% of the total value of aquaculture production in China ($US 148,963.1 million). This is mainly because tilapia is produced in China as a low-value food fish and used typically for local consumption in rural areas. On the other hand, the value of farmed tilapia in Egypt contributed 60.5% to total aquaculture value in 2017, whereas in Indonesia, it represented 16.3%. The values of farmed tilapia in selected major producer nations in 2017 are given in Fig. 1.8.

1.2.4 Major cultured species

Among cultured fishes of the world, tilapia rank second in terms of production, only after carps. According to FAO statistics, 16 tilapia/cichlid groups, in addition to unidentified cichlids, have been used for aquaculture production. However, commercial tilapia culture is currently restricted to about 10 species (Table 1.1). Nile tilapia is, by far, the most important farmed tilapia species in the world. It represented 70–>80% of total tilapia production during 2000–17. Nile tilapia is also ranked third in terms of global farmed fish production in 2017, only after grass carp and silver carp (Fig. 1.9), jumping two positions since 2002. Tilapia hybrids (particularly Blue–Nile hybrids) have played a significant role in global tilapia production since mid-2000s, contributing 6.7% in 2017. Unidentified tilapias

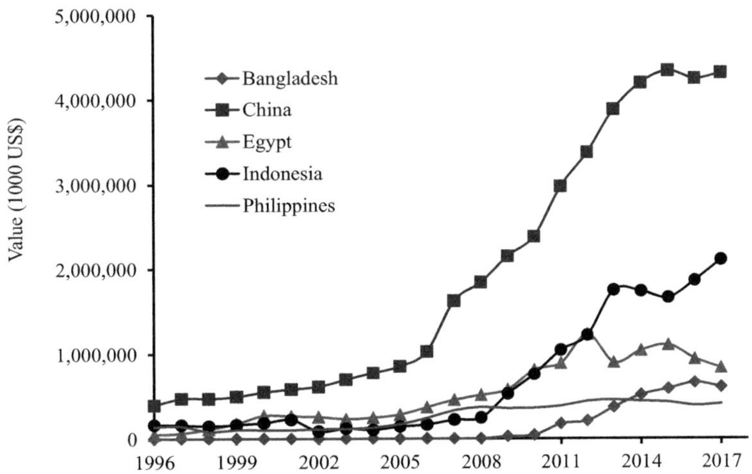

FIGURE 1.8 The value of farmed tilapia (US$ 1000) in selected major producers during 1996–2017. *From FAO Fisheries and Aquaculture Statistics (http://www.fao.org/fishery/statistics/en) 2019a.*

TABLE 1.1 Major cultured tilapia species and species production (t) in the world during 2000–17.

Species	Scientific name	2000	2002	2004	2006	2008	2010	2012	2014	2016	2017
Nile tilapia	*Oreochromis niloticus*	970,646	1,115,989	1,458,290	1,673,791	2,061,576	2,502,174	3,155,418	3,553,588	3,918,092	4,130,281
Blue-Nile tilapia hybrid	*Oreochromis aureus* x *O. niloticus*	0.	0.	0.	247,500	277,600	321,522	353,739	385,312	390,082	396,259
Mozambique tilapia	*Oreochromis mossambicus*	45,716	50,807	42,598	39,792	37,964	30,910	24,244	42,443	42,911	61,551
Tilapia shiranus	*Oreochromis shiranus*	0.	0.	0.	0.	0.	0.	820	1,754	4,851	5,311
Three spotted tilapia	*Oreochromis andersonii*	2,750	2,700	2,000	1,900	2,014	3,735	4,038	3,310	4,036	4,140
Blue tilapia	*O. aureus*	1,277	3,407	4,814	5,108	5,786	4,989	4,695	3,516	3,179	3,144
Longfin tilapia	*Oreochromis macrochir*	210	130	90	150	187	1,420	1,620	1,340	900	1000
Redbreast tilapia	*Tilapia rendalli*	853	210	136	165	160	1,001	1,617	2,770	3,142	5,593
Unidentified tilapias		168,095	243,852	287,175	296,129	440,807	627,966	875,782	1,160,793	1,213,509	1,272,468
Total		1,150,382	1,365,633	1,750,477	2,210,408	2,775,392	3,494,215	4,423,821	5,155,720	5,581,596	5,880,586

0., denotes an actual null value.
From FAO Fisheries and Aquaculture Statistics (http://www.fao.org/fishery/statistics/en) 2019a.

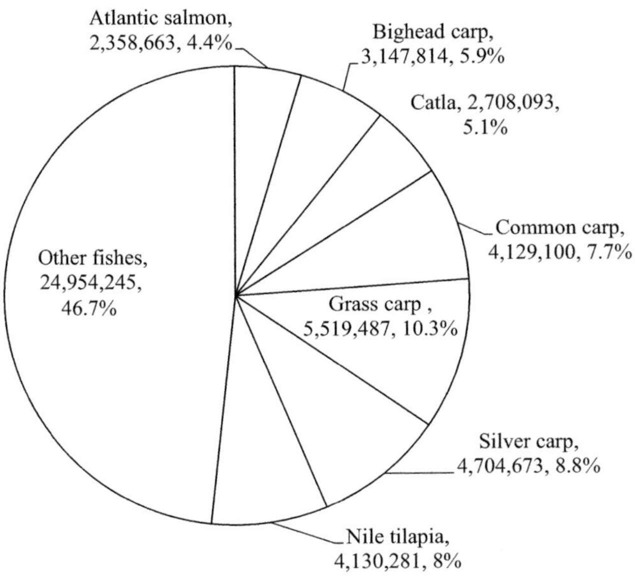

FIGURE 1.9 Global production of major farmed fish species (t, %) in 2017. *From FAO Fisheries and Aquaculture Statistics (http://www.fao.org/fishery/statistics/en) 2019a.*

also represent a significant proportion of the production. This category amounted 1,272,468 t in 2017, representing 21.6% of total tilapia production. The contribution of other tilapias, including Mozambique tilapia, blue tilapia, tilapia shiranus (*Oreochromis shiranus*), longfin tilapia (*Oreochromis macrochir*), three spotted tilapia (*Oreochromis andesonii*) and redbreast tilapia (*Tilapia rendalli*) is insignificant. They contributed only about 1% to total farmed tilapia production in 2017.

1.3 Tilapia production in Asia

Asia is the largest tilapia producer in the world, accounting for 70.4% of the production of global farmed tilapia in 2017. Tilapia is farmed mainly in freshwater environment in Asia. In 2017, about 96% of total farmed tilapia production came from freshwater environments. Thirty-one Asian countries, mainly in South Asia and the Far East, reported tilapia production in 2017. Tilapia culture in Asia has witnessed three developmental phases:

1. 1950–80: During that early period, tilapia culture was practiced at a very small scale and grew at slow rates. The production gradually increased from only 4810 t in 1950 to reach 88,011 t in 1980.
2. 1981–91: The production of tilapia witnessed a sharp increase from 109,301 t in 1981 to reach 353,686 t in 1991, with over 300% increase.
3. 1992–now: This period was characterized by an outstanding expansion and development of tilapia culture in Asia. As a result, tilapia production jumped from 421,649 t in 1992 to 4,140,896 t in 2017 (Table 1.2).

The growth rate in the production of farmed tilapia in Asia during 1950–2002 was among the fastest in world, with an overall average of 20.5% annually. During the period 2002–17, the annual growth rate of tilapia continued to increase, reaching an average of 21.4%. As mentioned above, it is noteworthy that the recorded production of tilapia in Asia is lower than the real production because considerable proportion of produced tilapia is consumed by fish farmers and their families, leading to underestimation of tilapia production in Asia.

1.3.1 Major producers

As stated earlier, Asia is the most important tilapia producer in the world. Currently, 61% of Asian countries practice tilapia culture, since 31 out of 51 countries reported tilapia production in 2017 (Table 1.3), with China being the largest producer. In 2017, China contributed about 38.3% to total Asian tilapia production. When the contribution of China is discounted, the contribution of Asia to global tilapia production declines from 70.4% to 44.1% in 2017. All the production of tilapia in China comes from freshwater culture, mainly from semi-intensive culture systems. The production trend in China can be divided into two phases (Fig. 1.10):

- 1950–89: During that period, the production of tilapia increased slowly from 660 t in 1950 to 39,000 t in 1988. China's production was exceeded by other Asian countries such as Taiwan, Indonesia and the Philippines.
- 1990–now: From 1990 onwards, the production of farmed tilapia in China increased at an exceptionally high rate, with an average annual growth rate of 12%. As a result, China currently dominates tilapia production in Asia.

In Indonesia, tilapia culture grew at a relatively slow rate from the 1970s through 2002. Afterwards, tilapia production witnessed a substantial increase, to jump from 139,651 t in 2004 to 1,319,200 t in 2017, with an annual growth rate of 20%. Indonesia is currently the second largest tilapia producer in the world, only after China. Tilapia culture is also growing at a very high rate in some other Asian countries including, Bangladesh, the Philippines, Thailand and Vietnam. Those six countries yielded 95.3% of Asian tilapia production in 2017.

The story of tilapia culture in Bangladesh and Vietnam is worth mentioning. Tilapia is not endemic to these two countries, and they do not have a long history in tilapia culture. Until 2008, no official tilapia production was reported in Bangladesh; the initial production started in 2009, with only 16,237 t. Since then, tilapia production in Bangladesh has been growing at an outstanding rate to reach 334,513 t in 2017, just in 9 years, with an exceptional

TABLE 1.2 Continental production of farmed tilapia during 1970–2017.

Continent	1970	1975	1980	1985	1990	1995	2000	2005	2010	2015	2017
Africa	4,723	6,735	12,456	28,724	33,094	35,706	176,963	244,416	644,383	1,080,724	1,220,320
Asia	23,337	39,938	86,934	175,014	328,546	616,670	911,795	1,566,283	2,521,555	3,943,248	4,140,896
Europe	0 -	0 -	0 -	120	203	320	180	453	308	779	334
N. America and Caribbean	200	1,032	3,856	9,322	13,514	14,335	34,010	66,158	68,784	122,777	130,848
Oceania	0 -	0 -	3	69	143	228	461	344	1,375	1,497	1,534
South America	0 -	19	103	366	2,307	30,658	66,995	113,926	257,807	308,167	386,649
Grand total	28,260	48,892	107,459	211,594	379,184	703,725	1,189,926	1,991,580	3,494,215	5,457,194	5,880,586

0-, denotes an actual null value.
From FAO Fisheries and Aquaculture Statistics (http://www.fao.org/fishery/statistics/en) 2019a.

TABLE 1.3 Production of farmed tilapia by country in Asia during 1970–2017.

Year	1970	1980	1990	2000	2002	2004	2006	2008	2010	2012	2014	2016	2017
Bangladesh	0.	0.	0.	0.	0.	0.	0.	0.	24,823	123,712	283,937	342,567	334,513
Cambodia	0.	0.	170	370	376	500	600	1,150	1,700	2,100	3,500	5,448	6,500
China	5,828	9,000	106,071	548,261	611,165	774,662	990,012	1,110,298	1,284,839	1,414,146	1,540,777	1,560,145	1,584,680
Hong Kong	450	2,120	1,195	613	411	480	351	391	297	266	368	261	250
Indonesia	1,191	14,901	53,768	85,179	109,768	139,651	218,934	328,831	458,752	717,831	1,040,594	1,154,849	1,319,200
Israel	1,400	2,512	4,795	7,059	7,819	9,270	8,235	6,751	7,662	7,215	7,797	7,559	7,350
Japan	0-	2,392	5,825	434	0.	0.	0-	0-	0-	0-	0.	0.	0.
Jordan	0.	0.	40	563	515	487	420	264	282	200	285	285	285
Republic of Korea	0-	0-	650	787	756	302	272	388	251	184	152	129	138
Kuwait	0.	0.	0-	30	16	275	557	274	300	299	295	186	175
Laos	20	176	1,250	18,928	26,872	29,205	15,050	16,129	20,580	25,500	27,000	25,000	28,000
Malaysia	12	366	1,145	18,471	20,757	25,642	29,810	34,823	38,886	52,295	38,924	36,998	32,526
Myanmar	0.	0.	0.	0.	9,200	18,500	26,300	32,794	40,583	43,684	47,699	33,134	33,755
Nepal	0.	0.	0.	0.	0.	0.	0.	0.	50	65	273	350	550
Philippines	1,417	13,214	76,142	92,579	122,399	145,869	202,040	257,133	258,839	260,536	259,198	259,045	267,735
Saudi Arabia	0.	0.	1,926	3,968	2,019	2,396	3,781	3,778	3,682	5,220	6,291	7,770	7,780
Singapore	0.	0.	0.	37	142	53	39	7	40	104	129	304	186
Sri Lanka	0.	20	30	60	90	680	1,260	2,180	850	1,825	19,985	15,468	15,188
Syria	0.	102	596	2,626	2,571	3,660	3,460	3,874	3,163	2,250	1,100	900	845
Taiwan	11,287	33,712	52,047	49,235	85,059	89,275	72,574	81,009	74,888	73,334	69,726	63,028	61,711
Thailand	1,732	8,419	22,895	82,581	83,837	160,407	205,568	217,313	179,355	203,074	190,016	200,824	203,696
Vietnam	0.	0.	0.	0.	0.	0.	0.	50,000	121,196	196,571	244,483	219,607	235,311
Total Asia	23,337	86,934	328,546	911,795	1,083,849	1,401,393	1,779,394	2,147,601	2,521,555	3,130,945	3,783,117	3,934,369	4,140,896

Countries with production less than 100 t per year were excluded.
0. and 0-, denote an actual null value.
From FAO Fisheries and Aquaculture Statistics (http://www.fao.org/fishery/statistics/en) 2019a.

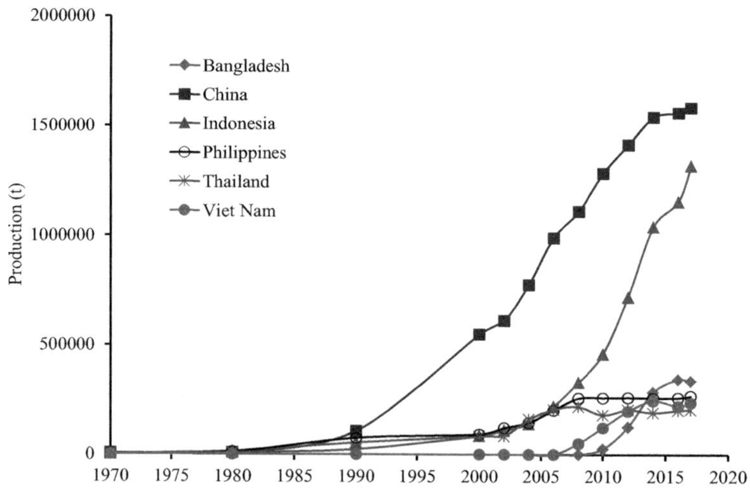

FIGURE 1.10 Major tilapia producers in Asia during 1970–2017. *From FAO Fisheries and Aquaculture Statistics (http://www.fao.org/fishery/statistics/en) 2019a.*

average annual growth rate of 80%. As a result, Bangladesh is currently ranked fourth, among the top tilapia producers in the world. Similarly, the first official recording of commercial tilapia production in Vietnam began in 2008. As in the case of Bangladesh, tilapia production in Vietnam witnessed a huge expansion during the last few years, to increase from 50,000 t in 2008 to 235,311 t in 2017, allowing it to occupy the eighth position among the top 10 tilapia producers in the world. These two success stories should motivate other producers in other regions to take the necessary steps towards development of tilapia culture industry. The lesson learnt is that such development can be quite fast, if the will and motivation exist.

The Philippines and Thailand are also among the top 10 global tilapia producers (sixth and eighth). Tilapia farming in other Asian countries, such as Laos, Malaysia, Myanmar, Sri Lanka, Israel and Saudi Arabia, has gained considerable attention in recent years. On the other hand, tilapia production in Taiwan has declined by 31% during the last 13 years (from 89,275 t in 2004 to 63,028 t in 2016). Similar decline in tilapia production was also observed in other countries, such as Jordan, Palestine, Syria and Qatar.

1.3.2 Major cultured species

It has been reported that Mozambique tilapia was the first tilapia species to be introduced to Asia, into the Indonesian island of Java, in 1939 (Guerrero, 2001). Subsequently, the species was introduced into other Asian countries during the 1940s through the 1960s of the last century and was considered as a prime candidate for aquaculture in Asia. Thus, the average annual production of this species increased at a rate of 26.7% during 1970–80, compared with 13.1% for Nile tilapia. However, Mozambique tilapia may have suffered from inbreeding problems due to the small number of original population of founder stocks. The acceptance of tilapia farmers to Mozambique tilapia was also limited because of the problem of overcrowding and poor growth. The dark colour of this fish also reduces its marketability and consumer's acceptance. Subsequently, Nile tilapia attracted the attention in the 1960s and early 1970s as an ideal aquaculture substitute for Mozambique tilapia. Therefore, commercial culture of Mozambique tilapia in Asia has almost stopped, except in Indonesia where it is still practiced, but at a very limited scale. The Indonesian supply of that species in 2017 was 59,200 t (4.5% of total tilapia production in the country) compared to 1,260,000 t of Nile tilapia.

Nile tilapia currently dominates tilapia culture in Asia, with a production of 2,868,103 t in 2017, representing 69.3% of total tilapia production in the continent (Table 1.4). In terms of countries, 21 Asian countries reported Nile tilapia production in 2017, compared to only six countries in 1980. The contribution of other tilapias, including blue tilapia, Galilean tilapia (mango tilapia) (*S. galilaeus*), Wami tilapia (*Oreochromis hornorum*), sabaki tilapia (*Oreochromis spilurus*), Zill's tilapia (redbelly tilapia) (*Tilapia zillii*) and red-breast tilapia (Congo tilapia) (*T. rendalli*) is negligible. These species have been introduced to Asia mainly for research and experimental purposes.

In addition to the tilapia species mentioned, introgressive hybridization between Nile tilapia and Mozambique tilapia has been reported in several Asian countries. All-male hybrids of Nile tilapia and blue tilapia are also widely cultured in China and Taiwan. Red tilapia, which is generally a hybrid of Mozambique tilapia and Nile tilapia and/or blue tilapia, is also commonly cultured in many Asian countries, including China, Taiwan, Thailand, Indonesia and the Philippines. The hybrids are characterized by high growth rates, preferred colour and high consumers' acceptance. The

TABLE 1.4 Major cultured tilapia species and species production reported in Asia during 1970–2017.

Species	Scientific name	1970	1975	1980	1985	1990	1995	2000	2005	2010	2012	2014	2016	2017
Blue tilapia	*Oreochromis aureus*	0.	0.	0.	0.	0 0	0 0	0-	2,690	2,530	1,800	900	600	645
Blue-Nile tilapia, hybrid	*O. aureus* x *O. niloticus*	0.	0.	0.	0.	0.	0.	0.	0.	321,200	353,600	385,200	390,000	396,200
Mozambique tilapia	*Oreochromis mossambicus*	1,186	3,530	12,637	22,216	41,813	53,307	44,831	38,581	29,833	22,863	41,040	40,958	59,405
Nile tilapia	*Oreochromis niloticus*	9,464	16,023	31,781	65,256	201,015	490,547	775,623	1,349,200	1,776,662	2,169,477	2,556,761	2,695,336	2,868,103
Sabaki tilapia	*Oreochromis spilurus*	0.	0.	0.	0.	0-	60	83	85	300	360	370	280	280
Unidentified tilapias		12,687	20,385	42,516	87,542	85,718	72,756	91,258	175,727	391,030	582,845	798,846	807,095	816,262
Grand total		23,337	39,938	86,934	175,014	328,546	616,670	911,795	1,566,283	2,521,555	3,130,945	3,783,117	3,934,369	4,140,896

0. and 0-, denote an actual null value; 0 0, more than zero but less than half of the unit used.
From FAO Fisheries and Aquaculture Statistics (http://www.fao.org/fishery/statistics/en) 2019a.

production of blue–Nile tilapia hybrids reached 396,200 t in 2017, contributing 9.6% to total tilapia production. In addition, the contribution of other 'unidentified' tilapia groups to tilapia production has also been sharply increasing since 2010, to reach 816,262 t in 2017, accounting for 19.7% of total Asian production of farmed tilapia.

1.4 Tilapia production in Africa

Despite the fact that tilapia are African fishes, tilapia culture in Africa is relatively new, with a relatively low contribution to world tilapia production, being 21% in 2017. Farmed tilapia production in Africa, however, has sharply increased during the past few years (Table 1.2). Generally, the trend in tilapia production in Africa can be divided into three phases:

1. 1950–98: During this 47-year period, the production of tilapia slowly grew from 908 t in 1950 to 67,424 t in 1998.
2. 1999–2009: The production increased from 119,299 t in 1999 to 454,110 t in 2009, with a relatively high growth rate (16% per year).
3. 2010–now: Tilapia production has dramatically increased from 644,403 t in 2010 to 1,220,320 t in 2017, with an annual growth rate of 20%.

1.4.1 Major producers

In 2017, 46 African countries reported production of farmed tilapia, compared to only 10 countries in 1980. Unlike Asia, most farmed tilapia production in Africa comes from brackish water environments. In 2017, tilapia production from brackish water amounted 855,789 t, representing 70% of total Africa's tilapia production. Farmed tilapia output in Africa is dominated by a single country, Egypt (Table 1.5). The production of farmed tilapia in Egypt accounted for 79% (967,301 t) of total production of farmed tilapia in Africa in 2017. If the contribution of Egypt is discounted, Africa's contribution to global tilapia output would decline from 21% in 2017 to only 4.3%. Tilapia culture in Egypt is practiced mainly in brackish water environments in the northern lakes areas along the Mediterranean coast. In 2017, the production of tilapia from brackish water systems in Egypt reached 854,808 t, representing 88.4% of total tilapia production in the country (and 70% in the continent).

Tilapia culture is also widely practiced in other countries, including Uganda, Ghana, Nigeria, Kenya, Zambia and Zimbabwe (Table 1.5). It is noteworthy that Uganda was among the top 10 producers in the world in 2017 (ranked ninth), with a production of 74,924 t. Significant attention has also been given to tilapia farming in Mali, Malawi, Tanzania, Benin, Burundi and Sudan during the last few years. The contribution of the rest of African countries is insignificant.

1.4.2 Major cultured species

Eleven tilapia species are currently used for aquaculture in Africa (Table 1.6), compared to only three species/species groups in 1980. Nile tilapia is, by far, the most widely cultured species. Nile tilapia was reportedly cultured in 23 African countries out of 32 countries that practiced tilapia culture in Africa in 2001. It also accounted for 95.1% of total tilapia production in Africa in 2017. The culture of other tilapia species namely, blue tilapia (*O. aureus*), longfin tilapia (*O. macrochir*), three spotted tilapia (*Oreochromis andersonii*), Mozambique tilapia (*O. mossambicus*), tilapia shiranus (*O. shiranus*), Tanganyika tilapia (*Oreochromis tanganicae*), mango tilapia (*S. galilaeus*), blackchin tilapia (*S. melanotheron*), redbelly tilapia (*T. zillii*) and redbreast tilapia (*T. rendalli*) was reported in 2017, though production was very limited. In addition to these species, a considerable proportion of tilapia production is reported under 'unidentified' tilapia and tilapia hybrids. That category comes second after Nile tilapia in terms of production. The production of unidentified tilapias in 2017 amounted to 40,942 t, representing 3.4% of total tilapia production in Africa.

1.5 Tilapia production in South America

Tilapia culture started in South America at a small scale, mainly for subsistence farming in the early 1970s. The first FAO record of tilapia production in the region was reported in Colombia in 1971, with only 1 t of Nile tilapia. The progress of tilapia culture in South America can be divided into three phases:

1. 1971–82: During that period, tilapia culture was practiced in only two countries, Colombia and Peru, with a very little production ranging from 1 t in 1971 to 182 t in 1982.
2. 1983–94: During that period, the number of countries practicing tilapia culture increased gradually to six countries in 1994. Nevertheless, tilapia production was still very low and was dominated by one country, Colombia (87.5%).
3. 1995–2017: The production of cultured tilapia in South America increased from 30,658 t in 1995 to 386,654 t in 2017, with an annual growth rate of 18.4%. During that period, the number of countries practicing tilapia culture increased to 11 countries (Table 1.7). More than 99% of tilapia production comes from freshwater environments.

TABLE 1.5 Production of farmed tilapia by country in Africa during 1970–2017.

Country	1970	1975	1980	1985	1990	1995	2000	2005	2010	2012	2014	2016	2017
Angola	0.	0.	0.	0.	0.	0.	5	120	300	300	305	653	1,299
Benin	0.	0.	0.	11	0.	0.	0.	320	220	305	1,165	1,042	2,774
Burkina Faso	0-	0-	0-	33	3	0	5	50	180	177	175	270	270
Burundi	0.	0.	0.	2	30	48	48	48	15	158	160	1,260	1,325
Cameroon	0.	0.	25	91	80	50	40	220	294	605	865	1,125	1,125
Central African Republic	0.	5	76	283	100	200	120	85	100	100	100	100	100
Congo	0-	0-	0-	61	240	139	66	80	55	95	130	173	202
Democratic Republic of Congo	0.	0.	0.	180	700	600	2,073	2,959	2,960	2,859	2,861	3,146	3,185
Côte d'Ivoire	0.	0.	0.	13	32	162	967	706	1,275	2,500	2,500	3,740	3,900
Egypt	2,500	4,000	9,000	22,346	24,916	21,969	157,425	217,019	557,049	768,752	759,601	940,309	967,301
Ghana	94	199	251	321	280	350	3,712	954	9,424	26,400	36,900	50,900	53,200
Kenya	0.	0.	70	113	405	536	222	622	9,115	16,115	18,072	11,962	9,885
Madagascar	0.	0.	0.	74	40	0 0	0 0	20	50	50	1,163	1,600	1,880
Malawi	0.	6	30	65	50	28	500	767	2,346	2,819	4,119	7,222	11,217
Mali	0.	0.	0.	5	10	58	19	708	616	277	1,414	3,669	3,424
Morocco	0-	0-	0-	0-	0-	0-	0-	0-	130	100	200	250	300
Mozambique	0.	0.	0.	0.	15	36	0	116	177	495	1,019	1,180	1,835
Niger	0.	0.	0.	7	36	35	15	40	50	85	219	200	230
Nigeria	2,129	2,525	2,952	4,573	3,795	6,020	2,705	6,144	11,989	16,872	27,987	23,706	22,534
Rwanda	0.	0.	23	35	154	70	252	18	98	494	1,453	1,453	3,200
Senegal	0-	0-	0-	1	5	40	9	18	37	202	754	859	436
South Africa	0.	0.	0.	0-	30	25	110	275	10	234	290	330	360
Sudan	0.	0.	0.	0.	0.	0.	0.	0.	0.	600	1,000	4,000	5,000
Sudan (former)	0.	0.	0.	30	234	1,000	1,000	1,000	2,000	0-	0-	0-	0.
Tanzania	0.	0.	0.	21	375	200	210	4	200	2,913	3,000	3,800	9,000
Uganda	0.	0.	0.	13	32	116	600	4,239	31,670	52,303	53,093	74,654	74,924
Zambia	0.	0.	27	354	1,400	3,770	4,020	5,080	10,208	12,956	19,195	28,500	30,100
Zimbabwe	0-	0-	0-	38	50	50	2,041	2,450	2,700	8,000	10,510	10,000	10,215
Grand total	4,723	6,735	12,456	28,724	33,094	35,706	176,963	244,416	644,383	917,575	949,099	1,176,992	1,220,320

Countries with production less than 100 t per year were excluded.
0. and 0-, denote an actual null value.
From FAO Fisheries and Aquaculture Statistics (http://www.fao.org/fishery/statistics/en) 2019a.

TABLE 1.6 Major cultured tilapia species and species production in Africa during 1970–2017.

Species	Scientific name	1970	1975	1980	1985	1990	1995	2000	2005	2010	2012	2014	2016	2017
Blackchin tilapia	*Sarotherodon melanotheron*	0-	0-	0-	0-	0-	0-	7	128	16	58	264	263	176
Blue tilapia	*Oreochromis aureus*	0.	0.	0.	0.	12	0.	0.	255	225	650	650	650	650
Longfin tilapia	*Oreochromis macrochir*	0.	0.	0.	0.	60	368	210	90	1,420	1,620	1,340	900	1,000
Mozambique tilapia	*Oreochromis mossambicus*	0.	0.	0.	0.	30	36	55	108	1,076	1,320	1,400	1,949	2,142
Nile tilapia	*Oreochromis niloticus*	2,594	4,204	9,447	23,424	26,996	25,228	165,406	229,067	616,671	878,139	893,766	1,121,226	1,160,059
Redbelly tilapia	*Tilapia zillii*	0-	0-	0-	0-	8	19	201	19	171	2	2	7	2
Redbreast tilapia	*Tilapia rendalli*	0.	0.	0.	0.	100	843	853	151	1,001	1,617	2,770	3,142	5,593
Three spotted tilapia	*Oreochromis andersonii*	0.	0.	27	314	1,000	2,217	2,750	2,000	3,735	4,038	3,310	4,036	4,140
Tilapia shiranus	*Oreochromis shiranus*	0.	0.	0.	0.	0.	0.	0.	0.	0.	820	1,754	4,851	5,311
Tanganyika tilapia	*Oreochromis tanganicae*	0.	0.	0.	0.	0.	0.	0.	0.	0.	0.	185	300	300
Unidentified tilapias	*Oreochromis* (=*Tilapia*) spp.	2,129	2,531	2,982	4,986	4,888	6,995	7,474	12,594	20,060	29,301	43,648	39,663	40,942
Total		4,723	6,735	12,456	28,724	33,094	35,706	176,963	244,416	644,383	917,575	949,099	1,176,992	1,220,320

0. and 0-, denote an actual null value.
From FAO Fisheries and Aquaculture Statistics (http://www.fao.org/fishery/statistics/en) 2019a.

TABLE 1.7 Production of farmed tilapia by country in South America during 1970–2017.

Country	1970	1975	1985	1990	1995	2000	2005	2010	2012	2014	2016	2017
Brazil	0-	0.	0.	0.	12,014	32,459	67,851	155,451	183,712	200,080	241,040	290,075
Colombia	0-	19	302	2,040	16,057	22,870	24,000	49,893	52,688	58,500	62,330	63,450
Ecuador	0.	0.	0.	21	626	9,201	19,142	47,735	39,820	23,902	22,620	23,050
Guyana	0.	0.	12	30	160	368	370	234	124	29	53	80
Paraguay	0.	0.	0 0	26	80	40	1,700	2,366	4,200	5,980	6,900	6,811
Peru	0-	0-	52	186	0 0	47	619	2,013	3,174	4,610	2,950	3,042
Venezuela	0.	0.	0.	4	1,650	970	168	61	55	178	38	35
Total	0-	19	366	2,307	30,658	66,125	113,926	257,810	283,868	293,383	336,027	386,654

0. and 0-, denote an actual null value.
Countries with production less than 100 t $year^{-1}$ were excluded. From FAO Fisheries and Aquaculture Statistics (http://www.fao.org/fishery/statistics/en) 2019a.

1.5.1 Major producers

As mentioned earlier, Colombia was the only country practicing tilapia culture in South America in the 1970s, while Peru reported tilapia production starting 1979. In 1980, the total production of tilapia was only 103 t, increased to 2307 t in 1990. In 2002, 10 countries reported tilapia production, increased to 11 countries in 2017. Interestingly, the first record of tilapia production in Brazil appeared in 1995. During 1995–2017, tilapia production in that country increased from 12,014 to 290,075 t, with an average annual growth rate of 15.4%. Tilapia production in Brazil represented 75% of total farmed tilapia in South America in 2017. This means that Brazil has one of the fastest growth rates of tilapia production in South America. As a result, Brazil was ranked fifth among the top 10 tilapia producers in the world in 2017.

Colombia and Ecuador are the second and third major tilapia producers, with a production amounting to 63,450 t (16.4%) and 23,050 t (6%) in 2017. Brazil, Colombia and Ecuador accounted for 97% of total tilapia production in South America in 2017. Tilapia culture in Paraguay also witnessed a significant growth during the last 10 years; increasing from 1900 t in 2007 to 6811 t in 2017, contributing 1.8% of total tilapia production in the continent. The current production of tilapia in the other South American countries is not significant (Table 1.7).

1.5.2 Major cultured species

One of the major problems associated with tilapia culture in South America is that most of cultured tilapias are not identified. Many tilapia strains and hybrids are currently used for aquaculture with minimal control and regulation. As a result, most of the tilapia production in South America is reported in the 'unidentified' category (Table 1.8). Out of the 386,654 t of tilapia produced in 2017, 340,626 t were 'unidentified' tilapias (88%). Nile tilapia is the second most important cultured category, where it accounted for 11.9% (45,953 t) of the total tilapia production in 2017.

1.6 Tilapia production in North America and the Caribbean

Mozambique tilapia were introduced into the Caribbean in 1947 and first came to the United States in 1954 (Fitzsimmons, 2001). Tilapia culture in North America and the Caribbean is therefore relatively new and began in the 1960s and 1970s, at small scale, mainly for subsistence objectives. The first FAO record of tilapia production appeared in 1970, with 200 t from Mexico. During 1980–2010, the production increased steadily at an annual growth rate of 8.8%, to reach 68,783 t in 2010 (Table 1.9). The production sharply increased during the following 7 years (2011–17) to reach 130,848 t in 2017, with an average annual growth rate of 12.4%. The contribution of tilapia production in North America and the Caribbean to global tilapia production is limited, only 2.2% in 2017. More than 99% of tilapia production in the region comes from freshwater environments.

1.6.1 Major producers

Twenty-three countries from North America, Central America and the Caribbean reported tilapia production in 2002. However, the annual production of 13 of these countries was less than 100 t each. Unlike Asia, Africa and South America, where a single country in each continent dominates tilapia production, no single country dominates the production in North America and the Caribbean (Table 1.9). Instead, Mexico, Honduras, Costa Rica, Guatemala, the United States and El Salvador together accounted for 98% of tilapia production in 2017 (42.3%, 22.9%, 12.4%, 7.5%, 6.6% and 6.4%, respectively). The production of the rest of the North American, Central American and Caribbean countries is not significant.

1.6.2 Major cultured species

As in South America, 'unidentified' tilapias dominate tilapia production in North America and the Caribbean. Out of the 130,848 t of tilapia produced in 2017, 74,445 t were 'unidentified' tilapias (56.9%). Nile tilapia came second, accounting for 41.6% (54,492 t) of total tilapia production in 2017, followed by blue tilapia (1.4%). The production of other tilapias was only 62 t in 2017 (Table 1.10).

1.7 Future potentials

1. The ever-increasing global growth rate of tilapia culture, accompanied with the continuous introductions of these fishes into new geographical areas, reflects a positive future for tilapia culture. Looking across aquaculture species, tilapia is expected to have the fastest aquaculture growth up to 2030 (Kobayashi et al., 2015). Global tilapia production is expected to be more than doubled during this period. Tilapia is currently playing a substantial role as a food fish and cash crop in developing countries, particularly in Asia. More value added of tilapia products will come from developing countries. This will encourage foreign companies to invest in joint ventures in the main producing countries. It is also expected that the increase in tilapia imports will continue.
2. The genetically improved Nile tilapia developed by the International Center for Living Aquatic Resources Management (ICLARM) (currently known as WorldFish Center) and the YY-males developed by the University

TABLE 1.8 Major cultured tilapia species and species production (t) in South America during 1970–2017.

Species	Scientific name	1970	1975	1980	1985	1990	1995	2000	2005	2010	2012	2014	2016	2017
Green terror	*Aequidens rivulatus*	0.	0.	0.	0.	3	0 0	0-	0-	2	2	2	0.	0.
Mozambique tilapia	*Oreochromis mossambicus*	0.	0.	0.	12	30	160	183	183	0-	0-	0-	0.	0.
Nile tilapia	*Oreochromis niloticus*	0-	19	103	352	2,244	4,443	13,182	28,009	61,111	58,302	46,538	45,501	45,953
Unidentified tilapias	*Oreochromis* (=*Tilapia*) spp.	0.	0.	0.	0-	30	26,055	52,760	85,734	196,697	224,149	246,782	290,486	340,626
Other cichlids	Cichla spp.	0.	0.	0.	0.	0.	0.	0.	0.	0.	1,415	60	40	75
Grand total		0-	19	103	366	2,307	30,658	66,125	113,926	257,810	283,868	293,383	336,654	386,654

0. and 0-, denote an actual null value.
From FAO Fisheries and Aquaculture Statistics (http://www.fao.org/fishery/statistics/en) 2019a.

TABLE 1.9 Production of farmed tilapia by countries in North America and the Caribbean during 1970–2017. Countries with production less than 100 t per year were excluded.

Land Area	1970	1975	1980	1985	1990	1995	2000	2005	2010	2012	2014	2016	2017
Cuba	0-	200	1,012	2,978	3,733	2,096	730	390	510	400	466	429	449
Belize	0.	0.	0.	0.	0.	14	0.	425	658	63	47	55	60
Costa Rica	0.	0.	18	50	232	3,800	8,100	17,626	23,034	23,355	22,650	16,200	16,200
Dominican Republic	0.	0.	0.	3	100	985	994	16	20	478	1,024	1,000	1,000
El Salvador	0.	0.	0.	15	4	196	56	1,955	4,090	4,100	832	6,811	6,821
Guatemala	0.	0.	0	70	161	774	2,361	2,000	846	5,455	7,500	8,500	9,773
Haiti	0.	0.	0.	0.	0.	0.	10	30	330	620	900	1,160	1,270
Honduras	0-	0-	6	35	120	172	1,900	28,376	16,455	20,500	29,750	30,100	30,000
Jamaica	0.	0.	20	834	3,364	3,500	4,500	4,795	3,800	582	864	927	1,091
Mexico	200	2,000	6,907	3,200	5,000	1,482	6,726	2,151	8,243	23,749	54,536	58,191	55,358
Nicaragua	0-	0-	0-	2	3	5	24	350	385	7	38	4	11
Panama	0-	0-	0-	73	49	186	900	179	391	285	200	149	120
USA	0.	0.	0.	5	2,041	6,838	8,051	7,803	9,979	9,979	8,618	8,618	8,618
Grand total	200	2,200	7,963	7,301	14,891	20,143	34,402	66,158	68,784	89,636	127,496	132,229	130,848

0. and 0-, denote an actual null value.
From FAO Fisheries and Aquaculture Statistics (http://www.fao.org/fishery/statistics/en) 2019a.

TABLE 1.10 Major cultured tilapia species and species production in North America and the Caribbean during 1970–2017.

Species	Scientific name	1970	1975	1980	1985	1990	1995	2000	2005	2010	2012	2014	2016	2017
Blackbelt cichlid	*Cichlasoma maculicauda*	0.	0.	0.	0.	6	140	30	0.	0.	0.	0.	0.	0.
Blue tilapia	*Oreochromis aureus*	0-	200	1,012	2,984	3,736	2,103	1,276	1,523	2,234	2,245	1,966	1,829	1,849
Blue-Nile tilapia, hybrid	*O. aureus* x *Oreochromis niloticus*	0.	0.	0.	0.	0.	0.	0.	0.	322	139	112	82	59
Jaguar guapote	*Cichlasoma managuense*	0-	0-	0-	0 0	6	40	40	1	0	0	0	0	1
Mozambique tilapia	*Oreochromis mossambicus*	0.	0.	0.	2	60	0 0	497	0.	0.	59	2	2	2
Nile tilapia	*O. niloticus*	0-	0-	26	954	3,530	3,868	16,126	51,817	46,068	47,751	54,040	54,323	54,492
Unidentified tilapias	*Oreochromis* (=Tilapia) spp.	200	2,000	6,925	3 361	7,548	13,971	16,422	12,817	20,159	39,442	71,376	75,992	74,445
Grand total		200	2,200	7,963	7,301	14,891	20,143	34,402	66,158	68,784	89,636	127,496	132,229	130,484

0. and 0-, denote an actual null value.
From FAO Fisheries and Aquaculture Statistics (http://www.fao.org/fishery/statistics/en) 2019a.

of Wales, Swansea, to produce genetically male tilapia (Mair et al., 1997) became a breakthrough in global tilapia culture, particularly in Asia. Those tilapia strains have already been widely distributed in many countries around the world.

3. China is still dominating global tilapia production. In addition, a significant expansion in tilapia farming in other Asian countries such as Bangladesh, Indonesia, the Philippines, Thailand and Vietnam occurred during the last two decades. It is also expected that the traditional nonacceptance of tilapia in some Asian countries such as India and Pakistan will change, and the interest in tilapia culture in those countries will increase. Therefore, the production of farmed tilapia in Asia is very likely to show a further bloom in the near future.
4. The availability of huge freshwater resources, environmental conditions suitable for tilapia culture and culture inputs in many countries in the Americas (Brazil and Mexico, for instance) make the future of tilapia culture in those countries very bright. While Brazil is currently ranked fifth among the top tilapia producers in the world, Mexico is very likely to become a major global tilapia producer in the near future. Nile tilapia (mainly sex-reversed, all-males) will dominate the production in the future.
5. More values will be added to produced tilapia, through processing, filleting, and addition of new tilapia products will likely emerge globally, especially in the Americas, for domestic consumption as well as for international markets.
6. Despite the great potential of tilapia culture in Africa, the production is still limited, with the exception of Egypt, Uganda, Ghana and Kenya. The shortage of freshwater resources, culture inputs and technical experience are the main handicaps for tilapia culture development in Africa. Those factors may limit the future expansion of tilapia culture in the continent. However, tilapia culture may still play a significant role in rural development in Africa if it is integrated with other plant/animal farming systems.

1.8 Constraints

Despite the bright future of tilapia culture in many parts of the world, there are a number of constraints which might restrict the development of this industry:

- The inadequate knowledge of tilapia farmers in many developing countries on biological, technical, environmental and social factors related to tilapia culture. Understanding those factors is critical for improving farmers' skills and increasing farm productivity and sustainability.
- Lack or shortage of funds and technical assistance in many developing countries, especially in Africa and Latin America.
- Insufficient quality seeds and processed feeds, especially in the Americas, where most of farmed tilapias are 'unidentified' strains and hybrids. Feeds and seeds are also a major challenge facing tilapia culture in Africa.
- Poor extension service programmes, especially in remote, rural areas, where tilapia culture is expected to expand.
- The continuous increase in the cost of culture inputs, such as fingerlings, feeds, fertilizer, fuel and labour, which reduces the profitability of tilapia culture enterprises.

References

Balarin, J.D., Hatton, J.P., 1979. Tilapia: A Guide to Their Biology and Culture in Africa. University of Stirling, Scotland.

FAO (Food and Agriculture Organization of the United Nations), 2019a. Global Aquaculture Production 1950–2016. http://www.fao.org/fishery/statistics/global-aquaculture-production/query/en.

FAO (Food and Agriculture Organization of the United Nations), 2019b. Global Capture Production 1950–2016. http://www.fao.org/fishery/statistics/global-capture-production/query/en.

Fitzsimmons, K., 2001. Tilapia production in the Americas. In: Subasinghe, S., Singh, T. (Eds.), Tilapia: Production, Marketing and Technical Developments. Proceedings of the Tilapia 2001 International Technical and Trade Conference on Tilapia. Infofish, Kuala Lumpur, Malaysia, pp. 7–16.

Guerrero III, R.D., 2001. Tilapia culture in Southeast Asia. In: Subasinghe, S., Singh, T. (Eds.), Tilapia: Production, Marketing and Technical Developments. Proceedings of the Tilapia 2001 International Technical and Trade Conference on Tilapia. Infofish, Kuala Lumpur, Malaysia, pp. 97–103.

Kobayashi, M., Msangi, S., Batka, M., Vannuccini, S., Dey, M.M., Anderson, J.L., 2015. Fish to 2030: the role and opportunity for aquaculture. Aquaculture Economics and Management 19 (3), 282–300.

Mair, G.C., Abucay, J.S., Skibinski, D.O.F., Abella, T.A., Beardmore, J.A., 1997. Genetic manipulation of sex ratio for the large-scale production of all-male tilapia, *Oreochromis niloticus*. Canadian Journal of Fisheries and Aquatic Sciences 54, 396–404.

Pillay, T.V.R., 1990. Aquaculture Principles and Practices. Blackwell Science Ltd, Fishing News books, Oxford, Edinburgh, London, p. 575.

Tacon, A.G.J., 2003. Aquaculture production trends analysis. In: Review of the State of World Aquaculture. FAO, Rome, pp. 5–29. FAO Fisheries Circular No. 886, Revision 2.

Chapter 2

Taxonomy and basic biology

Chapter outline

2.1 Introduction

Apart from the great economic importance of tilapias for aquaculture and fisheries, they play a significant role in the tropical aquatic ecosystems. This means that unplanned introductions and/or culture of tilapia are likely to cause severe ecological impacts. Therefore, the study of the basic biology and ecology of tilapia is necessary prior to their introduction into and/or culture in different geographical regions, in order to avoid, or at least minimize these impacts. This chapter discusses, from a broad perspective, the major aspects of tilapia biology and ecology, including taxonomy, external morphology, and feeding habits. Detailed information on these aspects is available in *The Biology and Culture of Tilapias* edited by Pullin and Lowe-Mcconnell (1982), *Cichlid Fishes* by Keenleyside (1991), and *Tilapias: Biology and Exploitation* edited by Beveridge and McAndrew (2000). Further information on the geographical distribution and transfer and introductions of tilapia is contained in Chapter 3. The ecological requirements of tilapia are also provided in Chapter 4.

2.2 Taxonomy

The name 'tilapia' was derived from the African Bushman word meaning 'fish' (Trewavas, 1982). Tilapias represent a large number of freshwater fish species within the family Cichlidae. According to Kaufman and Liem (1982), family Cichlidae is one of the four families (Cichlidae, Embiotocidae, Pomacentridae and Labridae) which the suborder Labroidei includes. Despite that over 70 species of tilapia have been described, yet, there is a considerable argument over whether these species are truly separate species. The taxonomic classification of tilapia is still confusing and a subject of continuous changes. This is mainly because of the similarity and overlap of their morphological characteristics, and also due to the fact that many species of tilapia freely hybridize in nature.

The genus *Tilapia* was first described by Smith (1840). It was later split, based on breeding behavior and feeding habits, into two subgenera: *Tilapia* (substrate spawners) (Fig. 2.1) and *Sarotherodon* 'brush toothed' (mouthbrooders). Mouthbrooders incubate the fertilized eggs and hatched fry in the mouth of the male or female parents or both male and female. Later, the subgenus *Sarotherodon* was raised to a genus and further subdivided into two genera: *Oreochromis* (mountain cichlids) (Figs 2.2 and 2.3) and *Sarotherodon* (Fig. 2.4) based on whether parental females (*Oreochromis*), males (*Sarotherodon*) or both parental sexes (*Sarotherodon*) perform the mouthbrooding

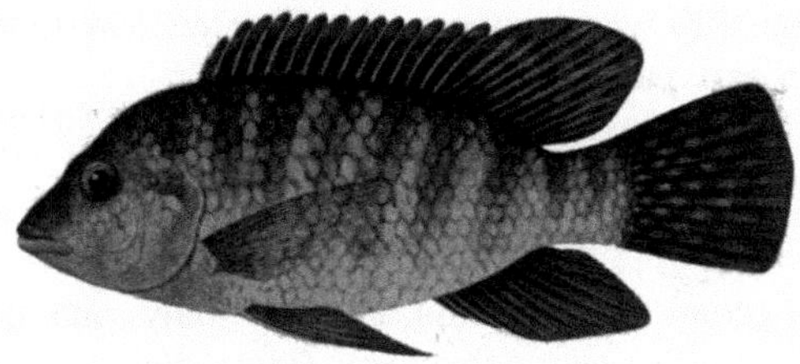

FIGURE 2.1 Redbelly tilapia (*Tilapia zillii*), a typical substrate spawner. *Photograph by A.-F. El-Sayed.*

Tilapia Culture. https://doi.org/10.1016/B978-0-12-816541-6.00002-7
Copyright © 2020 Elsevier Inc. All rights reserved.

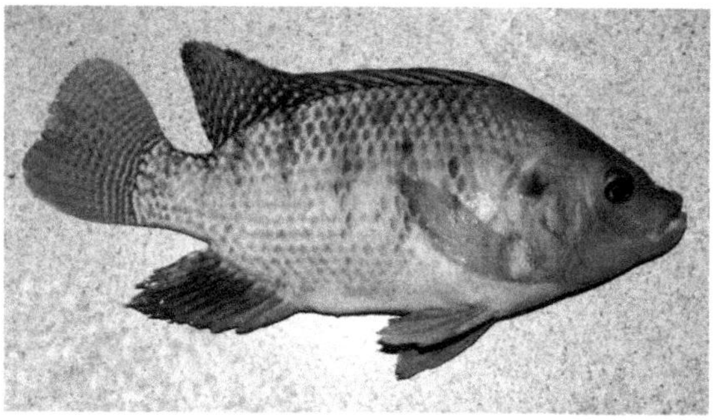

FIGURE 2.2 Nile tilapia (*Oreochromis niloticus*) is the most widely cultured tilapia species. *Photograph by A.-F. El-Sayed.*

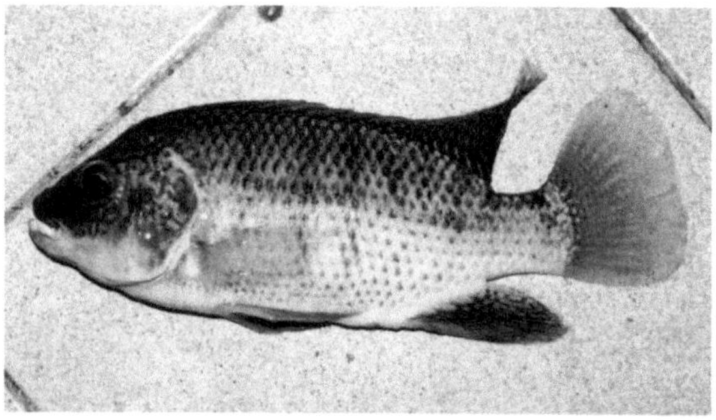

FIGURE 2.3 Blue tilapia (*Oreochromis aureus*) is another maternal mouthbrooder. It is also widely cultured. *Photograph by A.-F. El-Sayed.*

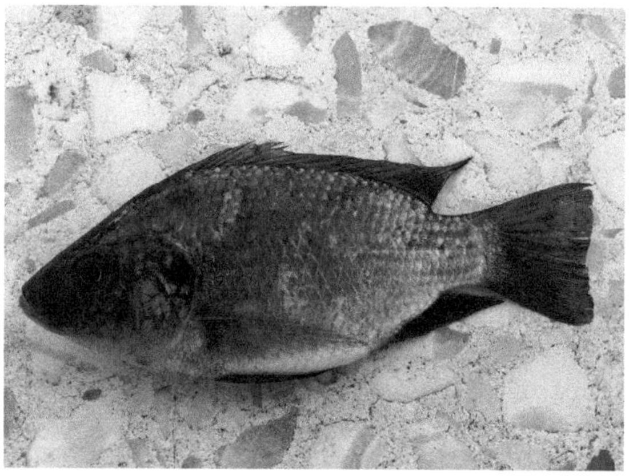

FIGURE 2.4 Galilee tilapia (*Sarotherodon galilaeus*) is a biparental mouthbrooder where both males and females incubate and defend fertilized eggs and hatched fry. *Photograph by A.-F. El-Sayed.*

behaviour. In early 1980s, two other alternative classifications of tilapia were proposed by E. Trewavas (cited in Fishelson and Yaron (1983):

1. The first classification includes five genera: *Tilapia*, *Sarotherodon*, *Oreochromis*, *Tristromella* and *Danakilia*.
2. The second classification includes only one genus, *Tilapia*, with seven subgenera: *Heterotilapia*, *Pelmatilapia*, *Sarotherodon*, *Oreochromis*, *Nyasalapia*, *Alcolapia* and *Neotilapia*.

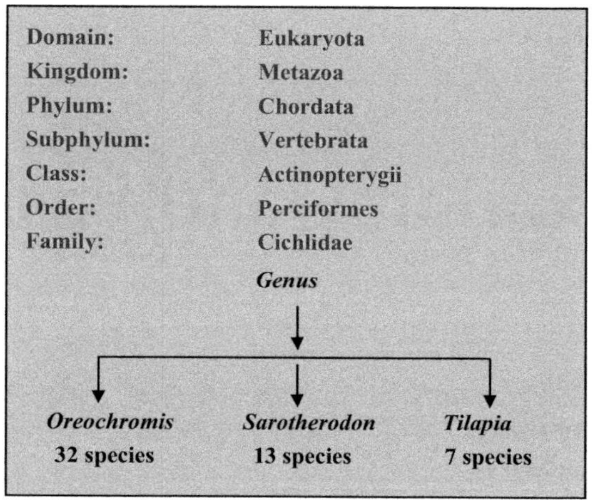

FIGURE 2.5 Taxonomy of tilapias.

According to Froese and Pauly (2018), genus *Oreochromis* includes 32 species, while genus *Sarotherodon* includes 13 species. In the meantime, seven species are included in genus *Tilapia* (Fig. 2.5 and Table 2.1). However, in 2013, a review of genus *Tilapia* resulted in the removal of most *Tilapia* species to the genera *Coelotilapia*, *Coptodon*, *Heterotilapia*, *Paracoptodon*, and *Pelmatolapia*, leaving only four species in genus *Tilapia* (Dunz and Schliewen, 2013). *Tilapia zillii* (Redbelly tilapia) is currently classified as *Coptodon zillii* by many authors.

All these revisions and changes in taxonomic classification of tilapia did not eliminate or resolve the current confusion. Therefore, some taxonomists and researchers still prefer to use the old genus *Tilapia* for all tilapia species.

2.3 Body shape and external morphology

Tilapias have fairly conventional, laterally compressed, deep body shapes (see Figs 2.1 and 2.3). The body is covered with relatively large, cycloid scales, which are not easily dislodged (Ross, 2000). The dorsal and anal fins have hard spines and soft rays. The pectoral and pelvic fins are large and more anterior in an advanced configuration. This character provides the fish with a great control over swimming and manoeuvring. The fins are also used for locomotion, and that is why cichlid fishes have red muscles designed for relatively low speed, but continuous movements (Ross, 2000). The numbers of scales, vertebrae, gill rakers and fin rays and spines are widely used for species distinction and identification. The fin formulas of different tilapias are presented in Table 2.2. It should be mentioned, however, that the number of fin spines and/or rays of the same species may vary from one strain to another and from one aquatic environment to another.

TABLE 2.1 Valid taxonomic position of tilapias.

No.	Valid name	English name	Author
Genus: *Oreochromis* (32 species)			
1.	*Oreochromis amphimelas*		Hilgendorf (1905)
2.	*Oreochromis andersonii*	Three spotted tilapia	Castelnau (1861)
3.	*Oreochromis angolensis*		Trewavas (1973)
4.	*Oreochromis aureus*	Blue tilapia	Steindachner (1864)
5.	*Oreochromis chungruruensis*		Ahl (1924)
6.	*Oreochromis esculentus*	Singida tilapia	Graham (1928)
7.	*Oreochromis hunteri*	Lake Chala tilapia	Günther (1889)
8.	*Oreochromis ismailiaensis*		Mekkawy (1995)
9.	*Oreochromis jipe*	Jipe tilapia	Lowe (1955)
10.	*Oreochromis karomo*	Karomo	Poll (1948)
11.	*Oreochromis karongae*		Trewavas (1941)
12.	*Oreochromis korogwe*	Korogwe tilapia	Lowe (1955)
13.	*Oreochromis lepidurus*		Boulenger (1899)
14.	*Oreochromis leucostictus*		Trewavas (1933)
15.	*Oreochromis lidole*		Trewavas (1941)
16.	*Oreochromis macrochir*	Longfin tilapia	Boulenger (1912)
17.	*Oreochromis mortimeri*	Kariba tilapia	Trewavas (1966)
18.	*Oreochromis mossambicus*	Mozambique tilapia	Peters (1852)
19.	*Oreochromis mweruensis*		Trewavas (1983)
20.	*Oreochromis niloticus*	Nile tilapia	Linnaeus (1758)
21.	*Oreochromis placidus*	Black tilapia	Trewavas (1941)
22.	*Oreochromis rukwaensis*	Lake Rukwa tilapia	Hilgendorf and Pappenheim (1903)
23.	*Oreochromis saka*		Lowe (1953)
24.	*Oreochromis salinicola*		Poll (1948)
25.	*Oreochromis schwebischi*		Sauvage (1884)
26.	*Oreochromis shiranus*	Tilapia shiranus	Boulenger (1897)
27.	*Oreochromis spilurus*	Sabaki tilapia	Günther (1894)
28.	*Oreochromis squamipinnis*		Günther (1864)
29.	*Oreochromis tanganicae*		Günther (1894)
30.	*Oreochromis upembae*		Thys van den Audenaerde (1964)
31.	*Oreochromis urolepis*	Wami tilapia	Norman (1922)
32.	*Oreochromis variabilis*	Victoria tilapia	Boulenger (1906)
Genus: *Sarotherodon* (13 species)			
1.	*Sarotherodon caroli*	Fissi	Holly (1930)
2.	*Sarotherodon caudomarginatus*		Boulenger (1916)
3.	*Sarotherodon galilaeus*	Mango tilapia	Linnaeus (1758)
4.	*Sarotherodon knauerae*		Neumann et al. (2011)

Continued

TABLE 2.1 Valid taxonomic position of tilapias.—cont'd

No.	Valid name	English name	Author
5.	*Sarotherodon lamprechti*		Neumann et al. (2011)
6.	*Sarotherodon linnellii*	Blackfin tilapia	Lönnberg (1903)
7.	*Sarotherodon lohbergeri*	Keppi	Holly (1930)
8.	*Sarotherodon melanotheron*	Blackchin tilapia	Rüppell (1852)
9.	*Sarotherodon mvogoi*		Thys van den Audenaerde (1965)
10.	*Sarotherodon nigripinnis*		Guichenot (1861)
11.	*Sarotherodon occidentalis*		Daget (1962)
12.	*Sarotherodon steinbachi*	Kululu	Trewavas (1962)
13.	*Sarotherodon tournieri*		Daget (1965)
Genus: *Tilapia* (7 species)			
1.	*Tilapia baloni*		Trewavas and Stewart (1975)
2.	*Tilapia brevimanus*		Boulenger (1911)
3.	*Tilapia busumana*		Günther (1903)
4.	*Tilapia guinasana*	Otjikoto tilapia	Trewavas (1936)
5.	*Tilapia pra*		Dunz and Schliewen (2010)
6.	*Tilapia ruweti*	Okavango tilapia	Poll and Thys van den Audenaerde (1965)
7.	*Tilapia sparrmanii*	Banded tilapia	Smith (1840)

Data from Froese, R., Pauly, D., 2018. FishBase. World Wide Web Electronic Publication. www.fishbase.org, version 06/2018.

TABLE 2.2 Fin formulas of various tilapia species.

Species	Location	Dorsal fin	Pectoral fin	Anal fin	References
Tilapia mariae	Umuoseriche Lake, Nigeria	XV–XVII, 10–14	11–15	9–12	Anene (1999)
Tilapia zillii	Umuoseriche Lake, Nigeria	XIII–XVII, 11–13	12–14	8–10	Anene (1999)
	Lake Edku, Egypt	XIV–XVI, 10–13	12–14	8–10	Abdalla (1995)
	Lake Mariut, Egypt	XIV–XVI, 9–13	12–14	7–9	Akel (1989)
Oreochromis niloticus	Lake Mariut, Egypt	XV–XVIII, 10–13	12–15	8–10	Akel (1989)
	Lake Edku, Egypt	XVI–XVIII, 12–14	12–15	9–10	Bakhoum (2002)
Oreochromis aureus	Lake Mariut, Egypt	XVI–XVII, 10–14	11–14	8–11	Akel (1989)
	Lake Edku, Egypt	XV–XVII, 12–13	12–14	9–10	Bakhoum (2002)
Sarotherodon galilaeus	Lake Mariut, Egypt	XV–XVIII, 11–13	11–14	9–11	Akel (1989)
Sarotherodon melanotheron	Lagos Lagoon, Nigeria	XV–XVII, 10–13	12–14	12–13	Omoniyi and Agbon (2008)
S. melanotheron	Badagry and Lagos Lagoon, Nigeria	XV–XVI, 10	11–12	12–13	Kuton and Adeniyi (2014)
Tilapia guineensis	Badagry and Lagos Lagoon, Nigeria	XVI, 11	12	11	Kuton and Adeniyi (2014)
T. guineensis	West Africa	XIV–XVI, 12–13		8–10	Teugels and Thys van den Audenaerde (2003)

Tilapia bodies are generally characterized by vertical bars, with relatively subdued colours, with little contrast over the body colours. This provides the fish with an ability to change their colours, in response to stress or environmental conditions, by controlling skin chromatophores. Tilapia have well-developed sense organs, represented by a prominent nares and clearly visible lateral line. The eyes are also relatively large, providing the fish with excellent visual capability.

2.4 Feeding habits

The increasing importance of tilapias as an aquaculture candidate makes it necessary to understand their food preferences and feeding regimes in their natural habitats, in order to prepare the suitable diets for them and adopt the appropriate feeding regimes under culture conditions. Tilapia are generally herbivorous/omnivorous (i.e. they are low on aquatic food chain) (Table 2.3). However, they possess many morphological features, including jaw structures, mouth size and shape, dentition, and size and number of gill rakers (Fryer and Iles, 1972). These features allow tilapia and other cichlids to occupy a wider variety of feeding niches.

Although they feed at low trophic levels and their feed costs are lower than for carnivorous fishes, yet tilapia are a source of high-quality protein suitable for human consumption, at a relatively low cost. Feeding habits and dietary preferences of tilapias depend, among other factors, on tilapia species and size, time of the day, photoperiod, water depth and geographical location. The feeding habits of tilapia in relation to these factors are briefly discussed in this section, with emphasis on economically important species.

During larval stages, tilapia feed initially on zooplankton, especially crustaceans (copepods) (Bowen, 1982; Harbott, 1982). When Florida red tilapia fry were stocked in fertilized seawater pools containing different food resources, copepods were selectively ingested (Grover et al., 1989). Frequent consumption of phytoplankton also takes place during early larval stages of some tilapia species.

The transition period from planktivore stage to a typical, specialized diet(s) is usually short (Bowen, 1976), but in some cases it occurs gradually over an extended period of a year or more (Whitefield and Blaber, 1978). The food of juvenile and adult tilapias consists of considerable variety of aquatic vegetation, phytoplankton, zooplankton, periphyton and detritus of plant origin, depending on tilapia species, as mentioned earlier. Many research studies have been carried out on the feeding habits of different tilapias, in their natural habitats, under a variety of environmental conditions.

Generally speaking, tilapia can be classified into one of the following broad categories according to their feeding patterns.

2.4.1 Genus: *Oreochromis*

Tilapia of the genus *Oreochromis* are primarily microphagous, feeding mainly on phytoplankton, periphyton, aquatic plants, benthic fauna and detritus, depending on food availability and fish species and size. *Oreochromis niloticus*, *Oreochromis aureus* and *Oreochromis mossambicus* are examples of this category (Table 2.3). These species can efficiently ingest the food sources mentioned through 'filter-feeding' or grazing.

a. Nile tilapia (*Oreochromis niloticus*)
Nile tilapia (*O. niloticus*) exhibit trophic plasticity according to the environment and the other species they coexist with (Bwanika et al., 2004). They are known to feed on phytoplankton, periphyton, aquatic plants, small invertebrates and benthic fauna, detritus and bacterial films (GISD, 2018a) and even other fish and fish eggs. They feed either via suspension filtering or surface grazing, depending on the food source. Harbott (1982) reported that all size classes of *O. niloticus* in Lake Turkana are primarily phytophagous, grazing on the dense algal plankton found in sheltered, inshore waters, while little selectivity of food items was recorded. *O. niloticus*, in Lake Hayq, Ethiopia, were found to feed on a wide variety of food items including various types of phytoplankton, zooplankton and macrophytes (Assefa and Getahun, 2015).

b. Blue tilapia (*Oreochromis aureus*)
Blue tilapia (*O. aureus*) have a wide variety of diets, including, phytoplankton, epiphytic algae, zooplankton, insects, vascular plants, copepods and cladocerans; depending on fish size (GISD, 2018b). Spataru and Zorn (1978) found that *O. aureus* in Lake Kinneret are mainly zooplankton feeders, while vegetable detritus, mixed with plankton and benthos forms, served as additional and alternative foods.

c. Mozambique tilapia (*Oreochromis mossambicus*)
Mozambique tilapia (*O. mossambicus*) feed on phytoplankton, zooplankton, zoobenthos, molluscs (gastropods), insects, benthic crustaceans, worms, fish and macrophytes (Sakhare and Jetithor, 2016; Froese and Pauly, 2018).

2.4.2 Genus: *Sarotherodon*

Tilapia of the genus *Sarotherodon* are also primarily phytoplankton feeders (Table 2.3), but they are more selective. However, feeding habits of this genus may vary considerably, depending on fish species and size, environmental

TABLE 2.3 Feeding habits of some economically important tilapias.

Species	Diet	Remarks	References
Oreochromis niloticus	Phytoplankton, zooplankton, benthic detritus, periphyton, aquatic plants, small invertebrates, benthic fauna and bacterial films.	Little selectivity of food items. The fish change food and feeding habit with size; increased preference for debris with increasing size.	Moriarty and Moriarty (1973), Dewan and Saha (1979), Harbott (1982), Northcott et al. (1991), GISD (2018a), Assefa and Getahun (2015)
Oreochromis aureus	Phytoplankton, zooplankton, detritus, vascular plant residues, epiphytic algae, insects, copepods and cladocerans.	Food preferences detected in juveniles and adults.	Spataru and Zorn (1978), Jiménez-Badillo and Nepita-Villanueva (2000), GISD (2018b)
Oreochromis mossambicus	Macrophytes, benthic algae, phytoplankton, zooplankton, detritus, periphyton, fish larvae, molluscs (gastropods), insects, benthic crustaceans, worms and fish.	Intraspecific variations in diet between environments and over time.	Bowen (1979), De Silva et al. (1984), de Moor et al. (1986), Sakhare and Jetithor (2016), Froese and Pauly (2018).
O. mossambicus x *O. niloticus*	Periphytic detritus, filamentous and colonial algae (periphytic epipelon).	Intraspecific variations in diet between environments.	Haroon et al. (1998)
Florida red tilapia	Macroalgae, phytoplankton.	Variations in diet between environments.	Grover et al. (1989)
Sarotherodon galilaeus	Phytoplankton (dinoflagellates).	Fish are highly selective.	Corbet et al. (1973), Spataru (1976)
S. galilaeus	Detritus, diatoms, desmids, blue-green algae, green algae, protozoan and unidentified plants	Euryphagous and can exploit a wide range of organisms.	Adeosun (2016)
Sarotherodon melanotheron	Macrophytes, blue-green and green algae, organic debris, aquatic insects and insect larvae, rotifers, diatoms, benthic invertebrates.	Plant materials more preferable than animal sources.	Fagade (1971), Oben et al. (1998)
S. melanotheron	Juveniles prefer cyanophyceae, chlorophyceae and rotifera, while adult fish prefer cladocera, bacillariophyceae and cyanophyceae	Feeding occurs mostly around 1200 noon and between 1500 and 1800 GMT.	Ofori-Danson and Kumi (2006)
Tilapia zillii	Macrophytes, blue-green and green algae, organic debris, zooplankton, aquatic insects and insect larvae and pupae, rotifers, diatoms, benthic invertebrates, arthropods.	Plant materials more preferable than animal sources. Variations in diet between seasons.	Buddington (1979), Spataru (1978), Oben et al. (1998)
T. zillii	Macrophytes, detritus, phytoplankton, zooplankton, insets and zoobenthos.	The importance of phytoplankton, detritus and insects declines, while the importance of macrophytes increases, with increasing fish size.	Shep et al. (2013), Dadebo et al. (2014)
Tilapia rendalli	Macrophytes, attached periphyton, zooplankton (cladocerans and copepods), insect larvae, fish eggs, detritus.	Feeding behaviour depends on fish size. Small fish are visual feeders, large fish are pump-filter feeders.	Caulton (1976), Lazzaro (1991)
Tilapia guineensis	Algae, detritus, sand, invertebrates.		Fagade (1971)
T. guineensis	Insects (*Diptera*) and macrophytes.	Molluscs, coleoptera and zooplankton represent some importance.	Shep et al. (2013)

conditions, food abundance and geographic locations. For example, Spataru (1976) found that the dinoflagellate *Peridinium cinctum* was the most abundant food in the stomachs of *Sarotherodon galilaeus* in Lake Kinneret, sometimes comprising >95% of the phytoplankton biomass, especially during the blooming season of these dinoflagellates (March–April). On the other hand, Adeosun (2016) reported that *S. galilaeus* in Oyan Lake (Nigeria) are euryphagous, opportunistic feeders, which can feed on a wide range of organisms, both on surface water and bottom sediments. Their food includes diatoms, desmids, blue-green and green algae, protozoan, detritus and unidentified plants. However, detritus is the most preferred food followed by filamentous blue-green algae.

Sarotherodon melanotheron are more selective, feeding mainly on phytoplankton and zooplankton throughout their life cycle (Froese and Pauly, 2018). Benthic algae, small fish and debris are also found occasionally in their stomachs. Ofori-Danson and Kumi (2006) found that *S. melanotheron* juveniles prefer the Cyanophyceae, Chlorophyceae and Rotifera, while adult fish prefer Cladocera, Bacillariophyceae and Cyanophyceae. The majority of these fish had 3/4 stomach fullness around noon (1200 GMT) and between 1500 and 1800 GMT, suggesting that they feed mostly at these times during the daytime.

2.4.3 Genus *Tilapia*

Tilapia of the genus *Tilapia* are generally macrophyte feeders (Abdel-Malek, 1972; Caulton, 1976; Lowe-Mcconnell, 1982). This explains why they are used for biological control of aquatic weeds. However, they cannot avoid ingesting the algae, phytoplankton, zooplankton, bacteria, benthic invertebrates, insect larvae, fish and vertebrate eggs and detritus which are attached to the macrophytes they feed on. These attached materials are therefore an important food component for *Tilapia* species (Bowen, 1982). Fagade (1971) found that the principal components in the stomachs of *Tilapia guineensis* and *Tilapia melanotheron melanotheron* in Lagos Lagoon (Nigeria) were algal filaments, diatoms, sand grains and unidentified organic material, and these components were very similar in both species. Adult *Tilapia rendalli* have also been found to consume a wide variety of food items, including macrophytes, phytoplankton, zooplankton, insect larvae, fish eggs and larvae and detritus (Caulton, 1976; Lazzaro, 1991).

Redbelly tilapia (*T. zillii*, also classified as *C. zillii*) feed mainly on macrophytes, detritus and phytoplankton, whereas the contribution of zooplankton, insects and zoobenthos is relatively low (Dadebo et al., 2014). However, the importance of phytoplankton, detritus and insects declines, while macrophytes become more important, with increasing fish size. Shep et al. (2013) found also that insect (*Diptera*) and macrophytes were the most important food items in the diet of *T. zillii* and *T. guineensis* and their hybrids in Ayamé man-made lake (Côte d'Ivoire). Molluscs, coleoptera and zooplankton also represented some importance.

2.5 Factors affecting feeding habits

It should be realized that the above-mentioned categories of feeding habits are not rigid, but extensive overlap may also occur in tilapia diets. Intraspecific variations may also occur in these diets between environments over time, as has been reported with *O. mossambicus* in Sri Lankan reservoirs (De Silva, 1985). In addition, tilapia introduced into new habitats can adjust their feeding strategy to reflect the relative abundance and composition of available food in their new habitat, to include even fish consumption. For example, blue tilapia (*O. aureus*) introduced into Muddy River system (Warm Springs area, Nevada, the United States) switched their diet from aquatic eelgrass (*Vallisneria*) to fish after the depletion of *Vallisneria* (Scoppettone et al., 2005). Consumed fishes included mosquitofish, shortfin molly, moapa dace and moapa White River springfish. Similarly, Bowen and Allanson (1982) observed that *O. mossambicus* which were moved to different habitats in South Africa had the ability to change their diets to fit with prevailing food availability. De Silva et al. (1984) reported also that the feeding habits of *O. mossambicus* from different lakes in Sri Lanka ranged from detritivory to herbivory, to total carnivory of small fish and invertebrates. The piscivory in *O. mossambicus* has also been confirmed by Doupé et al. (2009). The tilapia *Alcolapia grahami* (formerly *Oreochromis alkalicus*) of the alkaline Lake Magadi (pH 10) in Kenya were also found to feed on cyanobacteria (Bone and Moore, 2008).

Since light penetration in water column is affected by water depth and turbidity, natural food productivity in the water is likely to vary between different depths. Accordingly, the feeding patterns of tilapia may vary with varying water masses. Bowen (1982) stated that deposit feeders that feed in the littoral zone frequently ingest algae, detritus and bacteria, which cannot be distinguished from the material attached to macrophytes. On the other hand, deposit feeders that feed in deeper waters ingest a mixture of precipitated phytoplankton and detritus that are indistinguishable from the diets of suspension feeders. By this mechanism, tilapia can switch from one source of food to another with little change in diets composition (Moriarty et al., 1973).

Tilapia feeding patterns and efficiency may also be a subject of diurnal and seasonal changes. Extensive studies have considered the diel feeding patterns of tilapia, both in their natural habitats and under aquaculture conditions. Harbott (1982) found that all size classes of *O. niloticus* in Lake Turkana followed a daytime feeding cycle, but fish fry infrequently consumed invertebrates during the hours of darkness. Feeding activity of *O. niloticus* adults reared under conditions of self-feeding (using demand feeders) was also observed exclusively during the light phases (Toguyeni et al., 1997). Moreover, Nile tilapia in Lake Rudolf exhibited a regular diurnal feeding rhythm, commencing between 05.00 and 08.00 h and ceasing between 14.00 and 18.00 h, and the largest fish individuals appeared to feed longer (Harbott, 1975). On the other hand, Nile tilapia in Bangladesh ponds are reportedly continuous feeders, but they increase feeding activity from noon to midnight, with a peak immediately after dusk and reduced feeding activity after midnight (Dewan and Saha, 1979).

Fish size may also affect feeding rhythms in tilapia. For example, Richter et al. (1999) analyzed the diel feeding patterns and daily ration of *O. niloticus* in cages in Laguna de Bay, Philippines. They found that, in May, larger fish (31.5 g) feeding on natural food alone fed continuously from dawn to dusk, whereas smaller fish (9.8 g) exhibited two feeding periods per day, from sunrise to mid-morning and again from mid-afternoon until after sunset. In another study, Haroon et al. (1998) investigated the diel feeding patterns and ration of tilapia hybrids (*O. mossambicus* × *O. niloticus*) at two sizes (4.3–9.3 and 9.5–13.8 cm total length) in pond and paddy field in Bangladesh. Both small and large tilapia exhibited a single feeding peak around afternoon-dusk in the pond, but irregular feeding peaks in the rice field. However, small fish were more active feeders than large fish, and both feeding intensity and food consumption decreased with increasing fish size. Periphytic detritus was the principal food in the paddy field, while filamentous and colonial algae attached to sediments and mud (known as periphytic epipelon) were the main food in the pond. In the meantime, zooplankton was an insignificant dietary component in both habitats.

The feeding habits of *T. rendalli* in southern Brazilian lakes and reservoirs, in relation to fish size, have also been studied by Lazzaro (1991). Fish smaller than 30 mm in length were visual feeders, while fish with a size ranging from 30 to 50 mm were either visually feeders or pump-filter feeders, depending on zooplankton size. Fish larger than 70 mm were pump-filter feeders. Electivity and feeding rate increased with prey length. A difference in food preferences between juvenile and adult *O. aureus* in Mexico was also detected, in addition to a variation in the consumption of some food items during the rainy and dry seasons (Jiménez-Badillo and Nepita-Villanueva, 2000).

The time of the year may also have an influence on tilapia feeding habits. Spataru (1978) found that *T. zillii* in Lake Kinneret have great variations in their food in relation to season of the year. In winter and spring, *Chironomidae* pupae (Diptera) were prevalent in fish stomachs, while zooplankton forms were dominant in summer and autumn. Spataru and Zorn (1978) found also that *O. aureus* in the same lake feed more intensely on zooplankton in spring, where zooplankton forms are more abundant. Nile tilapia also showed seasonal variation in feeding activity in Bangladesh fish ponds (Dewan and Saha, 1979). The feeding activity was greater in summer than in winter. Greater amounts of phytoplankton were recorded in fish stomachs during winter, while debris was consumed more during summer.

From the above discussion, it appears that tilapia have irregular feeding patterns, depending, as mentioned earlier, on fish species and size, season of the year, time of the day, photoperiod, water depth, geographical location and type of habitat. It is crucially important that tilapia farmers, researchers and farm managers consider these factors in order to adopt the most suitable fertilization regimes, prepare the best pelleted diets and select the most convenient feeding regimes in terms of feeding frequency, timing and quantity.

2.6 Gut morphology

The digestive system of tilapias is characterized by certain modifications reflecting the types of food they ingest. It is relatively simple, unspecialized and consisting of a very short oesophagus connected to small, saclike stomach, and a very long, coiled intestine, which can reach up to 7–13 times the total fish length (Caulton, 1976; Balarin and Hatton, 1979). Such long intestines reflect the herbivorous feeding habits of these fishes, perhaps because vegetable foods are digested less readily than animal sources. Therefore, herbivorous fishes have amylase activities in the gut much higher than in carnivorous species.

Tilapia have two types of teeth: jaw teeth and pharyngeal teeth. Both types of teeth are varied in configuration from one tilapia species to another, to suit the different diet preferences. The jaw teeth are small, unicuspid, bicuspid or tricuspid structures that are arranged in 1–5 rows, and flattened distally to form blades that can be used as scrapers (Fryer and Iles, 1972; Lanzing and Higginbotham, 1976). The pharyngeal teeth of the phytoplanktivorous tilapia, such as *Sarotherodon esculentus*, are fine, thin and hooked on the pharyngeal bones, whereas these of macrophyte feeders, such as *T. rendalli*, are coarse and robust (Caulton, 1976). Microphagous tilapia are also characterized by numerous, long, thin, closely spaced gill rakers, while fish species that feed on large particles have fewer, large gill rakers. While gill rakers are specialized for feeding in many tilapia species, their role in feeding mechanism in some other tilapia species may not be significant. Drenner et al. (1987) found that the surgical removal of gill rakers did not affect phytoplankton ingestion rates of *S. galilaeus*. However, it may be unwise to adopt a firm conclusion based on only one study. Clearly, more work should be conducted on different tilapia species that employ different feeding strategies, before a concrete conclusion can be drawn on the role of gill rakers in feeding mechanisms of tilapia.

2.7 Closing remarks

1. The taxonomic classification of tilapia is still confusing and a subject of continuous modification. Currently, tilapia are divided into three genera, *Tilapia* (substrate spawners), *Sarotherodon* (maternal/paternal mouthbrooders) and *Oreochromis* (maternal mouthbrooders).
2. Tilapias are freshwater groups of fish species originated exclusively from Africa (excluding Madagascar) and from the Middle East (Jordan Valley and coastal rivers). They are distributed all over Africa, except the northern Atlas Mountains and South-West Africa.
3. Feeding and dietary preferences of tilapias depend on tilapia species and size, time of the day, photoperiod, water depth and location, with little selectivity.
4. Tilapia of the genus *Oreochromis* are primarily microphagous, feeding mainly on phytoplankton, periphyton and detritus.
5. Tilapia of the genus *Sarotherodon* are also primarily phytoplanktivorous, but they are more selective.
6. Tilapia of the genus *Tilapia* are generally macrophyte feeders. They also ingest algae, phytoplankton, zooplankton, invertebrate larvae, fish eggs, insects, bacteria and detritus which are attached to the macrophytes.
7. Tilapia introduced into new habitats can adjust their feeding habits to reflect the abundance and composition of available food in their new habitat, to include even fish consumption.
8. Feeding patterns and efficiency of tilapia may be a subject of diurnal and seasonal changes. Generally, tilapia feed intensively during early morning and late afternoon and reduce feeding during midday and at night.
9. The digestive system of tilapias is relatively simple, unspecialized, consisting of a very short oesophagus, small sac-like stomach and a very long intestine. Such a digestive tract reflects the herbivorous feeding habits of tilapia.
10. Tilapia have two types of teeth, jaw teeth and pharyngeal teeth. Both types of teeth are varied from one tilapia species to another to suit the different diet preferences.
11. Microphagous tilapia have numerous, long, thin, closely spaced gill rakers, while tilapia that feed on large particles have fewer, large gill rakers.

References

Abdalla, A., 1995. Age and Growth and Population Dynamics of Tilapia Species in the Egyptian Inland Water, Edku Lake (Ph.D. thesis). Assiut University, Egypt.

Abdel-Malek, S.A., 1972. Food and feeding habits of some Egyptian fishes in Lake Quarun. 1. *Tilapia zillii* (Gerv.) B. According to different length groups. Bulletin of the Institute of Oceanography and Fisheries 2, 204–213.

Adeosun, F.I., 2016. An investigation into the food and feeding ecology of *Sarotherodon galilaeus* in Oyan Lake, Ogun state, Nigeria. Nigerian Journal of Animal Science 18, 364–369.

Akel, E.H.K., 1989. Effect of Water Pollution on Tilapia Populations in Lake Mariout (M.Sc. thesis). Alexandria University, Alexandria, Egypt.

Anene, A., 1999. Morphometric and meristic description of *Tilapia mariae* (Boulenger, 1901) and *Tilapia zillii* (Gervais, 1848) from the Umuoseriche Lake in the freshwater reaches of the Niger delta floodplains. Acta Hydrobiologica 41, 211–218.

Assefa, W.W., Getahun, A., 2015. The food and feeding ecology of Nile tilapia, *Oreochromis niloticus*, in Lake Hayq, Ethiopia. International Journal of Fisheries and Aquatic Studies 2, 176–185.

Bakhoum, S.A., 2002. Occurrence of natural hybrids between nile tilapia, *Oreochromis niloticus* (L.) and blue tilapia, *O. aureus* (Steind.) in Lake Edku, Egypt. Egyptian Journal of Aquatic Biology and Fisheries 6, 143–162.

Balarin, J.D., Hatton, J.P., 1979. Tilapia: A Guide to Their Biology and Culture in Africa. University of Stirling, Scotland.

Beveridge, M.C.M., McAndrew, B.J. (Eds.), 2000. Tilapias: Biology and Exploitation. Kluwer Academic Publishers, Dordrecht/Boston/London, p. 505.

Bone, Q., Moore, R.H., 2008. Biology of Fishes, third ed. Taylor & Francis Group, New York, p. 478.

Bowen, S.H., 1976. Feeding Ecology of the Cichlid Fish Sarotherodon Mossambicus in Lake Sibaya, KwaZulu (Ph.D. thesis). Rhodes University, Grahamstown, South Africa.

Bowen, S.H., 1979. A nutritional constraint in detritivory by fishes: the stunted population of *Sarotherodon mossambicus* in Lake Sibaya, South Africa. Ecological Moneograph 49, 17–31.

Bowen, S.H., 1982. Feeding, digestion and growth- Qualitative considerations. In: Pullin, R.V.S., Lowe-McConnell, R.H. (Eds.), The Biology and Culture of Tilapias. ICLARM Conference Proceedings No. 7. ICLARM, Manila, Philippines, pp. 141–156.

Bowen, S.H., Allanson, B.R., 1982. Behavioral and trophic plasticity of juvenile *Tilapia mossambica* in utilization of the unstable littoral habitat. Environmental Biology of Fishes 7, 357–362.

Buddington, R.K., 1979. Digestion of an aquatic macrophyte by *Tilapia zillii* (Gervais). Journal of Fish Biology 15, 449–455.

Bwanika, G.N., Makanga, B., Kizito, Y., Chapman, L.J., Balirwa, J., 2004. Observations on the biology of Nile tilapia, *Oreochromis niloticus*, L., in two Ugandan crater lakes. African Journal of Ecology 42, 93–101.

Caulton, M.S., 1976. The importance of pre-digestive food preparation to *Tilapia rendalli* Boulenger when feeding on aquatic macrophytes. Transactions of the Rhodesia Scientific Association 57, 22–28.

Corbet, S.A., Green, J., Griffith, J., Betney, E., 1973. Ecological studies on crater lakes in west Cameroon lakes Kotto and Mboandong. Journal of Zoology 170, 309–324.

Dadebo, E., Kebtineh, N., Sorsa, S., Balkew, K., 2014. Food and feeding habits of the red-belly tilapia (*Tilapia zillii* Gervais, 1848) (Pisces: Cichlidae) in Lake Ziway, Ethiopia. Agriculture, Forestry and Fisheries 3, 17–23.

de Moor, F.C., Wilkinson, R.C., Herbst, H.M., 1986. Food and feeding habits of *Oreochromis mossambicus* (Peters) in hypertrophic Hartbeespoort Dam, South Africa. South African Journal of Zoology 21, 170–176.

De Silva, S.S., 1985. Body condition and nutritional ecology of *Oreochromis mossambicus* (Pisces, Cichlidae) populations of man-made lakes in Sri Lanka. Journal of Fish Biology 27, 621–633.

De Silva, S.S., Perera, M.K., Maitipe, P., 1984. The composition, nutritional status and digestibility of the diets of *Sarotherodon mossambicus* from nine man-made lakes in Srilanka. Environmental Biology of Fishes 11, 205–219.

Dewan, S., Saha, S.N., 1979. Food and feeding habits of *Tilapia nilotica* (L.) (Perciformes: Cichlidae). 2. Diel and seasonal patterns of feeding. Bangladesh Journal of Zoology 7, 75–80.

Doupé, R.G., Knott, M.J., Schaffer, J., Burrows, D.W., 2009. Investigational piscivory of some juvenile Australian freshwater fishes by the introduced Mozambique tilapia *Oreochromis mossambicus*. Journal of Fish Biology 74, 2386–2400.

Drenner, R.W., Vinyard, G.L., Hambright, K.D., Gophen, M., 1987. Ingestion by *Tilapia galilaea* is not affected by removal of gill rakers and microbranchiospines. Transactions of the American Fisheries Society 116, 272–276.

Dunz, A.R., Schliewen, U.K., 2013. Molecular phylogeny and revised classification of the haplotilapiine cichlid fishes formerly referred to as "Tilapia". Molecular Phylogenetics and Evolution 68, 64–80.

Fagade, S.O., 1971. The food and feeding habits of *Tilapia* species in the Lagos Lagoon. Journal of Fish Biology 3, 151–156.

Fishelson, L., Yaron, Z. (Eds.), 1983. Proceedings of the International Symposium on Tilapia in Aquaculture. Tel Aviv University, Israel, p. XI.

Froese, R., Pauly, D., 2018. FishBase. World Wide Web Electronic Publication. version (06/2018). www.fishbase.org.

Fryer, G., Iles, T.D., 1972. Alternative routes to evolutionary success as exhibited by African cichlid fishes of the genus Tilapia and the species flocks of the great lakes. Evolution 23, 359–369.

GISD (Global Invasive Species Database), 2018a. Oreochromis niloticus. Available from: http://www.iucngisd.org/gisd/speciesname/Oreochromis+niloticus.

GISD (Global Invasive Species Database), 2018b. Oreochromis aureus. Available from: http://www.iucngisd.org/gisd/speciesname/Oreochromis+aureus.

Grover, J.J., Olla, B.L., O'brien, M., Wicklund, R.I., 1989. Food habits of Florida red tilapia fry in manured seawater pools in the Bahamas. Progressive Fish-Culturist 51, 152–156.

Harbott, B.J., 1975. Preliminary observations on the feeding of *Tilapia nilotica* Linn. in Lake Rudolf. African Journal of Tropical Hydrobiology and Fisheries 4, 27–37.

Harbott, B.J., 1982. Studies on the feeding activity of *Sarotherodon niloticus* (L.) in Lake Turkana. In: A Report on the Findings of the Lake Turkana Project, 1972–1975, vol. 5. Government of Kenya and the Ministry of Overseas Development, London, pp. 1357–1368.

Haroon, A.K.Y., Pittman, K.A., Blom, G., 1998. Diel feeding pattern and ration of two sizes of tilapia, *Oreochromis* spp. in pond and paddy field. Asian Fisheries Science 10, 281–301.

Jiménez-Badillo, M.L., Nepita-Villanueva, M.R., 2000. Trophic spectrum of *Oreochromis aureus* (Perciformes: Cichlidae) in Infiernillo Dam, Michoacan-Guerrero, Mexico. Revista de Biologia Tropical 48, 487–494.

Kaufman, L., Liem, K.F., 1982. Fishes of the suborder Labroidei (pisces: Perciformes): phylogeny, ecology and evolutionary significance. Breviora 472, 1–19.

Keenleyside, M.H.A., 1991. Cichlid Fishes. Chapman & Hall, London, p. 378.

Kuton, M.P., Adeniyi, B.T., 2014. Morphological variations of *Tilapia guineensis* (Bleeker 1862) and *Sarotherodon melanotheron* (Ruppell1852) (Pisces: Cichlidea) from Badagry and Lagos Lagoon, South-West, Nigeria. Journal of Fisheries & Livestock Production 2, 112. https://doi.org/10.4172/2332-2608.1000112.

Lanzing, W.J.R., Higginbotham, D.R., 1976. Scanning microscopy of pharyngeal and oral teeth of the teleost *Tilapia mossambica*. Hydrobiologia 48, 137–139.

Lazzaro, X., 1991. Feeding convergence in South American and African zooplanktivorous cichlids *Geophagus brasiliensis* and *Tilapia rendalli*. Environmental Biology of Fishes 31, 283–293.

Lowe-Mcconnell, R.H., 1982. Tilapias in fish communities. In: Pullin, R.S.V., Lowe-McConnell, R.H. (Eds.), The Biology and Culture of Tilapias. ICLARM Conference Proceedings No. 7. ICLARM, Manila, Philippines, pp. 83–113.

Moriarty, C.M., Moriarty, D.J.W., 1973. Quantitative estimation of daily ingestion of phytoplankton by *Tilapia nilotica* and *Haplochromis nigripinnis* in Lake George, Uganda. Journal of Zoology 171, 15–24.

Moriarty, D.J.W., Darlington, P.E.C., Dunn, I.G., Moriarty, C.M., Tevlin, M.P., 1973. Feeding and grazing in Lake George, Uganda. Proceedings of Royal Society, Edinburgh (B) 184, 299–319.

Northcott, M.E., Beveridge, M.C.M., Ross, L.G., 1991. A laboratory investigation of the filtration and ingestion rates of the tilapia, *Oreochromis niloticus*, feeding on two species of blue-green algae. Environmental Biology of Fishes 31, 75–85.

Oben, B.O., Ugwumba, O.A., Oben, P.M., 1998. Food and feeding ecology of some tilapiine fishes from an inland tropical lake, Ibadan, Nigeria. In: Paper Presented at the International Conference for the Paradi Association and the Fisheries Society of Africa, Grahamstown (South Africa), 13–18 September, 1998.

Ofori-Danson, P.K., Kumi, G.N., 2006. Food and feeding habit of *Sarotherodon melanotheron*, Rüppell, 1852 (Pisces: Cichlidae) in Sakumo lagoon, Ghana. West African Journal of Applied Ecology 10, 9–18.

Omoniyi, T., Agbon, A.O., 2008. Morphometric variations in *Sarotherodon melanotheron* (Pisces: Cichlidae) from brackish and fresh water habitats in South-western Nigeria. West African Journal of Applied Ecology 12, 5.

Pullin, R.V.S., Lowe-Mcconnell, R.H. (Eds.), 1982. The Biology and Culture of Tilapias. ICLARM Conference Proceedings No. 7. ICLARM, Manila, Philippines, 432 pp.

Richter, H., Focken, U., Becker, K., Santiago, C.B., Afuang, W.B., 1999. Analysing the diel feeding patterns and daily ration of Nile tilapia, *Oreochromis niloticus* (L.), in Laguna de Bay, Philippines. Journal of Applied Ichthyology 15, 165–170.

Ross, L.G., 2000. Environmental physiology and energetics. In: Beveridge, M.C.M., McAndrew, B.J. (Eds.), Tilapias: Biology and Exploitation. Kluwer Academic Publishers, Dordrecht/Boston/London, pp. 89–128.

Sakhare, V.B., Jetithor, S.G., 2016. Food and feeding behaviour of Mozambique tilapia (*Oreochromis mossambicus* Peters) from Borna reservoir of Maharashtra, India. Journal of Fisheries 4, 431–434.

Scoppettone, G.G., Salgado, J., Nielsen, M.B., 2005. Blue tilapia (*Oreochromis aureus*) predation on fishes in the Muddy River system, Clark County, Nevada. Western North American Naturalist 65, 410–414.

Shep, H., Konan, M.K., Doumbia, L., Ouattara, M., Boussou, C.K., Ouattara, A., et al., 2013. Feeding relationships among *Tilapia zillii* (Gervais, 1848), *Tilapia guineensis* (Bleeker, 1862) and their hybrid in Ayamé man-made lake, Côte d'Ivoire. Pakistan Journal of Zoology 45, 1405–1414.

Smith, A., 1840. Illustration of the Zoology of South Africa. Volume 4, Pisces, p. 5. Smith, Elder and Co., London, p. 5.

Spataru, P., 1976. The feeding habits of *Tilapia galilaea* (Artedi) in Lake Kinneret (Israel). Aquaculture 9, 47–59.

Spataru, P., 1978. Food and feeding habits of *Tilapia zillii* (Gervais) (Cichlidae) in Lake Kinneret (Israel). Aquaculture 14, 327–338.

Spataru, P., Zorn, M., 1978. Food and feeding habits of *Tilapia aurea* (Steindachner) (Cichlidae) in Lake Kinneret (Israel). Aquaculture 13, 67–79.

Teugels, G.G., Thys van Den Audenaerde, D.F.E., 2003. Cichlidae. In: Paugy, D., Lévêque, C., Teugels, G.G. (Eds.), The fresh and Brackish Water Fishes of West Africa. Volume 2. Collection of Faune et flore tropicales 40. Institut de recherche de développement, Paris, France, Muséum national d'histoire naturelle, Paris, France and Musée royal de l'Afrique Central, Tervuren, Belgium, pp. 521–600.

Toguyeni, A., Fauconneau, B., Boujard, T., Fostier, A., Kuhn, E.R., Mol, K.A., et al., 1997. Feeding behaviour and food utilization in tilapia, *Oreochromis niloticus*: effects of sex ratio and relationship with the endocrine status. Physiology & Behavior 62, 273–279.

Trewavas, E., 1982. Tilapias: taxonomy and speciation. In: Pullin, R.V.S., Lowe-McConnell, R.H. (Eds.), The Biology and Culture of Tilapias. ICLARM Conference Proceedings No. 7. ICLARM, Manila, Philippines, pp. 3–13.

Whitefield, A.K., Blaber, S.J.M., 1978. Resource segregation among iliophagous fish in Lake St. Lucia, Zululand. Environmental Biology of Fishes 3, 293–296.

Chapter 3

Tilapia distribution, transfers and introductions

Chapter outline

3.1 Introduction

Tilapia are freshwater fishes belonging to Family 'Cichlidae'. According to FAO Fishbase (Froese and Pauly, 2018), Family Cichlidae includes 1699 species, widely distributed in Africa, Southeast Asia, the Middle East and South and Central America (Lagler et al., 1977). This chapter highlights the natural geographical distribution, transfer and introduction of tilapia, especially tilapia species that are either currently cultured or have aquaculture potential, or represent an important component in capture freshwater and brackish water fisheries. Special emphasis is given to Nile tilapia (*Oreochromis niloticus*), which is the most important farmed tilapia species in the world, representing 70% of total tilapia production in 2017, and Mozambique tilapia (*Oreochromis mossambicus*) (about 1% of total tilapia production) (FAO, 2019). These two species are the most widely distributed in the world. The introductions and transfers of other tilapia species are also briefly highlighted.

3.2 Natural geographical distribution of tilapia

Tilapias are a freshwater group of fish species originated exclusively from Africa (excluding Madagascar) and from Palestine (Jordan Valley and coastal rivers) (Philippart and Ruwet, 1982). They are distributed all over Africa, except the northern Atlas Mountains and South-West Africa (McAndrew, 2000). Outside Africa, they are also widely distributed in the South and Central America, Southern India, Sri Lanka (Philippart and Ruwet, 1982) and Lake Kinneret, Israel. Tilapias also inhabit a wide range of ecosystems (see Chapter 4 for details). They seem to have evolved as riverine fishes living in the marginal waters and floodplain pools, but they have been adapted to lacustrine conditions. This explains why they currently live in various ecological water systems, including slow-moving rivers and their floodplain pools and swamps, small shallow lakes, large deep lakes, impounded water bodies, isolated crater lakes, soda lakes, thermal springs and brackish water lakes (Philippart and Ruwet, 1982; Lowe-Mcconnell, 2000). These fishes are also highly adaptable to their environments, as reflected by their tolerance to a wide range of environmental conditions such as temperature, salinity, dissolved oxygen and ammonia (details on environmental requirements of tilapia are provided in Chapter 4).

Philippart and Ruwet (1982) suggested that the natural distribution of the two tilapia genera, *Tilapia* (substrate-

Tilapia Culture. https://doi.org/10.1016/B978-0-12-816541-6.00003-9
Copyright © 2020 Elsevier Inc. All rights reserved.

spawners) and *Oreochromis* (mouthbrooders), is a reflection of two types of factors:

1. Historical–geological factors which have led to geographical isolation and speciation (endemic species in lakes or stretches of rivers).
2. Ecological factors which represent the requirements of, and preferences to, the various environmental conditions such as temperature, salinity, water composition, in addition to the behavioural characteristics which reflect feeding and reproduction patterns.

Based on the historical factors, the genus *Tilapia* is widely distributed in West and Central Africa, but not in the eastern slope of the eastern Rift Valley and the river basins flowing into the Indian Ocean north of Zambesi River. These fish species are separated by ecological or behavioural barriers rather than by geographical or hydrographic barriers (Philippart and Ruwet, 1982). On the other hand, all species of the genus *Sarotherodon*, except *Sarotherodon galilaeus*, are restricted to West Africa. *S. galilaeus* have spread eastwards towards the Nile and the first Rift lakes. Meanwhile, the genus *Oreochromis* are widely distributed in the Rift Valley lakes and rivers and the rivers that drain into the Indian Ocean, but they are rare in Western Africa.

O. niloticus and *O. aureus* are distributed in the Nilo-Sudanian region. Moreover, *O. niloticus* is spreading eastwards into the Ethiopian Rift Valley, and moved southwards colonizing all the western Rift lakes (Lake Albert, Lake George, Lake Edward, Lake Kivu and Lake Tanganyika) and Lake Turkana in the eastern Rift Valley. This species is also spreading in Central and Western Africa (Senegal, Gambia, Volta, Niger, Benue and Chad), via the Chad and Niger basins. The following *O. niloticus* subspecies have been recognized: *Oreochromis niloticus baringoensis*, *Oreochromis niloticus cancellatus*, *Oreochromis niloticus eduardianus*, *Oreochromis niloticus filoa*, *Oreochromis niloticus niloticus*, *Oreochromis niloticus sugutae*, *Oreochromis niloticus tana* and *Oreochromis niloticus vulcani*. *O. mossambicus* is generally restricted to the eastward flowing streams, extending from the lower Zambezi River and its delta, the lower Shiré River and coastal plains from Zambezi delta southwards to Algoa Bay and the Bushmans River. Populations of this species are also found in the Hunyani and Shangani rivers and the middle Zambezi River tributaries, but it is not known whether they are native or introduced (Shelton and Popma, 2006).

It appears, therefore, that *Tilapia* and *Sarotherodon* species are more localized in West Africa, while *Oreochromis* species are more distributed in the Central and Eastern African regions. However, some species, such as *Tilapia zillii*, *S. galilaeus*, *O. niloticus* and, to a lesser extent, *O. aureus* have a larger and overlapping distribution. *T. zillii* and *S. galilaeus* are distributed far south to Lake Albert, suggesting that the Chad-Nile connection that enabled them to inhabit the Nile River must have occurred after *O. niloticus* had spread southwards and after the disappearance of the connection between Lake Albert and southerly lakes (McAndrew, 2000).

3.3 Factors affecting tilapia distribution

3.3.1 Habitat diversity

Habitat diversity is one of the major factors behind the wide distribution of tilapia. In Africa, for example, tilapia inhabit the following wide range of ecologically and geographically different habitats:

- Rivers: permanent and temporary rivers, rivers with rapids, large equatorial rivers (Zaire) and tropical and subtropical rivers (Nile, Niger, Senegal, Zambezi and Limpopo);
- Lakes:
  - shallow, swampy lakes (Lakes Bangweulu, Victoria, Kyoga, Rukwa and Chad),
  - deep lakes (Lakes Albert, Kivu, Tanganyika and Malawi),
  - man-made lakes (Lakes Nasser and Nobia),
  - alkaline and saline lakes (Lakes Magadi, Natron, Manyara, Mweru Wantipa, Chilwa, Chiuta, Turkana, Tana and Qarun),
  - crater lakes (Lakes Chala, Barombi, Mbo, Barombi ba Kotto and Bosumtwi),
  - lakes with low mineral contents (Lakes Bangweulu and Nabugabo),
  - acidic lakes (Tumba);
- Hot springs (Magadi);
- Open and closed estuaries and coastal lagoons (Lakes Maryut, Edku, Borullos, Manzalla), and
- Marine habitats (Gulf of Suez, Alexandria West Harbour, Abu Qir Bay in Alexandria).

3.3.2 Environmental conditions

The above-mentioned habitat diversity represents a wide range of environmental conditions, including physical parameters (temperature, photoperiod, depth, current velocity, turbidity, etc.), chemical parameters (salinity, pH, dissolved oxygen, mineral and gas contents) and biological factors (competition, food availability, productivity, etc.). This habitat diversity allows tilapia to tolerate an extremely varied range of these environmental conditions. The environmental requirements of tilapia are covered in detail in Chapter 4.

3.4 Tilapia transfers and introductions

Transfer of an aquatic species is the movement of that species within its geographical range. Transfers generally take place to support stressed populations, enhance genetic characteristics or re-establish a species that has failed locally (GESAMP, 1991). On the other hand, introductions are the movements of a species beyond its present geographical range. Introductions are intended to establish new taxa into the flora and fauna of an environment. Transfers and introductions can pose a wide variety of risks to the integrity of ecosystems, existing species, human health, agriculture, aquaculture and related primary industries.

Many tilapia species have been introduced into more than 100 countries; to become the most widely distributed group of exotic fish worldwide. They have been established in almost all water masses in which they were cultured or introduced into (Costa-Pierce, 2003). Some of these species are now widely distributed in most of Africa, Asia and the Americas (Costa-Pierce, 2003) and have become a part of the fish fauna of many tropical and subtropical freshwater environments.

Tilapia aquaculture has witnessed a rapid worldwide expansion during the past three decades. Despite that tilapia are tropical and subtropical freshwater fishes, originated in Africa and the Middle East, tilapia culture is currently practiced in over 120 countries all over the globe, even in countries beyond their ecological and geographical range. However, tilapia introductions for aquaculture or stocking in public waters in many countries were carried out without studying their potential ecological and socioeconomic impacts (Naylor et al., 2001; Azevedo-Santos et al., 2017; Cassemiro et al., 2017). Therefore, these introductions may have significant ecological, social and economic effects.

Philippart and Ruwet (1982) summarized the objectives of tilapia introductions as follows:

- Stocking natural lakes which are not inhabited naturally by tilapia (such as *Sarotherodon alcalicus grahami* into Lake Nakuru, *Oreochromis spilurus niger* and *T. zillii* into Lake Naivasha, *Oreochromis macrochir* and *Tilapia rendalli* into Lake Lusiwashi).
- Introductions into natural habitats to fill ecological niches that are not occupied by any of the tilapias present, to increase fisheries yields (such as *T. zillii* and *O. niloticus* into Lake Victoria and Lake Kyoga).
- Introductions into natural water bodies to develop tilapia-based new fisheries (such as *O. mossambicus* and *O. niloticus* in the reservoir of a southern Tunisian oasis).
- Introductions into natural water bodies to consume plankton production (*O. macrochir* into Lakes Kariba and Mcllwaine (Zimbabwe), *O. mossambicus* and *Sarotherodon mortimeri* into the lakes of the Zimbabwe eastern highlands).
- Biological aquatic weed control (such as *T. rendalli* into Sudanese irrigation canals) and the control of mosquitoes.
- Tilapia culture in rice fields, cages and ponds.
- Recreation (aquarium/ornamental fisheries).
- Providing sport fish to attract tourism.
- Accidental introductions occurring during the deliberate introduction of other tilapia species (such as *T. rendalli* into Lakes Victoria and Kyoga) or because of the confusion between sympatric species which have begun to differentiate (such as *O. niloticus* and *O. aureus*).

It should be emphasized that, because of the old, unrecorded introductions of tilapia, it is almost impossible in several cases to tell whether the presence of a given species is natural or introduced by man, accidently or deliberately.

Of the species transferred or introduced outside Africa, *O. mossambicus* and *O. niloticus* are by far the most important from both production and scientific points of view (De Silva et al., 2004). These species are now widely distributed in most of Asia and the Pacific, Latin America, Southern regions of North America (the United States and Mexico), the Caribbean and in many parts of Europe (Figs 3.1–3.3). In many cases, they have become a part of the fish fauna of most of tropical and subtropical freshwater and brackish water environments.

Among 114 global introductions of *O. niloticus*, 52 were established (45.6%) and 12 (10.5%) were 'probably established' (Froese and Pauly, 2018), with a total of 56.1%. However, 'probably established' introductions remain to be confirmed. For *O. mossambicus*, 128 introductions were recorded (Froese and Pauly, 2018). Out of this number 100 introductions were established (78%), 15 'probably established' (11.7%), while only 10.1% were 'not established'.

3.5 Pros and cons of tilapia introductions

The pros and cons of the impacts of tilapia introductions in natural waters, or for aquaculture, differ among societies, researchers and decision makers, depending on the objectives of these introductions. Deines et al. (2016) evaluated the trade-offs among ecosystem services associated with global tilapia introductions by analyzing 290 publications related to the presence or absence of ecological effects. They found that 152 papers reported presence of different ecological effects, while 53 publications reported both presence and absence of ecological effects. Additional 22 publications reported nonoccurrence of such effects. Accordingly, there are three scenarios describing these impacts.

1. The first scenario is that tilapia introduction causes adverse ecological impacts on native aquatic environments.

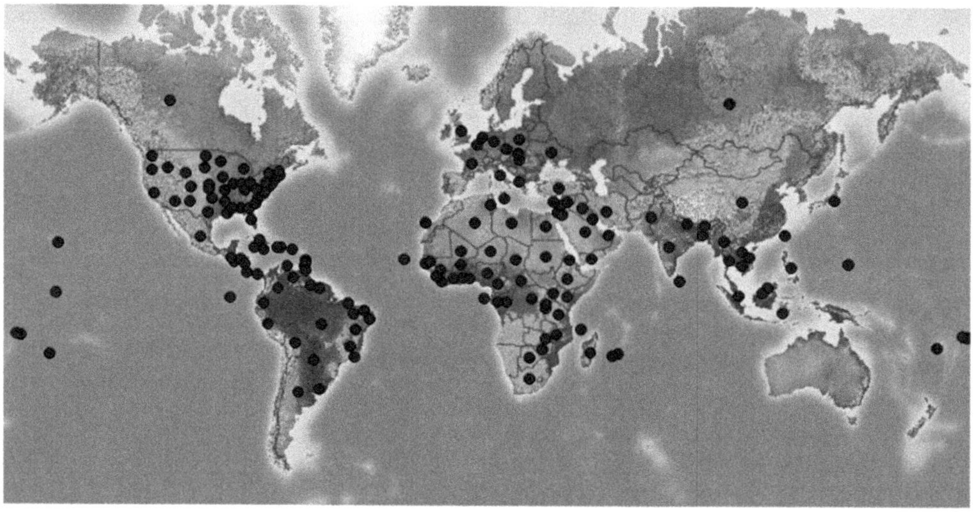

FIGURE 3.1 Global distribution of Nile tilapia. *From CABI Invasive Species Compendium (https://www.cabi.org/isc/datasheet/72086).*

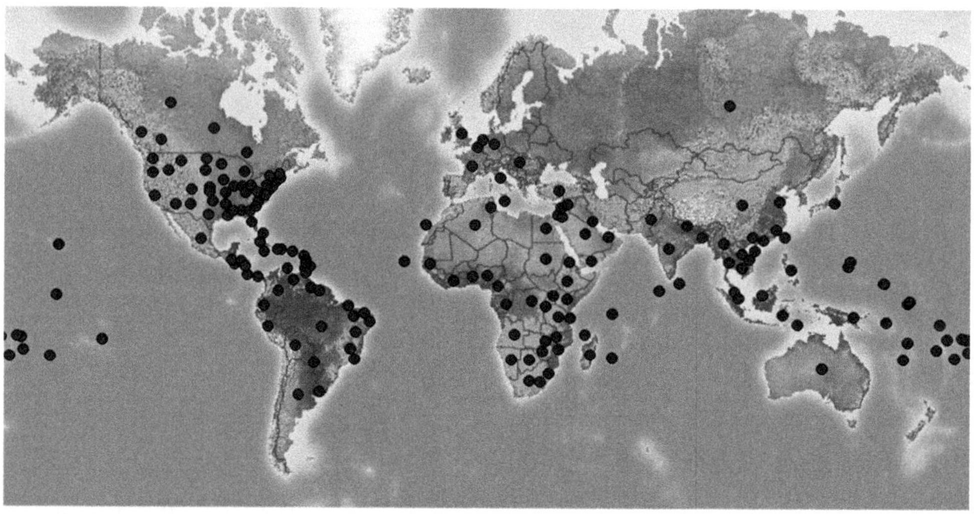

FIGURE 3.2 Global distribution of Mozambique tilapia (*Oreochromis mossambicus*). *From CABI Invasive Species Compendium (https://www.cabi.org/isc/datasheet/72085).*

2. The second scenario claims that despite the evidences of ecological impacts, the social and economic benefits of these fish introductions are more important.
3. The third scenario suggests that the impacts of tilapia introductions are controversial and not conclusive; and may even not occur.

3.5.1 Adverse ecological impacts

Aquatic biologists and conservationists are highly concerned about the potential threats and disturbances of tilapia introductions on the biodiversity and health of freshwater and brackish water ecosystems. Over 75% of published papers concluded that the impacts of tilapia introductions were negative (Deines et al., 2016). Twenty six percent of countries that have received tilapia introductions reported varying degrees of ecological effects (Deines et al., 2016); this figure is much higher than the most extreme 20% and the average 5% previously reported (Gozlan, 2008). These impacts include habitat loss and degradation, overexploitation, reduction or eradication of native species, hybridization with native species, spread of aquatic diseases and pollution. Sufficient evidences were provided supporting the assumption that the introduction of different tilapia species has already posed damage to the aquatic environments into which they were introduced (Sifa, 2005; Bittencourt et al., 2014; Gu et al., 2015; Ujjania et al., 2015; Zengeya et al., 2015).

The impacts of tilapia of the genus *Oreochromis* (e.g. *O. niloticus*, *O. mossambicus* and *O. aureus*), which were introduced mainly for aquaculture and/or fisheries support, are more devastating than those caused by other

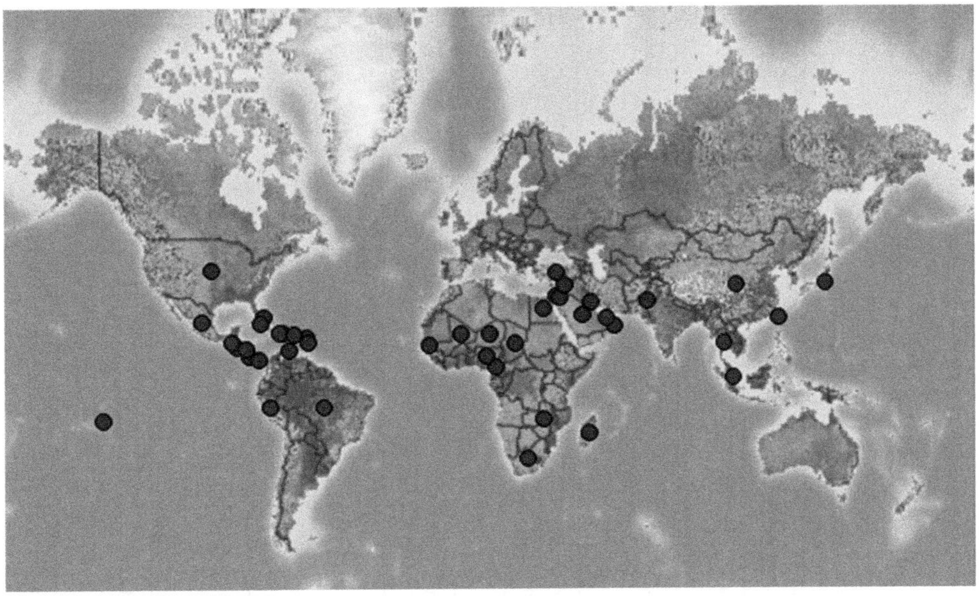

FIGURE 3.3 Global distribution of blue tilapia (*Oreochromis aureus*). *From CABI Invasive Species Compendium (https://www.cabi.org/isc/datasheet/72068).*

tilapia species. Table 3.1 summarizes the impacts of the introductions of these tilapia species (*Oreochromis* sp.) in selected countries, lakes, rivers and reservoirs worldwide. The recorded impacts include but not necessarily restricted to:

- reducing/endangering/displacement of native fish species (Athauda, 2010; Zengeya et al., 2011, 2015; Ujjania et al., 2015),
- competition for food and breeding sites with endemic species (Arthington and Blühdorn, 1996; Athauda, 2010; Khan et al., 2011),
- reduction of capture fisheries production (Sifa, 2005; Gu et al., 2015),
- eutrophication of freshwater reservoirs and alteration of the limnological parameters (Attayde et al., 2011),
- hybridization with other tilapias (Zengeya et al., 2013; Gu et al., 2015) and
- spreading pathogens and parasites (Arthur et al., 2010).

3.5.1.1 Loss of biodiversity and habitat degradation

The ecological impacts of introduced tilapia on freshwater ecosystems vary significantly depending on the invading species, the extent of the invasion and the vulnerability of the ecosystem to which they were introduced (Canonico et al., 2005). Loss and degradation of biodiversity caused by these species can occur throughout all levels of biological organization from the genetic and population levels to the species, community and habitat/ecosystem levels. It should also be recognized that tilapia introductions often occur simultaneously with other major factors affecting ecological changes in freshwater ecosystems; such as overfishing, flow modifications, habitat degradation and pollution (De Silva et al., 2009; Deines et al., 2016). But most of the studies conducted on the ecological impacts of tilapia introductions did not address these possibly confounding factors.

Almost all tilapia introductions into aquatic environments, either intentionally or accidently, led to some degrees of habitat degradation, loss and reduction or elimination of native ichthyfauna. For example, blue tilapia (*O. aureus*) were introduced into Muddy River, Nevada (USA), as sport fish, food source, forage for warm water predatory fish and aquatic plant control. But they caused significant changes in local fish community structure, reduction/elimination of native fishes and reduction of endemic fish habitat (Scoppettone et al., 2005). In Sri Lanka, the introduction of Mozambique tilapia into freshwater bodies led to displacement or extinction of the native fishes and competed for food with indigenous species (De Silva, 1985; Athauda, 2010). Similar impacts have also been reported in India (Ujjania et al., 2015), Brazil (Attayde et al., 2011; Bittencourt et al., 2014), South Africa (Zengeya et al., 2015) and many other countries (see Table 3.1 for more details).

3.5.1.2 Genetic pollution

3.5.1.2.1 Hybridization

One of the major risks of tilapia introductions is their ability to interbreed with closely related domestic species. Such uncontrolled hybridization is likely to cause a loss of genetic variability. As a result, the loss of pure tilapia

TABLE 3.1 Impacts of the introduction of tilapia (*Oreochromis* sp.) in selected countries and water masses.

Continent	Country/water body	Species	Positive impacts	Negative impacts	References
Africa	Uganda (Lake Victoria)	*Oreochromis niloticus*		Disappearance of native tilapias, due to hybridization and competition	Njiru et al. (2010)
	Uganda (Lake Bunyoni)	*O. niloticus*	Supplement declining endemics	Hybridization with other tilapias, retarded growth of Nile tilapia, infestation by parasites and poor fishery yields	Lowe-McConnell (1958), Beadle (1981)
	Southern Africa	*O. niloticus*	Aquaculture, stock enhancements, increase of fisheries yield and poverty alleviation	Reduction/displacement of indigenous species through competitive exclusion and hybridization	Zengeya et al. (2015)
	Zimbabwe (Lake Kariba, Zambezi River basins)	*O. niloticus*	Aquaculture, recreational and sport fishing	Reducing/endangering/displacing native tilapias (*Oreochromis mortimeri*)	Marshall (2000), Zengeya and Marshall (2007), Zengeya et al. (2011)
	Mozambique (Lake Chicamba)	*O. niloticus*	Significant contribution to the artisanal fishery	Potential impact on domestic species composition	Weyl (2008)
	South Africa (Limpopo River)	*O. niloticus*		Extinction risk of indigenous species (*Oreochromis mossambicus*) through hybridization and competition exclusion, loss of genetic integrity	van der Waal and Bills (2000), Zengeya et al. (2013)
	Madagascar	*O. mossambicus*, *O. niloticus*	Stock enhancement, support commercial fisheries	Decline of native fish species	Benstead et al. (2003)
Asia and the Pacific	Lao PDR	*O. niloticus* and major carps	Increases in total fish biomass		Arthur et al. (2010)
	Bangladesh (Kaptai Lake)	*O. niloticus*	Aquaculture and fisheries enhancement	Decline of the indigenous carp fishery	Hussain (1996)
	Bangladesh	*O. niloticus*	Sharp increase in total biomass, more fish protein to local communities	Reduction in the population number and biomass of small indigenous species	Shameem Ahmad et al. (2008)
	Malaysia	*O. niloticus* *O. mossambicus*	Aquaculture, recreational fisheries and stocks enhancement	Change of the structure of indigenous fish groups	Rahim et al. (2013)
	Pakistan	*O. aureus*	Aquaculture development	Compete for food and space with native fauna	Khan et al. (2011)
	India	*O. mossambicus*	Production enhancement and contribution to commercial catches	Reduction/elimination of endogenous fishes, change of production of local fishes and reduction in the average weight of Indian major carps	Ujjania et al. (2015)

	Thailand	*O. niloticus*	Aquaculture, increased per capita fish consumption and improved rural economy	Predation on eggs of indigenous cyprinids	Vidthayanon (2005)
	Cambodia	*O. mossambicus*	Fisheries enhancement	Decline of indigenous fishes, disturbance of the habitats and competition for space with endemic species	Nuov et al. (2005)
	China (Guangdong rivers)	*O. niloticus*	Aquaculture and fisheries enhancement	Reduction of the growth rates of native mud carp, decrease in catch per unit effort (CPUE) and income of native fishes and hybridization with other *Oreochromis* species (*O. aureus*)	Sifa (2005), Gu et al. (2015)
	Sri Lanka	*O. mossambicus*	Fisheries support	Displacement/extinction of the native fishes, compete for food with indigenous species	De Silva (1985), Athauda (2010)
	Australia (Murray—Darling basin)	*O. mossambicus*	Aquarium industry	Competition with indigenous species for food and breeding sites and exclusion of native fishes	Arthington and Blühdorn (1996)
The Americas	Nicaragua (lakes)	*Oreochromis* spp.	Aquaculture and fisheries support	Competitive displacement, decline of native cichlid populations	McCrary et al. (2007)
	Mexico (Laguna Chichancanab)	*O. mossambicus*		Microhabitat shifts, competitive exclusion of endemic pupfish (*Cyprinodon* spp.)	Fuselier (2001)
	Brazil	*O. niloticus*	Aquaculture and fisheries support	Reduction of the native fishes, competition with indigenous cichlids for food and breeding sites, reduction in CPUE of other commercial species and eutrophication of reservoirs	Figueredo and Giani (2005), Attayde et al. (2011), Bittencourt et al. (2014)
	USA (Muddy River, Nevada)	*O. aureus*	Sport fish, food source, forage for warm water predatory fish, aquatic plant control	Changes in local fish community structure, reduction/elimination of native fishes and reduction of endemic fish habitat	Scoppettone et al. (2005)
	USA (lower Colorado River and the Salton Sea)	*O. mossambicus* *O. aureus* *O. hornorum*	Sport fish, bait fish, mosquito and weed control	Reduction of native species (desert pupfish) and competition for food and nesting sites	Swift et al. (1993)
	Experimental (estuaries of the Gulf of Mexico)	*O. niloticus*	Aquaculture	Decline/displacement of native species	Martin et al. (2010)

species is gradually increasing. Unlimited numbers of hybridizations have been reported both in cultured and wild tilapia. In most cases, hybrids have morphometrically and biologically different characteristics from those of their parents. Natural hybridization between related tilapia species (either introduced or native) is also possible. For example, hybridization between *O. spilurus niger* x *Oreochromis leucosticte* (Lake Naivasha), *O. spilurus niger* x *O. niloticus* (Lake Bunyoni), *O. macrochir* x *O. niloticus* (Lake Itasy) has been reported (Moreau, 1983). The introduction of Nile tilapia into Limpopo River (South Africa) led to extinction risk of the indigenous species (*O. mossambicus*) through hybridization, competition exclusion and loss of genetic integrity (Zengeya et al., 2013). Similarly, the introduction of Nile tilapia into Lake Victoria (Uganda) resulted in the disappearance of native tilapias, due to hybridization and competition (Njiru et al., 2010). In Tanzania, hybridization occurred between the introduced Nile tilapia and blue-spotted tilapia (*Oreochromis leucostictus*) and the indigenous species (*Oreochromis esculentus*, *Oreochromis jipe* and *Oreochromis korogwe*) (Bradbeer et al., 2019). In the Pangani basin, several hybrids were recorded, including *O. niloticus* × *O. jipe*, *O. leucostictus* × *O. jipe* and *O. niloticus* × *O. korogwe*).

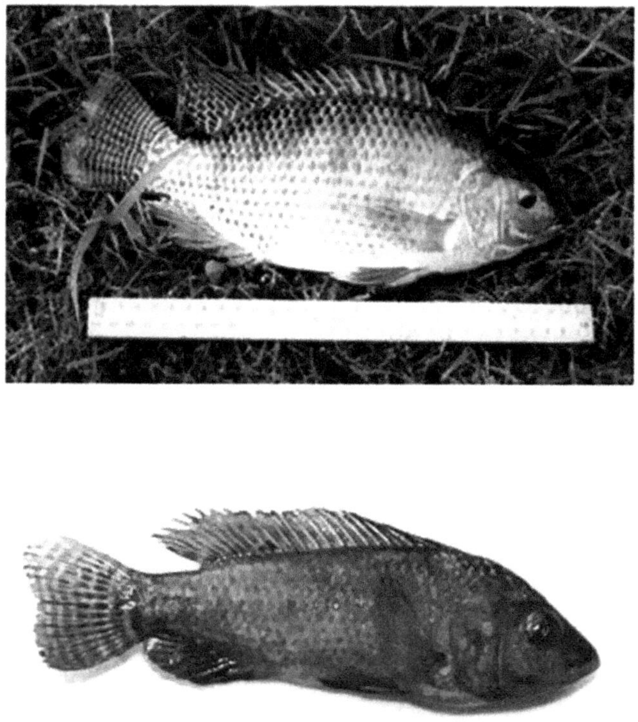

FIGURE 3.4 Normal and healthy Nile tilapia (top) and Nile tilapia showing body deformation because of inbreeding (bottom). *(top photo provided by M. Rizk; bottom photograph by A.-F. M. El-Sayed).*

3.5.1.2.2 Inbreeding

Inbreeding is defined as 'the mating or crossing of individuals more closely related than average pairs in the population'. The smaller the founder stock, the higher the chance of inbreeding. Inbreeding of tilapia has been a major problem both in wild populations established in new environments and farmed populations around the world. In most cases, the founder stocks which have been used for tilapia aquaculture were generally small. For example, it has been reported that the founder stock of Mozambique tilapia in Asia was only five individuals (three males and two females) introduced into Indonesia in the 1950s (Agustin, 1999). Those individuals were bred and their progenies formed the basis of tilapia culture and the establishment of feral stocks throughout much of Asia, except at higher latitudes, where they are not present. As expected, inbreeding of these fish was inevitable, leading to stunting, early sexual maturation, body deformation (Fig. 3.4), low survival and poor growth. As a result, Mozambique tilapia are no longer considered to be a desirable aquaculture candidate in many locations, and the species has been replaced by Nile tilapia or tilapia hybrids in many Asian countries. Inbreeding may also lead to the reduction of heterozygosity as has been suggested by Kocher (1997) who reported that some strains of farmed tilapia showed less than 10% of the heterozygosity of their wild counterparts.

3.5.1.2.3 Transgenesis

Despite that transgenesis offers several advantages for tilapia culture (see Chapter 14 for details), the rate of genetic change in transgenic tilapia is such that their phenotypic and behavioural properties cannot be easily predicted (Mair, 2002). When transgenic tilapia are introduced into new environments, they may have adverse effects both on the environment and on native species. Transgenic tilapia could also escape, and the transgene become a part of the gene pool, inducing artificial genetic diversity to native populations. This may increase or decrease fitness or have no phenotypic or ecological effects (Dunham, 1999). Negative impacts include overdominance and/or replacing the native populations. Guillen et al. (1999) found that transgenic tilapia had lower feeding motivation and dominance status than wild tilapia in Cuba. If large numbers of transgenic fish escape or are introduced, they could also reduce reproduction in natural populations through infertile matings (Dunham, 1999).

3.5.2 Beneficial impacts

On the contrary of the adverse impacts of tilapia introduction, the second scenario claims that the social and economic benefits of these fish introductions are sufficient to offset any negative ecological impacts they may cause.

Those who are in favour of this scenario believe that despite the necessity for protecting the aquatic environment and its biodiversity, feeding the poor and maintaining human well-being are more important. For example, it has been reported that tilapia culture and capture fisheries have made a significant contribution to food security in many developing countries in tropical and subtropical regions (De Silva et al., 2004; Canonico et al., 2005; Athauda, 2010; Deines et al., 2016). In addition, Shameem Ahmad et al. (2008) found that mixed-sex culture of Nile tilapia with selected small indigenous species (SIS) of Bangladesh and Nepal caused a reduction in the population number and biomass of these SIS. However, total fish production increased two to three times after tilapia introduction; providing more cheap protein source to the local communities that rely mainly on fish for their protein needs. It is evident that these benefits have direct and indirect socioeconomic impacts on various sectors, especially in rural areas. This would in turn lead to poverty alleviation, improvement of livelihood of rural households and sustainable access to an affordable animal protein source.

It should be emphasized that both socioeconomic contexts of tilapia introduction and ecological effects play a significant role in the perspective benefits or harm. Therefore, the relationship between socioeconomic choices and potential impacts on ecosystem health should be understood. This would help the stakeholders to use the economic outcomes to prevent or compensate the adverse impacts of invasive or introduced species and ensure that both ecosystems and socioeconomic benefits are secured and sustained. In this regard, De Silva et al. (2004) concluded that tilapia introductions to Asia and the Pacific have been positive. They reported the following social and economic benefits of introduced tilapias in these regions:

a. establishment of capture fisheries in certain countries (e.g. Sri Lanka, Indonesia and the Philippines);
b. an important aquaculture fish in most countries in the region, appropriate for a wide range of aquaculture operations;
c. a source of inexpensive animal protein in developing countries;
d. providing an opportunity for employment, especially in rural areas, and
e. a source of income through local and international marketing and trade.

According to FAO aquaculture database, the production of tilapia from freshwater capture fisheries and aquaculture has sharply increased in many countries to which they were introduced. This has contributed significantly to total fish production and food security, especially in rural societies. Table 3.2 shows the contribution of tilapia production to

TABLE 3.2 The contribution of introduced tilapia to total fish production in selected countries in 1970 and 2016.

Year	Production system	Brazil	Indonesia	Mexico	Philippines	Sri Lanka	Thailand
1970	Tilapia fisheries (t)	4300	15,109	400	0	8300	0
	Total freshwater (FW) fisheries (t)	83,800	297,895	5170	58,580	8300	78,080
	Percent of tilapia in total FW fisheries	5.13	5.07	7.74	0	100	0
	Tilapia aquaculture (t)	0	879	200	1417	0	1649
	Total FW aquaculture (t)	0	56,573	530	1417	0	19,829
	Percent of tilapia in total FW aquaculture	0	1.55	37.74	100	0	8.32
	Percent of tilapia in total FW fish production	5.13	4.51	10.53	2.36	100	1.48
2016	Tilapia fisheries (t)	22,860	48,714	122,633	41,677	43,836	20,700
	Total FW fisheries (t)	219,022	403,425	194,908	89,869	73,930	186,100
	Percent of tilapia in total FW fisheries	10.44	12.05	62.92	46.47	59.29	11.12
	Tilapia aquaculture (t)	239,131	1,103,812	58,191	241,379	15,468	208,144
	Total FW aquaculture (t)	505,395	3,382,390	66,255	263,005	24,334	398,597
	Percent of tilapia in total FW aquaculture	47.32	32.63	87.83	91.18	63.57	52.22
	Percent of tilapia in total FW fish production	36.17	30.44	69.24	80.21	60.35	39.14

Data from FAO Fisheries and Aquaculture Statistics (http://www.fao.org/fishery/statistics/en).

total inland water fish production in selected countries in Asia and Latin America (the major recipients of introduced tilapia). Tilapia currently represent 10% to over 60% of total freshwater fisheries in these countries; whereas farmed tilapia contribute between 35% and 90% to total inland water aquaculture. This clearly demonstrates the contribution of captured and farmed introduced tilapia to total fish production and food security in these countries.

3.5.3 Noneffect of tilapia introduction

A third category believes that the impact of alien species, including tilapia, is controversial and not conclusive; and it is premature to suggest that the introduction of these fishes have a significant negative effect on native aquatic biodiversity (Simberloff, 1981; Rahim, 2012). If environmental conditions are favourable, alien species can exploit unoccupied environmental space and coexist with native species (Simberloff, 1981), leading to increasing total species richness (Gido and Brown, 1999). De Silva et al. (2004) concluded also that there is neither explicit evidence nor an objective synthesis of available information to suggest that tilapias' introductions alone have caused negative ecological impacts on aquatic biodiversity in Asia and the Pacific. Guerrero (1999) also reported that tilapia introduction did not cause any adverse effects on the endemic fish fauna in the Philippine lakes and reservoirs. In addition, 23% of introduced species present no identified ecological risk (Gozlan, 2008).

Tilapia introduction may even increase total biomass without affecting species diversity and richness. In support, Arthur et al. (2010) found that stocking of nonnative Nile tilapia (*O. niloticus*) and major carps (mrigal *Cirrhinus cirrhosus*, rohu *Labeo rohita* and bighead carp *Hypophthalmichthys nobilis*) in freshwater wetlands in Lao PDR significantly increased the total biomass. No significant impacts on native fish species richness, diversity indices and species composition were detected. The main reason for this limited impact on native fish communities may have been due to the low niche overlap between nonnative and native species present in these wetlands.

Moreover, it has been hypothesized that native communities may reduce the biomass of invasive species or prevent their invasions through a different mechanism, known as 'biotic resistance' (Elton, 1958). Biotic resistance theory suggests that communities with high diversity will inhibit invasive species. In support, Gu et al. (2014) found that the biomass of nonnative Nile tilapia was significantly reduced with increasing native species richness in Pearl River and Jianjiang River (Guangdong Province, South China). These results suggest that species biodiversity represents an important defence against the invasion of Nile tilapia.

3.6 Management of tilapia introductions

Tilapia culture is expanding worldwide at an outstanding rate. Therefore, tilapia transfer and introduction for this purpose is inevitable. It will almost be impossible to ensure safe confinement; sooner or later the fish will escape from fish farms to natural waters, and may impact native biodiversity. This means that there should be conscious management measures to control tilapia introductions and combat their existing adverse ecological effects. This can be done through (Gozlan et al., 2010; Cassemiro et al., 2017) the following:

1. Prevention of tilapia introductions (if appropriate). If introductions are unavoidable, control and containment methods should be adopted. These may include:
   - selective removal,
   - prevention of transfers for other catchments,
   - environmental education to raise awareness of the risks of releasing nonnative fishes,
   - biocontrol programs and
   - effective public policies.
2. Implementation of government policies to address the problems linked to tilapia introductions. This would control both existing tilapia populations and introduction processes to minimize their impacts on aquatic biodiversity.
3. Culture of indigenous species should be encouraged; and supporting research and investment initiatives are highly recommended.
4. The development of aquaculture and fisheries enhancement using fish species that are not harmful to the natural ecosystem should be promoted. National governments and international organizations interested in fisheries and environmental sustainability must play a core role in this approach.
5. Stringent restrictions should be made to exclude nonnative tilapia from the areas where they have not yet been introduced into for aquaculture or fisheries programmes.
6. Prevention of the spread of tilapias to environmentally sensitive areas, or areas with significantly productive inland fisheries. This should go side by side with the prevention of further environmental deterioration.
7. With regard to the introductions of nonnative species, there is an urgent need for the development of national laws and legislation to comply with the international guidelines, and for effective local enforcement of such legislation.
8. Careful management procedures of tilapia culture facilities should be followed. These fish should be raised in contained facilities with no access to natural waters, or in regions where temperature barriers prohibit their spread and overwintering in case of escape.

3.7 Closing remarks

1. Tilapias are freshwater groups of fish species originated from Africa and the Middle East. The natural distribution of the two tilapia genera, *Tilapia* (substrate-spawners) and *Oreochromis* (mouthbrooders), is a reflection of historical—geological factors, and ecological factors, in addition to the behavioural characteristics which reflect feeding and reproduction patterns.
2. Tilapia have been introduced into more than 100 countries, to become the most widely distributed group of exotic fish worldwide. They have been established in almost all water masses in which they were cultured or introduced into in Africa, Asia and the Americas and have become a part of the fish fauna of many tropical and subtropical freshwater environments.
3. The impacts of tilapia introductions differ among societies, researchers and decision makers, depending on the objectives of these introductions. Three scenarios have been proposed to describe these impacts.
4. The first scenario insists that tilapia introduction causes adverse ecological impacts on native aquatic environments. Over 75% of published research concluded that the impacts of tilapia introductions were negative.
5. The second scenario claims that despite the evidences of ecological impacts, the social and economic benefits of these fish introductions are more important.
6. A third scenario suggests that the impacts of tilapia introductions are controversial and not conclusive, and may even not occur.
7. There should be conscious management measures to control tilapia introductions and combat their existing adverse ecological effects.

References

Agustin, L., 1999. Effects of Genetic Bottlenecks on Levels of Genetic Diversity and Differentiation in Feral Populations of *Oreochromis mossambicus* (Ph.D. thesis). Queensland University of Technology, Australia.

Arthington, A.H., Blühdorn, D.R., 1996. The effects of species interactions resulting from aquaculture operations. In: Baird, D.J., Beveridge, M.C.M., Kelly, L.A., Muir, J.F. (Eds.), Aquaculture and Water Resource Management. Blackwell Science, Oxford, pp. 114—139.

Arthur, R., Lorenzen, K., Homekingkeo, P., Sidavong, K., Sengvilaikham, B., Garaway, C.J., 2010. Assessing impacts of introduced aquaculture species on native fish communities: Nile tilapia and major carps in SE Asian freshwaters. Aquaculture 299, 81—88.

Athauda, S., 2010. Is tilapia becoming an invasive fish in Sri Lanka. In: Marambe, B., Silva, P., Wijesundara, S., Atapattu, N. (Eds.), Invasive Alien Species in Sri Lanka — Strengthening Capacity to Control Their Introduction and Spread. Biodiversity Secretariat of the Ministry of Environment, Sri Lanka, pp. 127—130.

Attayde, J.L., Brasil, J., Menescal, R.A., 2011. Impacts of introducing Nile tilapia on the fisheries of a tropical reservoir in North-eastern Brazil. Fisheries Management and Ecology 18, 437—443.

Azevedo-Santos, V.M., Fearniside, P.M., Oliveira, C.S., Padial, A.A., Pelicice, F.M., Lima Jr., D.P., et al., 2017. Removing the abyss between conservation science and policy decisions in Brazil. Biodiversity & Conservation 26, 1745—1752.

Beadle, L.C., 1981. The Inland Waters of Tropical Africa. Longman, London, 475 pp.

Benstead, J.P., De Rham, P.H., Gattolliat, J.-L., Gibon, F.-M., Loiselle, P.V., Sartori, M., et al., 2003. Conserving Madagascar's freshwater biodiversity. BioScience 53, 1101—1111.

Bittencourt, L.S., Silva, U.R.L., Silva, L.M.A., Dias, M.T., 2014. Impact of the invasion from nile tilapia on natives Cichlidae species in tributary of Amazonas river, Brazil. Biota Amazônia 4, 88—94.

Bradbeer, S.J., Harrington, J., Watson, H., Warraich, A., Shechonge, A., Smith, A., et al., 2019. Limited hybridization between introduced and critically endangered indigenous tilapia fishes in northern Tanzania. Hydrobiologia 832, 257—268.

Canonico, G.C., Arthington, A., McCrary, J.K., Thieme, M.L., 2005. The effects of introduced tilapias on native biodiversity. Aquatic Conservation: Marine and Freshwater Ecosystems 15, 463—483.

Cassemiro, F.A.S., Bailly, D., da Graça, W.J., Agostinho, A.A., 2017. The invasive potential of tilapias (Osteichthyes, Cichlidae) in the Americas. Hydrobiologia 817, 133—154.

Costa-Pierce, B.A., 2003. Rapid evolution of an established feral tilapia (*Oreochromis* spp.): the need to incorporate invasion science into regulatory structures. Biological Invasions 5, 71—84.

De Silva, S.S., 1985. Body condition and nutritional ecology of *Oreochromis mossambicus* (Pisces, Cichlidae) populations of man-made lakes in Sri Lanka. Journal of Fish Biology 27, 621—633.

De Silva, S.S., Subasinghe, R.P., Bartley, D.M., Lowther, A., 2004. Tilapias as Alien Aquatics in Asia and the Pacific: A Review. FAO Fisheries Technical Paper. No. 453. FAO, Rome, 65 pp.

De Silva, S.S., Nguyen, T.T.T., Turchini, G.M., Amarasinghe, U.S., Abery, N.W., 2009. Alien species in aquaculture and biodiversity: a paradox in food production. Ambio 38, 24—28.

Deines, A.M., Wittmann, M.E., Deines, J.M., Lodge, D.M., 2016. Tradeoffs among ecosystem services associated with global tilapia introductions. Reviews in Fisheries Science & Aquaculture 24, 178—191.

Dunham, R.A., 1999. Utilization of transgenic fish in developing countries: potential benefits and risks. Journal of the World Aquaculture Society 30, 1—11.

Elton, C.S., 1958. The Ecology of Invasions by Animals and Plants. Springer Science + Business Media, B.V., New York, 181 pp.

FAO, 2019. FAO Fisheries and Aquaculture Statistics. Global Aquaculture Production 1950—2017. http://www.fao.org/fishery/statistics/en.

Figueredo, C.C., Giani, A., 2005. Ecological interactions between nile tilapia (*Oreochromis niloticus*, L.) and the phytoplanktonic community of the Furnas reservoir (Brazil). Freshwater Biology 50, 1391—1403.

Froese, R., Pauly, D., 2018. FishBase. World Wide Web Electronic Publication. Version (06/2018). www.fishbase.org.

Fuselier, L., 2001. Impacts of *Oreochromis mossambicus* (Perciformes: Cichlidae) upon habitat segregation among cyprinodontids (Cyprinodontiformes) of a species flock in Mexico. Revista de Biologia Tropical 49, 647—656.

GESAMP (IMO/FAO/Unesco/WMO/WHO/IAEA/UN/UNEP (Joint Group of Experts on the Scientific Aspects of Marine Pollution), 1991. Reducing Environmental Impacts of Coastal Aquaculture. Reports and Studies, GESAMP, No. 47, Rome, Italy, 35 pp.

Gido, K.B., Brown, J.H., 1999. Invasion of North American drainages by alien fish species. Freshwater Biology 42, 387–399.

Gozlan, R.E., 2008. Introduction of non-native freshwater fish: is it all bad? Fish and Fisheries 9, 106–115.

Gozlan, R.E., Britton, J.R., Cowx, I., Copp, G.H., 2010. Current knowledge on non-native freshwater fish introductions. Journal of Fish Biology 76, 751–786.

Gu, D.E., Luo, D., Xu, M., Ma, G.M., Mu, X.D., Luo, J.R., et al., 2014. Species diversity defends against the invasion of Nile tilapia (*Oreochromis niloticus*). Knowledge and Management of Aquatic Ecosystems 414, 07.

Gu, D.E., Ma, G.M., Zhu, Y.J., Xu, M., Luo, D., Li, Y.Y., et al., 2015. The impacts of invasive Nile tilapia (*Oreochromis niloticus*) on the fisheries in the main rivers of Guangdong Province, China. Biochemical Systematics and Ecology 59, 1–7.

Guillen, I., Berlanga, J., Valenzuela, C.M., Morales, A., Toledo, J., Estrada, M.P., et al., 1999. Safety evaluation of transgenic tilapia with accelerated growth. Marine Biotechnology 1, 2–14.

Guerrero, R.D., 1999. Impacts of tilapia introductions on the endemic fishes in some Philippine lakes and reservoirs. In: van Densen, W.L.T., Morris, M.J. (Eds.), Fish and Fisheries of Lakes and Reservoirs in Southeast Asia and Africa. Westbury Publishing, Otley, UK, pp. 151–157.

Hussain, G.H., 1996. Progress of DEGITA project activities in Bangladesh. In: Paper Presented at the Third Steering Committee Meeting, International Network on Genetics in Aquaculture (INGA), July 1996, Cairo, Egypt, 17 pp. (unpublished).

Khan, A.M., Ali, Z., Shelly, S.Y., Ahmad, Z., Mirza, M.R., 2011. Aliens; a catastrophe for native fresh water fish diversity in Pakistan. The Journal of Animal and Plant Sciences 21 (2 Suppl. 1), 435–440.

Kocher, T., 1997. Introduction to the genetics of tilapia. In: Fitzsimmons, K. (Ed.), Proceedings from the Fourth International Symposium on Tilapia in Aquaculture. Northeast Regional Agriculture Engineering Service, Ithaca, New York, USA, pp. 61–64.

Lagler, K.F., Bardach, J.E., Miller, R.R., Passino, D.R.M., 1977. Ichthyology, second ed. John Wiley & Sons Inc., New York, London, Sydney. 506 pp.

Lowe-Mcconnell, R.H., 1958. Observations on the biology of *Tilapia nilotica* L. In East African waters. Revue de Zoologie et de Botanique Africaines 57, 129–170.

Lowe-Mcconnell, R.H., 2000. The role of tilapias in ecosystems. In: Beveridge, M.C.M., McAndrew, B.J. (Eds.), Tilapias: Biology and Exploitation. Kluwer Academic Publishers, Dordrecht/Boston/London, pp. 129–162.

Mair, G.C., 2002. Tilapia genetics and breeding in Asia. In: Guerrero III, R.D., Guerrero-del Castillo, M.R. (Eds.), Tilapia Farming in the 21st Century. Proceeding of the International Forum on Tilapia Farming in the 21st Century (Tilapia Forum 2002). Philippines Fisheries Association Inc., Los Banos, Laguna, Philippines, pp. 100–123.

Marshall, B.E., 2000. Freshwater fishes of the Zambezi basin. In: Timberlake, J. (Ed.), Biodiversity of the Zambezi Basin Wetlands. Occasional Publications in Biodiversity, No 8. Biodiversity Foundation for Africa, Bulawayo/Zambezi Society, Harare, Zimbabwe, pp. 393–459.

Martin, C.W., Valentine, M.M., Valentine, J.F., 2010. Competitive interactions between invasive Nile tilapia and native fish: the potential for altered trophic exchange and modification of food webs. PLoS One 5, e14395.

McAndrew, B.J., 2000. Evolution, phylogenetic relationships and biogeography. In: Beveridge, M.C.M., McAndrew, B.J. (Eds.), Tilapias: Biology and Exploitation. Kluwer Academic Publishers, Dordrecht/Boston/London, pp. 1–32.

McCrary, J.K., Murphy, B.R., Stauffer Jr., J.R., Hendrix, S.S., 2007. Tilapia (Teleostei: Cichlidae) status in Nicaraguan natural waters. Environmental Biology of Fishes 78, 107–114.

Moreau, J., 1983. Review of introductions of tilapia in open inland waters of Africa, their influence on ecology and fisheries. In: Fishelson, L., Yaron, Z. (Eds.), Proceedings of the International Symposium on Tilapia in Aquaculture. Tel-Aviv University, Israel, pp. 77–85.

Naylor, R.L., Williams, S.L., Strong, D.R., 2001. Aquaculture — a gateway for exotic species. Science 294, 1655–1656.

Njiru, M., Mkumbo, O.C., van der Knaap, M., 2010. Some possible factors leading to decline in fish species in Lake Victoria. Aquatic Ecosystem Health and Management 13, 3–10.

Nuov, S., Viseth, H., Ouk, V., 2005. Present status of alien species in aquaculture and aquatic ecosystem in Cambodia. In: Bartley, D.M., Bhujel, R.C., Funge-Smith, S., Olin, P.G., Phillips, M.J. (Comps./Eds.). International Mechanisms for the Control and Responsible Use of Alien Species in Aquatic Ecosystems. Report of an Ad Hoc Expert Consultation. Xishuangbanna, People's Republic of China, 27–30 August 2003. FAO, Rome, pp. 75–86.

Philippart, J.-C.L., Ruwet, J.-C.L., 1982. Ecology and distribution of tilapias. In: Pullin, R.S.V., Lowe-McConnell, R.H. (Eds.), The Biology and Culture of Tilapias. ICLARM Conference Proceedings No. 7. ICLARM, Manila, Philippines, pp. 15–59.

Rahim, K.A.A., 2012. Diversity, Ecology and Distribution of Non-indigenous Freshwater Fish in Malaysia (Ph.D. thesis). Universiti Putra Malaysia, Serdang Selangor.

Rahim, K.A.A., Esa, Y., Arshad, A., 2013. The influence of alien fish species on native fish community structure in Malaysian waters. Kuroshio Science 7–1, 81–93.

Scoppettone, G.G., Salgado, J., Nielsen, M.B., 2005. Blue tilapia (*Oreochromis aureus*) predation on fishes in the Muddy River system, Clark County, Nevada. Western North American Naturalist 65, 410–414.

Shameem Ahmad, S.A., Bart, A.N., Wahab, M.A., Shrestha, M.K., Rakocy, J.E., Diana, J.S., 2008. Impact of tilapia, *Oreochromis niloticus*, introduction on the indigenous species of Bangladesh and Nepal. In: Morrison, L., Egna, H. (Eds.), Twenty-Fifth Annual Technical Report, vol. I. Aquaculture CRSP, Oregon State University, Corvallis, Oregon, pp. 7–12.

Shelton, W.L., Popma, T.J., 2006. Biology. In: Lim, C., Webster, C.D. (Eds.), Tilapia: Biology, Culture, and Nutrition. Haworth Press, Inc., Binghamton, New York, pp. 1–49.

Sifa, L., 2005. Introduction and management of alien aquatic species in China. In: Bartley, D.M., Bhujel, R.C., Funge-Smith, S., Olin, P.G., Phillips, M.J. (Eds.), International Mechanisms for the Control and Responsible Use of Alien Species in Aquatic Ecosystems. Report of an Ad Hoc Expert Consultation. Xishuangbanna, People's Republic of China, 27–30 August 2003. FAO, Rome, pp. 87–98.

Simberloff, D., 1981. Community effects of introduced species. In: Nitecki, M. (Ed.), Biotic Crises in Ecological and Evolutionary Time. Academic Press, New York, pp. 53–81.

Swift, C.C., Haglund, T.R., Ruiz, M., Fisher, R.N., 1993. The status and distribution of the freshwater fishes of southern California. Bulletin Southern California Academy of Sciences 92, 101–167.

Ujjania, N.C., Dubey, M., Sharma, L.L., Balai, V.K., Srivastva, R.M., 2015. Bio-invasion of exotic fish tilapia (*Oreochromis mossambicus* P. 1852) in lake Jaisamand, India. International Journal of Fisheries and Aquatic Studies 3, 174–177.

van der Waal, B.C.W., Bills, R., 2000. *Oreochromis niloticus* (Teleostei: Cichlidae) now in the Limpopo River system. South African Journal of Science 96, 47–48.

Vidthayanon, C., 2005. Aquatic alien species in Thailand (Part 1): biodiversity. In: Bartley, D.M., Bhujel, R.C., Funge-Smith, S., Olin, P.G., Phillips, M.J. (Comps./Eds.). International Mechanisms for the Control and Responsible Use of Alien Species in Aquatic Ecosystems. Report of an Ad Hoc Expert Consultation. Xishuangbanna, People's Republic of China, 27–30 August 2003. FAO, Rome, pp. 113–118.

Weyl, O.L.F., 2008. Rapid invasion of a subtropical lake fishery in central Mozambique by Nile tilapia, *Oreochromis niloticus* (Pisces: Cichlidae). Aquatic Conservation: Marine and Freshwater Ecosystems 18, 839–851.

Zengeya, T.A., Marshall, B.E., 2007. Trophic interrelationships amongst cichlid fishes in a tropical African reservoir (Lake Chivero, Zimbabwe). Hydrobiologia 592, 175–182.

Zengeya, T.A., Booth, A.J., Bastos, A.D.S., Chimimba, C.T., 2011. Trophic interrelationships between the exotic Nile tilapia, *Oreochromis niloticus* and indigenous tilapiine cichlids in a subtropical African river system (Limpopo River, South Africa). Environmental Biology of Fishes 92, 479–489.

Zengeya, T.A., Robertson, M.P., Booth, A.J., Chimimba, C.T., 2013. A qualitative ecological risk assessment of the invasive Nile tilapia, *Oreochromis niloticus* in a sub-tropical African river system (Limpopo River, South Africa). Aquatic Conservation: Marine and Freshwater Ecosystems 23, 51–64.

Zengeya, T.A., Booth, A.J., Chimimba, C.T., 2015. Broad niche overlap between invasive Nile tilapia *Oreochromis niloticus* and indigenous congenerics in Southern Africa: should we be concerned? Entropy 17, 4959–4973.

Chapter 4

Environmental requirements

Chapter outline

4.1 Introduction

Tilapia are generally cultured semi-intensively or intensively under different culture and environmental conditions, stocking densities and management strategies. Water quality is very likely to be subjected to continuous changes, especially in intensive or super-intensive culture systems. Thus, water quality management becomes a key factor for successful aquaculture practices. It is necessary therefore to understand the major water quality parameters and their interrelationships, which affect fish growth and health and determine the failure or success of overall culture practices. Such understandings will enable fish farmers and farm managers to determine the chemical, biological and physical processes that take place in tilapia farms, and in turn, take the proper and correct supporting managerial decisions. In the meantime, tilapia have been introduced into many countries across the globe, mainly for aquaculture. The introduction of tilapia into many countries where the environmental conditions are outside their tolerance limits has made the traditional land-based systems unsuitable for their culture. Tilapia culture will certainly be affected by the varying environmental conditions in these geographically different regions.

This chapter discusses and analyzes the major environmental factors affecting tilapia in the wild or under aquaculture conditions. Special emphasis will be given to water temperature, salinity, dissolved oxygen (DO), ammonia and nitrites, pH, photoperiod and water turbidity.

4.2 Temperature

Temperature is one of the most important factors affecting the physiology, growth, reproduction and metabolism of tilapia. Temperature is of prime importance in temperate and subtropical regions, which are characterized by seasonal fluctuations in water temperature. Tilapia are thermophilic fish and known to tolerate a wide range of water temperature. Extensive research has been conducted on the effects of water temperature on tilapia performance. The temperature range for normal development, reproduction and growth of tilapia is about 20−35°C, depending on fish species, with an optimum range of about 25−30°C (Balarin and Haller, 1982; Chervinski, 1982; Philippart and Ruwet, 1982; El-Sayed and Kawanna, 2008; Xie et al., 2011). However, a tremendous difference in the growth and feed efficiency of tilapia may occur even within this narrow range of water temperature. El-Sayed and Kawanna (2008) evaluated the effects of three water temperatures (24, 28 and 32°C) (lying within the optimum range of tilapia tolerance) on the growth and feed conversion of Nile tilapia fry, reared in an indoor, recirculating system. The growth of the fish at 28°C was almost double the growth at 24 and 32°C. Fish performance at 24 and 32°C was not significantly different. It is clear that optimum water temperature (not only optimum temperature range) is essential for maximum fish growth. Similar results were also reported with Nile tilapia fingerlings (Xie et al., 2011). The maximum temperature for optimum growth and protein and

Tilapia Culture. https://doi.org/10.1016/B978-0-12-816541-6.00004-0
Copyright © 2020 Elsevier Inc. All rights reserved.

energy retention was 30°C, while increasing water temperature to 37°C resulted in a significant decrease in growth parameters.

Tilapia can also tolerate temperature as low as 7–10°C, but only for brief periods (Balarin and Haller, 1982; Jennings, 1991; Sifa et al., 2002). Longer exposure of tilapia to these low temperatures will certainly lead to mass mortality. Tilapia feeding is sharply reduced below 20°C, and they stop feeding at about 16°C, while severe mortality occurs at 12°C (Balarin and Haller, 1982). Of course, there are some variations among tilapia species in response to these temperature limits as shown in Table 4.1.

Contrary to the limited lower temperature tolerance of tilapia, they can tolerate relatively high water temperature. The upper lethal temperature limits for tilapia vary from species to another, but it has been reported that most tilapias cannot tolerate water temperature above 40–42°C for a long time (Balarin and Haller, 1982; Chervinski, 1982). The response of tilapia to varying water temperatures has been reviewed by Balarin and Hatton (1979) and Chervinski (1982). The influence of temperature on tilapia depends on species strain and size, duration of exposure, other environmental factors, culture systems and geographical location. These factors will be discussed in this section.

Since different tilapia species and strains have been introduced into many different geographic regions of the world, their response to water temperature in their new habitats should be of prime attention. It has been realized that the further the geographic location from the equator, the more tolerant are Nile tilapia strains to cold (Khater and Smitherman, 1988; Sifa et al., 2002). Sifa et al. (2002) related this phenomenon to 'natural selection' processes. These authors found also that Sudan and Egypt strains of Nile tilapia had better cold tolerance in China than genetically improved farmed tilapia (GIFT). They attributed this behaviour to the following:

(1) GIFT were introduced into China recently and had not been exposed to selective pressures for low water temperature for enough time.
(2) The Sudanese strain, introduced into China several years ago, has been subjected to cold tolerance and in turn has gone through some natural selection response to low water temperature.
(3) GIFT might have been contaminated with *Oreochromis mossambicus*, which have poor cold tolerance.

It is evident therefore that newly introduced tilapia have lower cold tolerance than those which have been introduced and adapted to local cold temperature for longer time.

The conditioning of tilapia at intermediate temperature before exposing to lower temperature may improve fish survival and tolerance to cold stress. Hofer and Watts (2002) reared genetically male tilapia at 28°C and exposed them to reduced temperatures of 20, 18, 16, 14, 13 or 12°C for 24 h, then returned them to 28°C. They found that 43% of the fish died at 14°C, and all of them died at 12°C. When the fish were pre-conditioned at 20°C, their survival was 72% and 23% when they were exposed to 14 and 12°C, respectively. In a similar study, Chervinski and Lahav (1976) found that *Oreochromis aureus* acclimated to 28°C for 2 weeks started to die at 11°C, while fish acclimated to 18°C for the same period began to die at 9°C.

It has been reported that decreased water temperature would stimulate the expression of antifreeze protein genes in tilapia. For example, El-Sayed (unpublished data) found that when Nile tilapia were exposed to cold stress they upregulated antifreeze gene, with high similarity to other type II antifreeze genes. The expression of this gene suggests that de novo synthesis of cold-induced proteins is necessary for adaptation and tolerance of Nile tilapia to low water temperature. In addition, Ammar et al. (2018) found that type IV antifreeze gene was upregulated in the intestine, gills, skin, spleen, liver, and brain of *Oreochromis niloticus* in response to cold stress. The expression of some immune-related genes was also significantly higher in winter which enables the fish to withstand cold stress.

Dietary lipids containing polyunsaturated fatty acids (UFAs) play a significant role in cold tolerance of fishes in temperate zones during winter times. This is mainly due to the unsaturation of membrane phospholipids and the reduction of saturated fatty acids. Thus, cold stress can modify the lipid metabolism in Nile tilapia by lowering total body saturated fatty acids and raising UFAs. Abdel-Ghany et al. (2019) studied the effects of dietary lipid sources on cold resistance of Nile tilapia subjected to decreasing water temperature. The fish were fed test diets containing fish oil (FO), corn oil (CO), coconut oil or a blend of FO and CO as lipid sources, for 8 weeks. At the termination of the feeding trial, the fish were exposed to gradually decreasing water temperature from 25 until death symptoms appeared. Fish fed on CO and blend oils contained higher body UFAs and had lower lethal temperature (8°C) than those fed on FO (9.5°C) and coconut (12°C) diets. This finding suggests that cold tolerance of Nile tilapia can be enhanced through dietary inclusion of dietary lipids rich in plant oils (n-6 UFAs).

Delta 9 desaturase (Δ9D) is one of the key enzymes involved in the process of cold acclimation through fatty acid unsaturation. This process reduces the rigidity of biological membranes caused by extreme cold and helps in the conformational flexibility of membrane-bound proteins. Δ9D expression in muscle and gill tissues of Nile tilapia was significantly increased in response to chronic cold stress (Zerai et al., 2010).

Fish species and size play a significant role in tilapia response to water temperature. Small fingerling tilapia were more susceptible to low temperature than larger fish (Hofer and Watts, 2002). The survival of large monosex Nile tilapia

TABLE 4.1 Temperature tolerance ranges of tilapia.

Species	Tolerance (°C)			References
	Lower lethal	Upper lethal	Optimum	
Oreochromis niloticus	10.5	42	27–30	Fukusho (1968), Denzer (1968), Beamish (1970)
O. niloticus (fry)			28	El-Sayed and Kawanna (2008)
O. niloticus			30	Xie et al. (2011)
O. niloticus	8.28		28–32	El Gamal (1988)
O. niloticus: GIFT Sudan strain Egypt strain	 11–8.4 7.4–9.8 7.4–11			Sifa et al. (2002)
O. niloticus: Egypt strain Ivory Coast strain Ghana strain	 10 12.2 14.1			Khater and Smitherman (1988)
Oreochromis aureus	6–8	41–42		Yashouv (1960), Philippart and Ruwet (1982), El Gamal (1988)
Oreochromis mossambicus	8–9.5	42		Kirk (1972), Chervinski (1982), Shafland and Pestrak (1982)
			28–30	Job (1969b)
Sarotherodon melanotheron	18	33		Pauly (1976)
	6.9–10.3			Shafland and Pestrak (1982), Jennings (1991)
			32	Philippart and Ruwet (1982)
Tilapia zillii	6.5	42.5	28.8–31.4	Kirk (1972), Platt and Hauser (1978), Philippart and Ruwet (1982)
Tilapia rendalli	11	41		Philippart and Ruwet (1982)
O. aureus × *O. mossambicus*	10			Behrends and Smitherman (1984)
Florida red tilapia			27 (at 0‰), 32 (at 18 or 36‰)	Watanabe et al. (1993)

fry during overwintering has also been reported to be higher than that of smaller fry (Dan and Little, 2000). This means that large fingerlings are preferred for transportation and culture if water temperature is expected to drop because of their higher cold tolerance. However, Cnaani et al. (2000) found that cold tolerance and fish size (2.3–10.5 cm) of *O. mossambicus* and *O. aureus* and their hybrids were not correlated, but *O. mossambicus* was the most cold-sensitive group, and genetic variations in cold tolerance had a large dominance component. Behrends et al. (1996) found also that *O. aureus* and their hybrids were more cold tolerant, and had better growth, than Nile tilapia when raised at suboptimal temperatures (17.2–21.2°C). Meanwhile, Chen et al. (2002) found that cold stress of *O. aureus* has led to an increase in the secretion of plasma norepinephrine, epinephrine and cortisol and a decrease in both phagocytic activity of leukocytes and plasma immunoglobulin. These fish can tolerate temperature as low as 6–7°C, but for few hours. Long exposure to such low temperature renders the fish unable to maintain body position.

It should be realized that other environmental conditions and farming systems may affect the response of tilapia to water temperature. These factors may have antagonistic or synergistic effects on farmed fish and may therefore negatively or positively affect fish performance. El-Sayed et al. (1996) found that the growth and survival of Nile tilapia reared in earthen ponds were significantly affected by pond depth and water temperature. Fish growth was poorest, and mortality highest, at pond depth of 50 cm, whereas the best performance and survival were achieved at 100–200 cm depth. At 50 cm pond depth, 85% of the fish died, while increasing the depth to 200–300 cm provided the fish with a refuge for escaping extreme temperatures during summer (escaping toward the bottom) and winter (escaping toward the surface) seasons, leading to a significant improvement in fish growth and survival. Similarly, Dan and Little (2000) overwintered Thai, GIFT, Egypt and Vietnam strains of Nile tilapia broodstock in deep and shallow ponds and in shallow and deep hapas suspended in deep ponds. They found that the survival was 99.6% and 100% in deep and shallow hapas in ponds, which was significantly higher than that of fish stocked in deep and shallow ponds (74.4%–90%).

The effects of water salinity on the response of tilapia to water temperature have also been investigated by a number of authors. Allanson et al. (1971) found that *O. mossambicus* tolerated 11°C at 5‰, while fish reared in freshwater (FW) did not survive at that temperature. These authors suggested that the ability of *O. mossambicus* to tolerate low water temperature is associated with the maintenance of high plasma sodium and chloride concentration. The effect of salinity on the growth and survival of tilapia at different temperatures is also evident. Watanabe et al. (1993) found that sex-reversed Florida red tilapia attained their best performance at 27°C when water salinity was 0‰. At 18 and 36‰, the best growth and feed efficiency were reached at 32°C. These results suggested that increasing water temperature above 27°C is only justifiable for tilapia reared in brackish water (BW), not in FW. Similar trends have been reported on Nile tilapia (Likongwe et al., 1996), where the growth of fish reared at 8, 12 and 16‰ increased with increasing water temperature from 24 to 32°C at all salinities. On the other hand, Jennings (1991) found that cold tolerance of *Sarotherodon melanotheron* did not differ with water salinity ranging from 5 to 35‰.

Hui et al. (2014) studied the effects of various combinations of water temperature (20–34°C), salinity (0–18‰) and pH (5–10) on reproductive performance of Nile tilapia. They found that the best egg fertilization and hatching rates were achieved at the combination of 27.3°C/9.2‰/7.4. The authors suggested that the application of these results would improve the tilapia seed production efficiency. The joint effect of temperature (16–36°C), salinity (0–22‰) and rearing density (200–1000 fish m^{-3}) on the specific growth rate (SGR) and feed conversion rate of Nile tilapia juveniles were also studied under laboratory conditions (Jun et al., 2012). The maximal fish growth and feed utilization were obtained at 29°C/6‰/500 fish m^{-3}. Choi et al. (2013) found also that rapid decrease in salinity, but not increase, leads to significant dysregulation of the immune system in Nile tilapia, making the fish more susceptible to infectious diseases. The message from this study is clear: farmed Nile tilapia should not be subjected to sudden decrease in water salinity.

Wang et al. (2017) evaluated the suitability of RNA/DNA ratio (as a bioindicator for growth) for assessing growth of Nile tilapia juveniles under temperature–salinity combinations, ranging from 16 to 36°C and 0–16‰. They found that the RNA/DNA ratio was significantly affected by these combinations in a nonlinear trend. Temperature had greater effect on RNA/DNA ratios than salinity, whereas the temperature × salinity interaction had a negative effect on the RNA/DNA ratio, especially at higher temperatures.

Tilapia are often subjected to abrupt or gradual transfer from FW to BW and vice versa, during transportation and culture practice, presumably because of their eurythermal and euryhaline nature. Understanding the response of these fishes to thermal and thermohaline shocks would be necessary for tilapia culture and farm managers in order to minimize thermal and thermohaline stresses, particularly during transportation. Al-Amoudi et al. (1996) studied the effects of thermal and thermohaline shocks on the tilapia *O. mossambicus* and *O. aureus* × *O. niloticus* hybrids transferred abruptly from 25°C freshwater to freshwater or saltwater (26‰) maintaining temperatures of 15, 20, 30 and 35°C. In FW, fish survival was not affected by thermal shock, but they suffered from coma and fungal infection at 15°C. In saltwater, the survival of *O. mossambicus* was not affected by thermohaline shocks, while tilapia hybrids maintained 7.6%, 100%, 100%, 70% and 59% survival at 15, 20, 25, 30 and 35°C, respectively. Plasma osmotic concentrations of *O. mossambicus* and tilapia hybrids transferred to 15 and 35°C saltwater were sharply increased, but gradually decreased to normal levels in *O. mossambicus*, while never returned to the initial low levels in tilapia hybrids. This study demonstrated that these fishes were more tolerant to high rather than low temperature shocks, and *O. mossambicus* are more resistant to thermohaline shocks than tilapia hybrids.

One of the factors that tilapia farmers, farm managers and researchers may not be aware of is the significant effects of water temperature on sex differentiation and morphological development during early larval stages of tilapia. Increased water temperature may limit larval growth and induce body deformation. Wang and Tsai (2000) studied the effects of water temperature on deformity and sex differentiation of *O. mossambicus* larvae. Zero- (day of hatch), five- and ten-day old larvae were reared at 20, 24, 28 and 32°C. The authors found that the percentage of deformity increased at higher water temperatures (28 and 32°C) before 5 days old, while low temperature (20°C) had no effects. The exposure of the larvae to low temperature before 10 days old induced a high proportion of females, while elevated temperature induced high percentage of males after 10 days old. The sex ratio of *O. niloticus* has also been found to be affected by water temperature. Baroiller et al. (1995) found that increasing water temperature to 34–36°C significantly increased the proportion of Nile tilapia males (69%–91%), while low temperature (19–23°C) had no effects on sex ratio. The same authors reported similar results with Florida red tilapia. These results suggest that a temperature–sex determination pattern could exist in tilapia with strong genotype–temperature interaction. It is also essential that water temperature during early larval stages be carefully monitored and optimized.

The effects of temperature on survival, growth and phenotypic sex of mixed (XX-XY) progenies of Nile tilapia have further been investigated (Baras et al., 2001). Fish larvae were exposed to different temperatures (20.4–39°C) during the first 28 days of their life. About 90% masculinizing efficiency was attained at 37.8–39.2°C, which was very close to the upper lethal temperature, and in turn resulted in high mortality (>70%). This result suggested that producing faster growing Nile tilapia males at high temperature may not compensate the high loss of production incurred during masculinizing processes. Further work is needed to select the most thermosensitive breeders or strains.

4.3 Salinity

The competition for FW with agriculture and other urban activities has increased the pressure to develop aquaculture in BW and seawater (SW). The first candidate to think of for aquaculture in BW is tilapia. These fishes, despite being FW fishes, are believed to have been evolved from marine ancestors (Kirk, 1972). This may explain the ability of most tilapia species and hybrids to tolerate a wide range of water salinity. They can normally grow and reproduce in BW. Some species can even grow and reproduce at very high water salinity. But salt tolerance does not necessarily indicate suitable conditions for maximum production. Extensive research has been conducted on the tolerance and adaptability of tilapia to water salinity. Available information indicates that salt tolerance depends on tilapia species, strains and size, adaptation time, environmental factors and geographic location (Balarin and Haller, 1982; Chervinski, 1982; Philippart and Ruwet, 1982; Suresh and Lin, 1992). The results of these studies will just be highlighted in this section (Table 4.2), while more detailed discussion will be devoted to the recent studies on this subject.

4.3.1 Species, sex and size

As indicated in Table 4.2, *O. mossambicus*, *O. spilurus*, *O. aureus* and *Tilapia zillii* are the most salinity-tolerant tilapia species. *O. mossambicus* have been reported to tolerate up to 120‰ water salinity (Whitefield and Blaber, 1979). Moreover, they can grow normally and reproduce at water salinity of 49‰, and their fry live and grow reasonably well at 69‰ (Whitefield and Blaber, 1979). *O. aureus* are less salinity tolerant but can grow well at a salinity of up to 36–44‰, while reproduction occurs at 19‰. With gradual acclimation, they can tolerate a salinity of up to 54‰ (Balarin and Haller, 1982). However, McMahon and Baca (1999) found that *O. aureus* reared at a salinity of 30‰ developed a toxic algae bloom and suffered from epithelia erosion caused by the dinoflagellate *Pfiesteria piscicida* and brighter flashing on the dorsal and pectoral fins and tail. The authors found also that higher salinity severely restricted fish reproduction despite increasing somatic growth. However, the authors did not mention whether the algae bloom occurred as a coincidence of suitable conditions, with or without the presence of the fish, and caused the problems that were observed. Similarly, McGeachin et al. (1987) found that *O. aureus* reared in SW cages (36‰) showed a sharp reduction in growth rates and were infected with *Bacillus* sp. which has led to severe mortality. *O. spilurus* grow and spawn normally in full strength sea water (>40‰) in Jeddah Fisheries Research Center (Saudi Arabia). Farming trials of this species in sea water in fiberglass tanks are also being

TABLE 4.2 Salinity tolerance of tilapia.

Species	Upper limit		Optimum limit	Remarks	References
	Direct transfer	Gradual transfer			
Oreochromis niloticus	18[1]	36[1]	5–10[2], 15[3]	Reproduce at 13.5–29‰[4]	[1]Al-Amoudi (1987a),[2]Payne and Collinson (1983),[3]Alfredo and Hector (2002),[4]Balarin and Haller (1982)
O. niloticus			8	Best survival and production compared with 15 and 25‰	Chowdhury et al. (2006)
Oreochromis mossambicus	27[5]	120[6]	17.5[7]	Spawn at up to 49‰[8]	[5]Al-Amoudi (1987b),[6]Whitefield and Blaber (1979),[7]Canagaratnam (1966),[8]Popper and Lichatowich (1975)
Oreochromis aureus	27[5]	54[4]	10–15[9]	Reproduce at 5–20‰, low growth and high mortality at 36‰[10]	[4]Balarin and Haller (1982),[9]Perry and Avault (1972),[10]McGeachin et al. (1987)
Oreochromis spilurus	33[4]	40[11]–44[12]	3–8[11]	Good growth and survival in seawater, but low fecundity.[11] They currently survive and spawn at 42‰ in Saudi Arabia (Red Sea water)[12]	[11]Al-Ahmed (2001);[12]A.-F.M. El-Sayed (personal observation, 2019).
Sarotherodon galilaeus		29[4]	19[4]	Reproduce in the wild at 29‰[4]	[4]Balarin and Haller (1982)
Tilapia rendalli		13–19[4]	0[13]		[13] Likongwe (2002)
Tilapia zillii		45[14]		Grow and reproduce naturally at 10–>30‰[15]	[14]Chervinski (1982),[15]A.-F.M. El-Sayed (personal observation)
O. niloticus × *O. mossambicus*		35[3]	15[3]	At 35‰, the fish failed to adapt	[3]Alfredo and Hector (2002)
Florida red tilapia			17.8[16]	Grow normally up to 36.2‰	[16]El-Ebiary et al. (1997)

carried out in a private aquaculture company (Tharawat Seas), with very promising results (Gialamas, Jeddah, 2019, personal communication).

Chowdhury et al. (2006) evaluated the effect of salinity on carrying capacity, growth performance and production of Nile tilapia reared in a recirculation system. Tilapia survival decreased with increasing water salinity from 8 to 15 or 25‰, regardless of fish stocking density (20 or 40 fish m^{-3}). Carrying capacity decreased significantly with increasing salinity. Growth rates and net production significantly declined beyond 8‰ water salinity.

T. zillii are also among the most salinity-tolerant tilapia species. They are found in Bardawil Lagoon (North Sinai, Egypt), Gulf of Suez, Lake Qarun (Faiyum Governorate, Egypt) and Abu Quir Bay (Alexandria, Egypt) which are highly saline water bodies (36–45‰) (Balarin and Hatton, 1979; El-Sayed, 1996, personal communication). *T. zillii* can also reproduce at 29‰, and even at higher salinities in Lake Qarun (>30‰). *Oreochromis spilurus* has also been successfully cultured in full SW in Kuwait, and trails are going on in Israel for their commercial culture in SW cages and tanks, with promising results (Carmelo, 2002).

Other tilapias are generally less euryhaline and can tolerate water salinities ranging from about 20 to 35‰ (see details in Table 4.2). Most of these tilapia grow, survive and reproduce at 0–29‰, depending on the species and acclimation period. On the other hand, some other tilapia species are considered 'stenohaline', since they tolerate only a narrow range of water salinity. *Tilapia rendalli*, *Tilapia sparrmanii* and *Oreochromis macrochir*, for example, have a maximum salinity tolerance of 19, 18 and 20‰, respectively (Whitefield and Blaber, 1976; Balarin and Haller, 1982; Philippart and Ruwet, 1982).

The salinity tolerance of tilapia is also affected by fish sex and size. Perschbacher and McGeachin (1988) evaluated the salinity tolerance of red tilapia (*O. mossambicus* × *Oreochromis urolepis hornorum*) fry, juveniles and adults. Adult fish were more salt tolerant than fry and juveniles. Fry and juveniles tolerated direct transfer to 19‰, without apparent stress and mortality, but 100% mortality occurred at 27‰. On the other hand, adult fish tolerated a direct transfer to 27‰, with a100% mortality at 37‰. Similarly, Watanabe et al. (1985) studied the ontogeny of salinity tolerance in Nile tilapia, blue tilapia and hybrids tilapia *O. mossambicus* female × *O. niloticus* male. The median lethal salinity-96 h (MLS-96) for Nile tilapia and blue tilapia over an age of 7–120 days post hatching (dph) was 18.9 and 19.2‰. In contrast, MLS-96 of tilapia hybrids changed with age and increased from 17.2‰ at 30 dph to 26.7‰ at 60 dph. The authors referred these ontogenetic changes in salinity tolerance to body size than to chronological age. Watanabe et al. (1985) reported also that male tilapia tend to be more salt tolerant than females.

It is also believed that tilapia hybrids descended from salt-tolerant parents (such as *O. mossambicus* and *O. aureus*) are highly salt tolerant (Suresh and Lin, 1992; Romana-Eguia and Eguia, 1999). This may explain why Taiwanese red tilapia (Liao and Chang, 1983) and Florida red tilapia (Watanabe et al., 1988a, 1988b) grow faster in SW and BW than in FW. Moreover, the tolerance of tilapia hybrids to salinity may be influenced by fish strain, as has been reported by Romana-Eguia and Eguia (1999). The authors studied the growth of five Asian red tilapia strains (BFS, NIFI, FAC, PF and HL) at 0, 17 and 34‰, for 10 weeks. The Philippines strain (PF) grew best in SW, while Thai strain (NIFI) grew well in BW. The authors concluded that some Asian tilapia strains can be developed for use in sustainable BW and SW culture systems. Tayamen et al. (2002) also evaluated progenies from 27 cross combinations of four *Oreochromis* species (5 pure breeds and 22 crossbreeds) for saline waters in the Philippines, in 10 environments with different water salinities. They found that *O. aureus* × *O. spilurus* gave the highest body growth, while *O. mossambicus* × *O. spilurus* produced the best survival.

Water salinity has also been reported to affect the reproduction of tilapia. Gonadal development and spawning of Nile tilapia occurred at salinities of 17–29‰, while the onset of reproduction was delayed with increasing water salinity from 25 to 50‰, and reproduction stopped completely at salinity above 30‰ (Fineman-Kalio, 1988). El-Sayed et al. (2003) found that spawning performance and protein requirements of Nile tilapia broodstock were significantly affected by water salinity. The fish were fed test diets containing 25%, 30%, 35% and 40% crude protein at three water salinities (0, 7 and 14‰). The size at first maturation increased with increasing dietary protein at all salinities. At 25% and 30% protein levels, broodstock reared at 0‰ reached their sexual maturity at bigger sizes than those reared at 7 and 14‰. At 0‰, spawning intervals were not significantly affected by dietary protein levels, while at 7 and 14‰, spawning intervals significantly decreased with increasing dietary protein levels. Spawning frequency and number of eggs per spawn were increased with increasing dietary protein levels. The total number of spawnings per female and absolute fecundity were better in fish fed 40% protein in FW than at 7 and 14‰ salinity. On the other hand, Watanabe et al. (1985) found that the total number of spawnings of Nile tilapia females was greater in BW (5–15‰) than in either full-strength SW (32‰) or FW.

A clear interaction between salinity and hardness on the one hand and eggs hatching and the larval survival of Nile tilapia on the other has been demonstrated by Bart et al. (2013). These authors tested the effects of water salinity (2–32‰) on the survival of yolk-sac larvae and swim-up fry of Nile tilapia (Chitralada strain), during artificial eggs incubation. Increasing salinity from 2 to 5‰ increased yolk-sac larval and swim-up fry survival when hardness was 50 mg L^{-1}, whereas survival remained similar at both salinity levels at water hardness ranging from 500 to 1000 mg L^{-1}. Salinity of 2‰ resulted in the highest hatching rates when water hardness was high. Furthermore, increasing water salinity to 9.0‰ decreased hatchability, but the decline was less at a water hardness of 1000 mg L^{-1} than at lower hardness (50 and 500 mg L^{-1}). This study suggested that high hardness levels may have increased the level of calcium in the incubation water, leading to the mitigation of adverse effects of increased salinity on hatchability and larval survival of Nile tilapia. The study also indicated that a salinity of 4‰ is optimum for egg incubation and larval survival.

4.3.2 Acclimation

Pre-acclimation to saltwater and gradual transfer to high salinity have a significant effect on tilapia growth and survival, as has been reported by Al-Amoudi (1987b). The author found that *O. aureus*, *O. mossambicus* and *O. spilurus* required shorter acclimation time (4 days) for a transfer to full-strength SW than *O. niloticus* and *O. aureus* × *O. niloticus* hybrids (8 days). These results indicated that the former tilapia group is more euryhaline than the latter group. Al-Amoudi et al. (1996) also found that *O. mossambicus* are more resistant to thermohaline shocks than *O. aureus* × *O. niloticus* hybrids. Similarly, the physiological and respiratory responses of *O. mossambicus* to salinity acclimation have been evaluated by Morgan et al. (1997). Fish reared in FW were transferred to FW, isotonic salinity (Iso, 12‰) and 75% SW (25‰), and a number of physiological parameters were measured. The authors found that plasma Na^+ and Cl^- were elevated 1 day after transfer to SW, but returned to FW levels on day 4. Plasma cortisol and glucose levels were higher, while growth hormone (GH), Na^+, K^+ ATPase activities and prolactins were lower in FW and ISO than in SW. These results suggested that the physiological changes associated with SW acclimation in tilapia are short term, energy demanding and may account for as much as 20% of total body metabolism after 4 days in SW. The increase in the metabolic energy diverted into osmoregulation, with increasing water salinity has also been reported in *O. mossambicus* and *O. spilurus* (Payne et al., 1988), *O. niloticus* × *O. aureus* and common carp (Payne, 1983).

Kammerer et al. (2010) evaluated plasma osmolytes and respiration of the FW Mozambique tilapia exposed to 25‰ SW. They found that cortisol increased rapidly by 3 h and remained elevated for 3 days, while plasma osmolality, Na^+ and Cl^- were elevated at 6–8 h, reaching a peak 24 h following SW exposure, and then decreased to near-FW levels after 3 days. Oxygen consumption rate increased at 24 h post exposure, while ventilation frequency increased by 3 h. The osmoregulatory and endocrine responses of Mozambique tilapia and Nile tilapia to acute changes in water salinity were also investigated by Breves et al. (2010). In both species, plasma osmolality sharply increased at 2 h after transfer from FW to BW or SW. Similar increases occurred also in plasma prolactin (PRL) and PRL receptor gene expression in both species. Transferring Nile tilapia from FW to BW and SW resulted in increased plasma GH and branchial GH receptor gene expression. Branchial gene expression of $Na^+/K^+/2\ Cl^-$ co-transporter (NKCC, an essential component in the recruitment of SW-type chloride cells) increased in Mozambique tilapia, while that of Nile tilapia was reduced, after transfer from BW to SW. The authors suggested that these differences in SW adaptability of the two species are attributed to a low capacity of Nile tilapia to upregulate NKCC gene expression. On the other hand, Mozambique tilapia are more euryhaline and can tolerate hypersaline water with a significant increase in Na^+, K^+-ATPase activity in the gill (Fiess et al., 2007).

Withyachumnarnkul et al. (2017) evaluated the survival, growth rates, haemato-immunological changes and susceptibility to pathogens of Nile tilapia reared under gradual increase in salinity, from 0 to 30‰. At 30‰ salinity, 50% of the fish died and fish growth rates were retarded by 40% compared to fish maintained at 0‰. Under increased salinity the fish also had significantly lower haematocrit, higher total white blood cell counts, higher numbers of lymphocytes and thrombocytes and higher serum lysozyme activity than those reared in FW. Sixty percent of Nile tilapia reared in full-strength SW were also infected by infectious spleen and kidney necrosis virus (ISKNV).

Feeding tilapia broodstock with diets containing higher salt levels may produce seeds with better adaptability to water salinity. Turingan and Kubaryk (1992) studied this assumption by feeding Taiwanese red tilapia (*O. mossambicus* × *O. niloticus*) broodstock diets containing 0.8, 3, 6, 9 or 12% salt for 2 months prior to spawning. They found that egg hatchability was higher in SW than in FW. The hatchability and larval growth were highest in fish fed 12% salt in SW and lowest in FW. In another study, Watanabe et al. (1985) found that the survival of fry produced from fertilized eggs of Nile tilapia spawned in FW and incubated at elevated salinities of 0, 5, 10, 15, 20, 25 and 32‰ was 85.5%, 84.4%, 82.5%, 56.3%, 37.9%, 20.0% and 0%, respectively. Fry salinity tolerance increased also with increasing the salinity of spawning, hatching or acclimatization. In addition, at equivalent salinity, early exposure of tilapia broodstock to high salinity produced progeny with high salinity tolerance than those spawned in FW and hatched at high salinity.

Steroid hormones may reduce the routine metabolism of euryhaline tilapia reared at high salinity and, in turn, improve fish growth. The growth of *O. mossambicus* continuously treated with 17α-methyltestosterone (MT) was faster than early or delayed MT-treated fish in FW and SW. The growth of continuously treated fish was 5−7 times higher in SW than in FW (Kuwaye et al., 1993). Similar results were reported by Ron et al. (1995) who studied the effects of MT treatment and feeding rate on the growth of *O. mossambicus* reared in FW and SW. The best growth was observed in MT-treated fish fed double ration in SW. Oxygen consumption (routine metabolism) was also much lower in SW than in FW. The authors suggested that the reduction in routine metabolism in fish reared in SW may have accounted for the increase in growth rates, compared to fish reared in FW.

4.4 Dissolved oxygen

DO is one of the limiting environmental factors affecting fish feeding, growth and metabolism. DO fluctuation is affected by photosynthesis, respiration and diel fluctuation. These factors must be fully considered where DO is concerned. Ambient DO range produces the best fish performance, while low DO levels limit respiration, growth and other metabolic activities of fish (Tsadik and Kutty, 1987).

Tilapia are known to withstand very low levels of DO. Most tilapias can tolerate as low DO levels as 0.1−0.5 mg L^{-1} for varying periods of time (Magid and Babiker, 1975; Tsadik and Kutty, 1987). They can even survive at zero DO concentration if they are allowed access to surface air. But tilapia usually suffer from high mortality if they fail to reach surface air. On the other hand, tilapia can tolerate conditions of high oxygen supersaturation (up to 400%), which usually occurs because of high photosynthesis resulting from phytoplankton and macrophytes blooming (Morgan, 1972).

Abdel-Tawwab et al. (2014) studied the effects of stocking density (0.2 or 0.4 g L^{-1}) and DO levels on the performance, body composition and immune response of Nile tilapia fingerlings (0.7 g). They found that the best performance was obtained at the lowest density and highest DO concentration (6.5 mg L^{-1}). At both densities, fish growth, feed utilization and body protein and lipid were reduced with decreasing DO from 6.5 to 1.5 mg L^{-1}. The lowest fish immunity was also observed at low DO/high stocking density combination. In a similar study, Abdel-Tawwab et al. (2015) found that DO significantly affected the performance, body composition and immune response of Nile tilapia of two sizes (3.7 and 12.9 g $fish^{-1}$). Fish growth, feed utilization and innate immunity were improved with increasing DO from low level (1.0−1.5 mg L^{-1}) to normal levels (6.0−6.5 mg L^{-1}) (Table 4.3). Smaller fish exhibited better performance than larger fish at normal DO concentration. At low DO levels, smaller fish were also more susceptible to bacterial infection, as indicated by heavy mortality, whereas no mortality occurred in larger fish after bacterial challenge. These results suggest that larger Nile tilapia are more tolerant to low DO than smaller fish.

Similarly, Tran-Duy et al. (2012) evaluated the effects of DO on feed intake and nitrogen and energy balances in all-male Nile tilapia of two size classes: large fish (>200 g) and small fish (<100 g). The feed intake of small fish levelled off at 3 mg DO L^{-1}. On the other hand, feed intake in larger fish increased with increasing DO from 2.6 to 6.0 mg L^{-1}, and the incipient DO for these fish was about 5.5 mg L^{-1}. The fish tended to reduce their energy requirement for maintenance as DO declined. The apparent digestibility coefficient (ADC) of dry matter, protein and energy of the large fish decreased significantly at 1.58 mg DO L^{-1}, compared to ADCs at higher DO levels. For large fish, gross energy (GE), digestible energy (DE) and metabolizable energy (ME) intake increased significantly with increasing DO levels from 1.6 to 6.1 mg L^{-1}. Energy in branchial and urinary excretory products, heat production and retained energy followed the same trend up to 4 mg DO L^{-1}, then levelled off. For small fish, GE, FE,

TABLE 4.3 Environmental tolerance of tilapia to dissolved oxygen, ammonia and pH.

	Oxygen (mg L^{-1})		Ammonia (mg L^{-1})		pH	
Tilapia species	Minimum	Optimum	Range	Optimum	Range	Optimum
Oreochromis niloticus	0.1−0.5	6.0−6.5[1], 5.5[2]	Up to 7.4*[3], 1.0**[1]	<0.1	3.7−11.0	5.5−9.0[4]
Oreochromis aureus		>3.0	1.93−3.14*[5]			
Oreochromis mossambicus × *O. niloticus*			6.6⁺, 4.07⁺⁺, 2.88⁺⁺⁺[6]			

*Median lethal (LC_{50}) of unionized ammonia (NH_3) for fingerlings; **LC_{50} for larvae; ⁺LC_{50} for larvae at 48 h; ⁺⁺LC_{50} for larvae at 72 h; ⁺⁺⁺LC_{50} for larvae at 96 h. [1]Abdel-Tawwab et al. (2105); [2]Tran-Duy et al. (2012); [3]Benli and Köksal (2005); [4]Rebouças et al. (2016); [5]Küçük (2014); [6]Daud et al. (1988).

DE and ME also increased with increasing DO levels from 1.3 mg L^{-1} to 2.3 mg L^{-1} and levelled off with further increase in DO concentration to 3.66 mg L^{-1}.

The interaction between feed composition and DO concentration may also have a significant effect on tilapia performance, as reported by Tran-Ngoc et al. (2016). These authors fed Nile tilapia (35 g) with two diets: a fishmeal (FM)-based diet (control) and soybean meal (SBM)-based diet at normoxia (100% oxygen saturation, 6.9 mg L^{-1}) and hypoxia (50% saturation, 3.5 mg L^{-1}). The best growth rates were attained in the FM 'control' diet under normoxia, while no interaction between oxygen and diet composition was found. ADC of dry matter, crude protein, ash and carbohydrate were higher in normoxia than in hypoxia. For the plant-based diet, the decline in digestibility was larger than for the FM diet. In addition, diet composition and oxygen level induced changes in intestinal morphology, where low DO enhanced the negative effect of SBM diet on intestinal morphology.

It is well known that increasing water temperature reduces the rate of DO in the water. This leads to increased respiration rate and oxygen consumption in tilapia because under increased water temperature the rate of metabolism and, in turn, the tissue demand for oxygen increase. Franklin et al. (1995) found that the rate of oxygen consumption in tilapia increased from 0.74 to 0.97 mg L^{-1} per hour with increasing water temperature from 37 to 42°C. Similar results were reported with a number of tilapia species and their hybrids (Becker and Fishelson, 1986). Moreover, early studies of Job (1969a; 1969b) indicated that the respiration of tilapia was independent of DO at oxygen saturation of 25%–32% (at temperature ranging from 15 to 30°C), while below these saturation levels the metabolic rate became dependent on oxygen availability, and mortality occurred when DO remained below 20% saturation for more than 2–3 days. On the contrary, Teichert-Coddington and Green (1993) found that reducing the aeration in tilapia ponds in Honduras from 30% to 10% of oxygen saturation did not affect fish growth and water quality, and both aeration levels produced better growth than unaerated ponds. Nevertheless, the authors reported that aeration leads to the suspension of settled particulate matter and causes water turbidity and suggested that more research is needed to improve aeration techniques in order to reduce such turbidity.

Handling stress has a significant effect on oxygen consumption in tilapia. Ross and Ross (1983) found that handling stress of Nile tilapia has increased oxygen consumption rate from +150% to +300% of the resting value and did not fully return, in many cases, to the resting value after 3 h. The authors suggested that following handling stress, the fish should be returned to water containing high levels of DO, and should not be fed for at least 1 h. The message from this result is clear: 'handling stress should be minimized'. The respiration rate of the fish increased also curvilinearly with increasing body weight.

Increases in carbon dioxide tension in the water lead to decreased oxygen consumption (but increased ventilation rate). However, in addition to their tolerance of low levels of DO, tilapia can also withstand very high levels of CO_2, ranging from 50 to 72.6 ppm (Fish, 1956). It has been suggested that high CO_2 water supplies caused nephrocalcinosis in tilapia (R.J. Roberts, cited in Chervinski, 1982). This means that CO_2 concentration should also be kept minimal in tilapia culture water.

4.5 Ammonia and nitrite

4.5.1 Ammonia

Most of the nitrogenous wastes of fishes are excreted via gills in the form of ammonia. Excreted ammonia exists in unionized NH_3 form (UIA-N), which is toxic to fish, and ionized NH_4^+, which is nontoxic (Chervinski, 1982). The toxicity of ammonia depends on DO, CO_2 and pH. The toxicity increases with decreasing DO and decreases with increasing CO_2 (Chervinski, 1982). Fish species and size, acclimation time and culture systems also affect the toxicity of ammonia to fish.

The toxicity of ammonia to tilapia has been related to different physiological changes. Ahmed et al. (1992) found that Nile tilapia exposed to ammonia had lower red blood cells and haemolytic anaemia leading to a significant reduction in blood oxygen content which enhances ammonia toxicity. Oxygen saturation of arterial blood of *T. zillii* was also decreased after exposure to sublethal ammonia concentration (1.1–3.3 mg L^{-1}) for 2 weeks (El-Shafey, 1998). El-Shafai et al. (2004) also evaluated the effect of prolonged exposure to sublethal UIA-N on the growth performance of Nile tilapia fed on fresh duckweed. They found that the toxic level of NH_3-N and its negative effect on the growth performance ranges from 0.07 to 0.14 mg UIA-N L^{-1}. They further recommended that the NH_3-N concentration should be maintained below 0.1 mg UAI-N L^{-1}.

The median lethal concentration (LC_{50}) of NH_3 has also been studied in a number of tilapia species and hybrids. Redner and Stickney (1979) found that the 48 h LC_{50} for *O. aureus* was 2.46 ppm. When the fish were acclimatized to the sublethal concentration of 0.43–0.53 ppm for 35 days, they were able to withstand a concentration of 3.4 ppm NH_3 without any mortality for 48 h. Daud et al. (1988) also reported that the LC_{50} of unionized ammonia at 48 h, 72 h and 96 h in red tilapia (*O. mossambicus* × *O. niloticus*) fry was 6.6, 4.07 and 2.88 ppm, respectively. The authors related the relatively high resistance of fish fry to unionized ammonia to the high levels of DO (7–10.1 mg L^{-1}). The threshold lethal concentration was

0.24 ppm. Prior to death, fry swam erratically and exhibited haemorrhage of gill filaments. Küçük (2014) also found that the medial lethal concentrations (24 h, LC_{50}) of unionized ammonia for blue tilapia reared under different water salinities were 2.83, 2.26, 3.14, 3.11 and 1.93 mg L^{-1} at 1, 8, 12, 16 and 20‰, respectively. However, these values of LC_{50} were not significantly different, indicating that the tolerance of blue tilapia to acute unionized ammonia was not affected by water salinity (Table 4.3).

On the other hand, Benli and Köksal (2005) found that the median lethal concentrations (48 h, LC_{50}) of unionized ammonia (NH_3) for larval and fingerling Nile tilapia exposed to different levels of ammonia were 1.0 and 7.40 mg L^{-1}, respectively. Exposed larvae showed very rapid movement, swimming on their sides and losing equilibrium. When fingerlings were exposed to ammonia concentrations, they exhibited an increase in their movements, ventilation, convulsions and spiral swimming. They also had excessive mucous secretion in the gills and on the body surface, haemorrhage in the gills and darkening on their eyes and skin.

The effect of ammonia on tilapia performance is also related to water pH and exposure period, in addition to ammonia concentration. Hargreaves and Kucuk (2001) found that a brief daily exposure of *O. aureus* to up to 0.91 mg L^{-1} NH_3-N at pH 9 did not affect fish growth and feed utilization, while a brief daily exposure to 1.81 mg L^{-1} NH_3-N reduced SGR. At a concentration of 3.23 mg L^{-1} NH_3-N at pH 9.5, SGR was only 35% that of the control fish. These results suggested that brief sublethal ammonia exposure in aquaculture has little effect on tilapia performance.

Hegazi and Hasanein (2010) evaluated the effects of chronic exposure of juvenile Nile tilapia (10 g) to sublethal total ammonia nitrogen (TAN) at low (5 mg L^{-1}) or high (10 mg L^{-1}) levels. They found that oxidative stress indices (lipid peroxidation and protein carbonylation) and antioxidant enzyme activities, including xanthine oxidase, aldehyde oxidase, superoxide dismutase, catalase, glutathione peroxidase (GPx), glutathione S-transferase, glutathione reductase, γ-glutamyl cysteinyl synthetase and γ-glutamyl transpeptidase, were significantly increased in liver and white muscle of fish exposed to both low and high TAN levels. These results demonstrate that these ammonia levels induce reactive oxygen species generation in fish liver and muscles, as a mediator of ammonia toxicity. This was indicated by the significant increase in both oxidative stress biomarkers and activities of antioxidant enzymes. In another study, Hegazi et al. (2010) investigated the mechanism of chronic sublethal ammonia exposure in the brain of Nile tilapia (18 g) exposed to low (5 mg L^{-1}) or high (10 mg L^{-1}) TAN. The activities of cytosolic and mitochondrial enzymes related to ammonia detoxification were examined. The activities of c-alanine aminotransferase (c-ALT), c-aspartate aminotransferase (c-AST), c-malic enzyme (c-ME), m-malic enzyme (m-ME), glutamate dehydrogenase (GDH) in the amination direction and glutamine synthetase (GSase) in fish exposed to TAN were significantly increased with increasing TAN level. Similar trends in the concentrations of free amino acids, such as alanine, glutamine, glycine, histidine, serine and γ-aminobutyric acid were observed. On the other hand, the activity of m-ALT and glutaminase (GLase) was significantly decreased.

Alongside the same line, Benli et al. (2008) investigated the effects of exposure to sublethal TAN (control, 1, 2, 5, 10 mg L^{-1}) on the histology of Nile tilapia (*O. niloticus* L.) The exposure to ammonia concentrations, especially at high levels (5 and 10 mg L^{-1}) resulted in histopathologic alterations in fish gills, liver and kidney. Gill tissues displayed hyperaemia, chloride cell proliferation, fusion in secondary lamella and telangiectasia. Liver tissue revealed cloudy swelling and hydropic degeneration, whereas kidney tissues exhibited hyperaemia and glomerulonephritis. El-Greisy et al. (2016) found also that unionized ammonia has a significant effect on fertilized eggs, egg hatchability and newly hatched larvae of Nile tilapia. The lethal dose (LC_{50}, 96 h) on yolk-sac fry was 0.8 mg L^{-1}. The mortality rate increased with increasing ammonia concentration from 0.7 to 1.5 mg L^{-1}, and all the fish died at 1.5 mg L^{-1}. Fertilized eggs deformation, egg hatchability rates and larval growth and survival also decreased with increasing ammonia concentration to 0.6 mg NH_3-N L^{-1}.

4.5.2 Nitrite

Ammonia is oxidized into nitrite (NO_2) and then into nitrate (NO_3) through nitrifying bacteria grown on suspended organic matter. The bacteria remove the organic matter from the culture system by using it as food, while the bacteria itself can be used as natural food for filter-feeding fishes such as tilapia and carps. Nitrate is relatively nontoxic to tilapia; however, prolonged exposure to elevated levels of nitrate may decrease immune response and induce mortality (Plumb, 1997).

On the other hand, nitrite is highly toxic to fish including tilapia because it disturbs multiple physiological functions, including immune, respiratory, endocrine, ion regulatory, antioxidant, excretory processes and growth retardation (Sun et al., 2014). The mechanisms of nitrite toxicity includes (1) its competition with chloride (Cl^-) for uptake in gill epithelia; (2) the elevation of extracellular K^+ levels which affect skeletal muscle contractions and membrane potentials and (3) it impairs oxygen binding with haemoglobin due to the oxidation of Fe^{2+} to Fe^{3+}, resulting in methaemoglobin (MHb) production, and causing hypoxia due to the reduction of the oxygen-carrying capacity of the blood (Jensen, 2003; Yildiz et al., 2006).

A number of studies have considered the lethal and sublethal effects of nitrite on Nile tilapia. Yildiz et al. (2006) assessed the response of Nile tilapia (55.7 g) exposed to two sublethal NO_2—N concentrations (0.50 and 1.38 mg L^{-1}) for 24 and 48 h. They found that nitrite exposure caused an increase in MHb levels. However, MHb levels were unrelated to environmental and plasmatic nitrite concentrations. Nitrite exposure has also resulted in a marked reduction in blood haemoglobin and haematocrit levels. On the other hand, the time of exposure (24 and 48 h) did not affect nitrite concentration in fish blood. Similar results were observed in Nile tilapia exposed to different nitrite concentrations (0, 10, 18, 32, 56 and 100 mg L^{-1}) at two sodium chloride (NaCl) levels (35.0 and 70.0 mg L^{-1}) for 96 h (Yanbo et al., 2006). The LC_{50} of nitrite were 28.18 and 44.67 mg L^{-1} at low and high chloride content, respectively, indicating that high concentrations of chloride ions could reduce the toxicity of nitrite. Nitrite exposure also produced high MHb levels but did not cause mortality. The MHb level increased with increasing nitrite concentration but decreased with increasing chloride concentration. Abnormal behaviour and nitrite toxicity symptoms were observed in nitrite-exposed fish, especially at low NaCl concentrations. Toxicity signs included an increase in fish movement, convulsions, sideways and spiral swimming, disbalance, brown gills, haemorrhage in the muscles, skin darkening and death. It should be emphasized, however, that tested NaCl levels (35.0 and 70.0 mg L^{-1}) were low, while tilapia are generally reared in BW with much higher salinity. Therefore, further work is needed to elucidate the effects of nitrite on tilapia performance, physiological functions and behaviour at higher NaCl concentrations.

The tolerance of tilapia to nitrite is also influenced by fish size. Atwood et al. (2001) found that small-sized Nile tilapia (4.4 g) were more tolerant to nitrite than large fish (90.7 g). The 96-h LC_{50} of NO_2 - N was 81 and 8 mg L^{-1} in small and large fish, respectively. The addition of chloride source (500 mg L^{-1} $CaCl_2$ or NaCl) to culture water protected both small and large fish from nitrite toxicity. Such protection was achieved at a chloride:nitrite ratio of 1.5:1 (by weight).

The toxicity of nitrite exposure at molecular and physiological levels has also been investigated in tilapia. Sudharsan et al. (2000) studied the effect of nitrite toxicity on the dehydrogenases in Mozambique tilapia (*O. mossambicus*). The activity of dehydrogenases, LDH, SDH and GDH, were estimated in various tissues of the fish exposed to sublethal concentrations of nitrite for 24, 48, 72 and 96 h. The activities of these dehydrogenases were tissue specific and time-dependent. A significant decrease in the activity levels of LDH occurred while SDH and GDH showed increase in their activity when compared with the control. Xu et al. (2016) studied the effects of nitrite stress on energy metabolism in Nile tilapia at the molecular and physiological levels. The fish were challenged with nitrite (1.43 mmol L^{-1} NO_2^- − N) for 48 h, followed by a recovery period in nitrite-free water for 48 h. The levels of the adenosine monophosphate-activated protein kinase (AMPK) were examined and the protein activity of AMPK was quantified. The authors found that both AMPKα1 and AMPKα2 isoforms have structural features similar to mammalian AMPKα. mRNA encoding the AMPKα isoforms was also highly expressed in various tissues with clear patterns. Under acute nitrite challenge, both mRNA encoding the AMPKα isoforms and AMPK activity changed with time. The plasma glucose, lactic acid and triglycerides (TGs), as well as the energy in the hepatopancreas and muscle were also altered over time; confirming changes in energy metabolism. These results suggest that AMPK acts as an energy metabolism sensor in Nile tilapia.

4.6 pH

Some tilapias are known to tolerate a very wide range of water pH. For example, the tilapia *Oreochromis alcalicus grahami* live successfully in Lake Magadi (Kenya) which has a pH of 10.5 (Randall et al., 1989). These fish were reported to tolerate a pH range of 5—11 for at least 24 h, but die at pH <3.5 and >12 (Reite et al., 1974). They overcome the problem of ammonia excretion by excreting >90% of their nitrogenous wastes as urea. This process is facilitated by SW-type gill chloride cells (Wilkie and Wood, 1996). Nile tilapia can also survive at a pH range of 4—11 (Balarin and Hatton, 1979; Wangead et al., 1988). In the meantime, *Tilapia congica* live in the very acidic water (4.5—5.0) of Lake Tumba (Zaire).

Wangead et al. (1988) studied the effects of acid water on survival, behaviour and growth of Nile tilapia fingerlings (0.4—1.0 g) and adults (45.4—46.3 g). They found that both fingerlings and adults died at pH 2-3 within 1—3 days. Both size groups tolerated pH 4—5 very successfully and attained survival and growth rates similar to the control group (pH 7) after 60—70 days. However, adult fish were more resistant to low pH, with a survival rate of 86.6%, 100% and 100% at pH 4, 5 and 7, respectively, whereas the survival of fingerlings was 57.8%, 82.2% and 84.5%, respectively, at the same pH values. Similarly, Rebouças et al. (2016) assessed the optimum range of water pH for Nile tilapia culture. The fish (1.37 g) were reared at a water pH ranging from 4.5 to 9.5 for 8 weeks. The results revealed that a pH of 5.5—9.0 is suitable for rearing these fish (Table 4.3).

Other tilapias are less tolerant to water pH and may develop physiological changes following transfer from neutral water to acidic water. Yada and Ito (1997) studied the effects of transferring *O. niloticus* and *O. mossambicus* from neutral water to acidic water with a pH of 4.5, 4.0 and 3.5. After 3 days, *O. niloticus* showed the lowest level of plasma Na^+ at pH below 4.5, while the lowest level of plasma Na^+ in *O. mossambicus* occurred only at pH 3.5. Plasma Na^+ of *O. mossambicus* tended to get back to normal, while that of *O. niloticus* continued to decrease after the exposure to pH 3.5. In both species, gill Na, K-ATPase activity increased after the exposure to acidic water. These results indicated that *O. mossambicus* have greater ability to maintain plasma Na^+ in acidic water than *O. niloticus*. On the other hand, low or high water pH may lead to behavioural changes, damage of gill epithelial cells, reduction in the efficiency of nitrogenous excretion and increased mortality. In support, Wangead et al. (1988) reported that fingerling and adult Nile tilapia exposed to pH 2–3 showed rapid swimming and opercular movements, surfacing and gulping of air, lack of body position and mass mortality within 1–3 days. Similarly, Chen et al. (2001) found that *O. mossambicus* exposed to high pH for 7 days decreased ammonia nitrogen excretion, but increased urea nitrogen excretion. This situation was reversed at low pH (i.e. increased ammonia excretion and decreased urea excretion). The authors reported also that the LDO_{50} increased significantly at low pH (7.14, 4.02, 3.36, 0.84 and 0.32 mg L^{-1} at pH 4, 5, 6, 8.3 and 9.6, respectively).

Bonga et al. (1987) found that the short-term effects of acid exposure on prolactin secretion in *O. mossambicus* depend on pH and rate of acidification. Rapid acidification to pH 4 has resulted in necrosis of the integumental epithelium and caused damage of the skin, high plasma electrolyte loss and impaired the response of prolactin cells. At lower acidification rate (0.5 pH unit minute^{-1}), these symptoms hardly occurred and branchial permeability to water and ions increased and prolactin secretion increased by threefold. Slow acclimation of tilapia to low pH may enable the fish to withstand long-term exposure to low environmental pH and prevent epithelial cell damage. Van Ginneken et al. (1997) exposed *O. mossambicus* to water gradually acidified to pH 4 for 37 days. The fish successfully withstood this low pH without any mortality or significant changes in energy-rich compounds and plasma Na^+, Cl^-, cortisol and glucose between the control and acidified groups. This result indicated that the fish were able to maintain ionic balance and there was no activation in the pituitary–interrenal axis. The effects of gradual acidification on metabolic rates of *O. mossambicus* and common carp (*Cyprinus carpio*) have also been investigated by van Dijk et al. (1993). They found that standard metabolic rate, maximum metabolic rate and oxygen consumption in tilapia decreased in acidic water (pH 4), whereas these metabolic parameters did not decrease in carp. Wokoma and Marioghae (1996) also studied the lethal time (LT_{50}) and physiological changes in *Tilapia guineensis* in relation to varying water pH. They found that LT_{50} increased from 1.2 to 62 h with increasing the pH from 2 to 3, whereas the critical lethal pH was 3.3. They also found that the routine metabolic rate of small fish (1.4 g) was higher than that of larger fish (10.6 g) at high ambient oxygen concentration (6.3 mg L^{-1}) and the metabolic rate decreased at low ambient oxygen concentration.

4.7 Alkalinity and hardness

Alkalinity (measured as mg $CaCO_3$ L^{-1}) is the buffering capacity of the water to changes in pH (i.e. water ability to neutralize acids). Alkaline water (AW) generally has relatively high pH and bicarbonate (HCO_3^-) and carbonate (CO_3^{2-}) concentrations. High-carbonate alkalinity is a major stressor on fishes which inhabit AWs. High pH may decrease ammonia excretion and increase CO_2 excretion in these fishes (Parra and Baldisserotto, 2007). This means that water alkalinity should be maintained at appropriate levels in order to maintain the pH at the favourable level. Moderately AW is generally better for aquaculture, as it minimizes the changes in water pH, and in turn reduces the acidic or alkaline fish stress (Torres Rojas and Rocha, 2004).

Very few studies have considered the effects of water alkalinity on farmed tilapia. These studies indicated that tilapia performance is significantly affected by water alkalinity. Torres Rojas and Rocha (2004) found that Nile tilapia larvae reared under three levels of alkalinity ($CaCO_3$), low, medium and high (15.5, 32.6 and 56.8 mg L^{-1}, respectively), for 42 days attained the best growth rates and condition factor at the medium level (32.6 mg L^{-1}). Zhao et al. (2015) identified the potential genes responsible for alkalinity stress response in Nile tilapia using RNA sequencing (RNA-Seq). The analysis was performed on gill transcriptome profiles from fish exposed to FW and AW. The results revealed that alkalinity stress induced transcriptome changes in Nile tilapia. Several genes that displayed distinct differences in their expression in fish gills were identified. Differentially expressed genes encoding important modulators of alkalinity stress adaptation were also identified, including carbonic anhydrases, glutamine synthetase and cytochrome P450.

Bart et al. (2013) examined the effects of water hardness (55–4239 mg L^{-1} $CaCO_3$) on survival of eggs during artificial incubation, yolk-sac larvae and swim-up fry of Nile tilapia (Chitralada strain). They found that high water hardness (500–4200 mg L^{-1}) resulted in better survival of yolk-sac larvae and swim-up fry than low water hardness (50 and 132 mg L^{-1}).

4.8 Photoperiod

Photoperiod is a key artificial factor in regulating the daily activity rhythms of fish (Biswas and Takeuchi, 2002; Fortes-Silva et al., 2010; Costa et al., 2016a, 2016b), promoting fish growth, metabolic rates, body pigmentation, sexual maturation and reproduction (Biswas and Takeuchi, 2002; Trippel and Neil, 2002; El-Sayed and Kawanna, 2004). The effects of photoperiods on the growth, reproduction and other physiological functions of tilapia have been investigated by several researchers (Biswas and Takeuchi, 2002; El-Sayed and Kawanna, 2004, 2007; Carvalho et al., 2012, 2013; El-Sayed et al., 2013; Hornsby et al., 2013; Guerra-Santos et al., 2017).

Tilapia, like other fishes, may possess an endogenous molecular clock, which makes the daily rhythms persist under constant conditions. This means that the duration of the light phase photoperiod may affect fish performance and hepatic insulin-like growth factor-I (IGF-I) gene expression. This assumption was tested by a number of authors (Vera Cruz and Brown, 2009; Costa et al., 2016a, 2016b). The effects of the short duration (8 h) or long duration (16 h) of the light phase photoperiod on the growth, feed conversion and hepatic IGF-I gene expression in Nile tilapia (16 g) were evaluated (Vera Cruz and Brown, 2009). Long duration improved growth rate and feed conversion compared with the short light phase. Significant positive correlations also existed between IGF-I concentrations and growth rates.

Costa et al. (2016a) also investigated clock gene expression rhythms in tilapia, their endogenous origin, and how they are synchronized by light and feeding cycles. They found that all the clock genes analyzed in brain regions showed daily rhythms; with *clock1*, *bmal1a*, and *cry2a* showing the peak at the end of the light, whereas *per1b* and *cry5* showed acrophase between the end of the dark phase and the beginning of the light phase. In another study, the same authors (Costa et al., 2016b) tested the presence of daily rhythms in the somatotropic axis of tilapia fed at midlight (ML) or middark (MD) times, and the effect of the time of day of GH injection on the response of this axis. The mRNA expression levels of hypothalamic pituitary adenylate cyclase-activating polypeptide (PACAP), pituitary GH, liver IGF-I and IGF2a, liver and muscle GH receptors (ghr1 and ghr2) and IGF receptors (igf1ra and igf2r) were evaluated. Daily rhythms in fish fed at ML were observed in the liver for ghr1, ghr2 and igf2r, with the acrophases shown in the light phase. The time of both GH injection and feeding influenced the response to GH injection. ML-fed fish injected with GH, 3 h after lights off, showed a significant increase in liver igf1, igf2a and ghr2, and muscle ghr2 expression.

It is evident from these studies that photoperiod is one of the most important factors acting as synchronizers of biological rhythms in fishes. Fish may prefer feeding and behaviour in certain phases of the light–dark cycle, if they are allowed to self-feed. This assumption was tested in tilapia by a number of authors. For example, Guerra-Santos et al. (2017) tested the synchronization to feeding schedule of daily rhythms of locomotor activity and digestive enzymes of Nile tilapia fed once a day at 11:00 and 23:00 h. The results revealed that feeding time and light cycle synchronize the daily rhythms of behaviour, digestive physiology and plasma glucose. Fish fed at 11:00 h exhibited a diurnal locomotor activity and synchronization to the feeding schedule, whereas fish fed at 23:00 were less diurnal, and their pattern of locomotor activity was disrupted. Also, alkaline protease activity in the midgut showed daily rhythm with the maximum expression (acrophase) at the beginning of the dark phase in both 11:00 and 23:00 h groups, while the acrophase in the daily rhythm of plasma glucose was shifted by 12 h.

It has been reported that the response of Nile tilapia to photoperiod cycles depends on fish developmental stage and sex (El-Sayed and Kawanna, 2004). Larval stage was more sensitive to photoperiod than fingerling and juvenile stages. Fish fry subjected to long photoperiods (24 and 18 h) had significantly better performance than those exposed to intermediate or short photoperiods (12 or 6 h). One possible explanation of the decreased larval growth during shorter photoperiods is that during short light phases insufficient time will be available for the establishment of a robust rhythmicity, as has been reported by Biswas and Takeuchi (2002). The effect of photoperiod on synchronizing an endogenous rhythm to the external environment may also require more energy in the shorter photoperiods, leading to a reduction of somatic fish growth (Biswas and Takeuchi, 2002).

On the other hand, it has been suggested that the improvement in the growth of fingerling Nile tilapia with increasing photoperiod is related to the reduction of standard metabolic rate (Biswas and Takeuchi, 2002). Therefore, the adoption of the optimum photoperiod in tilapia culture systems, especially in closed systems, is essential since it will reduce the amount of energy used for standard metabolism, and in turn increase the energy spared for somatic growth, leading to increased fish production and profitability.

Very few studies have considered the effects of light intensity and photoperiod on reproductive performance of tilapia. The information reported, despite being limited, indicated that low light intensity leads to low spawning activity (Ridha and Cruz, 2000). Ridha and Cruz (2000) recommended a light intensity of 2500 lux and a photoperiod of 18 h day^{-1} for optimum seed production of Nile tilapia. Gonads development, fecundity and spawning frequencies also tend to improve with increasing photoperiod (Behrends and Smitherman, 1983). It appears that the best reproductive performance is achieved under normal day length (12 h light:12 h dark cycles) (Campos-Mendoza et al., 2004; El-Sayed and Kawanna, 2007).

Light intensity may affect the behaviour and social hierarchy of tilapia, depending on fish size. Carvalho et al.

(2013) studied the effects of light intensity on the aggression and social stability of Nile tilapia adult males. Fish behaviour was observed for 11 days under low (280.75 lx) and high (1394.14 lx) light intensities. The results indicated that higher light intensity increased the frequency of aggressive interactions, but the dominance of the fish was not affected by light intensity. The authors concluded that the effect of light intensity is not strong enough to destabilize the social hierarchy. On the other hand, high light intensity increased the response time to fighting (and decreased aggressive behaviour) in juvenile Nile tilapias (Carvalho et al., 2012). This behaviour of juvenile fish under intense light is probably a natural mechanism to reduce predation risk. On the contrary, adult fish are generally more aggressive under high light intensity because they need to defend their territory and attract females for mating (Carvalho and Gonçalves-De-Freitas, 2008).

Environmental light plays a significant role in shaping signal reception and visual sensitivity in Nile tilapia, depending on fish size. For example, Hornsby et al. (2013) measured spectral sensitivity, lens transmission and body pattern reflectance from juvenile and adult Nile tilapia held under two environmental light treatments (broad-spectrum light and red-shifted light). Spectral sensitivity in juveniles reared under both light treatments differed mainly at short wavelengths, where the irradiance of the two light treatments was the most differed. On the other hand, adult fish held under the same two light regimes did not differ in spectral sensitivity. These results indicate that environmental light can influence fish communication, suggesting that the characteristics of environmental light should be considered in relevant ecological studies. In support, El-Sayed et al. (2013) reported that Nile tilapia larvae are visual feeders at the onset of exogenous feeding. They prefer dark-coloured feed, while fingerling fish showed no preference to diet colours, since they depend on other chemical and physical stimulators. The visual-based behaviour of Nile tilapia larvae could also be related to the development of eye retina during larval stages, which plays a significant role in colour vision.

4.9 Water turbidity

Water turbidity can be a major problem in semi-intensive, fertilized FW fish ponds. According to Yi et al. (2003), this turbidity originates from a number of sources, namely (1) turbid source water, (2) rainwater run-off from pond dikes containing clay materials and (3) resuspension of bottom mud by water and fish movements. The high suspended colloidal particles reduce fertilizer effect, cause water acidity and inhibit light penetration, and in turn adversely affect primary productivity in fish ponds (Boyd, 1990). The influence of turbidity on growth, feed conversion and survival of all-male, sex-reversed Jamaica red tilapia fry has been studied by Ardjosoediro and Ramnarine (2002). The fish were reared in water at clay turbidity levels of 0, 50, 100, 150 and 200 mg L^{-1} for 7 weeks. Fish growth, feed efficiency and survival were all significantly reduced with increase in water turbidity, but the differences at the higher levels of 100–200 mg L^{-1} were not significant. The authors suggested that clay turbidity levels in earthen ponds should be kept below 100 mg L^{-1}.

It is essential that proper mitigation techniques must be applied in order to minimize the adverse effects of turbidity on pond productivity and fish growth. Yi et al. (2003) described the source of clay turbidity and evaluated different clay turbidity mitigation techniques and their effects on the growth of sex-reversed all-male Nile tilapia, and on water quality, in order to find a suitable mitigation method for controlling turbidity during the rainy season, for 149 days. Five mitigation treatments were adopted: (1) control; (2) covering upper 50 cm of pond dikes with black plastic material to prevent turbidity from run-off (edge covered); (3) covering pond bottoms with green manure (terrestrial weeds) to alter soil texture (weed-covered); (4) covering pond bottoms with small mesh (1 cm) net to prevent turbidity from fish disturbance (bottom-covered) and (5) covering pond dikes with rice straw (straw-covered). The ponds were fertilized with chicken manure at a rate of 500 kg ha^{-1} per week, in addition to supplemental urea and triple superphosphate to provide 28 kg N ha^{-1} per week and 7 kg P ha^{-1} per week. The authors found that the run-off of pond dikes represented the main clay turbidity and covering pond dikes was effective in mitigating this turbidity. The straw- and weed-covered treatments produced the best growth rates and yield. The authors referred the better performance and effective control of turbidity in straw- and weed-covered treatments to the following: (1) the increased natural food availability; (2) metabolic and decomposition products from plant materials cleared pond water and reduced the shading effect of turbid water; (3) the aggregation of clay particles and algal cells may have led to the sedimentation of larger particles and (4) the adsorption of clay on weed and straw. However, covering pond dikes with rice straw significantly reduced clay turbidity caused by run-off and enhanced fish growth through microbial biofilm developed on the rice straw. Therefore, the authors suggested that covering pond dikes with rice straw can be a cost-effective tool for clay turbidity mitigation in tilapia ponds during rainy seasons.

4.10 Closing remarks

1. Water quality management has become a key factor for successful aquaculture practices. It is necessary therefore to understand the major water quality parameters and their interrelationships, which affect fish

growth and health and determine the failure or success of overall culture practices.
2. A temperature of about 28–30°C appears optimal for growth performance of Nile tilapia under recirculating culture systems.
3. The further the geographic location from the equator, the more tolerant are Nile tilapia strains to cold.
4. The conditioning of tilapia at intermediate temperature before exposing them to lower temperatures may improve fish survival and tolerance to cold stress.
5. Small fingerling tilapia appear more susceptible to low temperature than larger fish. Large fingerlings must be used if water temperature is expected to drop.
6. The resistance of tilapia to cold stress may be better in brackish water than in freshwater.
7. Increased water temperature may limit larval growth and induce body deformation. The exposure of the larvae to low temperature before 10 days old may induce a high proportion of females, while elevated temperature may induce high percentage of males.
8. Most tilapia species and hybrids tolerate a wide range of water salinity and can normally grow and reproduce in brackish water environments.
9. *O. mossambicus*, *O. aureus*, *O. spilurus* and *T. zillii* are the most salinity-tolerant tilapia species, while other tilapias are generally less euryhaline and can grow, survive and reproduce at 0–29‰, depending on the species, size and sex and acclimation period.
10. Pre-acclimation to saltwater and gradual transfer to high salinity significantly improve tilapia growth and survival. Feeding tilapia broodstock with diets containing higher salt levels may also produce seeds with better adaptability to water salinity.
11. Handling stress increases oxygen consumption in tilapia and therefore, should be minimized.
12. Ammonia is very toxic to tilapia and therefore, the UIA-N concentration should be maintained below 0.1 mg L^{-1}.
13. Nitrite is also toxic to tilapia. The addition of chloride source (500 mg L^{-1} $CaCl_2$ or NaCl) (at a chloride:nitrite ratio of 1.5:1) to culture water may protect tilapia from nitrite toxicity.
14. Larval stages of tilapia (Nile tilapia) may be more sensitive to photoperiod than fingerling and juvenile stages. Long photoperiods (18L:6D and 24L:0D cycle) produce better performance than short photoperiods (6L:18D cycle). A 12L:12D cycle has been recommended for optimum reproduction performance of Nile tilapia.
15. Water turbidity can be a major problem in semi-intensive, fertilized freshwater fish ponds. Covering pond dikes with rice straw (or similar plant materials like wheat straw) or covering pond bottoms with terrestrial weeds are cost-effective tools for clay turbidity mitigation in tilapia ponds, especially during rainy seasons.

References

Abdel-Ghany, H.M., El-Sayed, A.F.M., Ezzat, A., Essa, M.A., Helal, A.M., 2019. Dietary lipid sources affect cold tolerance of Nile tilapia (*Oreochromis niloticus*). Journal of Thermal Biology 79, 50–55.

Abdel-Tawwab, M., Hagras, A.E., Elbaghdady, H.M., Monier, M.N., 2014. Dissolved oxygen level and stocking density effects on growth, feed utilization, physiology, and innate immunity of Nile tilapia, *Oreochromis niloticus*. Journal of Applied Aquaculture 26, 340–355.

Abdel-Tawwab, M., Hagras, A.E., Elbaghdady, H.M., Monier, M.N., 2015. Effects of dissolved oxygen and fish size on Nile tilapia, *Oreochromis niloticus* (L.): growth performance, whole body composition, and innate immunity. Aquaculture International 23, 1261–1274.

Ahmed, N.A., El-Serafy, S.S., El-Shafey, A.A.M., Abdel-Hamid, N.H., 1992. Effect of ammonia on some haematological parameters of *Oreochromis niloticus*. Proceedings of Zoological Society of Arab Republic of Egypt 23, 155–160.

Al-Ahmed, A.A., 2001. A review of tilapia culture in Kuwait. World Aquaculture 32, 47–48.

Al-Amoudi, M.M., 1987a. Acclimation of commercially cultured *Oreochromis* species to sea water – an experimental study. Aquaculture 65, 333–342.

Al-Amoudi, M.M., 1987b. The effect of high salt diet on the direct transfer of *Oreochromis mossambicus, O. spilurus* and *O. aureus/O. niloticus* hybrids to seawater. Aquaculture 64, 333–338.

Al-Amoudi, M.M., El-Sayed, A.-F.M., El-Ghobashy, A., 1996. Effects of thermal and thermo-haline shocks on survival and osmotic concentration of the tilapias *Oreochromis mossambicus* and *Oreochromis aureus* x *Oreochromis niloticus* hybrids. Journal of the World Aquaculture Society 27, 456–461.

Alfredo, M.H., Hector, S.L., 2002. Blood gasometric in hybrid red tilapia *Oreochromis niloticus* (Linnaeus) x *O. mossambicus* (Peters) while adapting to increasing salinity. Journal of Aquaculture in the Tropics 17, 101–112.

Allanson, B.R., Bok, A., Vanwyk, N.I., 1971. The influence of exposure to low temperature on *Tilapia mossambica* Peters (Cichlidae). 2. Changes in serum osmolarity, sodium and chloride ion concentrations. Journal of Fish Biology 3, 181–185.

Ammar, A.Y., El Nahas, A.F., Mahmoud, S., Barakat, M.E., Hassan, A.M., 2018. Characterization of type IV antifreeze gene in Nile tilapia (*Oreochromis niloticus*) and influence of cold and hot weather on its expression and some immune-related genes. Fish Physiology and Biochemistry 44, 515–525.

Ardjosoediro, I., Ramnarine, I.W., 2002. The influence of turbidity on growth, feed conversion and survivorship of the Jamaica red tilapia strain. Aquaculture 212, 159–165.

Atwood, H.L., Fontenot, Q.C., Tomasso, J.R., Isely, J.J., 2001. Toxicity of nitrite to Nile tilapia: effect of fish size and environmental chloride. North American Journal of Aquaculture 63, 49–51.

Balarin, J.D., Hatton, J.P., 1979. Tilapia: A Guide to Their Biology and Culture in Africa. University of Stirling, Scotland.

Balarin, J.D., Haller, R.D., 1982. The intensive culture of tilapia in tanks, raceways and cages. In: Muir, J.F., Roberts, R.J. (Eds.), Recent Advances in Aquaculture. Croom Helm, London and Canberra. Westview Press, Boulder, CO, pp. 267–355.

Baras, E., Jacobs, B., Melard, C., 2001. Effect of water temperature on survival, growth and phenotypic sex of mixed (XX-XY) progenies of Nile tilapia *Oreochromis niloticus*. Aquaculture 192, 187–199.

Baroiller, J.F., Clota, F., Geraz, E., 1995. Temperature sex determination in two tilapia, *Oreochromis niloticus* and the red tilapia (red Florida strain): effect of high or low temperature. In: Goetz, F.W., Thomas, P. (Eds.), Proceedings of the Fifth International Symposium on the Reproductive Physiology of Fish. University of Texas, Austin, TX, pp. 158–160.

Bart, A.N., Prasad, B., Thakur, D.P., 2013. Effects of incubation water hardness and salinity on egg hatch and fry survival of Nile tilapia *Oreochromis niloticus* (Linnaeus). Aquaculture Research 44, 1085–1092.

Beamish, F.W.H., 1970. Influence of temperature and salinity acclimation on temperature preferenda of the euryhaline fish *T. nilotica*. Journal of the Fisheries Research Board of Canada 27, 1209–1214.

Becker, K., Fishelson, L., 1986. Standard and routine metabolic rate, critical oxygen tension and spontaneous scope for activity of tilapias. In: Maclean, J.L., Dizon, L.B., Hosillos, L.V. (Eds.), Proceedings of the First Asian Fisheries Forum. Asian Fisheries Society, Manila, Philippines, pp. 623–628.

Behrends, L.L., Smitherman, R.O., 1983. Use of warm water effluents to induce winter spawning of tilapia in a temperate climate. In: Fishelson, L., Yaron, Z. (Eds.), Proceedings of the International Symposium on Tilapia in Aquaculture. Tel-Aviv University, Israel, pp. 446–454.

Behrends, L.L., Smitherman, R.O., 1984. Development of a cold-tolerant population of red tilapia through introgressive hybridization. Journal of the World Mariculture Society 14, 172–178.

Behrends, L.L., Kingsley, J.B., Bulls, M.J., 1996. Cold tolerance in maternal mouthbrooding tilapias: heritability estimates and correlated growth responses at suboptimal temperatures. In: Pullin, R.S.V., Lazard, J., Legendre, M., Amon Kottias, J.B., Pauly, D. (Eds.), Proceedings of the Third International Symposium on Tilapia in Aquaculture. ICLARM Conference Proceedings No. 41. ICLARM, Penang, Malaysia, pp. 257–265.

Benli, A.Ç.K., Köksal, G., 2005. The acute toxicity of ammonia on tilapia (*Oreochromis niloticus* L.) larvae and fingerlings. Turkish Journal of Veterinary and Animal Sciences 29, 339–344.

Benli, A.Ç.K., Köksal, G., Özkul, A., 2008. Sublethal ammonia exposure of Nile tilapia (*Oreochromis niloticus* L.): effects on gill, liver and kidney histology. Chemosphere 72, 1355–1358.

Biswas, A.K., Takeuchi, T., 2002. Effect of different photoperiod cycles on metabolic rate and energy loss of both fed and unfed adult tilapia *Oreochromis niloticus*: Part II. Fisheries Science 68, 543–553.

Bonga, S.E.W., Flike, G., Balm, P.H.M., 1987. Physiological adaptation to acid stress in fish. In: Witters, H., Vanderborght, O. (Eds.), Symposium on Ecophysiology of Acid Stress in Aquatic Organisms. Annales de Société Royale Zoologique de Belgique, Belgique, pp. 243–254.

Boyd, C.E., 1990. Water Quality in Ponds for Aquaculture. Auburn University, Auburn, AL, USA, 482 pp.

Breves, J.P., Hasegawa, S., Yoshioka, M., Fox, B.K., Davis, L.K., Lerner, D.T., et al., 2010. Acute salinity challenges in Mozambique and Nile tilapia: differential responses of plasma prolactin, growth hormone and branchial expression of ion transporters. General and Comparative Endocrinology 167, 135–142.

Campos-Mendoza, A., Mcandrew, B.J., Coward, K., Bromage, N., 2004. Reproductive response of Nile tilapia (*Oreochromis niloticus*) to photoperiodic manipulation; effects on spawning periodicity, fecundity and egg size. Aquaculture 231, 299–314.

Canagaratnam, P., 1966. Growth of *Tilapia mossambica* Peters in different salinities. Bulletin of the Fisheries Research Station Ceylon 19, 1–2.

Carmelo, A., 2002. Commercial culture of *Oreochromis spilurus* in open seawater cages and onshore tanks. Israeli Journal of Aquaculture – Bamidgeh 54, 27–33.

Carvalho, T.B., Gonçalves-De-Freitas, E., 2008. Sex group composition, social interaction, and metabolism in the fish Nile tilapia. Brazilian Journal of Biology 68, 807–812.

Carvalho, T.B., Ha, J.C., Gonçalves-De-Freitas, E., 2012. Light intensity can trigger different agonistic responses in juveniles of three cichlid species. Marine and Freshwater Behaviour and Physiology 45, 91–100.

Carvalho, T.B., Mendonça, F.Z., Costa-Ferreira, R.S., Gonçalves-De-Freitas, E., 2013. The effect of increased light intensity on the aggressive behavior of the Nile tilapia, *Oreochromis niloticus* (Teleostei: Cichlidae). The Zoologist 30, 125–129.

Chen, S.-M., Chen, P.-C., Hsiao, I.-C., Chen, J.-C., 2001. Effects of pH on the nitrogenous excretion and lethal DO of tilapia *Oreochromis mossambica*. In: Sixth Asian Fisheries Forum. Book of Abstracts. Asian Fisheries Society, Manila, Philippines, p. 51.

Chen, W., Sun, L., Tsai, C., Song, Y., Chang, C., 2002. Cold-stress induced the modulation of catecholamines, cortisol, immunoglobulin M and leukocyte phagocytosis in tilapia. General and Comparative Endocrinology 126, 90–100.

Chervinski, J., Lahav, M., 1976. The effect of exposure to low temperature on fingerlings of local Tilapia (*Tilapia aurea*) (Steindachner) and imported Tilapia (*Tilapia vulcani*) (Trewavas) and *Tilapia nilotica* (Linne) in Israel. Bamidgeh 28, 25–29.

Chervinski, J., 1982. Environmental physiology of tilapias. In: Pullin, R.V.S., Lowe-McConnell, R.H. (Eds.), The Biology and Culture of Tilapias. ICLARM Conference Proceedings No. 7. ICLARM, Manila, Philippines, pp. 119–128.

Choi, K., Cope, W.G., Harms, C.A., Law, J.M., 2013. Rapid decreases in salinity, but not increases, lead to immune dysregulation in Nile tilapia, *Oreochromis niloticus* (L.). Journal of Fish Diseases 36, 389–399.

Chowdhury, M.A.K., Yi, Y., Lin, C.K., El-Haroun, E.R., 2006. Effect of salinity on carrying capacity of adult Nile tilapia *Oreochromis niloticus* L. in recirculating systems. Aquaculture Research 37, 1627–1635.

Cnaani, A., Gall, G.A.E., Hulata, G., 2000. Cold tolerance of tilapia species and hybrids. Aquaculture International 8, 289–298.

Costa, L.S., Rosa, P.V., Fortes-Silva, R., Sanchez-Vazquez, F.J., Lopez-Olmeda, J.F., 2016a. Daily rhythms of the expression of genes from the somatotropic axis: the influence on tilapia (*Oreochromis niloticus*) of feeding and growth hormone administration at different times. Comparative Biochemistry and Physiology - Part C: Toxicology & Pharmacology 181–182, 27–34.

Costa, L.S., Serrano, I., Sanchez-Vazquez, F.J., Lopez-Olmeda, J.F., 2016b. Circadian rhythms of clock gene expression in Nile tilapia (*Oreochromis niloticus*) central and peripheral tissues: influence of different lighting and feeding conditions. Journal of Comparative Physiology B 186, 775–785.

Dan, N.C., Little, D.C., 2000. The culture performance of monosex and mixed-sex new season and over-wintered fry in two strains of Nile tilapia (*Oreochromis niloticus*) in Northern Vietnam. Aquaculture 184, 221–231.

Daud, S.K., Hasbollah, A., Law, A.T., 1988. Effect of unionized ammonia on red tilapia (*Oreochromis mossambicus/O. niloticus* hybrids) fry. In: Pullin, R.S.V., Bhukaswan, T., Tonguthai, K., Maclean, J.L. (Eds.), Proceedings of the Second International Symposium on Tilapia in Aquaculture. ICLARM Conference Proceedings No. 15. Department of Fisheries, Bangkok, Thailand, and ICLARM, Manila, Philippines, pp. 411–414.

Denzer, H.W., 1968. Studies on the physiology of young Tilapia. FAO Fisheries Report 44 (4), 356–366.

El-Ebiary, E.H., Zaki, M.A., Mourad, M.H., 1997. Effect of salinity on growth, feed utilization and haematological parameters of Florida red tilapia fingerlings. Bulletin of the National Institute of Oceanography and Fisheries 23, 203–216.

El-Greisy, Z.A.E.-B., Elgamal, A.E.E., Ahmed, N.A.M., 2016. Effect of prolonged ammonia toxicity on fertilized eggs, hatchability and size of newly hatched larvae of Nile tilapia, *Oreochromis niloticus*. The Egyptian Journal of Aquatic Research 42, 215–222.

El-Sayed, A.-F.M., El-Ghobashy, A., Al-Amoudi, M.M., 1996. Effects of pond depth and water temperature on the growth, mortality and body composition of Nile tilapia, *Oreochromis niloticus* (L.). Aquaculture Research 27, 681–687.

El-Sayed, A.-F.M., Mansour, C.R., Ezzat, A.A., 2003. Effects of dietary protein levels on spawning performance of Nile tilapia (*Oreochromis niloticus*) broodstock reared at different water salinities. Aquaculture 220, 619–632.

El-Sayed, A.-F.M., Kawanna, M., 2004. Effects of photoperiod on the performance of farmed Nile tilapia *Oreochromis niloticus*: I. Growth, feed utilization efficiency and survival of fry and fingerlings. Aquaculture 231, 393–402.

El-Sayed, A.-F.M., Kawanna, M., 2007. Effects of photoperiod on growth and spawning efficiency of Nile tilapia (L.) broodstock in a recycling system. Aquaculture Research 38, 1242–1247.

El-Sayed, A.-F.M., Kawanna, M., 2008. Ambient water temperature boosts growth rates of Nile tilapia Fry reared in recycling systems. Aquaculture Research 39, 670–672.

El-Sayed, A.F.M., El-Ghobashy, A.E., El-Mezayen, M.M., 2013. Effect of feed colour on growth and feed utilization of Nile tilapia (*Oreochromis niloticus* L.) larvae and fingerlings. Aquaculture Nutrition 19, 870–876.

El-Shafai, S.A., El-Gohary, F.A., Nasr, F.A., van der Steen, N.P., Gijzen, H.J., 2004. Chronic ammonia toxicity to duckweed-fed tilapia (*Oreochromis niloticus*). Aquaculture 232, 117–127.

El-Shafey, A.A.M., 1998. Effect of ammonia on respiratory functions of blood of *Tilapia zillii*. Comparative Biochemistry and Physiology 121A, 305–313.

El Gamal, A.-R., 1988. Reproductive Performance, Sex Ratios, Gonadal Development, Cold Tolerance, Viability and Growth of Red and Normally Pigmented Hybrids of Tilapia aurea and T. nilotica (Ph.D. thesis). Auburn University, Auburn, Alabama, USA.

Fiess, J.C., Kunkel-Patterson, A., Mathias, M., Riley, L.G., Yancey, P.H., Hirano, T., et al., 2007. Effects of environmental salinity and temperature on osmoregulatory ability, organic osmolytes, and plasma hormone profiles in the Mozambique tilapia (*Oreochromis mossambicus*). Comparative Biochemistry and Physiology 146A, 252–264.

Fineman-Kalio, A.S., 1988. Preliminary observations on the effect of salinity on the reproduction and growth of freshwater Nile tilapia, *Oreochromis niloticus* (L.), cultured in brackishwater ponds. Aquaculture and Fisheries Management 19, 313–320.

Fish, G.R., 1956. Some aspects of the respiration of six species of fish from Uganda. Journal of Experimental Biology 33, 186–195.

Fortes-Silva, R., Martinez, F.J., Villarroel, M., Sanchez-Vazquez, F.J., 2010. Daily rhythms of locomotor activity, feeding behavior and dietary selection in Nile tilapia (*Oreochromis niloticus*). Comparative Biochemistry and Physiology 156A, 445–450.

Franklin, C.E., Johnston, I.A., Crockford, T., Kamunde, C., 1995. Scaling of oxygen consumption of Lake Magadi tilapia, a fish living at 37°C. Journal of Fish Biology 46, 829–834.

Fukusho, K., 1968. The specific difference of temperature response among cichlid fishes of genus *Tilapia*. Bulletin of the Japanese Society of Scientific Fisheries 34, 103–111.

Guerra-Santos, B., Lopez-Olmeda, J.F., De Mattos, B.O., Baiao, A.B., Pereira, D.S.P., Sanchez-Vazquez, F.J., et al., 2017. Synchronization to light and mealtime of daily rhythms of locomotor activity, plasma glucose and digestive enzymes in the Nile tilapia (*Oreochromis niloticus*). Comparative Biochemistry and Physiology, Part A Molecular and Integrated Physiology 204, 40–47.

Hargreaves, J.A., Kucuk, S., 2001. Effects of diel un-ionized ammonia fluctuation on juvenile hybrid striped bass, channel catfish, and blue tilapia. Aquaculture 195, 163–181.

Hegazi, M.M., Hasanein, S.S., 2010. Effects of chronic exposure to ammonia concentrations on brain monoamines and ATPases of Nile tilapia (*Oreochromis niloticus*). Comparative Biochemistry and Physiology - Part C: Toxicology & Pharmacology 151, 420–425.

Hegazi, M.M., Attia, Z.I., Hegazi, M.A.M., Hasanein, S.S., 2010. Metabolic consequences of chronic sublethal ammonia exposure at cellular and subcellular levels in Nile tilapia brain. Aquaculture 299, 149–156.

Hofer, S.C., Watts, S.A., 2002. Cold tolerance in genetically male tilapia (GMT registered), *Oreochromis niloticus*. World Aquaculture 33, 19–21.

Hornsby, M.A., Sabbah, S., Robertson, R.M., Hawryshyn, C.W., 2013. Modulation of environmental light alters reception and production of visual signals in Nile tilapia. Journal of Experimental Biology 216, 3110–3122.

Hui, W., Xiaowen, Z., Haizhen, W., Jun, Q., Pao, X., Ruiwei, L., 2014. Joint effect of temperature, salinity and pH on the percentage fertilization and hatching of Nile tilapia (*Oreochromis niloticus*). Aquaculture Research 45, 259–269.

Jennings, D.P., 1991. Behavioural aspects of cold tolerance in blackchin tilapia, *Sarotherodon melanotheron*, at different salinities. Environmental Biology of Fishes 31, 185–195.

Jensen, F.B., 2003. Nitrite disrupts multiple physiological functions in aquatic animals. Comparative Biochemistry and Physiology, Part A Molecular and Integrated Physiology 135, 9–24.

Job, S.V., 1969a. The respiratory metabolism of *Tilapia mossambica* (Teleostei). I. The effect of size, temperature and salinity. Marine Biology 2, 121–126.

Job, S.V., 1969b. The respiratory metabolism of *Tilapia mossambica* (Teleostei). II. The effect of size, temperature, salinity and partial pressure of oxygen. Marine Biology 3, 222–226.

Jun, Q., Pao, X., Haizhen, W., Ruiwei, L., Hui, W., 2012. Combined effect of temperature, salinity and density on the growth and feed utilization of Nile tilapia juveniles (*Oreochromis niloticus*). Aquaculture Research 43, 1344–1356.

Kammerer, B.D., Cech Jr., J.J., Kultz, D., 2010. Rapid changes in plasma cortisol, osmolality, and respiration in response to salinity stress in tilapia (*Oreochromis mossambicus*). Comparative Biochemistry and Physiology, Part A Molecular and Integrated Physiology 157, 260–265.

Khater, A., Smitherman, R.O., 1988. Cold tolerance and growth of three strains of *Oreochromis niloticus*. In: Pullin, R.S.V., Bhukaswan, T., Tonguthai, K., Maclean, J.L. (Eds.), Proceedings of the Second International Symposium on Tilapia in Aquaculture. ICLARM Conference Proceedings No. 15. Department of Fisheries, Bangkok, Thailand, and ICLARM, Manila, Philippines, pp. 215–218.

Kirk, R.G., 1972. A review of the recent development in tilapia culture with special reference to fish farming in the heated effluents of power stations. Aquaculture 1, 45–60.

Küçük, S., 2014. Acute toxicity of ammonia to blue tilapia, *Oreochromis aureus*, in saline water. African Journal of Biotechnology 13, 1550–1553.

Kuwaye, T.T., Okimoto, D.K., Shimoda, S.K., Howerton, R.D., Lin, H.-R., Pang, P.K.T., et al., 1993. Effect of 17 α-methyltestosterone on the growth of the euryhaline tilapia, *Oreochromis mossambicus*, in fresh water and in sea water. Aquaculture 113, 137–152.

Liao, I.C., Chang, S.L., 1983. Studies on the feasibility of red tilapia culture in saline water. In: Fishelson, L., Yaron, Z. (Eds.), Proceedings of the International Symposium on Tilapia in Aquaculture. Tel Aviv University, Tel Aviv, Israel, pp. 524–533.

Likongwe, J.S., Stecko, T.D., Stauffer, J.R., Carline, R.F., 1996. Combined effects of water temperature and salinity on growth and feed utilisation of juvenile Nile tilapia *Oreochromis niloticus* (Linnaeus). Aquaculture 146, 37–46.

Likongwe, J.S., 2002. Studies on potential use of salinity to increase growth of tilapia in aquaculture in Mali. In: McElwee, K., Lewis, K., Nidiffer, M., Buitrago, P. (Eds.), Nineteenth Annual Technical Report. Pond Dynamics/Aquaculture CRSP. Oregon State University, Corvallis, OR, USA, pp. 167–174.

Magid, A.M.A., Babiker, M.M., 1975. Oxygen consumption and respiratory behaviour of three Nile fishes. Hydrobiologia 46, 359–367.

McGeachin, R.B., Wicklund, R.I., Olla, B.L., Winton, J.R., 1987. Growth of *Tilapia aurea* in seawater cages. Journal of the World Aquaculture Society 18, 31–34.

McMahon, D.Z., Baca, B., 1999. The Effects of Various Salinities on the Growth, Pathology and Reproduction of Blue tilapia *Oreochromis aureus*. In: World Aquaculture '99- Book of Abstracts. World Aquaculture Society, Baton Rouge, LA, USA, 508 pp.

Morgan, J.D., Sakamoto, T., Grau, E.G., Iwama, G.K., 1997. Physiological and respiratory responses of the Mozambique tilapia (*Oreochromis mossambicus*) to salinity acclimation. Comparative Biochemistry and Physiology 117A, 391–398.

Morgan, P.R., 1972. Causes of mortality in the endemic tilapia of Lake Chilwa (Malawi). Hydrobiologia 40, 101–119.

Parra, J.E.G., Baldisserotto, B., 2007. Effect of water pH and hardness on survival and growth of freshwater Teleosts. In: Kapoor, B.G. (Ed.), Fish Osmoregulation. Science Publishers, Enfield, pp. 135–150.

Pauly, D., 1976. The biology, fishery and potential for aquaculture of *Tilapia melanotheron* in a small west African lagoon. Aquaculture 7, 33–49.

Payne, A.I., 1983. Estuarine and salt tolerant tilapias. In: Fishelson, L., Yaron, Z. (Eds.), Proceedings of the International Symposium on Tilapia in Aquaculture. Tel-Aviv University, Israel, pp. 534–543.

Payne, A.I., Collinson, R.I., 1983. A comparison of the biological characteristics of *Sarotherodon niloticus* (L.) with those of *S. aureus* (Steindachner) and other tilapia of the delta and lower Nile. Aquaculture 30, 335–351.

Payne, A.I., Ridgway, J., Hamer, J.L., 1988. The influence of salt (NaCl) concentration and temperature on the growth of *Oreochromis spilurus*, *O. mossambicus* and a red tilapia hybrid. In: Pullin, R.S.V., Bhukaswan, T., Tonguthai, K., Maclean, J.L. (Eds.), Proceedings of the Second International Symposium on Tilapia in Aquaculture. ICLARM Conference Proceedings No. 15. Department of Fisheries, Thailand, and ICLARM, Manila, Philippines, pp. 481–487.

Perry, W.G., Avault, J.W., 1972. Comparisons of stripped mullet and tilapia for added production in caged catfish studies. Progressive Fish-Culturist 34, 229–232.

Perschbacher, P.W., McGeachin, R.B., 1988. Salinity tolerance of red hybrid tilapia fry, juvenile and adults. In: Pullin, R.S.V., Bhukaswan, T., Tonguthai, K., Maclean, J.L. (Eds.), Proceedings of the Second International Symposium on Tilapia in Aquaculture. ICLARM Conference Proceedings No. 15. Department of Fisheries, Thailand, and ICLARM, Manila, Philippines, pp. 415–420.

Philippart, J.-C.L., Ruwet, J.-C.L., 1982. Ecology and distribution of tilapias. In: Pullin, R.S.V., Lowe-McConnell, R.H. (Eds.), The Biology and Culture of Tilapias. ICLARM Conference Proceedings No. 7. ICLARM, Manila, Philippines, pp. 15–59.

Platt, S., Hauser, W.J., 1978. Optimum temperature for feeding and growth of *Tilapia zillii*. Progressive Fish-Culturist 40, 105–107.

Plumb, J.A., 1997. Infectious diseases of tilapia. In: Costa-Pierce, B.A., Rakocy, J.E. (Eds.), Tilapia Aquaculture in the Americas, vol. 1. World Aquaculture Society, Baton Rouge, LA, USA, pp. 212–228.

Popper, D., Lichatowich, T., 1975. Preliminary success in predator control of *Tilapia mossambica*. Aquaculture 5, 213–214.

Randall, D.J., Wood, C.M., Perry, S.F., Bergman, H., Maloiy, G.M.O., Mommsen, T.P., et al., 1989. Urea excretion as a strategy for survival in a fish living in a very alkaline environment. Nature 337, 165–166.

Rebouças, V.T., Lima, F.R.D., Cavalcante, D.D.H., Sá, M.V.D.C.E., 2016. Reassessment of the suitable range of water pH for culture of Nile tilapia *Oreochromis niloticus* L. in eutrophic water. Acta Scientiarum. Animal Sciences 38, 361–368.

Redner, B.D., Stickney, R.R., 1979. Acclimation to ammonia by *Tilapia aurea*. Transactions of the American Fisheries Society 108, 383–388.

Reite, O.B., Maloiy, G.M.O., Aasehaug, B., 1974. pH, salinity and temperature tolerance of Lake Magadi Tilapia. Nature 247, 315.

Ridha, M.T., Cruz, E.M., 2000. Effect of light intensity and photoperiod on Nile tilapia *Oreochromis niloticus*. Aquaculture Research 31, 609–617.

Romana-Eguia, M.R.R., Eguia, R.V., 1999. Growth of five Asian red tilapia strains in saline environments. Aquaculture 173, 161–170.

Ron, B., Shimoda, S.K., Iwama, G.K., Gordon Grau, E., 1995. Relationships among ration, salinity, 17 α-methyltestosterone and growth in the euryhaline tilapia, *Oreochromis mossambicus*. Aquaculture 135, 185–193.

Ross, B., Ross, L.G., 1983. The oxygen requirements of *Oreochromis niloticus* under adverse conditions. In: Fishelson, L., Yaron, Z. (Eds.), Proceedings of the International Symposium on Tilapia in Aquaculture. Tel-Aviv University, Israel, pp. 134–143.

Shafland, P.L., Pestrak, J.M., 1982. Lower lethal temperatures for fourteen non-native fishes in Florida. Environmental Biology of Fishes 7, 149–156.

Sifa, L., Chenhong, L., Dey, M., Gagalac, F., Dunham, R., 2002. Cold tolerance of three strains of Nile tilapia, *Oreochromis niloticus*, in China. Aquaculture 213, 123–129.

Sudharsan, R., Rani, A.S., Reddy, T.N., Reddy, P.U.M., Raju, T.N., 2000. Effect of nitrite toxicity on the dehydrogenases in the fish *Tilapia mossambica*. Journal of Environment and Pollution 7, 127–130.

Sun, L.N., Jiang, X.L., Xie, Q.P., Yuan, J., Huang, B.F., Tao, W.J., et al., 2014. Transdifferentiation of differentiated ovary into functional testis by long-term treatment of aromatase inhibitor in Nile tilapia. Endocrinology 155, 1476–1488.

Suresh, A.V., Lin, C.K., 1992. Tilapia culture in saline waters: a review. Aquaculture 106, 201–226.

Tayamen, M.M., Reyes, R.A., Danting, M.J., Mendoza, A.M., Marquez, E.B., Salguet, A.C., et al., 2002. Tilapia broodstock development for saline waters in the Philippines. Naga 25, 32–36.

Teichert-Coddington, D., Green, B.W., 1993. Tilapia yield improvement through maintenance of minimal oxygen concentrations in experimental grow-out ponds in Honduras. Aquaculture 118, 63–71.

Torres Rojas, N.E., Rocha, Ö., 2004. Water alkalinity influence on the growth of nile Tilapia larvae, *Oreochromis niloticus* Linnaeus, 1758 (Perciformes, Cichlidae). Acta Scientiarum. Biological Sciences 26, 163–167.

Tran-Duy, A., van Dam, A.A., Schrama, J.W., 2012. Feed intake, growth and metabolism of Nile tilapia (*Oreochromis niloticus*) in relation to dissolved oxygen concentration. Aquaculture Research 43, 730–744.

Tran-Ngoc, K.T., Dinh, N.T., Nguyen, T.H., Roem, A.J., Schrama, J.W., Verreth, J.A.J., 2016. Interaction between dissolved oxygen concentration and diet composition on growth, digestibility and intestinal health of Nile tilapia (*Oreochromis niloticus*). Aquaculture 462, 101–108.

Trippel, E.A., Neil, S.R.E., 2002. Effect of photoperiod and light intensity on growth and activity of juvenile haddock (*Melanogrammus aeglefinus*). Aquaculture 217, 633–645.

Tsadik, G.G., Kutty, M.N., 1987. Influence of Ambient Oxygen on Feeding and Growth of the Tilapia, Oreochromis niloticus (Linnaeus). UNDP/FAO/NIOMR, Port Harcourt (Nigeria), 13 pp.

Turingan, J.E., Kubaryk, J.M., 1992. The effect of high salt diet on survival and hatchability of Taiwanese red tilapia (*Oreochromis mossambicus x Oreochromis niloticus*) eggs upon direct transfer to seawater. In: Aquaculture'92 - Book of Abstracts. World Aquaculture Society, Baton Rouge, LA, USA, 220 pp.

van Dijk, P.L.M., van den Thillart, G., Balm, P., Wendelaar Bonga, S., 1993. The influence of gradual water acidification on the acid/base status and plasma hormone levels in carp. Journal of Fish Biology 42, 661–671.

Van Ginneken, V.J.T., Van Eersel, R., Balm, P., Nieveen, M., Van Den Thillart, G., 1997. Tilapia are able to withstand long-term exposure to low environmental pH, judged by their energy status, ionic balance and plasma cortisol. Journal of Fish Biology 51, 795–806.

Vera Cruz, E.M., Brown, C.L., 2009. Influence of the photoperiod on growth rate and insulin-like growth factor-I gene expression in Nile tilapia *Oreochromis niloticus*. Journal of Fish Biology 75, 130–141.

Wang, H., Chang, G., Qiang, J., Xu, P., 2017. Relationship of RNA/DNA ratio to somatic growth of Nile tilapia juveniles (*Oreochromis niloticus*) under joint effects of temperature and salinity. Aquaculture Research 48, 2663–2671.

Wang, L.-H., Tsai, C.-L., 2000. Effects of temperature on the deformity and sex differentiation of tilapia, *Oreochromis mossambicus*. Journal of Experimental Zoology 286, 534–537.

Wangead, C., Greater, A., Tansakul, R., 1988. Effects of acid water on survival and growth rate of Nile tilapia (*Oreochromis niloticus*). In: Pullin, R.S.V., Bhukaswan, T., Tonguthai, K., Maclean, J.L. (Eds.), Proceedings of the Second International Symposium on Tilapia in Aquaculture. ICLARM Conference Proceedings No. 15. Department of Fisheries, Thailand, and ICLARM, Manila, Philippines, pp. 433–438.

Watanabe, W.O., Kuo, C.-M., Huang, M.-C., 1985. The ontogeny of salinity tolerance in the tilapias *Oreochromis aureus, O. niloticus* and *O. mossambicus* x *O. niloticus* hybrids, spawned and reared in freshwater. Aquaculture 47, 353–367.

Watanabe, W.O., Ellingson, L.J., Wicklund, R.I., Olla, B.L., 1988a. The effects of salinity on growth, food consumption and conversion in juvenile, monosex male Florida red tilapia. In: Pullin, R.S.V., Bhukaswan, T., Tonguthai, K., Maclean, J.L. (Eds.), Proceedings of the Second International Symposium on Tilapia in Aquaculture. ICLARM Conference Proceedings No. 15. Department of Fisheries, Thailand, and ICLARM, Manila, Philippines, pp. 515–523.

Watanabe, W.O., French, K.E., Ellingson, L.J., Wicklund, R.I., 1988b. Further investigations on the effects of salinity on growth in Florida red tilapia: evidence for the influence of behaviour. In: Pullin, R.S.V., Bhukaswan, T., Tonguthai, K., Maclean, J.L. (Eds.), Proceedings of the Second International Symposium on Tilapia in Aquaculture. ICLARM Conference Proceedings No. 15. Department of Fisheries, Thailand, and ICLARM, Manila, Philippines, pp. 525–530.

Watanabe, W.O., Wicklund, R.I., Olla, B.L., 1993. Saltwater culture of Florida red tilapia: a summary of research at the Caribbean marine research Centre (1985-1991). Proceedings of the First International Symposium on Aquaculture: Technology and Investment Opportunities. Ministry of Agriculture and Water, Riyadh, Saudi Arabia, pp. 49–68.

Whitefield, A.K., Blaber, S.J.M., 1976. The effects of temperature and salinity on *Tilapia rendalli* Boulenger 1896. Journal of Fish Biology 9, 99–104.

Whitefield, A.K., Blaber, S.J.M., 1979. The distribution of the freshwater cichlid *Sarotherodon mossambicus* in estuarine systems. Environmental Biology of Fishes 4, 77–81.

Wilkie, M.P., Wood, C.M., 1996. The adaptations of fish to extremely alkaline environments. Comparative Biochemistry and Physiology 113B, 665–673.

Withyachumnarnkul, B., Palang, I., Reungsri, J., Sirithammajak, S., Jitrakorn, S., Kiatpathomchai, W., et al., 2017. Nile tilapia reared under full-strength seawater: hemato-immunological changes and susceptibility to pathogens. Aquaculture 480, 42–50.

Wokoma, K., Marioghae, I.E., 1996. Survival of *Tilapia guineensis* under conditions of low dissolved oxygen and low pH. In: Pullin, R.S.V., Lazard, J., Legendre, M., Amon Kottias, J.B., Pauly, D. (Eds.), Proceedings of the Third International Symposium on Tilapia in Aquaculture. ICLARM Conference Proceedings No. 41, Penang, Malaysia, pp. 442–448.

Xie, S., Zheng, K., Chen, J., Zhang, Z., Zhu, X., Yang, Y., 2011. Effect of water temperature on energy budget of Nile tilapia, *Oreochromis niloticus*. Aquaculture Nutrition 17, e683–e690.

Xu, Z., Li, E., Xu, C., Gan, L., Qin, J.G., Chen, L., 2016. Response of AMP-activated protein kinase and energy metabolism to acute nitrite exposure in the Nile tilapia *Oreochromis niloticus*. Aquatic Toxicology 177, 86–97.

Yada, T., Ito, F., 1997. Difference in tolerance to acidic environments between two species of tilapia, *Oreochromis niloticus* and

O. mossambicus. Bulletin of the National Research Institute of Fisheries Science 9, 11–18.

Yanbo, W., Wenju, Z., Weifen, L., Zirong, X., 2006. Acute toxicity of nitrite on tilapia (*Oreochromis niloticus*) at different external chloride concentrations. Fish Physiology and Biochemistry 32, 49–54.

Yashouv, A., 1960. Effect of low temperatures on *Tilapia nilotica* and *Tilapia galilaea*. Bamidgeh 12, 62–66.

Yi, Y., Lin, C.K., Diana, J.S., 2003. Hybrid catfish (*Clarias macrocephalus x C. gariepinus*) and Nile tilapia (*Oreochromis niloticus*) culture in an integrated pen-cum-pond system: growth performance and nutrient budget. Aquaculture 217, 395–408.

Yildiz, H.Y., Köksal, G., Borazan, G., Benli, Ç.K., 2006. Nitrite-induced methemoglobinemia in nile tilapia, *Oreochromis niloticus*. Journal of Applied Ichthyology 22, 427–429.

Zerai, D.B., Fitzsimmons, K.M., Collier, R.J., 2010. Transcriptional response of delta-9-desaturase gene to acute and chronic cold stress in Nile tilapia, *Oreochromis niloticus*. Journal of the World Aquaculture Society 41, 800–806.

Zhao, Y., Wang, J., Thammaratsuntorn, J., Wu, J.W., Wei, J.H., Wang, Y., et al., 2015. Comparative transcriptome analysis of Nile tilapia (*Oreochromis niloticus*) in response to alkalinity stress. Genetics and Molecular Research 14, 17916–17926.

Chapter 5

Semi-intensive culture

Chapter outline

5.1 Introduction

The world has been facing a continuous increase in human population, together with decreasing per capita food supply and increasing the cost of food/feed sources. Therefore, the search for more efficient food production systems has become a must (Diana, 2012). Semi-intensive fish culture (SIC) has been widely adopted as a simple and cheap method of fish production. SIC system is simply the production of fish, and other aquatic animals, using natural food, through pond fertilization, or fertilization and supplemental feeding. In other words, SIC is a means of producing low-cost fish, through low production inputs, that contribute to hunger alleviation and food security, especially in rural areas in developing countries. It is no surprise, therefore, that SIC systems are adopted mainly in herbivorous and omnivorous fishes that feed low down in the food chain, such as tilapias and carps. The production of SIC systems is usually lower than of intensive systems due to the lower stocking density and production inputs. Keeping into account the input/output (cost–benefit) ratio, this system could become more convenient and cost-effective for small-scale farmers than intensive farming systems.

Semi-intensive farming of tilapia has been practiced for many years in different parts of the world, particularly in Southeast Asia, either in monoculture or polyculture systems. Over the past three decades, SIC of tilapia with other herbivorous fishes such as carps has witnessed increased popularity in several countries in the world, particularly among small-scale farmers in Asia, Africa and Latin America. This chapter discusses the different aspects of SIC of tilapia, including pond fertilization, monoculture, polyculture and integrated culture under different culture and environmental conditions.

5.2 An overview of pond fertilization

The main objective of pond fertilization is to stimulate the primary productivity in fish ponds, enhance autotrophic and heterotrophic food production and improve water quality as well. Increased primary productivity generally stimulates secondary production in fish ponds, increasing trophic levels and food abundance. Although several nutrients can become limiting in fish ponds, nitrogen (N), phosphorus (P) and carbon (C) are the most common inputs in pond fertilization, and the ratio between them is also of prime

Tilapia Culture. https://doi.org/10.1016/B978-0-12-816541-6.00005-2
Copyright © 2020 Elsevier Inc. All rights reserved.

importance. Potassium (K) is generally not considered as fertilizer element, since earlier studies revealed that K fertilization did not affect pond production (Hickling, 1962). However, K may be required if K content and alkalinity of culture water are low. In high alkalinity ponds, nitrogen and phosphorus must be added to stimulate productivity, and the ratio of these nutrients depends on local conditions, such as water and soil chemistry. The average nutrient composition of phytoplankton in fish ponds ranges from 45% to 50% C, 8%–10% N and 1% P, giving a ratio of about 50:10:1 (Edwards et al., 2000). Efficient fertilization requires a number of measures that should be taken into account. These are the following:

- Availability of considerable amounts of carbon.
- Alkalinity should be >20 mg L^{-1} (Boyd, 1974). If the water is relatively soft, acidic, with low alkalinity (<20 mg L^{-1}), liming may be necessary to raise alkalinity before the application of inorganic fertilizer.
- Fertilization history of the pond. Understanding fertilization history, water quality, bottom composition and overall pond dynamics is extremely important for efficient and sustainable fertilization. For example, available P in fish ponds is rapidly removed by reaction with divalent cations such as Fe^{2+}, Ca^{2+} and Mg^{2+}, forming inactive precipitation. Pond bottom mud also adsorbs P and leads to its removal from culture water. The more mud the bottom contains, the more P it adsorbs (Shrestha and Lin, 1996a, 1996b). Therefore, P requirement for pond fertilization depends on the type of bottom soils and their P saturation (Knud-Hansen, 1992). It has been reported that maximum N and P fertilization rates of ponds in acid sulphate soil with high P binding capacity were 4 and 2 kg ha^{-1} d^{-1}, respectively (Asian Institute of Technology (AIT), unpublished data, cited in Yakupitiyage (1995). Further increase in N loading may lead to ammonia toxicity. There was a negative relationship between the ability of pond sediments to remove soluble P from water and organic matter and P contents of pond bottoms (Knud-Hansen, 1992).
- Season of the year has also a significant effect on fertilization effectiveness of fish ponds. Green et al. (1990) found that the production of Nile tilapia in ponds fertilized with chicken manure in Panama was better in dry seasons than in rainy seasons. Similarly, the production of blue tilapia (*Oreochromis aureus*) in ponds fertilized with chicken manure in addition to 0–20–0 inorganic fertilizer was 48% less in wet season than in dry season (Ledgerwood et al., 1978). Low production during rainy season was attributed to the increased turbidity resulting from bank erosion following heavy rains, which reduces light penetration and decreases photosynthesis process.
- Cost-efficiency analysis. Fertilization strategies are often evaluated based on their ability to enhance fish growth and pond yield. Nevertheless, fertilization regime that produces the best yield may not necessarily be the most cost-effective. It is therefore essential that the farmers understand the dynamic processes in the ponds, and how fertilization efficiency is affected by light penetration, pond depth, bottom soil composition and nutrient contents of the water. Economic and ecological analyses of fertilization application are also appreciated, so that the farmer can choose the best fertilization strategy (more discussion on the economic consideration is provided in Section 5.7).

5.3 Fertilization of tilapia ponds

5.3.1 Organic fertilizers

An organic fertilizer is a fertilizer that is derived from organic sources, including organic compost, cattle manures, poultry droppings and domestic sewage. Organic fertilizers have been widely used in tilapia ponds, especially in Asia (Edwards et al., 1994a, 1994b; Shevgoor et al., 1994; Diana, 2012), Central America (Green et al., 1990; Watanabe et al., 2002) and Africa (Njoku and Ejiogu, 1999; Abdelghany and Ahmad, 2002; Mataka and Kang'ombe, 2007; Longwe et al., 2010; El-Sayed, 2013a, 2013b). A wide variety of organic fertilizers, including poultry manure, cattle manure, domestic sewage (sludge), green manure and composted agricultural wastes, are currently in use in tilapia pond fertilization.

Organic manures enhance secondary production in fish ponds more than inorganic fertilizers. This is mainly because the organic matters in these manures stimulate heterotrophic bacteria, and, in turn, enhance the decomposition of organic matters in the pond (Diana et al., 1994; Diana, 2012). Diana (2012) suggested that animal manures should be used for the basic productivity, while nitrogen or phosphorus can be added as needed to gain nutrient balance in the pond. This approach is very appropriate due to its ecological efficiency and cost-effectiveness. However, this scenario may not be easily applied in some countries. For example, current certification rules and best practices consider animal manures as potential problems to human health (Boyd, 2003).

The effectiveness of fertilization depends on type and composition of fertilizer (Table 5.1), culture systems (monoculture vs. polyculture), fish species and species combinations, stocking size and density and environmental conditions. Nutrient contents in soil and water (particularly P and N), local climate, weather patterns and rainfall also influence pond conditions and productivity, and in turn, affect fish production from fertilization regimes (Diana, 2012). The density of higher aquatic plants and large

TABLE 5.1 Feed and fertilization strategies suggested for optimum yield of tilapia in semi-intensive culture systems (*O. n* = *Oreochromis niloticus*).

Cultured fish								
Species (country)	Size (g)	Density ha^{-1}	Fertilization regime	Feeding	Culture Period (days)	Yield (t ha^{-1})	Remarks	References
O. n (Honduras)		10,000	Chicken manure, 1000 kg ha^{-1}/wk		152	1.76	During rainy season.	Green et al. (1990)
O. n (Honduras)		10,000	Chicken manure, 1000 kg ha^{-1}/wk		150	1.71	During dry season.	Green et al. (1990)
O. n (Panama)		10,000	Chicken manure, 1000 kg ha^{-1}/wk		149	2.07	During dry season.	Green et al. (1990)
O. n (Panama)		10,000	Chicken manure, 1000 kg ha^{-1}/wk		141	1.68	During rainy season.	Green et al. (1990)
O. n (The Philippines)		20,000	Chicken manure, 500 kg ha^{-1}/wk	23% cp diet, 1.5% bw d^{-1}	151	4.35	Based on cost–benefit analysis.	Green (1992)
O. n (Cameroon)	202–222	7600	Cattle manure, daily, 226 kg dry wt. ha^{-1}/day	CSC: 3% bw d^{-1} 6% bw d^{-1}	100	4.80 yr^{-1} 6.50 yr^{-1}	Polyculture with *Clarias gariepinus* (1100 fish ha^{-1}) as Police-fish.	Middendorp (1995)
♂ *O. n* (Thailand)	15	20,000	280 kg chicken manure + 56.3 kg urea + 17.5 TSP ha^{-1}/wk		234	4.0–4.2	2.5-m deep ponds, no water addition. Weekly fertilization produced best growth.	Diana and Lin (1998)
♂ *O. n* (Philippines)	0.05	40,000	AP (28 kg N + 5.6 kg P) ha^{-1}/wk	28.6% cp diet: - 100% satiation - 67% satiation	120	3.14 3.58	Survival 57%. Survival 65%.	Brown et al. (2002)
♂ *O. n* (Kenya)	16.9	1000	DAP + urea, 20 kg ha^{-1} N wk^{-1}		147	2.95	During cool season (22.5–26.4 °C).	Veverica et al. (2001)
♂*O. n* (Egypt)	1–3	20,000	Chicken manure, 1000 kg ha^{-1}/wk, for 60 days	30% cp diet, 3% bw d^{-1}, starts day 60.	145	7.40 yr^{-1}	African catfish (59 g) were used for seed control.	Green et al. (2002)
			54.4 kg urea +92.4 kg SP ha^{-1}/wk	No feeding	145	3.20 yr^{-1}	Same regime.	
Nile tilapia	13.8	30,000	750 kg chicken litter ha^{-1}, biweekly application, 100 kg TP and 20 kg urea ha^{-1}	25% cp diet, 3% bw d^{-1}, 6 wks after stocking	133	4.75	Feeding at 6-wk delay was comparable to no delay, and better than at 13-wk delay.	Abdelghany et al. (2002)
Silver carp	1.9							
Common carp (Egypt)	10.7							
Red tilapia (Thailand)	33	62.5 m^{-3}	Urea + TSP; 4 kg N + 2.18 kg P ha^{-1}/day	Commercial diet, 0%–100% satiation	90	13.5 kg m^{-3}	Cages in fertilized ponds, 50% satiation was economically best.	Yi et al. (2004a)

Continued

TABLE 5.1 Feed and fertilization strategies suggested for optimum yield of tilapia in semi-intensive culture systems (*O. n* = *Oreochromis niloticus*).—cont'd

Cultured fish								
Species (country)	Size (g)	Density ha^{-1}	Fertilization regime	Feeding	Culture Period (days)	Yield (t ha^{-1})	Remarks	References
♂ *O. n* (Thailand)	23–24	30,000	Urea + TSP; 28 kg N + 7 kg P ha^{-1}/wk, N:*P* = 4:1	30% cp diet: • Fertilization + feeding at d 80 • Fertilization until d 80, followed by feeding.	160	16.7 yr^{-1} 13.0 yr^{-1}	Fertilization plus feeding was better than fertilization followed by feeding.	Thankur et al. (2004)
♂ *O. niloticus* (Kenya)	21	20,000	Urea (20 kg N ha^{-1}) and DAP (8 kg P ha^{-1}) weekly	Wheat bran, local diets, pig diets; twice per day, 2% bw d^{-1}	258	6.2–7.7 yr^{-1}	*C. gariepinus* (1000 fish ha) used as police-fish; formulated feed was best; wheat bran was most economic; FCR: 2.6–3.0	Liti et al. (2005)
♂ *O. niloticus* (Kenya)	14	19,462	Urea (20 kg N ha^{-1}), DAP (8 kg P ha^{-1}) weekly	Rice bran, wheat bran, maize bran	250	6.2–7.7	*C. gariepinus* (250 fish ha^{-1}); maize bran produced highest yield; wheat bran was most cost-effective.	Liti et al. (2006)
O. n (85%)	0.3	30,000 –50,000	Chicken litter (550 kg ha^{-1}/week) or MSP (72.5 kg ha^{-1}/week) and urea (45 kg ha^{-1}/week)	25% cp floating pellets, twice a day, to satiation, 60 days after stocking	190	4.9–8.6	With equal nutrient inputs and stocking densities, manure-fertilized ponds could perform equally well as pellet-fed ponds.	El-Naggar et al. (2008)
Catfish (15%)	132							
300 silver carp (Egypt)	100							
Nile tilapia	5.0	35,000	Weekly; compost at 300 kg ha^{-1}; cattle manure at 425 kg ha^{-1}; chicken litter at 425 kg ha^{-1} or 5 kg urea +20 kg TSP ha^{-1}	Supplemental feed (25% cp) was added to all treatments at 5% bw d^{-1}	150	4.75		Ahmed and Hassan (2011)
Silver carp	5.0	5000						
Mullet (Egypt)	5.0	10,000						
Nile tilapia	10	24,000	Weekly, poultry manure at 500 kg ha^{-1}	Supplemental feed (25% cp) was added (ad libitum)	180	7.2	African catfish (100 g) were used for controlling over-population of tilapia.	El-Sayed, personal survey (2013)
Thinlip mullet (Egypt)	40	5200						
O. n (Nepal)	6.2	10,000	Weekly, DAP and organic manure or urea at 4 kg N ha^{-1} and 1 kg P ha^{-1}	**1** Feed only (25%–30% cp) at 3% bw d^{-1} **2** Fertilization + feeding **3** Fertilization + feeding at 1.5% bw d^{-1}	120 –150	1.5–4.3	The best growth, yield and profitability were achieved by fertilization with feeding at 1.5% bw d^{-1}	Manyala et al. (2015)
O. n (Thailand)	95	30,000	Weekly, 0–7 kg TSP (46% P_2O_5) + 28 kg N (urea) ha^{-1}	Floating feed (30% cp), 50% ad libitum	130	9.6–10.6	About 1.75 kg P and 28 kg N per week were best in terms of economic return and nutrient loss.	Oo et al. (2015)

AP, ammonium phosphate; *SP*, superphosphate; *TSP*, triple superphosphate; *DAP*, diammonium phosphate; *MSP*, mono superphosphate; *bw*, body weight.

filamentous algae should also be fully considered since they may compete with phytoplankton for nutrients. Therefore, fertilization of ponds infested with higher plants may reduce the development of phytoplankton blooms. In this regard, water depth in tilapia ponds should be more than 1 metre in order to limit light penetration and macrophyte growth (Boyd et al., 2016).

Water quality, particularly alkalinity and ammonia concentration, should be considered when applying organic fertilization in tilapia ponds. McGeachin and Stickney (1982) found that 70–140 kg ha^{-1} dry, laying hen manure produced the best growth and survival of *O. aureus* reared in simulated sewage lagoons, depending on water alkalinity. About 70 kg ha^{-1} per day was suggested at high alkalinity, while 140 kg ha^{-1} per day produced the best yield at low alkalinity. The levels of unionized ammonia also increased with increasing manuring rate, due to the increase in water alkalinity. Significant amount of this ammonia is also lost from pond water through volatilization to the atmosphere at high alkalinity (>8.5).

Organic fertilization should also be applied at proper rates because insufficient fertilizer will result in low yield, while excessive fertilization may lead to significant deterioration in water quality, dissolved oxygen (DO) deficiency, and in turn will result in a reduction in fish yield. Massive mortality of Nile tilapia has been reported in a number of farms at Kafr El-Shaikh Governorate in Egypt, due to excessive application of organic fertilizer (El-Sayed, Alexandria, 2004; personal communication). Anuta (1995) found that the best yield of *Tilapia guineensis* reared in tanks fertilized with 0, 100 and 150 kg chicken manure ha^{-1} per day was achieved at 100 kg ha^{-1}/day. The NH_4-N, NO_3 and chemical oxygen demand (COD) were all increased with increasing fertilization rates. Organic manure stimulates food production by adding organic detritus that stimulates heterotrophic food chains and increase primary productivity. Produced phytoplankton provides oxygen for respiration of aerobic organisms present in the pond.

Fresh manure may be preferred to dry manure for pond fertilization. Hepher and Pruginin (1982) suggested that fresh manure be used for tilapia pond fertilization and stated that fresh manure disintegrates in water into colloidal particles which are easily attacked by bacteria and readily incorporated into food web. Some semi-intensive tilapia farmers in Egypt pile the dry animal manure on farm dikes and spray it with water for few days, before washing it into the ponds (El-Sayed, Alexandria, 1998; personal communication). This process increases fermentation rate and reduces the time needed for achieving maximal primary production in the ponds, compared with dry manure. However, fermentation may reduce nitrogen content of the manure and in turn would reduce its potential effectiveness.

Animal manures are also better applied in tilapia ponds in fine particulate or colloidal state. Small-sized particles stimulate the growth of bacteria by providing enough surface areas for the attachment and mineralization, where minerals are used for photosynthesis and phytoplankton production. In this regard, buffalo manure has not been recommended as a major organic fertilizer in tilapia ponds, as it causes a reduction in DO, due to the respiratory demand of the bacteria (Edwards et al., 1994b). The presence of tannin in buffalo manure stains pond water brown, which reduces light penetration and in turn inhibits phytoplankton productivity. Buffalo manure is also characterized by large-size particles, high C:N ratio (about 26:1) and poor soluble nutrients. Shevgoor et al. (1994) reported that only 6% of buffalo manure nitrogen was released as dissolved nitrogen and 35% of total P was released as soluble reactive P. Fertilization rate higher than 100 kg dry matter (DM) ha^{-1} per day caused water quality deterioration, high suspended solids and reduced light penetration and phytoplankton production. Under such conditions, DO declined to near 0 at dawn. Therefore, buffalo manure rate should not exceed 50 kg ha^{-1} per day (Edwards et al., 1994a). It is also recommended that buffalo manure be supplemented with urea (Edwards et al., 1996).

On the other hand, poultry manure is a better source of manure in tilapia ponds than that of large ruminants as it has a higher N (and P) content. Indeed, poultry manure is widely used for tilapia pond fertilization, and the main reasons are it is readily available from feedlots and in a convenient dry form for transportation and application. It is also characterized by small-size particles and better C:N ratio (about 10:1) and also by its solubility in water. Generally speaking, a fertilizing rate of <100 kg ha^{-1} d^{-1} of poultry manure increases phytoplankton productivity and improves fish production (see Table 5.1). However, controversial results have been reported on the use of poultry manure for tilapia pond fertilization.

Hopkins and Cruz (1982) reported that the yield of Nile tilapia reared in polyculture with common carp and snakehead murrel *Channa striata* or *Clarias batrachus* in the Philippines was better with pig manure or chicken manure than with duck manure. Green et al. (1989) compared the effects of chicken manure, dairy cow manure and inorganic fertilizer on the production of male Nile tilapia. They found that chicken litter produced the best net fish production (see details in Table 5.1). Similar results have also been reported by Green et al. (1990, 2002); Green (1992). These authors referred better tilapia growth and yields in pond fertilized with organic fertilizer (poultry manure), compared to inorganically fertilized ponds, to increased heterotrophic production and/or direct consumption of organic manure by the fish. Moreover, it has been suggested that diel oxygen stratification is more pronounced in inorganically fertilized ponds, presumably due to the greater water clarity and the more even distribution of primary production in organically fertilized ponds (Diana et al., 1991).

In contrast, Ledgerwood et al. (1978) found that chicken manure was not a very effective fertilizer in blue tilapia ponds in El-Salvador, and the addition of inorganic P (but not N) increased fish yields. Knud-Hansen et al. (1993) found that the addition of urea and triple superphosphate (TSP) into Nile tilapia ponds increased N and P inputs in the ponds and improved primary productivity, while the addition of chicken manure to these inorganic fertilizers did not enhance fish yield. The effectiveness of chicken manure-P was only 10% of TSP-P. Economic analyses of that study discouraged the use of chicken manure as a source of N and P in tilapia ponds in Thailand.

It appears from these discrepancies concerning pond fertilization that this subject is more complex, confusing and wider than we could imagine. Indeed, the types and quantities of nutrients required and the relative amounts of fertilizers needed to provide such nutrients are varying, depending on the type of fertilizer used, nutrient contents of the water, types of bottom soil, water quality, environmental climatic conditions and geographical location. This means that the effectiveness of certain fertilizer is probably site-specific, and fertilizer requirements should be evaluated on a farm-by-farm basis, and even on a pond-by-pond basis.

It has been assumed that supplemental and complete processed feeds are better-quality inputs than organic fertilizers in semi-intensive fish ponds. This assumption was tested by Muendo et al. (2006) who explored the trophic structure in organically fertilized and feed-supplied Nile tilapia ponds using multivariate analyses. The fish (18 g) were fed 25% crude protein (cp) floating pellets, fertilized with chicken manure or with partially composted field grass. Average tilapia weights at harvest were much higher in chicken manure-fertilized ponds (252 g) than in pellet-fed (174 g) and grass-fertilized (172 g) ponds, while the net yield was higher in pellet-fed ponds, due to their higher stocking density. The authors concluded that organically fertilized ponds can perform equally well as pellet-driven ponds, or even better.

5.3.2 Inorganic fertilizers

As stated earlier, N, P and C are the most important nutrients required for optimum pond management and fish production in semi-intensive systems. Not only is that, but the ratios between them are also important. Boyd (1976) studied the effects of N and N:P:K ratios in blue tilapia ponds fertilized with 22.5 kg ha^{-1} of 0–20–5, 5–20–5 and 20–20–5 (N–P–K). He found that the best fish yield was obtained at 5–20–5 kg ha^{-1}. Excessive nitrogen fertilization is not recommended, as it may lead to waste of resources without improving fish yields. Veverica et al. (2001) fertilized sex-reversed Nile tilapia ponds with diammonium phosphate (DAP) during cool and warm seasons in Kenya for 147 and 133 days. Triple phosphate and sodium carbonate were also applied to the ponds to maintain sufficient P and C levels. The authors found that increasing N levels beyond 20 kg ha^{-1} wk^{-1} did not improve tilapia yield. Gross profit was also higher at 20 kg ha^{-1}per week than at 30 kg ha^{-1} per week during both cold and warm seasons. Meanwhile, optimal fertilization rate in tilapia ponds in Thailand was reported to be about 28 kg N ha^{-1} per week at a N:P ratio of 4:1 by weight (Knud-Hansen et al., 1993).

In conclusion, about 4 kg of N and 1–2 kg of P ha^{-1} per day is required to maintain a green pond optimum plankton productivity. However, farmers should be careful when calculating amounts of fertilizer to add, keeping in mind that urea (46–0–0) is actually 46% N, whilst TSP (0–46–0) is 46% P_2O_5 and only 20% P. Table 5.2, which contains a list of the major inorganic fertilizers commonly used in tilapia culture, can be used as a guideline for the application of inorganic fertilizers.

Alkalinity and pH of pond water have a significant effect on the efficiency of applied fertilizer. Pond fertilization is more effective in high alkalinity water (>40 mg L^{-1}) than in waters of lower alkalinity (Boyd et al., 2016). Thus, low alkalinity water should be limed before pond fertilization in order to increase alkalinity and bottom pH, and improve the efficiency of nutrient absorption. In alkaline environment (soil pH of 7–8), phosphate becomes more available to the water column. On the other hand, urea and ammonium-containing fertilizers are acid-forming, causing alkalinity to decline.

The frequency of fertilization may, or may not, affect the production of tilapia in fertilized ponds. Knud-Hansen and Batterson (1994) investigated the most efficient frequency of urea and TSP application on phytoplankton productivity in Nile tilapia ponds. The ponds were fertilized daily, twice a week, weekly, twice every 3 weeks or once every 2 weeks, for 5 months. No relationship was found between the frequency of fertilization and either phytoplankton production or fish yields. However, primary productivity and fish yield were linearly correlated. Light availability, nutrients and temperature were the main factors affecting primary productivity. The highest productivity was achieved in water with low turbidity and relatively high alkalinity. This means that nutrient uptake by phytoplankton decreases as inorganic turbidity increases, due to low light penetration. Thus, frequency of application should be adjusted according to phytoplankton abundance and water 'greenness'. When the water is rich in phytoplankton, pond fertilization may be delayed.

Tilapia farmers should consider the following remarks for efficient pond fertilization and optimum performance:

TABLE 5.2 List of the major inorganic fertilizers commonly used in tilapia culture (% of pure salt).

Fertilizer	Formula	Common name	N	P	K
Nitrogenous fertilizers					
Urea	$CO(NH_2)_2$	Carbamide	46.7	0	0
Sodium nitrate	$(NaNO_3)$	Chile saltpetre	16.5	0	0
Ammonium nitrate	NH_4NO_3	Nitrate of ammonia	35.0	0	0
Ammonium sulphate	$(NH_4)_2SO_4$	–	21.2	0	0
Ammonium phosphate, monobasic	$NH_4H_2PO_4$	MAP	12.2	27.0	0
Ammonium phosphate, dibasic	$(NH_4)_2HPO_4$	DAP	21.2	23.5	0
Phosphate fertilizers					
Di-calcium phosphate, anhydrous	$CaHPO_4$	Double superphosphate	0	22.8	0
Single superphosphate	$Ca(H_2PO_4)_2 + CaSO_4$	Superphosphate	0	7.0–8.7	0
Triple superphosphate	$Ca(H_2PO_4)_2$	TSP	0	19.2–23.6	0
Bone meal			0	15.0	0
Rock phosphate	$Ca_3(PO_4)_2CaF_2$	Fluroapatite	0	13.0	0
Potassium fertilizers					
Potassium nitrate	KNO_3	Saltpetre	13.8	0	38.7
Potassium chloride	KCl	Muriate of potash	0	0	52.4
Potassium sulphate	K_2SO_4	Glaser's salt (Sulphate of potash)	0	0	44.9

After Tacon (1987).

- Fertilizing ponds on a weekly basis is better than on daily basis.
- Fertilizer requirements will increase as the fish grow towards the critical standing crop (CSC).
- Fertilizer should be used according to the needs of the pond, based on water greenness. Fertilization should be increased if tilapia pond water is getting clear (less green) and decreased or stopped when the pond becomes over green and fish start to die.
- Secchi disk visibility (SDV) is a simple method of measuring the greenness and primary productivity of pond water. A lower SDV ($<$20 cm) indicates eutrophication and means that the water is 'over green', which may cause fish mortality due to low DO in early morning, and high oscillation in water pH.
- The use of supplemental feeds may reduce or even eliminate the need for fertilizer, as feeds also contain the required N and P, especially when the CSC is approached.
- Inorganic fertilizers are better dissolved in water and sprayed on water surface, or suspended in bags near the water intake or paddle wheels.
- Organic fertilizers are generally cheaper than inorganic fertilizers and keep the water much greener for longer time, but they may cause DO depletion in early morning.
- Organic fertilizers are better applied more regularly and distributed in small amounts at many spots in the pond.
- Chicken manure is rich in P and can be cheaper when used in combination with urea.
- Pond water should not be exchanged unless there is a problem with water quality (e.g. eutrophication, sharp oscillation in oxygen and pH); otherwise fertilizer will be lost from the pond, causing economic loss.
- Organic fertilizers must not be used in nursery ponds with hapas because it will increase mortality, and the water will cause skin irritation to labourers working in the pond.
- During rainy season and cloudy weather, primary productivity of fertilized ponds may decrease due to the lack or shortage of sunlight. In this case, farmers should not add too much fertilizer because when the sun comes out, the pond may become over green, leading to eutrophication and causing fish mortality.
- Inorganic fertilizer may not lead to green water due to another limiting nutrient or inappropriate water hardness or pH. In this case, liming may also be necessary before fertilization if the water is acidic.

5.3.3 Periphyton-based tilapia culture

Periphyton-based pond culture (also known as 'acadja') is a simple and cheap way of producing natural food for herbivorous and omnivorous fishes, such as tilapia and carps. In this culture system, woody branches, bamboo poles or any other hard substrates are planted or fixed in shallow waters such as ponds, lagoons, reservoirs, etc., to allow the growth of sessile autotrophic and heterotrophic aquatic biota known as periphyton (Fig. 5.1). Periphyton community comprises bacteria, fungi, protozoa, phytoplankton, zooplankton, benthic organisms and a wide range of invertebrates (Milstein, 1997; Azim et al., 2001). This system enhances natural productivity, which provides natural food for herbivorous and omnivorous fishes. Maximum periphyton biomass colonization in the pond occurs within 15–30 days after substrates installation (Richard et al., 2009). Herbivorous fishes such as tilapia and carps have been reported to graze efficiently on periphyton communities in fish ponds, leading to significant enhancement of fish production and reduction of production costs (Wahab et al., 1999a, 1999b).

Several trials have been carried out during the past two decades on raising fish and crustaceans in periphyton-based pond systems, with promising results. Species studied included tilapias (Hem and Avit, 1994; Huchette et al., 2000; Huchette and Beveridge, 2003; Haque et al., 2016), carps (Wahab et al., 1999a, 1999b; Azim et al., 2002; Azim and Wahab., 2005; Keshavanath and Gangadhar., 2005), mullet (*Liza aurata*) (Richard et al., 2010) and freshwater prawn (*Macrobrachium rosenbergii*) (Tidwell et al., 2000; van Dam et al., 2002; Tidwell and Bratvold, 2005; Uddin et al., 2006). Polyculture of freshwater prawn with tilapia has also been studied (Keshavanath et al., 2004; Uddin et al., 2007a, 2009). These studies indicated that periphyton can be used as a natural food source in fish ponds, depending on fish species, size, stocking density, culture systems and periphyton substrates. Economic analyses of these research studies revealed that this practice can be highly profitable.

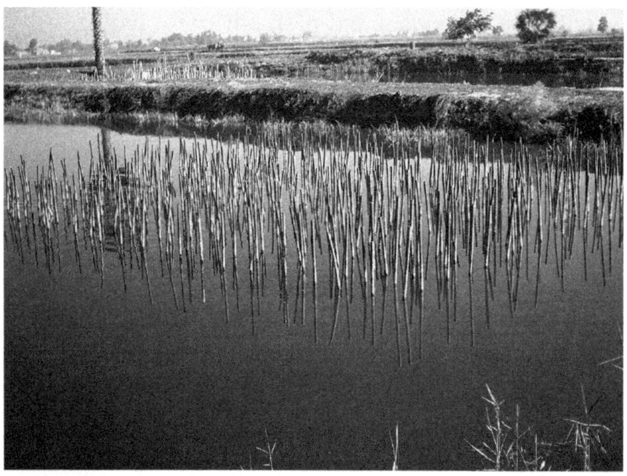

FIGURE 5.1 Periphyton-based tilapia culture. *Photograph by A.-F. El-Sayed.*

It has been reported that 10 bamboo poles m^{-2} increased fish yield 20%–100%. The quantity and quality of periphyton produced varied with substrate type, grazing pressure and fertilization level. Azim et al. (2001) found that bamboo poles produced more and better periphyton than jute sticks and branches of hizol tree.

Manipulation of the carbon:nitrogen (C/N) ratio is necessary for the optimization and enhancement of pond productivity and increasing the nutrient use efficiency in periphyton-controlled pond aquaculture. A C/N ratio of 20:1 has been suggested for best nutrient utilization efficiency, with maize flour being a cheap, locally available and effective source of carbon (Asaduzzaman et al., 2010; Haque et al., 2015). The combined effects of C/N and controlled periphyton (CP)-based polyculture systems (known as C/N-CP) have been evaluated by a number of authors (Asaduzzaman et al., 2008, 2009; 2010; Haque et al., 2015). When C/N balance was achieved in the presence of periphyton substrate, fish and shrimp growth rates, net yields and profitability were all improved.

Periphyton can also partially or totally replace supplemental feed in fish ponds. Studies on hybrid tilapia (Milstein, 1997; Keshavanath et al., 2004; Milstein et al., 2005, 2009) and Nile tilapia (Uddin et al., 2007a, 2009) indicated that periphyton can replace or complement supplemental feeding in tilapia culture in earthen ponds, without reducing fish yield, but with substantial reduction in production costs. Similarly, substantial improvement in growth rates of hybrid red tilapia (*Oreochromis mossambicus* × *Oreochromis niloticus*) fry was achieved in a periphyton-based system compared to substrate-free tanks (Keshavanath et al., 2004). In addition, Milstein and Lev (2004) found that blue tilapia reared on natural periphyton showed similar growth, survival and yield to fish fed on pelleted diets. However, periphyton-based system resulted in considerable reduction in production costs. Thus, periphyton-based aquaculture can be an excellent alternative to reduce the costs of production inputs and allow an economically profitable tilapia production, particularly in rural, resource-limited regions in developing countries.

Periphyton-based cage culture of tilapia has also been considered by a number of authors (Norberg, 1999; Huchette et al., 2000; Huchette and Beveridge, 2003). These studies indicated that this system could be profitable if proper species and sizes, stoking densities, cage design, substrate materials, supplemental feeding and management techniques are adopted. However, the viability of this system, according to these studies, was not certain. On the other hand, recent studies indicated that periphyton-based cage system could be highly viable and cost-effective. Sakr et al. (2015) evaluated periphyton as a natural food source of fingerling Nile tilapia (2.37 g) fed reduced dietary protein levels in cages for 70 days. The results revealed that periphyton provided an additional natural food source for caged fish and positively affected growth performance and feed efficiency. In the presence of periphyton, dietary protein could also be reduced from 25% to 15%, without any adverse effects on fish performance. In the meantime, the diet containing the lowest protein level (15%) with periphyton was the most cost-effective. Feed efficiency cost (cost of food consumed kg^{-1} of fish produced) was about 19% less at this diet than at the control, periphyton-free diet.

The potential of periphyton-based cage culture of Nile tilapia (46.6 g) in a hydroelectric reservoir in Brazil was also evaluated at three stocking densities (55, 82 and 110 fish m^{-3} equivalent to 2.5, 3.75 and 5 kg m^{-3}, respectively) and two feeding regimes: 100% of daily ration (control, without periphyton substrate) or 50% of daily ration (in the presence of periphyton) (Garcia et al., 2016). The proposed final biomasses were 40, 60, and 80 kg m^{-3}, respectively. The presence of bamboo, as periphyton substrate, improved fish growth, but the carrying capacity of the cages was reduced at the highest density. Periphyton also improved DO concentration inside the cages between 50 and 140 days of the trial and reduced it after 155 days of culture. These results demonstrated that Nile tilapia can benefit from periphyton in cages until they reach, at least, 500 g. The authors concluded that inclusion of bamboo substrates inside the cages can result in producing up to 52 kg m^{-3} of Nile tilapia using 32% less diet in a period almost 20% shorter than in the control, periphyton-free group. However, if tilapia farmers prefer to produce 80 kg m^{-3}, they can still use 30% less diet, but the production period would be 20% longer.

Alongside the same line, Garcia et al. (2017) evaluated the profitability of adopting periphyton system in Nile tilapia cages, in combination with a restricted diet and reduced stocking densities in Brazil. The fish (46.56 g) were stocked in the cages at three densities to reach final biomasses of 40, 60, and 80 kg m^{-3} and fed either 100% ration (control, without periphyton substrate) or 50% of daily ration, in the presence of periphyton. The inclusion of the bamboo substrates in cages enhanced periphyton production and improved fish growth and feed conversion ratio (FCR) and shortened the farming cycle length. The profitability index of periphyton-based systems was also up to 87% higher than the traditional system which is currently used by Brazilian tilapia farmers.

It is clear from the above discussion that periphyton-based aquaculture can be an appropriate technology to reduce production costs and allow an economically viable tilapia production in monoculture and polyculture systems. This approach can be an ideal alternative in resource-limited regions in Asia, Africa and Latin America, where small-scale, rural tilapia culture is commonly practiced.

5.4 Supplemental feeding

5.4.1 Rationale

Pond fertilization in semi-intensive tilapia culture is often associated with supplemental feeding, especially during the later grow-out stages. The adoption and effectiveness of supplemental feeding in semi-intensive culture depends on economic, social, biological and technical factors. It has been reported that tilapia can rely totally on natural food, produced through fertilization, up to certain size (CSC). Beyond this CSC, fish growth will slow down because natural food would be insufficient to meet their requirement. At this size, supplemental feed becomes necessary to sustain fish growth (Fig. 5.2). Thus, supplemental feeding at smaller fish size will lead to the waste of resources and increase in operating costs unnecessarily. In the meantime, further delay in supplemental feeding will result in a reduction in fish growth and total yield.

Relying on natural food during early stages of SI culture, and delaying feeding with commercial formulated feed or supplemental feed sources to latter stages, has been a common practice for small-scale farmers in many developing countries for decades. Large-scale fish producers usually raise their fish intensively using commercial, high-protein pellets, with low feeding levels, while small-scale farmers use locally available sources at higher rates. Tilapia are produced mainly for local consumption, where their gate prices in most of the developing countries are relatively low. Therefore, the use of high-quality commercial feed is not recommended in small-scale farming systems (Yakupitiyage, 1995). Instead, pond fertilization and supplemental feeding would be more productive and cost-effective.

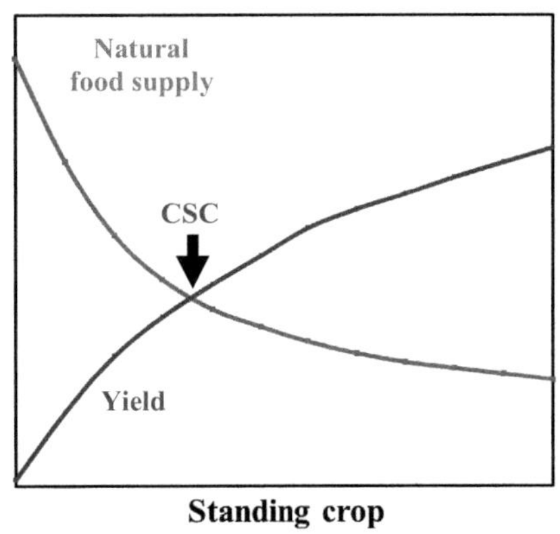

FIGURE 5.2 Changes in natural food in the pond and fish yield, in relation to standing crop of cultured organisms and supplemental feeds. *CSC*, critical standing crop. *Modified from De Silva (1995).*

This assumption was tested by several authors, where different fertilization and supplemental feeding regimes were evaluated in order to develop low-cost tilapia production systems. For example, Diana et al. (1994) evaluated the effects of addition of supplemental feed to fertilized Nile tilapia ponds by adding feed alone, feed plus fertilizer or fertilizer alone. The combination of feed and fertilizer was more efficient in growing tilapia than feeding or fertilizing alone. In a similar study, Green et al. (2002) found that Nile tilapia raised in ponds fertilized with chicken manure at 1000 kg ha^{-1} for the first 60 days, followed by supplemental feed beginning day 61, produced better yield (7.4 t ha^{-1} per year) than feeding only (4.4 t ha^{-1} per year) and fertilizer only (3.7 t ha^{-1} per year).

The effect of fertilization and feeding rates on growth performance, economic returns and water quality in a cage-cum-pond system for production of Nile tilapia was also evaluated by Waidbacher et al. (2006). All-male fish were stocked in cages installed into ponds and in open ponds at 150 fish per cage and 2 fish m^{-2}. Caged fish were fed a 24% protein diet at 3% and 6% bw d^{-1} without pond fertilization and 6% BWD with pond fertilization. The open water treatment was not stocked with fish but contained only caged fish, which were fed 6% bw d^{-1} for the first 57 days followed by 3% bw d^{-1} for the rest of the study. The results indicated that both feeding rate and pond fertilization had a significant effect on fish growth, profitability and water quality. Pond fertilization and feeding at 6% bw d^{-1} resulted in the best fish performance and yield, water quality and economic profits. Manyala et al. (2015) developed a low-cost tilapia production with fertilization and supplementary feeding, in a study carried out in three countries: Nepal, Cambodia and Kenya. The overall objective was to increase profitability, improve the supply of cheap, high-quality animal protein source to local communities with limited food resources and contribute to the overall development of national aquaculture sectors. The following treatments were used to raise Nile tilapia fingerlings (6.2 g) in the three countries: (1) fertilization only with DAP and organic manure or urea at 4 kg ha^{-1} N and 1 kg ha^{-1} P weekly; (2) feed only with 25%–30% cp diets, at a daily feeding rate of 3% of fish body weight; and (3) fertilization and feeding at 1.5% body weight daily. The best tilapia growth, yield and economic profitability were achieved by fertilization with feeding at 50% of the satiation level.

5.4.2 Timing of supplemental feeding

A number of studies have been conducted to investigate the most suitable timing for supplemental feeding in semi-intensive tilapia culture. The most comprehensive study in this regard was conducted by Diana et al. (1996). These authors found that the most efficient system is to grow the fish up to 100–150 g with fertilizers alone. Feeding the fish before they reach this size was wasteful. The authors found also that the best annual revenue was achieved when the fish were fed 50% *ad libitum* once they reached 100 g (Fig. 5.3). In another study, Lin et al. (1997) studied the effects of different fertilizers and feeding regimes on nutrient budget and growth in Nile tilapia ponds in Thailand, in two experiments, each lasted for 160 days. All-male Nile tilapia (23–24 g) were stocked at 3 fish m^{-2} and reared under continuous urea fertilization (60.7 kg ha^{-1} per week + 35.7 kg TSP ha^{-1} per week), while commercial feed (30% cp) was added beginning on day 80. In the other trial, ponds were fertilized until day 80 and followed by feeding commercial feed only. The final weight and net yield were better in the ponds receiving the fertilization throughout the study and feeding on day 80 than the other treatment. Fish harvest removed 15.45%–20.04% N and 10.02%–15.10% P from the total inputs, with no significant difference between the experiments. The major portions of N and P were not accounted for in the estimated losses. These N and P losses ranged between 70.66%–78.01% and 81.88%–87.25%, respectively.

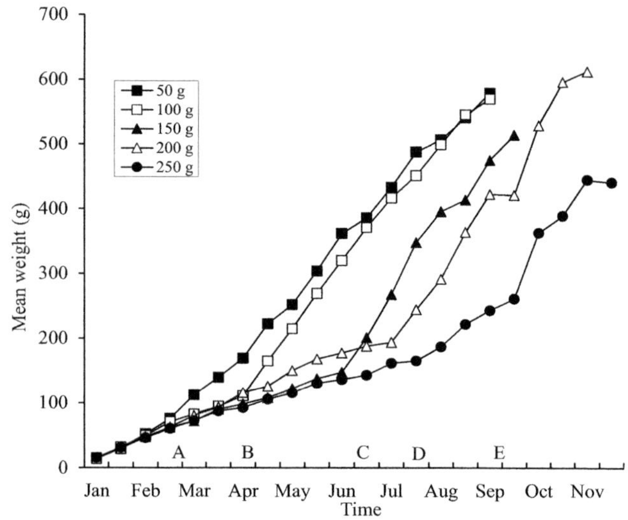

FIGURE 5.3 The effects of timing of supplemental feeding on the weight gain of Nile tilapia fed with pelleted feed at 50% satiation level in fertilized ponds. All ponds were fertilized with inorganic fertilizers at the same optimal rate. Treatments were first feeding at 50 g (■), 100 g (□), 150 g (▲), 200 g (△) and 250 g (●). The letters on the X-axis indicate the dates when supplementary feeding was initiated for each treatment. *From Diana et al. (1996), with permission from the World Aquaculture Society.*

Brown et al. (2000) studied the timing of supplemental feeding of Nile tilapia in fertilized ponds in seven different fish farms in the Philippines. Sex-reversed fish fingerlings (1.1 g) stocked in ponds (at 4 fish m^{-2}) fertilized with ammonia and ammonium phosphate at a weekly rate of 28 and 5.6 kg ha^{-1}. The fish were fed a farm-made diet beginning day 45 or day 75. No significant differences in fish growth and net yield were found between the two feeding timings; however, fish fed at day 45 consumed significantly more food. Abdelghany and Ahmad (2002) studied the effects of timing of supplemental feed on growth and production of Nile tilapia in polyculture with common carp and silver carp in fertilized ponds for 19 weeks. A commercial diet (25% cp) was provided to the fishes at the beginning of the study, after 6 weeks and after 13 weeks, while the control group received no feeding. The authors found that providing the feed after 6 weeks led to better performance and lower feed consumption than the rest of the diet-fed groups. Similarly, El-Naggar et al. (2008) raised Nile tilapia with African catfish and silver carp in a polyculture system in earthen ponds fertilized with chicken manure (550 kg ha^{-1} per week) or mono superphosphate (MSP) (72.5 kg ha^{-1} per week) and urea (45 kg ha^{-1} per week) for 190 days. Supplemental feeding with 25% cp floating pellets started 60 days after stocking. With equal nutrient inputs and stocking densities, manure-fertilized ponds performed equally well as pellet-fed ponds.

It is clear from the foregoing discussion that delaying supplemental feeding in well-fertilized ponds does not reduce fish yield but reduces feed cost significantly. This simply means that small-scale tilapia farmers who adopt semi-intensive farming system must not feed their fish immediately after stocking, but rely on fertilization as far as natural food supports fish growth during the early stages of fish life.

Feeding rates is also another important factor affecting the economic return of tilapia in semi-intensive culture systems. Since natural food is the main food input in the ponds, excessive supplemental feeding may result in a considerable economic loss, in addition to a severe environmental impact. In support, Lin and Yi (2003) found that Nile tilapia reared in fertilized ponds and fed supplemental diets at 50%, 75%, and 100% satiation, produced comparable yields. However, considerable reduction in production costs and in nutrient loading was achieved at the 50% level. This means that at this feeding level, about 50% of the feed can be saved. Similar results were reported with red tilapia fed supplemental feeds in fertilized, brackish water ponds (Yi et al., 2004a). Abdelghany and Ahmad (2002) reported also that the highest production and net income of Nile tilapia polycultured with common carp and silver carp in fertilized ponds and fed 0%, 1%, 3%, 5% biomass and to apparent satiation were achieved at 2.67% of fish biomass day^{-1} (equivalent to apparent satiation). These results clearly demonstrate that an optimal feeding regime will reduce both feed costs and nutrient loading in the ponds.

5.4.3 On-farm feed resources

As mentioned in Chapter 6, intensively farmed tilapia depend exclusively on high-quality, commercial pelleted feeds. These feeds are produced by both small-scale and large-scale feed mills. Therefore, I intentionally did not cover feed formulation and processing in this chapter, since farmers buy their feed from feed mills and need not to worry about feed formulation and manufacturing. On the contrary, farmers who raise tilapia in semi-intensive systems often adopt fertilization and supplemental feed strategies, as discussed earlier. These farmers can produce the supplemental feeds on-farm, using locally available inputs, in order to minimize feed and production costs. It would be appropriate here to provide tilapia farmers with some vital information on farm-made tilapia feeds.

Feed ingredients such as wheat bran, rice bran, cotton seed cake (CSC), etc. (Table 5.3), can be used solely as supplemental feed sources for tilapia in semi-intensive systems. This approach can substantially reduce feed cost and improve fish yields, depending on feed source, feeding rate and fertilization effectiveness. Middendorp (1995) found that the net production of Nile tilapia reared in ponds receiving daily cattle manure and CSC at a daily rate of 3% or 6% of their body weight was significantly high (4.8 and 6.5 t ha^{-1} per year, respectively), while the use of cow manure alone resulted in negative net production. The use of on-farm resources as pond inputs to cultured *Tilapia rendalli* and *Oreochromis shiranus* on smallholder farms in Malawi in monoculture and polyculture systems has also been investigated (Chikafumbwa, 1998). The ponds received daily applications of Napier grass (NP) and maize bran (MB) or isonitrogenous combinations (0.7 kg N ha^{-1} per day) of NP, MB, wood ash and urea for 126 and 112 days. The application of NP/MB produced the best performance.

Most farmed tilapia is produced in resources-limited, rural areas in Africa, Asia and Latin America. At the same time, many households produce tilapia for subsistence using very low inputs. It is necessary therefore that unconventional, locally available and cheap feed sources be used as feed/food inputs for semi-intensive culture of tilapia in earthen ponds. Plant sources and agricultural by-products which are of little or no economic values, such as sugarcane bagasse and water hyacinth, have been successfully incorporated in tilapia feeds (El-Sayed, 2003). The chemical composition of some feed ingredients commonly used for aquafeed manufacturing in Egypt is given in Table 5.3, while Table 5.4 contains a list of some unconventional feed sources which are of potential use for farm-made tilapia feed in Egypt.

Plant materials and agricultural by-products are generally used without processing (or with minimal processing, such as sun drying) because it may not be economic to

TABLE 5.3 Chemical composition (% dry weight, as-fed bases) of feed ingredients of potential use for on-farm feed production for tilapia in Egypt.

Ingredient	Moisture	Crude protein	Crude lipids	Crude fibre	NFE	Ash
Plant sources						
Corn plant	78.72	1.45	0.54	4.41	12.73	2.15
Sweet corn (first cut)	92.51	0.64	0.15	2.13	3.83	0.75
Sweet corn (second cut)	76.95	1.87	0.61	5.48	12.65	2.44
Sugarcane leaves	71.13	1.32	0.24	7.66	15.54	4.11
White corn	10.33	9.14	4.82	7.21	67.10	1.40
Yellow corn	7.90	8.30	2.90	2.11	82.50	2.10
Sorghum	11.00	9.16	4.22	2.93	82.71	1.20
Barely	13.20	10.11	1.60	8.20	77.11	3.00
Kidney beans	9.75	27.97	0.95	5.65	50.71	5.51
Agricultural products						
Soybean meal	13.55	45.45	16.92	7.67	24.62	5.51
Cottonseed meal (with hulls)	7.50	27.10	8.50	21.44	27.2	6.9
Cotton seed meal (no hulls)	7.06	44.41	10.06	5.22	25.73	7.53
Sesame seeds (hulls)	9.00	30.21	14.40	18.09	20.10	17.40
Lentils seed cake	18.51	13.33	10.73	7.08	35.22	7.49
Rice bran	10.63	13.07	12.06	10.32	57.2	7.65
Rice mill run	9.22	11.07	7.81	1.14	75.93	4.21
Coarse wheat bran	12.11	11.09	3.56	17.83	63.78	4.33
Fine wheat bran	12.19	17.05	3.12	9.44	65.51	4.50
Animal sources						
Blood meal	9.33	81.22	1.12	–	–	5.33
Fishmeal (local)	10.3	65.25	10.5	–	–	16.56
Fishmeal (imported)	9.00	70.04	6.11	–	–	11.62
Animal gelatin	11.41	85.69	3.09	–	–	–
Meat and bone meal	4.56	61.82	6.16	–	–	26.00
Poultry by-product meal	13	53.85	23.37	–	–	18.22
Shrimp meal (local)	12.71	51.67	5.55	–	–	26.93

NFE, nitrogen-free extract.
After El-Sayed (1999).

process these sources into the supplemental feed. For example, sugarcane bagasse is essentially carbon, whereas water hyacinth contains very high amounts of water, and therefore, processing them may not be cost-effective to the fish farmers. It should also be emphasized that the quality, sustainable availability, composition and costs of these feed inputs must be determined before the farmer decides whether or not to use them as food inputs. Field trials of these sources are also necessary because a big gap sometimes exists between the results obtained based on laboratory research and these achieved under field practices.

The majority of noncommercial, semi-intensive tilapia farms, particularly in sub-Saharan Africa (SSA) depend mostly on farm-made fish feeds. For example, about 70% of the tilapia feeds used in Nigeria are farm-made, in the form of dry mash, dough balls and meat mincer pellets, fed

TABLE 5.4 Selected unconventional feedstuffs that can be used as feed inputs for semi-intensive culture of tilapia in Egypt.

Feedstuff	Description	Nutritional value/composition (%)	Processing and use
Bakery waste	Includes flour waste, bread rejects, bran	Depends on the source of flour	Fed directly or ground or mixed with other ingredients
Brewers' waste	The residues of sugar and starch extraction from barely. It is relatively rich in fibre and digestible carbohydrates	CP = 15; EE = 8.2; CF = 18.9; ash = 23	Included either wet or dried in the feeds
Poultry manure	Dried poultry excreta collected from poultry farms, usually contain undigested food particles and grains	CP = 7–11; Ca = 4.4–11.7; P = 1.3–3.2	Dried and used directly as a feed ingredient or mineral source at about 5% in the feeds
Buffalo and cow manure	Dried or wet excreta collected from buffaloes farms	CP = 5–9; Ca = 4–13; P = 2.3–3.4	Used fresh or dried as feed ingredient for herbivorous fish
Restaurants wastes and rejects	Plant-and animal-based wastes and rejects rich in carbohydrates and ash	Varying according to the source	Sorted and used directly or dried and grinded
Fruit and vegetable market wastes and rejects	Consist of leaves, roots, stems and rejects of fruits and vegetables collected from auction and whole sale markets	CP = 8–13; CF = 15–20; ash = 22-28	Used fresh, dried or as silage for cattle, poultry or fish
Rice polishing wastes	Rice grains, middling, bran and hulls	Varying according to the source	Thrown directly into fish ponds, or mixed with the feed
Sugarcane bagasse	Residues of sugarcane pressing	>40% digestible carbohydrate, >45 fibre contents	Dried, grinded and incorporated into the feed (at low levels)
Duckweed	Grown naturally in freshwater lakes, canals, reservoirs and drainage	CP 42%	Fed fresh to tilapia and carps
Starch and yeast industry wastes	Residues of starch and yeast industry	CF = 37; NFE = 40	Incorporated in animal feed
Aquatic weeds	Freshwater weeds and macrophytes	Varies according to species and location	Used fresh or dried as feed sources for herbivorous fishes
Water hyacinth	A macrophyte heavily grown in freshwater canals, reservoirs and drainages	CP = 21.1; EE = 1; CF = 19; ash = 18.2; NFE = 40.7	Cut into small pieces and used fresh or dried and included in the feed (at 10%–20%)

CP, crude protein; *EE*, ether extract; *CF*, crude fibre; *Ca*, calcium; *P*, phosphorus.

in moist or sun-dried form (Ayinla, 2007; El-Sayed, 2013a, 2013b). This is mainly because small-scale commercial farmers cannot afford manufactured pelleted feeds, which are usually imported at very high prices. The main protein sources of farm-made feeds in SSA are oilseed cakes (cotton, soybean and sunflower), fishmeal, blood meal, carcass meal, brewer's waste, groundnut cake, palm kernel cake, and poultry by-product meal (El-Sayed, 2013a); whereas energy sources include cereal bran, corn, kitchen waste and vegetables. Farm-made feed formulations vary by country and season, depending on availability and prices of ingredients and the culture system adopted. These formulations range from single feed ingredients such as wheat bran, rice bran or ground corn to formulated mixes, moist feed cakes and processed, dry pellets.

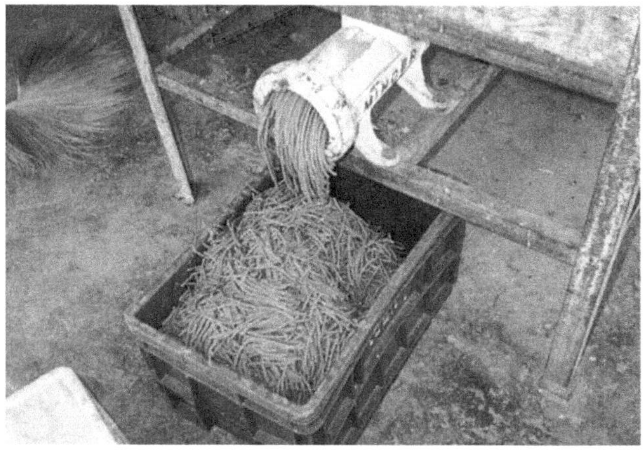

FIGURE 5.4 Extrusion of farm-made tilapia feed in Thailand. *Photo provided by T. Samrit.*

5.4.4 On-farm feed formulation and preparation

In addition to feed ingredients, formulated supplemental feeds are often used to feed tilapia in semi-intensive systems. These feeds must be low in protein, but high in energy contents, since the fish get some of their protein requirement from natural food available in fish ponds. On-farm feed formulation depends on a number of factors, including the following:

1. The fund resources of the farmers to purchase feed ingredients and feed manufacturing equipment, electricity, fuel, etc.
2. Available feed ingredients, sources, composition and costs. This includes seasonal availability, current usage, proximate composition, quality control, digestibility and assimilation, handling and processing costs prior to mixing or pelleting (Tacon, 1995).
3. Intended processes employed, such as sorting, grinding, mixing and pelleting (steam pelleting, cold pelleting, expansion pelleting, flaking, mash, crumple, paste, ball, moist or dry pellets).
4. Production targets, stocking density of fish and natural food availability in fish ponds.

The value chain of farm-made aquafeed is very simple and short. This feed is generally produced using easy and simple techniques, at small quantities and for self-use and not for sale. The feed is processed by grinding raw ingredients and mixing them at certain ratios to make a balanced diet. Mixing is carried out manually or with the use of mechanical mixers. In order to produce their feeds on farm, fish farmers should follow the following steps.

1. Prepare the equipment needed for feed preparation, such as weighing scale, sieves, mixer, 10–20 kg-capacity meat grinder, corn or soybean meal grinder and a steamer (if cooking is intended).
2. Sort the ingredients to assure that they do not contain any spoilt or rotten parts and hard objects such as nails, rubbles, etc.
3. Dry the ingredients separately (sun drying is recommended in tropical and subtropical regions to save energy costs).
4. Mix the ingredients at the predetermined levels.
5. Add water or cooked carbohydrate sources such as starch to make a paste.
6. Use simple meat grinder to extrude the pellets (Fig. 5.4).
7. Dry the pellets (sun drying is recommended in tropical and subtropical regions). After drying the pellets should be broken into appropriate sizes suitable for the developmental stages of farmed fishes.
8. Store the feed in clean, shaded and aerated stores.

The vast majority of fish farms in Africa rely on farm-made feeds, fed in moist or sun-dried form. These feeds are produced by fish farmers themselves, involving home-based operations with simple and mostly primitive facilities (Alagoa et al., 2011). As mentioned above, this is mainly because small-scale commercial farmers cannot afford manufactured pelleted feeds. The farmers also have minimal access to quality feed ingredients, finance, storage facilities, etc. They also lack the basic knowledge on on-farm feed management (El-Sayed, 2013a). Therefore, farm-made feeds in many countries, especially in SSA, are characterized by their high price, poor quality and inconsistency in production rates. Micronutrients, such as vitamin and mineral mixes and antioxidants are generally not added to diet formulations by most small-scale farmers. This practice leads to further deterioration in feed quality, reduction in storage time and the acceleration of spoilage. Farm-made feeds also contain high levels of fines, which results in feed wastage and poor feed efficiency. It is no surprise therefore that FCR of these feeds is generally poor, ranging from 1.5 to > 3.8 (Liti et al., 2005; El-Sayed, 2013a).

It appears from the above discussion that farm-made feeds in many countries, especially in Africa, suffer from several constraints, summarized as follows:

1. The use of inappropriate formulations, due to the lack of scientific background and unawareness of the nutritional requirements of the farmed species;
2. Inconsistent supply of raw materials;
3. Poor-quality ingredients and finished feeds (high content of fines, low nutrient contents, wrong pellet size, high FCR, etc.);
4. Inconsistent production rates;
5. High price of raw materials and processed feeds;
6. Poor storage facilities, leading to quality deterioration and acceleration of spoilage and;
7. Unavailability of electricity in many rural areas, which is essential for grinding the ingredients and pelletizing the diets.

5.5 Polyculture

Tilapia can produce high yields in monoculture systems because they can fill several feeding niches, compared to selective feeders such as carps. However, the production of tilapia with other fish or crustacean species in a polyculture system is spreading widely in many parts of the world. This system results in higher net yield and better water quality than monoculture system, due to the full exploitation of multiple niches. Polyculture also reduces the environmental impact of aquaculture, increases farmers' profitability and provides ecological benefits by optimizing the use of available pond resources (McKinnon et al., 2002; Wang and Lu, 2016). In other words, polyculture is more sustainable and environmentally friendly than monoculture system.

For maximizing tilapia production in polyculture systems, it is essential to fully understand operating characteristics of the system, such as stocked fish and shellfish (species, sizes, stocking densities and ratios), timing of culture and fish–environment relationships (Junior et al., 2012; Simão et al., 2013). Understanding such complicated relationships will enable fish farmers and farm managers to select the suitable species, sizes, stocking densities, fertilization regimes, nutritional inputs and other management practices. The culture of fish species which have different feeding habits in the same pond will result in more efficient utilization of pond resources. If different feeding niches are adopted in such a way that the wastes of one species are used as food for another, higher production efficiency is expected to be achieved (Milstein, 1997; Shoko et al., 2016; Sri-Uam et al., 2016).

The selection of proper species for polyculture will also minimize antagonistic and maximize synergistic relationships in fish ponds, leading to increasing available food resources for cultured species and improving environmental conditions. Such fish–fish and fish–environment relationship is exemplified by tilapia and common carp culture in Israel. Monoculture of tilapia and carp usually results in the accumulation and decomposition of organic matter, leading to increasing ammonia and nitrite levels in the pond. Blooming of blue green algae and other small algae is also developed in monocultured tilapia ponds, where the fish feed on these algae. In tilapia–carp polyculture system, a synergistic relationship occurs, where carp stir up the mud and facilitate the efficient utilization of organic and inorganic matter. This process significantly reduces the accumulation of ammonia, nitrite and organic loading. Stirring also makes nutrients more available for large-size algae, which can be used as fish food. Higher photosynthesis leads also to increased oxygenation and pH and reduced nitrification.

5.5.1 Tilapia polyculture with other fishes

Tilapia are generally cultured with a number of freshwater or brackish water species including carps, mullets, catfishes, prawns and shrimps. The culture of tilapia with other aquatic species has been a traditional practice in Southeast Asia, Africa and Latin America for many years. In China, for example, polyculture of tilapia in semi-intensive systems with different combinations of fishes has been practiced for decades. However, farming tilapia with carps remains the most common (Yang and Huang, 2011; Wang and Lu, 2016). The culture of tilapia with carps may not affect tilapia growth, but it improves the survival rate, water quality and total net production of the pond (Yang and Huang, 2011). The net production from polyculture of tilapia with other fish species in China is generally higher than that reported in other countries.

Several studies have considered the ecological and economic efficiency of different combinations of tilapia and other fish species, including carps, catfish, mullets and other cichlids, in polyculture systems. These research studies indicate that fish growth, yield and profitability are significantly higher than that obtained when tilapia are cultured alone. Edirisinghe (1990) stocked common carp, bighead carp and Nile tilapia in fertilized ponds at a density of 18,000 fish ha^{-1} at a ratio of 2:1 or 1:2 bighead carp:tilapia and 2:3:4 bighead carp:common carp:tilapia, for 154 days. The inclusion of common carp significantly increased the growth rate of bighead carp and tilapia, indicating that the incorporation of a bottom feeder was beneficial. Similarly, Wang et al. (1998) studied the effects of rearing different combinations of aquatic animals in polyculture systems. They found that the polyculture of common sea perch–Chinese shrimp–tilapia hybrids converted nitrogen more efficiently than other fish combinations. In another study, the effects of the structure of tri-species polyculture of Chinese shrimp, Taiwan red tilapia (*O. mossambicus* x *O. niloticus*) and constricted tagelus (*Sinonovacula constricta*) stocked at different combinations, on the profitability and ecological efficiency of the system was investigated (Tian et al., 2001). The COD and *chlorophyll-a* were higher, while transparency was lower in the control (shrimp monoculture) than in polyculture treatments, indicating the efficiency of polyculture systems in N and P conversion. The best stocking density for optimum performance was 7.2:0.08:14.0 shrimp: tilapia:tagelus m^{-2}. The total conversion efficiency of N and P in the system was 23.4% and 14.7%.

Shoko et al. (2016) raised mixed-sex Nile tilapia either solely or in combination with North African catfish (*Clarias gariepinus*), with a catfish: tilapia ratio of 1:3, at three densities (30,000, 60,000 and 90,000 fish ha^{-1}) for 240 days. Significantly higher growth rates, net yield and profitability were attained in the polyculture than in monoculture system. The highest growth, yield and economic benefits were achieved at high and medium densities than at low densities. This result demonstrates that Nile tilapia and African catfish can be farmed in a polyculture system at very high stocking densities without adversely affecting their growth, yield and economic profitability. However, the results of this particular study may not be reliable because the growth rates at all densities were relatively low and the feed conversion was extremely poor (2.83–3.55 for tilapia and 2.63–3.52 for catfish).

Tilapia–mullet polyculture is a common practice in many areas in Egypt. This practice has been reported to improve the efficiency with which natural food resources are used within the pond, resulting in better feed utilization, environmental quality, system sustainability and net economic profits. Tahoun et al. (2013) evaluated the performance and profitability of tilapia–mullets polycultured at different combinations. Nile Tilapia were stocked with striped mullet (*Mugil cephalus*) and thinlip grey mullet (*Liza ramada*) at 100% tilapia, 75% tilapia + 25% *M. cephalus* or *L. ramada*, and 75% tilapia + 12.5% *M. cephalus* + 12.5% *L. ramada*. The highest yield, best feed utilization and highest economic return were achieved at 75% tilapia with 25% striped mullet. In tilapia–mullet polyculture in Israel, tilapia represent about 90%. In case of tilapia–mullet–common carp integration, the ratio is generally 75–10–15, respectively (Milstein, 1997). About 2% grass carp and/or namsif (hybrid of silver carp with bighead carp) are stocked in the ponds to control plankton and macrophytes. Red drum (*Sciaenops ocellata*) are sometimes included as a predator to get rid of tilapia seeds. Total yield in this co-culture system ranges from 10 to 30 t ha^{-1} per year.

5.5.2 Tilapia polyculture with crustaceans

The polyculture of tilapia with freshwater prawns and marine shrimp is now a common practice in many countries, especially in Southeast Asia (Uddin et al., 2007b; Tidwell et al., 2010; Jatobá et al., 2011). Freshwater prawn (*M. rosenbergii*) and tilapia can be polycultured year-round (Garcia-Pérez et al., 2000). Tilapia and prawns have different feeding habits and can live together synergistically. Tilapia are generally herbivorous or filter feeders occupying the water column, while prawns are benthic and omnivorous consuming benthic organisms, processed feeds, wastes, detritus and even tilapia faeces (D'Abramo and New, 2010). In addition, prawns bioturbate at the pond bottom bringing back nutrients to the water column, enhancing primary productivity and increasing natural food availability for tilapia (Kimpara et al., 2011). Therefore, coculture of these two groups improves pond production and the water quality and increases economic returns (New and Valenti, 2017).

Extensive research has been conducted on tilapia–prawn polyculture, particularly in Asia. Results were site-specific, and oscillated significantly, depending on soil nature, climate conditions, water source, appropriate feed availability, and management practices (New and Valenti, 2017). However, published research on this topic has mainly considered aspects such as stocking density (Uddin et al., 2007b), profitability (Garcia-Pérez et al., 2000) and the effects of confined and unconfined tilapia on water quality (Danaher et al., 2007; Tidwell et al., 2010). For example, from an economical point of view, a stocking density of tilapia and freshwater prawn (*M. rosenbergii*) at 30,000 ha^{-1} with a ratio of 3:1 showed the best result (Uddin et al., 2007b). The growth, survival and yield of tilapia stocked at one fish m^{-2} with 0, 2, 4 and 6 freshwater prawn post larvae were not affected by the stocking density of the prawn (Dos Santos and Valenti, 2002). A stocking density of up to six prawn larvae m^{-2} did not affect tilapia production and required neither additional feeding nor significant changes in management. This polyculture system allowed increased production with the same amount of feed. Tidwell et al. (2010) compared the effects of confined and unconfined tilapia on water quality, growth and survival of prawn and tilapia polycultured in earthen ponds. Juvenile prawns (0.8 g) were stocked into earthen ponds at 62,000 ha^{-1}, alone or with either unconfined all-male Nile tilapia (89.2 g) at 4400 fish ha^{-1}, or confined in 1 m^3 cages at 100 fish $cage^{-1}$. Prawns were fed a sinking pellet (28% protein) while tilapia were fed a floating pellet (32% protein). Confined and unconfined tilapia performed almost similar, while the growth and production of prawn grown with caged tilapia were better than those reared with free, unconfined fish.

Hernandez Barraza et al. (2012) demonstrate that integrated shrimp–tilapia farming, at different stocking ratios (20: 0, 20:2, 20:4 and 20:8) in a polyculture tank system was more productive than monoculture of shrimp, without any adverse effects on fish and shrimp. The best growth and FCR were obtained in shrimp polyculture treatment with highest tilapia density (20:8). Tilapia has also been proven to improve shrimp farms in Negros, the Philippines (Cruz et al., 2008). For example, black tiger shrimp were not affected by vibriosis disease when cultured in plankton-rich tilapia effluent water due to the presence of the green algae *Chlorella*, which is known to inhibit the luminous bacteria (Tendencia et al., 2004, 2005). This is because tilapia effluent water produces substances which can act antagonistically to pathogenic bacteria and effectively prevent their growth and propagation (Tendencia et al., 2004, 2005). In support, Makridis et al. (2006) reported that *Chlorella* and *Tetraselmis* cultures inhibit the growth of *Vibrio,* suggesting that these microalgae produce superoxide which is used as bacterial inhibitor. To take advantage of the bioremediation effect of tilapia, many farmers stock tilapia in cages within the shrimp ponds (Cruz et al., 2008).

The survival, growth and yield of both *O. niloticus* and tiger shrimp (*Penaeus monodon*) reared at different combinations of stocking densities, in a polyculture brackish water system were significantly affected by stocking densities and competition for food (Gonzales-Corre, 1988). The best performance of shrimp was attained at a stocking density of 6000 shrimp and 6000 tilapia ha^{-1}, compared to monoculture systems. However, tilapia had low survival and slow growth in all treatments, due to the competition for food between Nile tilapia and tiger shrimp. It is, therefore, worth mentioning that in polyculture systems there is a degree of competition even between species with completely different feeding niches, especially at high stocking densities.

5.5.3 The use of predator fish to control tilapia breeding

One of the serious drawbacks associated with tilapia culture in semi-intensive systems is their continuous and excessive breeding in culture ponds, especially at low stocking densities. This phenomenon often results in overpopulation and low production of marketable fish, mainly due to the competition for food and space. Controlling the reproduction and recruitment of tilapia in ponds is, therefore, essential for successful and profitable tilapia culture. There are a number of methods which are used for tilapia seed control, including monosex culture, the use of predators and stock manipulation. The production of monosex tilapia was highlighted in Chapter 8. The use of carnivorous fishes including walking catfishes, *C. gariepinus*, *Clarias macrocephalus* and catfish hybrids, for controlling overpopulation of tilapia has been a common practice in many parts of the world.

Lazard and Oswald (1995) found that the addition of 260, 150 g African catfish controlled the population of Nile tilapia in 10- acre ponds. The authors found also that other carnivorous fishes such as banded jewelfish, *Hemichromis fasciatus* and catfish *Heterobranchus isopterus* have been successful in controlling tilapia seeds. Similarly, the inclusion of catfish fingerlings with blue tilapia significantly controlled their reproduction and improved their growth, in addition to the improvement in catfish growth (Morrison et al., 1995). The initial stocking size of predatory African catfish has a significant effect on tilapia recruitment and growth rates. Limbu et al. (2015) assessed the effects of different sizes of African walking catfish (small, 40 g and large, 62.5 g) on recruitment, growth rates, survival and yield of mixed-sex Nile tilapia for 126 days. Large catfish were more effective in reducing tilapia recruitment than small catfish. Larger African catfish also resulted in significantly higher growth performance and yield of Nile tilapia. The authors concluded that tilapia farmers can reduce tilapia breeding and obtain higher growth and larger size of marketable tilapia by stocking their ponds with large African catfish predator of about 60 g or more.

Nile perch, *Lates niloticus* (Ofori, 1988) and tarpon, *Megalops cyprinoides* (Fortes, 1985) have also been successful in controlling tilapia population in monoculture and polyculture systems, respectively. A prey:predator ratio of 1:20 to 1:250 for *L. niloticus* with tilapia has been suggested for controlling tilapia seed production (Ofori, 1988). In addition to controlling fish population, the use of these predators improves the growth and yield of cultured fishes. The snakehead (*C. striata*) can also be successfully used for controlling tilapia recruitment in Asia, even at very low predator:prey ratios. Yi et al. (2004b) reported that snakehead stocked with monoculture or polycultured mixed-sex tilapia completely controlled fish recruitment at a predator:prey ratio of 1:80. However, the addition of snakehead into tilapia ponds did not result in any improvement in tilapia growth, but significantly reduced tilapia yields.

Sahar (*Tor putitora*), which is a carnivorous fish, native to Southeast Asia (Afghanistan, Pakistan, India, Nepal, Bangladesh, Bhutan and Myanmar), has been used to control tilapia recruitment and improve their performance. In Nepal, Nile tilapia–sahar polyculture reduced tilapia recruitment and resulted in a better growth and higher production than tilapia monoculture. The best tilapia growth and yield, growth of sahar and gross income were obtained at a stocking ratio of 1:16 sahar:tilapia (Shrestha et al., 2011). Polyculture of Nile tilapia and Mayan cichlid (*Cichlasoma urophthalmus*), which is native in Mexico, was investigated as a means of reducing tilapia recruitment (Hernández et al., 2014). The presence of this cichlid did not affect tilapia performance. Cichlid performance was inversely proportional to their stocking density because they competed for available tilapia larvae.

5.6 Integrated culture

Integrated aquaculture is the practice of farming fish and shellfish with land crops and domestic animals. In another word, it is a means of diversification of farm outputs, through the full utilization of available resources and wastes. This farming system depends mainly on available resources with minimum use of inputs from outside the farm. Integrated aquaculture has been an ancient practice in China and many other Southeast Asian countries (Pillay, 1990). The most popular integrated farming systems of tilapia are their culture in rice fields and their integration with domestic animals. The pen-cum-pond system is also a promising integrated system. The research conducted at the Asian Institute of Technology (AIT) revealed that this production system has a great production potential, in addition to its ability to reduce the environmental impacts resulting from culture effluents (see Chapter 14). The common integrated systems of tilapia are discussed in the following sections.

5.6.1 Tilapia culture in rice fields

According to FAOStat (2018) (http://www.fao.org/faostat/en/#data/QC), the world rice crop area was 160 million ha in 2016, about 88% of which is in Asia. This huge area can be a substantial source of fish for rural households worldwide. Fish culture in rice field has received great attention in recent years as a means of sustainable rural development, food security and poverty alleviation in several developing countries, especially in Asia. In fact, rice–fish farming has evolved in Southeast Asia for centuries (Defu and Maoxing, 1995). Therefore, the traditional rice–fish farming system has been selected by FAO, United Nations Development Programme (UNDP), and Global Environment Facility (GEF) as a 'globally important agricultural heritage system' (GIAHS) (Koohanfkan and Furtado, 2004).

Raising fish in rice fields has many advantages:

1. The recycling of nutrients by the fish through feeding and depositing faeces in the soil, which can be used as a fertilizer for rice, reducing the dependence on commercial fertilizers. In this process, the uptake of nutrients such as phosphorus and nitrogen by the rice is usually increased.
2. The increase in rice yields.
3. The increase in revenue from both rice and fish production.
4. An additional source of protein for rural households, especially in countries facing shortage in captured fish.
5. An effective method of insect pest control (such as leafhoppers, stem-borers and aphids).
6. An effective method of controlling weeds, which herbivorous fishes consume.

5.6.1.1 Tilapia culture in rice fields in Asia

Tilapia culture in rice fields is widely practiced in many Asian countries and has also gained considerable momentum in some countries in Africa and Latin America. Tilapia can be raised in rice fields in monoculture systems; however, this approach is not very common. Instead, polyculture of tilapia with carps is widely practiced in Southeast Asia and Africa (Fig. 5.5). Stocking densities of target species are varying, depending on geographical location, fish sizes and culture objectives (market size vs. fingerling production). The fish can also be grown with or without fertilization or supplemental feed, and therefore the yield varies considerably. Accordingly, the profitability of tilapia culture in rice fields depends on the inputs pumped into the system.

A number of research studies have been conducted on monoculture of tilapia in rice fields, with varying results. Stocking sizes of cultured fishes appear to play an important role in fish growth and rice yield. When tilapia was stocked at 7500 fish ha^{-1}, at two sizes; small (2.9–3.5 g) and large sizes (28.2–33 g), the growth rates of small fish (12.8 g $fish^{-1}$) was better than that of large fish (33.76 g $fish^{-1}$) (Haroon and Pittman, 1997). In a 78-d culture period, the net yields were 37.2 and −58.3 kg ha^{-1} $crop^{-1}$ for small and large tilapia, respectively, whereas survival rate was 66%. The low tilapia growth, survival and yield in that particular study has been attributed to (1) slower swimming of the fish which were entangled in aquatic macrophytes leading to predation by frogs, snakes and birds and (2) lower nutrient ingestion and digestion. Zooplankton in the ponds had little contribution to filter

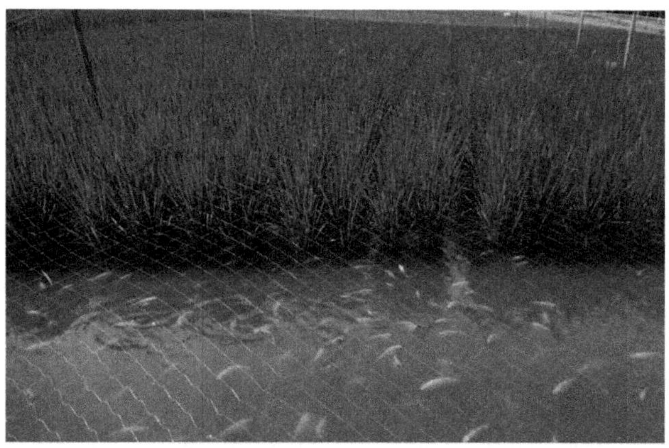

FIGURE 5.5 Raising red tilapia in a rice field in Indonesia. *Photo from Shutterstock.*

feeding mechanism of tilapia, and ontogenetic shifts in tilapia diets were also minimal or absent. Similar results on poor survival, growth and yields of tilapia monocultured in rice fields have also been reported by other authors (Haroon and Alam, 1992; Sevilleja et al., 1992; Torres et al., 1992).

Because tilapia reach their sexual maturity at an early age (3–6 mo), stocking large tilapia in rice field may result in fish reproduction, which will lead to overpopulation and fish stunting because of the increased competition for food and space. In rice–fish culture, if large tilapia are to be monocultured, all-male populations are preferable. All-male culture overcomes the problem of early spawning, and is likely to improve fish growth and yield. However, more research is needed alongside this line, before any concrete conclusion can be drawn.

The polyculture of tilapia in rice fields has become a common practice in Southeast Asia. In China, for example, the polyculture of Nile tilapia, common carp, grass carp (*Ctenopharyngodon idella*) and Crucian carp (*Carassius auratus*) in rice fields is very common, productive and profitable. This culture system is practiced mainly in Guangxi, Sichuan and Hunan provinces (Ming and Yi, 2004). All-male Nile tilapia or hybrid tilapia fingerlings (5 cm) are generally stocked in rice fields, mainly with carps, at a density of 4500–7500 fish ha^{-1}, about 10 days after transplanting rice seedlings (Yi, Pathum Thani, Thailand, 2004; personal communication). The fish depends exclusively on natural food available in rice fields, and no supplemental feed is provided. After 100 days of culture, the fish reach about 150 g in average, yielding about 500–1100 kg ha^{-1}. Produced fish are generally marketed in local rural markets. Even in countries such as Vietnam, Bangladesh and India, where tilapia culture has not been very popular, their polyculture in rice fields started to gain considerable grounds. As a result, polyculture of tilapia with carps in rice filed has become established extensively in some bheries of West Bengal (India) (Natarajan and Aravindan, 2002).

The growth and yield of Nile tilapia and common carp in integrated rice–fish system were investigated in Bangladesh (Frei et al., 2007). Tilapia and carp were raised in single culture and in polyculture with supplemental feeding at 2× (twice) maintenance level. The highest fish yield was obtained in the carp–tilapia mixed culture (586 ± 125 kg ha^{-1}), followed by tilapia alone and carp alone. Based on this result, a carp–tilapia combination was tested with different inputs, including regular urea fertilization and two different feeding levels; continuous feeding at 2× maintenance level (Feed Level I) and 4× maintenance level reduced to 2× at later growth stage (Feed Level II). The best yield was obtained in Feed Level II (935 ± 29 kg ha^{-1}). The highest rice production (4.2 t ha^{-1}) was obtained from rice–fish with urea fertilization. DO and pH values decreased in rice–fish ponds compared to rice only, especially when supplementary feed was provided. Kunda et al. (2009) also evaluated the effects of raising catla (*Catla catla*) and Nile tilapia in a prawn-mola (*Amblypharyngodon mola*) polyculture in rice fields after rice harvesting, in a rotational practice in Bangladesh. The inclusion of tilapia (10 g) or catla (41 g) at 2500 fish ha^{-1} increased total yield and profit. Despite the fact that tilapia did not improve prawn size, survival or productivity, they significantly reduced phytoplankton concentration in the water.

Hossain et al. (2015) assessed the effects of ditch size (5%, 10% and 15% of the total cultivable rice field) on growth, production and economic return of all-male Nile tilapia in rice–fish system. The fish fingerlings (19 g) were stocked at a density of 5000 ha^{-1} and raised for 4 months. Larger ditch size (15% of the total land area) resulted in significantly better performance, survival and fish production than smaller (5%) and medium (10%) ditch sizes. But rice production decreased with increasing ditch size. However, economic return was better in medium ditch size than in the smaller and larger ditches.

Rice field may also be a suitable environment for small-scale tilapia seed production, which can be used as a source of income for poor households. Barman and Little (2006) assessed the production of Nile tilapia seed in irrigated spring rice–fields in Northwest Bangladesh. Farmers were supplied with mature GIFT strain Nile tilapia to stock in their rice plots. The majority of farmers succeeded in producing fingerlings in their plots, with an average harvest weight of 21 g. Most fingerlings were sold (43%) and/or stocked in farmers' own grow-out ponds (39%), while some fingerlings were used for direct household consumption (17%). This simply means that rice–fish farming can be a sustainable source of fingerling fish, income and food fish production for rural, poor communities.

Many variables, including fish species and sizes, stocking densities, culture inputs (such as inorganic fertilizer, manure and supplemental feed), season, rice vegetative phase, rice reproductive and ripening phase affect the growth and yield of cultured tilapia. Accordingly, the net production and profitability of tilapia culture in rice fields vary strongly from one geographical region to another and even from one season to another in the same region. In Vietnam, for example, Nile tilapia has been successfully raised with silver barb and common carp in rice fields at a total density of 20,000 fishes ha^{-1}, at different combinations of sizes and stocking densities, for 149 days (Rothuis et al., 1998). Small tilapia (1.8 g) were stocked at 6600, 5400, 3400 and 1400 fish ha^{-1}, while silver barb stocked at 0, 4000, 10,000 and 16,000 fish ha^{-1}, whereas common carp was stocked at 13,400, 10,600, 6600 and 2600. Large tilapia (28.8 g), silver barb and common carp were stocked at 3800, 4500 and 0 fish ha^{-1}. Tilapia survival was about 64%, and the growth was inversely correlated with initial stocking density. The best growth of tilapia (89 g) was achieved at 1400 tilapia, 16,000 large silver barb (80 g) and 2600 common carp ha^{-1}. The good growth of tilapia was attributed to the availability of natural food at low stocking density and the synergistic effect of cultured species, where the digested plants contained in the excretes of silver barb may have been utilized by tilapia.

The effects of stocking density on the growth, production and economic return of all-male tilapia were investigated in a rain-fed rice–fish ecosystem in southwestern part of Bangladesh, for a period of 120 days (Mridha et al., 2014). Fish fingerlings (18 g) were stocked in rice fields at a density of 4000, 5000, and 6000 fish ha^{-1} and relied completely on the natural food without any supplemental feeding. Rice and straw production slightly (but not significantly) increased with increasing fish density. On the other hand, the best fish survival and growth rates were achieved at 4000 fish ha^{-1}, while the highest production (457.21 kg ha^{-1}) and net profit were recorded at 5000 fish ha^{-1}, followed by 4000 and 6000 fish ha^{-1}, respectively. Once again, this study demonstrated that tilapia culture in rice fields is technically feasible and economically profitable.

The use of fertilizer and/or supplemental feed in rice–fish culture is disputable, and not fully understood. Some researchers found that the growth and yield of Nile tilapia raised in rice field were low and not affected by the source of fertilizer (organic or inorganic) (Mang-Umphan and Arce, 1988). Vromant et al. (2002) found also that the growth and yield of Nile tilapia raised in polyculture system with Java barb *Barbodes gonionotus* and common carp in rice fields were significantly improved when supplemental fertilizer and artificial feed were provided. However, growth, yield and survival values were still low compared to that of Java barb. The author concluded that Nile tilapia are not well suited for culture in rice fields.

In contrast, Dela Cruz and Lopez (1980) reported that the culture of Nile tilapia in rice field supplemented with feed and fertilizer in the Philippines was profitable. About 480 kg of Nile tilapia and 222 kg of common carp ha^{-1} were produced from rice fields stocked with 10,000 fish ha^{-1} and supplemented with feed and fertilizer. The application of fertilizer increases primary productivity in the fields and, in turn, enhances food consumption by the fish. Similar positive effects of rice fertilization on tilapia growth and yield have been reported by Sevilleja et al. (1992).

Once again, it is clear from the above studies that the suitability of tilapia culture in rice fields is still controversial, and more research is needed to further investigate the potential of these fishes as a candidate for this system. More research is also needed on whether fertilization, supplemental feeding or a combination of both would be more biologically and economically appropriate. More information should also be gathered on fish and crustacean species that are commonly cultured with tilapia in rice fields in order to adopt the most suitable species which occupy different trophic niches from that of tilapia. The growth and yield of tilapia raised in rice fields are summarized in Table 5.5.

One of the crucial factors that rice–fish farmer should be aware about is the time at which the fish must be stocked in rice fields. The frequent fertilization of the rice fields after transplantation and the low plant density at this early

TABLE 5.5 The growth and yield of Nile tilapia raised in rice fields.

Culture system	Initial weight (g)	Final weight (g)	Net yield (kg ha^{-1})	Period (days)	References
Monoculture	2.2	15	43	65	Torres et al. (1992)
Monoculture	3.1	13	37	78	Haroon and Pittman (1997)
Polyculture	1.8	56	117	149	Rothuis et al. (1998)
Polyculture	28.8	66	62	149	Rothuis et al. (1998)
Polyculture	5 cm	150	500–1500	100	Ming and Yi (2004)
Monoculture	20	56.8	132.4	77	Rasowo and Auma (2006)
Monoculture	11.7	83.2	425	111	Frei et al. (2007)
Polyculture	11.7	107	460	111	Frei et al. (2007)
Polyculture	3.9	51.5	–	60	Nnaji et al. (2013)
Monoculture	18.2	82.5–111	317–388	120	Mridha et al. (2014)
Monoculture	19.7	111–126	349–407	115	Hossain et al. (2015)

stage, which allows high light penetration to the water, enhances plankton productivity. Progressive growth of the rice is accompanied by progressive shading, low nutrient availability and decreased primary productivity. Accordingly, the average daily food consumption by cultured fish is expected to be higher during the rice vegetative phase (early stage) than during the rest of the cropping season. Therefore, it is essential that the farmer stocks his tilapia as early as possible after rice transplantation.

Along with the additional fish crop obtained from rice fields, rice yield can be increased up to 20% (Lightfoot et al., 1992). Tilapia culture and rice farming are also complementary systems, since the fish can feed on rice pests and play a significant role in integrated pest management (Halwart, 1998). The fish have also been reported to control caseworms *Nymphula depunctalis* (Vromant et al., 1998). The saving of pesticides cost and earning from fish sales have been reported to increase the net income from rice–fish farming by 7%–65%, compared to rice monoculture (Halwart, 1998).

5.6.1.2 Tilapia culture in rice fields in Africa

Tilapia culture in rice fields in Africa has gained considerable attention during the past two decades and appears promising, especially in countries like Egypt, Mali, Burkina Faso, Senegal, Côte d'Ivoire and Ghana (Ofori et al., 2005; Miller, 2006; Sanni and Juanich, 2006). Available results indicated that the presence of the fish with rice crop does not reduce rice harvest, but increases revenue over rice monoculture. This suggests that rice–fish integration could be a viable option for income generation for small rice farmers in many African regions.

Rice is widely cultivated in Egypt as a major food crop. According to the Central Agency for Public Mobilization and Statistics (CAPMAS), about 0.6 million ha of agricultural land were cultivated with rice in 2015/2016 (http://www.capmas.gov.eg/Pages/IndicatorsPage.aspx?page_id=6151&ind_id=2361). The potential of rearing fish in rice fields in an integrated system is increasing. In fact, rice–fish farming has been a common practice among rice farmers in many areas in the Nile Delta region for many years. The total production of fish in rice fields increased from 10,000 t in 1999 to 34,000 t in 2014, with tilapia representing about 48% of this production (GAFRD, 2016). However, the production declined drastically to reach 13,535 t in 2016 (GAFRD, 2018); probably due to the continuous shrinking of the lands allocated to rice cropping. One or more ditches (about 50 cm deep and 100 cm wide) are generally dug along the rice field and used as a nursery and refuge for the fish. Because the rice-growing period is not sufficient to produce market-size fish, juvenile fish reared in rice fields are subsequently transferred to other aquaculture systems for fattening. When the rice field is drained for harvesting, the fish are segregated in the ditches where they can be easily collected.

The profitability of integrating fish culture into rice farming was determined in north central Nigeria ((Nnaji et al., 2013). Nile tilapia (3.9 g) and African catfish (*C. gariepinus*) (2.2 g) fingerlings were raised in rice plots for 60 days. Tilapia and catfish were stocked at a density of 2 fish m^{-2} (20,000 fish ha^{-1}), with a ratio of 2:1, and were fed with compounded feed and wheat offal. At the end of the study, the weight gain of Nile tilapia and catfish fingerlings were 47.60 and 110.80 g, respectively. These results showed that the integration of tilapia and catfish into the rice system appears highly profitable, compared to rice monoculture. The performance and economic feasibility of tilapia–rice co-culture in Ghana was also evaluated by Ofori et al. (2005). Rice was grown either solely or in combination with tilapia, with or without fertilization with organic manure. Nile tilapia fingerlings (25 g) were stocked at 3000 fish ha^{-1}. The yield of rice crop was significantly affected by the presence of tilapia, while fertilization did not affect rice or fish performance. However, the net return from the rice–tilapia integration was 5%–11% higher than the rice monoculture. The viability of integrating rice farming with Nile tilapia culture in the West Kano Rice Irrigation Scheme in Kenya was also investigated for 77 days (Rasowo and Auma, 2006). Mixed-sex tilapia fingerlings (20 g) were stocked at a rate of 6000 fish ha^{-1}, 2 weeks after transplanting the rice. Phosphate and nitrogen fertilizers were applied, but no supplemental feeding was provided. An average fish production of 132.4 kg ha^{-1} was obtained. The mean recovery rate of tilapia was 43%. Total rice yield from the fields stocked with fish was lower than from unstocked fields, whereas the net return was not significantly different.

5.6.2 Tilapia–wheat rotation farming

In Egypt, most pond-farmed tilapia are harvested in November and December because the water temperature drops during the winter and becomes unfavourable for tilapia survival. The ponds remain abandoned from December until March or April. Tilapia farmers in some areas, especially in Kafr El Shaikh Governorate, use their ponds during the winter months to grow wheat. After fish harvest, wheat seeds are sown on pond bottoms in about November, and the crop is generally harvested in early May. This practice is highly productive and water efficient (Fig. 5.6). It has been reported that wheat growth at harvest produced an average yield of 5.4 t ha^{-1}, using only the water remaining in the pond bottom without any fertilization (van der Heijden, 2012). Fath El-Bab et al. (2014) evaluated the technical and economic performance of Nile tilapia and wheat in a rotational farming system. The fish were first raised in earthen ponds for a full production

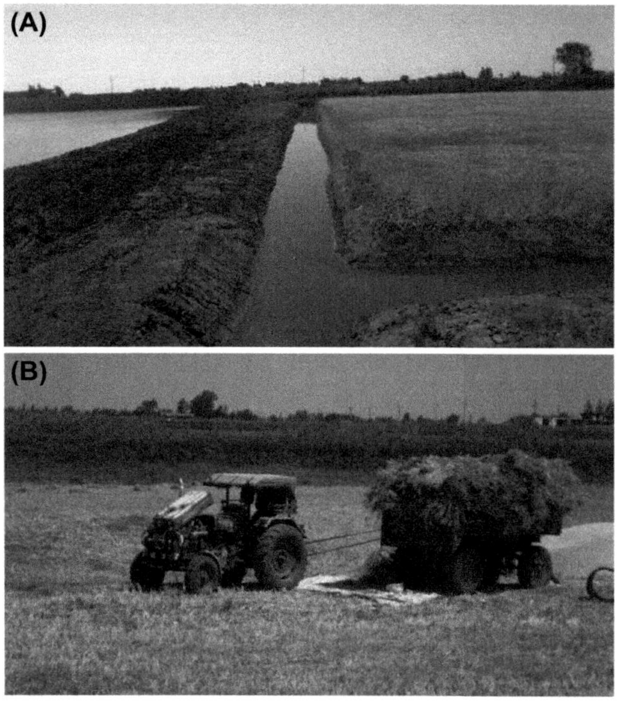

FIGURE 5.6 Growing (A) and harvesting and threshing (B) wheat crop in tilapia ponds in Kafr El-Shaikh, Egypt. *Photographs by A.-F. El-Sayed.*

cycle, followed by growing wheat in the harvested ponds. After wheat harvest, the ponds were used again for farming tilapia. Artificial feed (25% cp) and fertilization with organic or inorganic fertilizers were applied during tilapia farming. The best economic profit was obtained when Nile tilapia were grown in ponds fertilized with poultry manure followed by wheat cultivation; where the return increased by 16.6%, compared to the same ponds receiving the same inputs but without wheat cultivation.

5.6.3 Animal–tilapia culture

Farming tilapia with domestic animals, including pigs, ducks, chicken and cattle has become a common practice in many parts of the world, particularly in developing countries (Table 5.6). Ducks and pigs are probably the most successful candidates for farming with fish. In China, which is the largest fish producer from aquaculture, pig raising is widely integrated with Chinese and common carp culture, while tilapia/pig farming is practiced in certain provinces in southwest China (e.g. Sichuan) (Yi, Pathum Thani, Thailand, 2004; personal communication). Tilapia–duck farming is very popular and mutually beneficial in some coastal provinces such as Guangdong (south China). The ducks can feed on unwanted organisms in and around fish ponds, while their excreta fertilize these ponds. The following sections throw more light on these integrated animal–tilapia culture systems.

5.6.3.1 Tilapia–duck culture

As mentioned above, tilapia–duck farming (Fig. 5.7) is a promising and profitable integrated culture system, compared to other integrated farming systems (Pillay, 1990). The major fish species integrated with duck raising in China are silver carp, bighead carp and Tilapia. The number of ducks to be raised in the fish pond depends on duck species, the quality and quantity of feeds provided and the method of raising. The stocking density of ducks depends also on the environmental conditions and the stocking ratio and density of fish species polycultured in the pond. Generally, between 2000 and 4000 ducks ha^{-1} are raised in fish ponds. Fish performance and yield decrease if the ducks number exceeds 4000 ha^{-1}, due to the higher manure load, low oxygen and high ammonia concentrations, and increased biological oxygen demand (BOD) (Bao-tong and Hua-zhu, 1984).

The effect of the number of ducks on fish production is controversial. Delmendo (1980) reported that increasing the number of ducks to 1000–2000 duck ha^{-1} yielded only 1.5 t fish ha^{-1} yr^{-1}, while Hopkins and Cruz (1982) achieved a total yield of 5.48 t ha^{-1} per year of tilapia and carp (4.7 t tilapia) when the number of ducks was only 750 ha^{-1}, with a manure load of 81 kg DM ha^{-1} per day, at a stocking density of 20,000 fish ha^{-1}. Even a very low number of ducks with tilapia farming can make a big difference in fish growth, yield and system profitability. Similarly, Sin (1980) reported that raising 1000–2000 ducks ha^{-1} increased annual fish yield to 5 t ha^{-1}, compared with only 1 t ha^{-1} per year produced from nonintegrated ponds. This controversy may have been related to the type of ducks, the quality of feed and excreta, as stated above. Gopalakrishnan (1988) found that 'Muscovy' ducks were not suitable for integrated farming with tilapia (*Oreochromis andersonii*) in Zambia because they do not stay in the water long enough to produce sufficient manure. When 'Peking' ducks were used, fish production significantly improved (3.5–4.5 t ha^{-1} per year).

Soliman et al. (2000) studied the effects of raising ducks at low intensity (298 ducks ha^{-1}) on the production and profitability of Nile tilapia, blue tilapia, silver carp, common carp and grey mullet. The fishes were stocked at equal numbers in a polyculture system, in earthen ponds fertilized with cow manure and superphosphate and supplemented with a 10.6% cp diet, in Egypt. Integrated ponds resulted in better growth, FCR, yield and profitability than nonintegrated ponds. However, only common carp and silver carp showed significantly higher weight gain in integrated system, while tilapia growth was similar in both systems, presumably due to the sufficient food availability resulted from fertilization and supplemental feeding.

TABLE 5.6 Summary of integrated animal/tilapia culture in some countries.

	Fish		Animal		Harvest data			
Country	Species (size)	# ha^{-1}	Type	# ha^{-1}	FW (g)	Yield (mt ha^{-1}/yr)	Remarks	References
Egypt	*Mugil cephalus* (6.5)		Ducks	298	146.9	1.6 (total)	Better growth and yield than nonintegrated system	Soliman et al. (2000)
	Cyprinus carpio (3.6)				270.6			
	Silver carp (3.3)				519.5			
	Tilapia (3.1)				274			
Philippines	Nile tilapia	8,500	Pigs	20	184	1.7 (total)	Tilapia survival 78%, increasing fish density to 20,000 reduced average harvest weight, but did not increase total yield	Hopkins and Cruz (1982)
	Common carp	1,000			505			
	Channa striata	100						
Philippines	Nile tilapia	8,500	Pigs	100	118	2.3 (total)	Tilapia survival >100%, increasing fish density to 2000 reduced average harvest weight, but did not increase total yield	Hopkins and Cruz (1982)
	Common carp	1,400			183			
	C. striata	100			385			
Philippines	Nile tilapia	5,000–20,000	Broiler chicken	900		0.34–0.67	Best tilapia yield at a density of 15,000 ha^{-1}	Pudadera et al. (1986)
	Milkfish	2,000				0.075–0.12		
	Penaeus indicus	50,000				0.19–0.28		
Nigeria	Nile tilapia (15)	20,000	Chicken	1,000	575	14.9	Indigenous chicken were better than exotic chicken	Njoku and Ejiogu (1999)
	Catfish (5)	10,000			1,375	13.8		
Rwanda	Nile tilapia (14)	20,000	Rabbit	200–1,600	31–71	1.1–3.3	The highest yield (3.3 t ha^{-1} per year) was obtained at a density of 1200 rabbits ha^{-1}	Tabaro et al. (2012b)

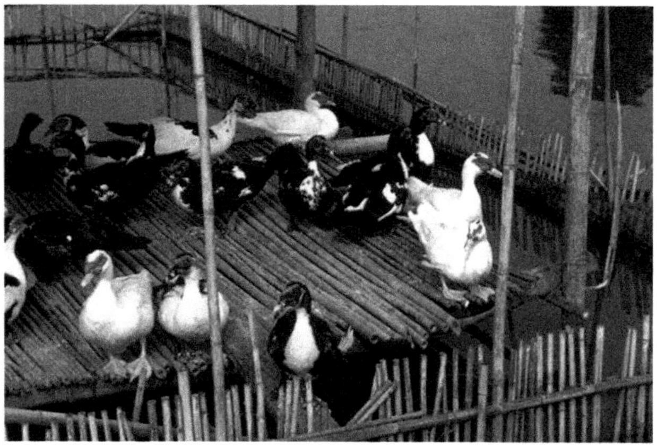

FIGURE 5.7 Duck–tilapia integrated culture in Thailand. *Photo provided by P. Edwards.*

5.6.3.2 Tilapia–chicken culture

As in case of ducks–fish farming, the performance of fish raised with chicken in an integrated system depends on the species and number of chicken, the quality and quantity of their feeds and excreta and water quality. Higher chicken density (i.e. higher manure load) may increase ammonia and BOD and decrease DO and water transparency, and finally leads to reduced fish yield (Hopkins and Cruz, 1982; Njoku and Ejiogu, 1999). Therefore, the integration of tilapia with poultry should be carefully managed because the adoption of improper poultry type and density could lead to significant economic loss.

A number of studies have been conducted on integrated fish–chicken farming (Fig. 5.8), with varying results. Pudadera et al. (1986) evaluated the integrated culture of Nile tilapia, milkfish (*Chanos chanos*) and shrimp (*Penaeus indicus*) with broiler chicken, in brackish water ponds in the Philippines. Tilapia were stocked at 5000, 10,000, 15,000 and 20,000 fish ha^{-1}, while the densities of milkfish, shrimp and chicken were kept constant at 2000, 50,000 and 900, respectively. Tilapia production ranged from 333.8 to 669.7 kg ha^{-1}, and the best net production of tilapia was obtained at 15,000 fish ha^{-1}. Njoku and Ejiogu (1999) raised 15-g Nile tilapia and 5-g African mud catfish (*Heterobranchus longifilis*) in ponds in Nigeria, at a stocking density of 30,000 fish ha^{-1}, with a ratio of 2:1. The ponds were integrated with 1000, 1500 and 2000 indigenous chicken ha^{-1} or 1500 exogenous broiler chicken ha^{-1} (control) for 270 days. The best daily weight gain (2 g d^{-1}) and yield (14.9 t ha^{-1}) were attained at 1000 chicken (3.6 t dry manure ha^{-1}), compared to 0.5 g d^{-1} and 3.09 t ha^{-1}, when exotic broilers were used. That particular study emphasizes that the type of fertilizer adopted for pond fertilization should be carefully considered.

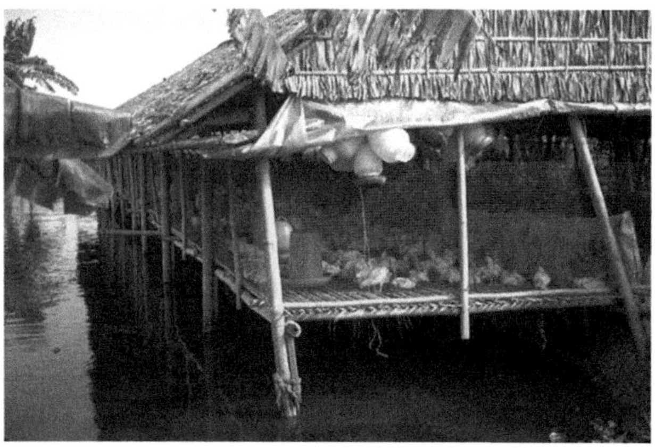

FIGURE 5.8 Chicken–tilapia integrated culture in Thailand. *Photo provided by P. Edwards.*

5.6.3.3 Tilapia–rabbit culture

Rabbit manure contains more nutrients than the manure of other farm animals, such as cattle, pigs and poultry (Lukefahr, 2007). The gradual nutrient release of rabbit excreta suggests that rabbit can be integrated with fish culture. However, only a few studies have considered the use of rabbit manure in aquaculture (Breine et al., 1996; Tabaro et al., 2012a, 2012b). Tabaro et al. (2012a) assessed the effects of rabbit droppings on water quality and growth performance of Nile tilapia in Rwanda for 152 days. Nile tilapia fingerlings (14 g) were stocked in 400 m^2 ponds at a density of 2 fish m^{-2}. The ponds were fertilized with rabbit droppings from rabbits reared over fish ponds at three densities (1, 2 and 4 rabbits per 100 m^2). The results indicated that rabbit droppings increased all nutrient contents, except nitrates; which decreased with time. Average fish weight at harvest was higher at the highest rabbit density than at lower densities; but the yield was relatively low (460–635 kg ha^{-1}). The same authors (Tabaro et al., 2012b) evaluated the effects of varying rabbit densities (200, 400, 800, 1200 and 1600 rabbits ha^{-1}) over fish ponds on water quality, plankton productivity and Nile tilapia growth. Fish growth and yield were positively correlated with rabbit density up to 800 rabbits ha^{-1} and decreased at higher densities. It should be mentioned that at 1200 rabbit ha^{-1} the average final weight and yield were much higher than those at other treatments because the initial weight in that treatment was 32.8 g, much higher than other treatments (12–14.7 g). Phytoplankton biomass and daily primary productivity also increased with increasing rabbit densities. These results suggest that a density of 800–1200 rabbits ha^{-1} appears optimum for best performance and water quality.

5.6.3.4 Pen-cum-pond system

Pen-cum-pond system is a system in which one or more fish species are reared semi-intensively in ponds and fed naturally on the wastes resulting from other intensively cage (pen)-cultured fish species. This system has been developed and used successfully by a number of researchers (Lin and Diana, 1995; Yi and Lin, 2001; Yi et al., 2003). Tilapia co-culture in in-pond raceways was reviewed by Masser (2017).

Yi et al. (2003) studied the ability of Nile tilapia reared in a semi-intensive system in ponds to utilize the wastes resulting from intensive culture of hybrid catfish (*C. macrocephalus* x *C. gariepinus*). They found that tilapia yield from catfish-waste system was comparable to that obtained from fertilized ponds. Tilapia recovered considerable amounts of N and P contained in the wastes of intensive catfish culture. The authors suggested that water circulation between catfish pen and tilapia ponds is cost-effective, as it can sharply reduce nutrient contents in pond effluent. Similar results have been reported with walking catfish (*C. macrocephalus*) and catfish hybrids (Lin and Diana, 1995), where the wastes from caged catfish increased phytoplankton productivity in the ponds, which supported the growth of Nile tilapia in the same ponds containing the cages. Moreover, tilapia reared in cages, feeding only on phytoplankton in intensive channel catfish ponds grew reasonably well and improved the water quality in the ponds (Perschbacher, 1995).

In Nepal, the cage-cum-pond integration with Nile tilapia (30 fish m^{-3}) and African catfish (100 fish m^{-3}) in cages and carps (silver carp, common carp, bighead carp, rohu, mrigal and grass carps at 4:2:1.5:1:1:0.5 ratio, respectively) (10,000 fish ha^{-1}) in open pond was evaluated (Mandal et al., 2014). Four treatments were tested: (1) carps in ponds without cage, (2) tilapia in cage and carps in open pond, (3) catfish in cage and carps in open pond and (4) tilapia and catfish in separate cages and carps in open pond. Caged tilapia and catfish were fed on locally made feeds (24% cp), while the control ponds were fertilized biweekly with DAP and urea at a rate of 4.0 kg N and 2.0 kg P ha^{-1} per day. The cage–pond integration of Nile tilapia and African catfish with carps produced the highest yield (9.4 t ha^{-1} per year), whereas the best net return was obtained from the integration of tilapia and carp.

Yi and Lin (2000) stated the advantages of integrated cage culture in ponds as follows:

1. Wastes derived from high-protein diets of caged fish can be used as food source for open pond fish.
2. Nutrients in wastes derived from cages are recovered, reducing the concentration of nutrients contained in the effluents, which are usually released directly or indirectly to the surrounding environment, causing increased eutrophication in the waters.
3. It is used in polyculture ponds to confine costly high-protein diets to caged high-valued species, to achieve higher economic returns.
4. It is used in subtropical or temperate regions, where tropical fish species cannot overwinter, to make full use of growing seasons and make management, such as fish harvest, easy and convenient.
5. This system makes it possible to fatten large fingerlings with high-protein diets in cages and nurse fry with natural food derived from cage wastes in open water of the same pond.

5.7 Economic efficiency of integrated culture

Although integrated fish–animal farming sounds, in most cases, biologically profitable, it may not be economically so, since several factors affect the profitability of this integration system. The economic effectiveness of fish–livestock production systems varies sharply among farming communities. For example, conventional fish–livestock farming may be inappropriate in urban areas because of the large areas needed for the construction and integration of fish and animal facilities. Processing of livestock wastes into feed ingredients or fertilizer for aquaculture may also not be viable. Other culture inputs, such as agricultural by-products (rice bran, wheat bran, corn bran, etc.), labour and transportation, may also not be available in urban areas, or available but at high costs. This means that the cost of fish–animal integration in urban areas can be very expensive and may not be cost-effective.

In rural areas, where livestock is generally produced, the wastes are usually available at very low costs. Agricultural by-products and labour are also available at sustainable levels and low cost. Fish–livestock integration in rural areas is, therefore, very likely to be more sustainable and profitable. Small-scale tilapia culture in earthen ponds in Africa, in integration with crop farming (e.g. vegetables, rice and other field crops), was economically feasible and environmentally friendly, compared to traditional nonintegrated systems (Jamu, 2001). The introduction of tilapia into existing integrated farming systems in Bangladesh using the pond–dike and associated systems enhanced livelihoods and reduced poverty of rural households (Karim et al., 2011). The effectiveness of integrated farming systems is thus location specific. This means that the comparisons between integration practices in different locations are difficult and, sometimes, unreliable. Another important factor that affects the economic return of feedlot livestock–fish farming is the cost of livestock feeds, which may render the system unprofitable, especially in resource-poor areas.

As mentioned earlier, fertilizer is a key element in integrated fish–livestock farming. Understanding pond dynamics and conducting a broad economic analysis are necessary for successful and cost-effective fertilization regimes. The farmers should be aware of the following economic factors before they decide which fertilization strategy they will adopt (Knud-Hansen, 1998):

1. Market cost of biologically available N, P and C (purchasing versus on-farm production).
2. Transport and labour cost, including the lost opportunity costs and aquaculture integration with other activities.
3. The need for additional capital expenses, such as water aeration, mixing or exchange.
4. Market value of culture organisms (e.g. social acceptance, marketability of manure-raised fish).
5. Ecological impacts, including water quality (e.g. DO, ammonia, pH, turbidity, diseases, etc.) and increased organic loads.

Based on the above criteria, getting the best economic fertilizer is location specific. Again, comparison between farms in terms of fertilizer requirement, quality and productivity may be inappropriate unless these farms are ecologically, socially and economically similar. Evaluation and comparisons should, therefore, be conducted on farm-by-farm basis, taking into account the 'uniqueness' of each farm.

As mentioned earlier, the tilapia–livestock integrated farming can be 'biologically' excellent, but economically 'failure'. For example, when Nile tilapia and African mud catfish were raised in ponds in Nigeria, in integration with indigenous chicken or exogenous broiler chicken, economic analyses indicated that the use of indigenous chicken resulted in substantial economic return, whereas the use of exotic broilers has led to a net deficit (Njoku and Ejiogu, 1999). The high profitability with indigenous chickens was attributed to input saving on variable costs, which in turn decreased total production costs, as opposed to the extremely high production costs when exogenous chicken were used. Similarly, Nitithamyong et al. (1990) found that the growth of Nile tilapia reared with snakehead and pig in an integrated system for 7 months was significantly higher than in monoculture or polyculture with snakehead. However, the integrated system resulted in significantly lower economic return than the other two systems.

It is obvious from the above discussion that if the farmer/farm operator does not understand the ecological and dynamic processes occurring in the pond, the performance and yield could be very poor. For example, Ayinla et al. (1994) found that when broiler birds were integrated with Nile tilapia and bagrid catfish *Chrysichthys nigrodigitatus* at 1500 birds ha^{-1}, fish mortality reached 40% in tilapia and 70% in catfish. These high mortality rates have been related to high organic loads, which may have led to deterioration in water quality. The mortality could have been sharply reduced if some management interactions such as reducing bird number, partial changing of culture water and aeration have been taken.

5.8 Closing remarks

1. Organic fertilizers stimulate natural food production through adding detritus, which in turn, stimulates heterotrophic food chains and produces more phytoplankton and zooplankton. This natural food can be consumed by microphagous tilapias leading to considerable improvements in fish yield. Organic manure is better applied in fine particles or colloidal state.
2. Tilapia should rely completely on natural food produced through fertilization till they reach 'a critical standing crop'; then supplemental feed should be applied. Timing of supplemental feeding ranges from 40 to about 150 days after stocking, depending on tilapia species, stocking size and fertilization regimes.
3. The history of the ponds and water quality, especially alkalinity, ammonia and turbidity should be fully considered before pond fertilization.
4. Semi-intensive, polyculture of tilapia may be preferred to monoculture due to the full utilization of food niches in the ponds. However, understanding the complicated relationships between cultured species and the surrounding environment is essential in order to enable the fish farmers to select the most appropriate species, sizes and stocking densities.
5. Carnivorous fish species such as Nile perch (*L. niloticus*) and catfishes are successfully used for controlling tilapia seed production. The stock ratio varies according to the species and sizes used. A ratio of 1:50 Nile perch:tilapia, for example, has been suggested.
6. The suitability of tilapia culture in rice fields is questionable, and extensive research is needed to verify whether or not tilapia should be considered as a candidate for rice–fish culture, and whether monoculture or polyculture is preferable.
7. Duck–tilapia culture has been the most successful; however, 'Muscovy' ducks may not be a good candidate. The type and density of ducks and chicken significantly affect fish growth and yield as well as water quality.
8. Rabbit–tilapia culture may be economically feasible. About 800–120 rabbits ha^{-1} have been suggested. However, more research is needed to consolidate the reported results.
9. Pen-cum-pond system could be an excellent system for tilapia culture, since tilapia can use the waste of other fishes raised in cages/pens, leading to both economic and environmental benefits.
10. Understanding pond dynamics and conducting a broad economic analysis are necessary for successful and cost-effective fish–livestock farming.
11. For successful and sustainable integrated fish–animal farming, the farmers should consider the economic

and social factors, including market cost, variable costs, transport and labour cost, any additional capital expenses, market value of cultured species and ecological impacts of the system.

References

Abdelghany, A.E., Ahmad, M.H., 2002. Effects of feeding rates on growth and production of Nile tilapia, common carp and silver carp polycultured in fertilized ponds. Aquaculture Research 33, 415–423.

Abdelghany, A.E., Ayyat, M.-S., Ahmad, M.H., 2002. Appropriate timing of supplemental feeding for production of Nile tilapia, silver carp, and common carp in fertilized polyculture ponds. Journal of the World Aquaculture Society 33, 307–315.

Ahmed, M.H., Hassan, A.A., 2011. Effect of using different types of organic manure (chicken; cattle; compost and mineral fertilizer) in polyculture on water quality, plankton abundance and on growth performance of fish in earthen ponds. Proceedings of the 4th Global Fisheries and Aquaculture Research Conference. The Egyptian International Center for Agriculture, Giza, Egypt, 3–5 October 2011. Massive Conferences and Trade Fairs, pp. 451–465.

Alagoa, Y., Elo, O., Andrew, U., Ojukulli, A., 2011. A Report on Aquaculture Value Chain Analysis in the Niger Delta. Partnership Initiatives in the Niger Delta (PIND), p. 57.

Anuta, J.D., 1995. Effects of chicken manure application on water quality and production of *Tilapia guineensis* in freshwater concrete tanks. Journal of Aquaculture in the Tropics 10, 167–176.

Asaduzzaman, M., Wahab, M.A., Verdegem, M.C.J., Azim, M.E., Haque, S., Salam, M.A., 2008. C/N ratio control and substrate addition for periphyton development jointly enhance freshwater prawn *Macrobrachium rosenbergii* production in ponds. Aquaculture 280, 117–123.

Asaduzzaman, M., Wahab, M.A., Verdegem, M.C.J., Mondal, M.N., Azim, M.E., 2009. Effect of stocking density of fresh water prawn *Macrobrachium rosenbergii* and addition of different levels of tilapia *Oreochromis niloticus* on production in C/N controlled periphyton based system. Aquaculture 286, 72–79.

Asaduzzaman, M., Wahab, M.A., Verdegem, M.C.J., Adhikary, R.K., Rahman, S.M.S., Azim, M.E., et al., 2010. Effects of carbohydrate source for maintaining a high C:N ratio and fish driven re-suspension on pond ecology and production in periphyton-based freshwater prawn culture systems. Aquaculture 301, 37–46.

Ayinla, O.A., Oladosu, G.A., Ajiboye, M.O., Ansa, E.J., 1994. Pollution and hazards of integrated livestock-cum-fish farming systems as observed in Nigeria. Paper presented at the CIFA Seminar on African Inland Fisheries, Aquaculture and Environment. Harare, Zimbabwe, 5–7 December, 1994.

Ayinla, O.A., 2007. Analysis of feeds and fertilizers for sustainable aquaculture development in Nigeria. In: Hasan, M.R., Hecht, T., De Silva, S.S., Tacon, A.G.J. (Eds.), Study and Analysis of Feeds and Fertilizers for Sustainable Aquaculture Development. FAO Fisheries Technical Paper No. 497. FAO, Rome, pp. 453–470.

Azim, M.E., Verdegem, M.C.J., Wahab, M.A., van Dam, A.A., Beveridge, M.C.M., 2001. Periphyton boosts production in pond aquaculture systems. World Aquaculture 32, 57–61.

Azim, M.E., Verdegem, M.C.J., Rahman, M.M., Wahab, M.A., van Dam, A.A., Beveridge, M.C.M., 2002. Evaluation of polyculture of Indian major carps in periphyton-based ponds. Aquaculture 213, 131–149.

Azim, M.E., Wahab, M.A., 2005. Periphyton-based pond polyculture. In: Azim, M.E., Verdegem, M.C.J., van Dam, A.A., Beveridge, M.C.M. (Eds.), Periphyton: Ecology, Exploitation and Management. CABI Publishing, Wallingford, UK, pp. 207–222.

Bao-Tong, H., Hua-Zhu, Y., 1984. Integrated Management of Fish-Cum-Duck Forming and its Economic Efficiency and Revenue. Network of Aquaculture Centres in Asia (NACA), Bangkok, Thailand. NACA/WP/84/14.

Barman, B.K., Little, D.C., 2006. Nile tilapia (*Oreochromis niloticus*) seed production in irrigated rice-fields in Northwest Bangladesh—an approach appropriate for poorer farmers? Aquaculture 261, 72–79.

Boyd, C.E., 1974. Lime requirements of Alabama fish ponds. In: Alabama Agricultural Experimental Station, Bulletin, vol. 459. Auburn University, Alabama, USA.

Boyd, C.E., 1976. Nitrogen fertilizer effects on production of tilapia in ponds fertilized with phosphorus and potassium. Aquaculture 7, 385–390.

Boyd, C.E., 2003. Guidelines for aquaculture effluent management at the farm level. Aquaculture 226, 101–112.

Boyd, C.E., Tucker, C.S., Somridhivej, B., 2016. Alkalinity and Hardness: critical but elusive concepts in aquaculture. Journal of the World Aquaculture Society 47, 6–41.

Breine, J.J., Teugels, G.G., Podoor, N., Ollevier, F., 1996. First data on rabbit dung as a water fertilizer in tropical fish culture and its effect on the growth of *Oreochromis niloticus* (Teleostei, Cichlidae). Hydrobiologia 321, 101–107.

Brown, C.L., Bolivar, R.B., Jimenez, E.T., Szyper, J., 2000. Timing of the onset of supplemental feeding of Nile tilapia (*Oreochromis niloticus*) in ponds. In: Fitzsimmons, K., Filho, J.C. (Eds.), Tilapia Culture in the 21st Century. Proceedings from the Fifth International Symposium on Tilapia Aquaculture. American Tilapia Association and ICLARM, Rio de Janeiro, Brazil, pp. 237–240.

Brown, C.L., Bolivar, R.B., Jimenez, E.B.T., Szyper, J.P., 2002. Reduction of feed rations below satiation levels in tilapia pond production. In: McElwee, K., Lewis, K., Nidiffer, M., Buitrago, P. (Eds.), Nineteenth Annual Technical Report. Pond Dynamics/Aquaculture CRSP. Oregon State University, Corvallis, Oregon, pp. 21–23.

Chikafumbwa, F.J.K., 1998. Use of different fishpond inputs on pond mud nutrient levels in integrated crop fish culture. In: Coetzee, L., Gon, J., Kulongowski, C. (Eds.), International Conference for the Paradi Association and the Fisheries Society of Africa. FSA/Paradi, Grahamstown, South Africa, p. 201.

Cruz, P.S., Andalecio, M.N., Bolivar, R.B., Fitzsimmons, K., 2008. Tilapia–Shrimp polyculture in Negros Island, Philippines: a review. Journal of the World Aquaculture Society 39, 713–725.

D'Abramo, L.R., New, M.B., 2010. Nutrition, feeds and feeding. In: New, M.B., Valenti, W.C., Tidwell, J.H., D'Abramo, L.R., Kutty, M.N. (Eds.), Freshwater Prawn: Biology and Farming. Willey-Blackwell, Oxford, UK, pp. 239–255.

Danaher, J.J., Tidwell, J.H., Shawn, D., Coyle, S.D., Dasgupta, S., 2007. Effects of two densities of caged monosex Nile tilapia, *Oreochromis niloticus*, on water quality, phytoplankton populations, and production when polycultured with *Macrobrachium rosenbergii* in temperate ponds. Journal of the World Aquaculture Society 38, 367–382.

De Silva, S.S., 1995. Supplementary feeding in semiintensive aquaculture systems. In: New, M.B., Tacon, A.G.J., Csavas, I. (Eds.), Farm-made

Aquafeeds. FAO Fisheries Technical Paper No. 434. FAO, Rome, pp. 24–60.

Defu, C., Maoxing, S., 1995. Rice–fish culture in China: present and future. In: Mackay, K.T. (Ed.), Rice–Fish Culture in China. International Development Research Center (IDRC), Ottawa, ON, Canada, pp. 15–21.

Dela Cruz, C.R., Lopez, E.A., 1980. Rotational farming of rice and fish in paddies. Fishery Research Philippines 5, 39–52.

Delmendo, M.N., 1980. A review of integrated livestock-fowl-fish farming systems. In: Pullin, R.S.V., Shehadeh, Z.H. (Eds.), Proceedings of Integrated Agriculture-Aquaculture Farming Systems. ICLARM Conference Proceedings No. 4, ICLARM, Manila, Philippines, pp. 59–71.

Diana, J.S., Lin, C.K., Schneeberger, P.J., 1991. Relationships among nutrient inputs, primary production, and yield of *Oreochromis niloticus* in ponds. Aquaculture 92, 323–342.

Diana, J.S., Lin, C.K., Jaiyen, K., 1994. Supplemental feeding of tilapia in fertilized ponds. Journal of the World Aquaculture Society 25, 497–506.

Diana, J.S., Lin, C.K., Yi, Y., 1996. Timing of supplemental feeding for tilapia production. Journal of the World Aquaculture Society 27, 410–419.

Diana, J.S., Lin, C.K., 1998. The effects of fertilization and water management on growth and production of Nile tilapia in deep ponds during the dry season. Journal of the World Aquaculture Society 29, 405–413.

Diana, J.S., 2012. Some principles of pond fertilization for Nile tilapia using organic and inorganic inputs. In: Mischke, C.C. (Ed.), Aquaculture Pond Fertilization: Impacts of Nutrient Input on Production, first ed. John Wiley & Sons, Inc, pp. 163–177.

Dos Santos, M.J.M., Valenti, W.C., 2002. Production of Nile tilapia *Oreochromis niloticus* and freshwater prawn *Macrobrachium rosenbergii* stocked at different densities in polyculture systems. Journal of the World Aquaculture Society 33, 369–376.

Edirisinghe, U., 1990. Suitability of common carp for inclusion in bighead carp-Nile tilapia polyculture systems in ponds fertilized with duck litter. In: Hirano, R., Hanyu, I. (Eds.), The Second Asian Fisheries Forum. Asian Fisheries Society, Manila, Philippines, pp. 201–204.

Edwards, P., Pacharaprakiti, C., Yomjinda, M., 1994a. An assessment of the role of buffalo manure for pond culture of tilapia. I. On-station experiment. Aquaculture 126, 83–95.

Edwards, P., Kaewpaitoon, K., Little, D.C., Siripandh, N., 1994b. An assessment of the role of buffalo manure for pond culture of tilapia. II. Field trial. Aquaculture 126, 97–106.

Edwards, P., Demaine, H., Innes-Taylor, N., Turongruang, D., 1996. Sustainable aquaculture for small-scale farmers: need for a balanced model. Outlook on Agriculture 25, 19–26.

Edwards, P., Lin, C.K., Yakupitiyage, A., 2000. Semi-intensive pond aquaculture. In: Beveridge, M.C.M., McAndrew, B.J. (Eds.), Tilapias: Biology and Exploitation. Kluwer Academic Publishers, Dordrecht/Boston/London, pp. 377–403.

El-Naggar, G., Ibrahim, N.A., Abou Zead, M.Y., 2008. Influence of fertilizer type and stocking density on water quality and growth performance of Nile tilapia-African catfish in polyculture system. In: Elghobashy, H., Fitzsimmons, K., Diab, A. (Eds.), Proceedings of the Eighth International Symposium on Tilapia in Aquaculture. Central Laboratory for Aquaculture Research, Abbasa, pp. 157–170.

El-Sayed, A.-F.M., 1999. Aquaculture Feed and Fertilizer Resource Atlas of Egypt. FAO, Regional Office for the Near East, Cairo, Egypt, p. 105. FIRI/670.

El-Sayed, A.-F.M., 2003. Effects of fermentation methods on the nutritive value of water hyacinth for Nile tilapia, *Oreochromis niloticus* (L.) fingerlings. Aquaculture 218, 471–478.

El-Sayed, A.-F.M., 2013a. Tilapia feed management practices in Sub-Saharan Africa. In: Hasan, M.R., New, M.B. (Eds.), *On-farm Feeding and Feed Management in Aquaculture.* FAO Fisheries and Aquaculture Technical Paper No. 583. FAO, Rome, pp. 377–405.

El-Sayed, A.-F.M., 2013b. On-farm feed management practices for Nile tilapia (*Oreochromis niloticus*) in Egypt. In: Hasan, M.R., New, M.B. (Eds.), *On-farm Feeding and Feed Management in Aquaculture.* FAO Fisheries and Aquaculture Technical Paper No. 583. FAO, Rome, pp. 101–129.

Fath El-Bab, A., Mostafa, M., Hassan, A., 2014. Effect of exploitation of fish ponds in the cultivation of wheat in the winter season on growth performance and total yield of *Oreochromis niloticus.* Egyptian Journal of Aquatic Biology and Fisheries 18, 53–66.

Frei, M., Razzak, M.A., Hossain, M.M., Oehme, M., Dewan, S., Becker, K., 2007. Performance of common carp, *Cyprinus carpio* L. and Nile tilapia, *Oreochromis niloticus* (L.) in integrated rice–fish culture in Bangladesh. Aquaculture 262, 250–259.

GAFRD (General Authority for Fish Resources Development), 2016. Fish Statistics Year Book-2014, 24th Edition. Ministry of Agriculture and Land Reclamation, Cairo.

GAFRD (General Authority for Fish Resources Development), 2018. Fish Statistics Year Book-2016, 26th Edition. Ministry of Agriculture and Land Reclamation, Cairo.

Garcia-Pérez, A., Alston, D.E., Cortés-Maldonado, R., 2000. Growth, survival, yield, and size distributions of freshwater prawn *Macrobrachium rosenbergii* and tilapia *Oreochromis niloticus* in polyculture and monoculture systems in Puerto Rico. Journal of the World Aquaculture Society 31, 446–451.

Garcia, F., Romera, D.M., Sousa, N.S., Paiva-Ramos, I., Onaka, E.M., 2016. The potential of periphyton-based cage culture of Nile tilapia in a Brazilian reservoir. Aquaculture 464, 229–235.

Garcia, F., Sabbag, O.J., Kimpara, J.M., Romera, D.M., Sousa, N.S., Onaka, E.M., et al., 2017. Periphyton-based cage culture of Nile tilapia: an interesting model for small-scale farming. Aquaculture 479, 838–844.

Gonzales-Corre, K., 1988. Polyculture of tiger shrimp (*Penaeus monodon*) with Nile tilapia (*Oreochromis niloticus*) in brackishwater fishponds. In: Pullin, R.S.V., Bhukaswan, T., Tonguthai, K., Maclean, J.L. (Eds.), Proceedings of the Second International Symposium on Tilapia in Aquaculture. ICLARM Conference Proceedings No. 15. Department of Fisheries, Bangkok, Thailand, and ICLARM, Manila, Philippines, pp. 15–20.

Gopalakrishnan, V., 1988. Role of tilapia (*Oreochromis andersonii*) in integrated farming systems in Zambia. In: Pullin, R.S.V., Bhukaswan, T., Tonguthai, K., Maclean, J.L. (Eds.), Proceedings of the Second International Symposium on Tilapia in Aquaculture. ICLARM Conference Proceedings No. 15. Department of Fisheries, Thailand, and ICLARM, Manila, Philippines, pp. 21–28.

Green, B.W., Phelps, R.P., Alvarenga, H.R., 1989. The effect of manures and chemical fertilizers on the production of *Oreochromis niloticus* in earthen ponds. Aquaculture 76, 37–42.

Green, B.W., Teichert-Coddington, D.R., Phelps, R.P., 1990. Response of tilapia yield and economics to varying rates of organic fertilization and season in two Central American countries. Aquaculture 90, 279–290.

Green, B.W., 1992. Substitution of organic manure for pelleted feed in tilapia production. Aquaculture 101, 213–222.

Green, B.W., El Nagdy, Z., Hebicha, H., 2002. Evaluation of Nile tilapia pond management strategies in Egypt. Aquaculture Research 33, 1037–1048.

Halwart, M., 1998. Trends in rice-fish farming. FAO Aquaculture Newsletter 18, 3–11.

Haque, M.R., Islam, M.A., Rahman, M.M., Shirin, M.F., Wahab, M.A., Azim, M.E., 2015. Effects of C/N ratio and periphyton substrates on pond ecology and production performance in giant freshwater prawn *Macrobrachium rosenbergii* (De Man, 1879) and tilapia *Oreochromis niloticus* (Linnaeus, 1758) polyculture system. Aquaculture Research 46, 1139–1155.

Haque, M.R., Islam, M.A., Wahab, M.A., Hoq, M.E., Rahman, M.M., Azim, M.E., 2016. Evaluation of production performance and profitability of hybrid red tilapia and genetically improved farmed tilapia (GIFT) strains in the carbon/nitrogen controlled periphyton-based (C/N- CP) on-farm prawn culture system in Bangladesh. Aquaculture Reports 4, 101–111.

Haroon, A.K.Y., Alam, M., 1992. Integrated Paddy-Cum-Fish/shrimp Farming. Fisheries Research Institute, Mymensingh-2201, p. 41. Final Report.

Haroon, A.K.Y., Pittman, K.A., 1997. Rice-fish culture: feeding, growth and yield of two size classes of *Puntius gonionotus* Bleeker and *Oreochromis* spp. in Bangladesh. Aquaculture 154, 261–281.

Hem, S., Avit, J.L.B., 1994. First results on "acadja enclose" as an extensive aquaculture system (West Africa). Bulletin of Marine Science 55, 1038–1049.

Hepher, B., Pruginin, Y., 1982. Tilapia culture in ponds under controlled conditions. In: Pullin, R.S.V., Lowe-McConnell, R.H. (Eds.), The Biology and Culture of Tilapias. ICLARM Conference Proceedings No.7, ICLARM, Manila, Philippines, pp. 185–203.

Hernandez Barraza, C., Loredo, J., Adame, J., Fitzsimmons, K.M., 2012. Effect of Nile tilapia (*Oreochromis niloticus*) on the growth performance of Pacific white shrimp (*Litopenaeus vannamei*) in a sequential polyculture system. Latin American Journal of Aquatic Research 40, 936–942.

Hernández, M., Gasca-Leyva, E., Milstein, A., 2014. Polyculture of mixed-sex and male populations of Nile tilapia (*Oreochromis niloticus*) with the Mayan cichlid (*Cichlasoma urophthalmus*). Aquaculture 418–419, 26–31.

Hickling, C.E., 1962. Fish Culture. Faber and Faber Ltd, London, p. 295.

Hopkins, K.D., Cruz, E.M., 1982. The ICLARM-CLSU Integrated Animal-Fish Farming Project: Final Report. ICLARM Technical Report 5. ICLARM, Manila, Philippines.

Hossain, M.A., Mridha, M.A.R., Shah, A.K.M.A., Nahiduzzaman, M., Uddin, M.S., 2015. Performance of mono-sex tilapia (*Oreochromis niloticus*) in rice field with different ditch size. Aquaculture Research 46, 1891–1901.

Huchette, S.M.H., Beveridge, M.C.M., Baird, D.J., Ireland, M., 2000. The impacts of grazing by tilapias (*Oreochromis niloticus* L.) on periphyton communities growing on artificial substrate in cages. Aquaculture 186, 45–60.

Huchette, S.M.H., Beveridge, M.C.M., 2003. Technical and economical evaluation of periphyton-based cage culture of tilapia (*Oreochromis niloticus*) in tropical freshwater cages. Aquaculture 218, 219–234.

Jamu, D., 2001. Opportunities and challenges for African aquaculture. In: Subasinghe, R., Tarlochan, S. (Eds.), Tilapia: Production, Marketing and Technological Developments. Proceedings of the Tilapia 2001 International Technical and Trade Conference on Tilapia. Kuala Lumpur, Malaysia, pp. 105–112.

Jatobá, A., Vieira, F.D.N., Buglione-Neto, C.C., Mouriño, J.L., Silva, B.C., Seiftter, W.Q., et al., 2011. Diet supplemented with probiotic for Nile tilapia in polyculture system with marine shrimp. Fish Physiology and Biochemistry 37, 725–732.

Junior, B., Paula, A., Azevedo, C.M.D.B., Pontes, F.S., Henry-Silva, G.G., 2012. Polyculture of Nile tilapia and shrimp at different stocking densities. Revista Brasileira de Zootecnia 41, 1561–1569.

Karim, M., Little, D.C., Kabir, M.S., Verdegem, M.J.C., Telfer, T., Wahab, M.A., 2011. Enhancing benefits from polycultures including tilapia (*Oreochromis niloticus*) within integrated pond-dike systems: a participatory trial with households of varying socio-economic level in rural and peri-urban areas of Bangladesh. Aquaculture 314, 225–235.

Keshavanath, P., Gangadhar, B., Ramesh, T.J., van Dam, A.A., Beveridge, M.C.M., Verdegem, M.C.J., 2004. Effects of bamboo substrate and supplemental feeding on growth and production of hybrid red tilapia fingerlings (*Oreochromis mossambicus x Oreochromis niloticus*). Aquaculture 235, 303–314.

Keshavanath, P., Gangadhar, B., 2005. Research on periphyton-based aquaculture in India. In: Azim, M.E., Verdegem, M.C.J., van Dam, A.A., Beveridge, M.C.M. (Eds.), Periphyton: Ecology, Exploitation and Management. CABI Publishing, Wallingford, UK, pp. 223–236.

Kimpara, J.M., Tito Rosa, F.R., De Lima Preto, B., Valenti, W.C., 2011. Limnology of *Macrobrachium amazonicum* grow-out ponds subject to high inflow of nutrient-rich water and different stocking and harvest management. Aquaculture Research 42, 1289–1297.

Knud-Hansen, C.F., 1992. Pond history as a source of error in fish culture experiments: a quantitative assessment using covariance analysis. Aquaculture 105, 21–36.

Knud-Hansen, C.F., Batterson, T.R., Mcnab, C.D., 1993. The role of chicken manure in the production of Nile tilapia, *Oreochromis niloticus* (L.). Aquaculture and Fisheries Management 24, 483–493.

Knud-Hansen, C.F., Batterson, T.R., 1994. Effect of fertilization frequency on the production of Nile tilapia (*Oreochromis niloticus*). Aquaculture 123, 271–280.

Knud-Hansen, C.F., 1998. Pond Fertilization: Ecological Approach and Practical Applications. Pond Dynamics/Aquaculture CRSP, Oregon State University, Corvallis, Oregon, p. 125.

Koohanfkan, P., Furtado, J., 2004. Traditional rice-fish systems as globally indigenous agricultural heritage systems (GIAHS). International Rice Commission Newsletter 53, 66–74.

Kunda, M., Azim, M.E., Wahab, M.A., Dewan, S., Majid, M.A., Thilsted, S.H., 2009. Effects of including catla and tilapia in a freshwater prawn-mola polyculture in a rotational rice-fish culture systems. Aquaculture Research 40, 1089–1098.

Lazard, J., Oswald, M., 1995. Mixed culture of African catfish-tilapia: polyculture or police fish system. Aquatic Living Resources 8, 455–463.

Ledgerwood, R.D., Hughes, D.G., Ortis, V., 1978. Wet and Dry Season Comparison of *Tilapia Aurea* Production in El Salvador in New Fertilized and Unfertilized Earthen Ponds. Paper Presented at the 9th Annual Meeting of the World Mariculture Society, Atlanta, Georgia, USA, 3 January, 1978.

Lightfoot, C., Costa-Pierce, B.A., Bimbao, M.A.P., Dela Cruz, C.R., 1992. Introduction to rice-fish research and development in Asia. In: Dela Cruz, C.R., Lightfoot, C., Costa-Pierce, B.A., Carangal, V.R., Bimbao, M.A.P. (Eds.), Rice-fish Research and Development in Asia. ICLARM Conference Proceedings No. 24, ICLARM, Manila, Philippines, pp. 1–10.

Limbu, S.M., Shoko, A.P., Lamtane, H.A., Shirima, E.D., Kishe-Machumu, M.A., Mgana, H.F., et al., 2015. Effect of initial stocking size of the predatory African sharptooth catfish (*Clarias gariepinus*) on recruits, growth performance, survival and yield of mixed-sex Nile tilapia (*Oreochromis niloticus*) in concrete tank culture system. International Aquatic Research 7, 63–73.

Lin, C.K., Diana, J., 1995. Co-culture of Nile tilapia (*Oreochromis niloticus*) and hybrid catfish (*Clarias macrocephalus* x *C. gariepinus*) in ponds. Aquatic Living Resources 8, 449–454.

Lin, C.K., Yi, Y., Diana, J., 1997. The effects of pond management strategies on nutrient budgets: Thailand. In: Fourteenth Annual Technical Report. Pond Dynamics/Aquaculture CRSP. Oregon State University, Corvallis, Oregon, USA, pp. 19–24.

Lin, C.K., Yi, Y., 2003. Minimizing environmental impacts of freshwater aquaculture and reuse of pond effluents and mud. Aquaculture 226, 57–68.

Liti, D., Cherop, L., Munguti, J., Chhorn, L., 2005. Growth and economic performance of Nile tilapia (*Oreochromis niloticus* L.) fed on two formulated diets and two locally available feeds in fertilized ponds. Aquaculture Research 36, 746–752.

Liti, D.M., Mugo, R.M., Munguti, J.M., Waidbacher, H., 2006. Growth and economic performance of Nile tilapia (*Oreochromis niloticus* L.) fed on three brans (maize, wheat and rice) in fertilized ponds. Aquaculture Nutrition 12, 239–245.

Longwe, P.M., Kang'ombe, J., Kaunda, E.K.W., 2010. A case study of GK Aqua farms in Chikwawa District, Malawi. EC: FP7 Project, SARNISSA, p. 21.

Lukefahr, S.D., 2007. Strategies for the development of small- and medium-scale rabbit farming in South-East Asia. Livestock Research for Rural Development 19 (9). http://www.lrrd.org/lrrd19/9/luke19138.htm.

Makridis, P., Costa, R.A., Dinis, M.T., 2006. Microbial conditions and antimicrobial activity in cultures of two microalgae species, *Tetraselmis chuii* and *Chlorella minutissima*, and effect on bacterial load of enriched *Artemia metanauplii*. Aquaculture 255, 76–81.

Mandal, R.B., Jha, D.K., Shrestha, M.K., Pant, J., Rai, S., Pandit, N.P., 2014. Cage-pond integration of African catfish (*Clarias gariepinus*) and Nile tilapia (*Oreochromis niloticus*) with carps. Aquaculture Research 45, 1311–1318.

Mang-Umphan, K., Arce, R.G., 1988. Culture of Nile tilapia (*Oreochromis niloticus*) in a rice-fish culture system using chemical and commercial organic fertilizers. In: Pullin, R.S.V., Bhukaswan, T., Tonguthai, K., Maclean, J.L. (Eds.), Proceedings of the Second International Symposium on Tilapia in Aquaculture. ICLARM Conference Proceedings No. 15. Department of Fisheries, Thailand, and ICLARM, Manila, Philippines, pp. 59–62.

Manyala, J.O., Pomeroy, R.S., Nen, P., Fitzsimmons, K., Shrestha, M.K., Diana, J.S., 2015. Low-cost tilapia production with fertilization and supplementary feeding. World Aquaculture 1, 43–46.

Masser, M., 2017. Tilapia co-culture in cages and in-pond raceways. In: Perschbacher, P.W., Stickney, R.R. (Eds.), Tilapia in Intensive Co-culture. Willey-Blackwell, Oxford, UK, pp. 148–155.

Mataka, L., Kang'ombe, J., 2007. Effect of substitution of maize bran with chicken manure in semi-intensive pond culture of *Tilapia rendalli* (Boulenger). Aquaculture Research 38, 940–946.

McGeachin, R.B., Stickney, R.R., 1982. Manuring rates for production of blue tilapia in simulated sewage lagoons receiving laying hen waste. Progressive Fish-Culturist 44, 25–28.

McKinnon, A.D., Trott, L.A., Alongi, D.M., Davidson, A., 2002. Water column production and nutrient characteristics in mangrove creeks receiving shrimp farm effluent. Aquaculture Research 33, 55–73.

Middendorp, A.J., 1995. Pond farming of Nile tilapia *Oreochromis niloticus* L. in northern Cameroon. Mixed culture of large tilapia (>200 g) with cattle manure and cottonseed cake as pond inputs, and African catfish, *Clarias gariepinus* (Burchell), as police-fish. Aquaculture Research 26, 723–730.

Miller, J., 2006. The potential of development of aquaculture and its integration with irrigation within the context of the FAO Special Programme for Food Security in the Sahel. In: Halwart, M., van Dam, A. (Eds.), Integrated Irrigation and Aquaculture in West Africa-Concept, Practices and Potential, vol. 5. FAO, Rome, pp. 61–74.

Milstein, A., 1997. Do management procedures affect the ecology of warm water polyculture ponds. World Aquaculture 28, 12–19.

Milstein, A., Lev, O., 2004. Organic tilapia culture in Israel. In: Bolivar, R., Mair, G., Fitzsimmons, K. (Eds.), Proceedings of the Sixth International Symposium on Tilapia in Aquaculture. Manila, Philippines, pp. 657–660.

Milstein, A., Joseph, D., Peretz, Y., Harpaz, S., 2005. Evaluation of organic tilapia culture in periphyton-based ponds. Israeli Journal of Aquaculture Bamidgeh 57, 143–155.

Milstein, A., Peretz, Y., Harpaz, S., 2009. Culture of organic tilapia to market size in periphyton-based ponds with reduced feed inputs. Aquaculture Research 40, 55–59.

Ming, L.Q., Yi, Y., 2004. Tilapia culture in China. In: Bolivar, R., Mair, G., Fitzsimmons, K. (Eds.), Proceedings of the Sixth International Symposium on Tilapia Aquaculture. Manila, Philippines, pp. 18–27.

Morrison, J.R., Deavours, W.L., Jones, J.C., Tabb, M.A., 1995. Maximizing first–year growth of mixed-sex blue tilapia *Oreochromis aureus* in polyculture with catfish *Ictalurus* spp. Journal of the World Aquaculture Society 26, 447–452.

Mridha, M.A.R., Hossain, M.A., Azad Shah, A.K.M., Uddin, M.S., Nahiduzzaman, M., 2014. Effects of stocking density on production and economics of all-male tilapia (*Oreochromis niloticus*) culture in a rain fed rice-fish ecosystem. Journal of Applied Aquaculture 26, 60–70.

Muendo, P.N., Milstein, A., van Dam, A.A., El-Naggar, G., Stoorvogel, J.J., Verdegem, M.C.J., 2006. Exploring the trophic structure in organically fertilized and feed-driven tilapia culture environments using multivariate analyses. Aquaculture Research 37, 151–163.

Natarajan, P., Aravindan, C.M., 2002. Status of tilapia farming and its prospects in India. In: Guerrero III, R.D., Guerrero-del Castillo, M.R. (Eds.), Tilapia Farming in the 21st Century. Proceedings of the

International Forum on Tilapia Farming in the 21st Century (Tilapia Forum 2002). The Philippine Fisheries Association, Inc., Los Banos, Laguna, Philippines, pp. 78–86.

New, M.B., Valenti, W.C., 2017. Tilapia-*Macrobrachium* polyculture. In: Perschbacher, P.W., Stickney, R.R. (Eds.), Tilapia in Intensive Co-culture. Willey-Blackwell, Oxford, UK, pp. 156–185.

Nitithamyong, C., Chiayvareesajja, J., Chiayvareesajja, S., Tansakul, R., Wongwit, C., 1990. Growth and production of Nile tilapia (*Oreochromis niloticus*) in monoculture and polyculture with snakehead (*Channa striata*), and in integrated culture with pig and snakehead. In: De Silva, S.S. (Ed.), Fish Nutrition Research in Asia. Proceedings of the Fourth Asian Fish Nutrition Workshop. Special Publication No. 5. Asian Fisheries Society, Manila, Philippines, pp. 175–180.

Njoku, D.C., Ejiogu, C.O., 1999. On-farm trials of an integrated fish-cum-poultry farming system using indigenous chickens. Aquaculture Research 30, 399–408.

Nnaji, J.C., Madu, C.T., Raji, A., 2013. Profitability of rice-fish arming in Bida, North Central Nigeria. Journal of Fisheries and Aquatic Science 8, 148–153.

Norberg, J., 1999. Periphyton fouling as a marginal energy source in tropical tilapia cage farming. Aquaculture Research 30, 427–430.

Ofori, J.K., 1988. The effect of predation by *Lates niloticus* on overpopulation and stunting in mixed sex culture of tilapia species in ponds. In: Pullin, R.S.V., Bhukaswan, T., Tonguthai, K., Maclean, J.L. (Eds.), Proceedings of the Second International Symposium on Tilapia in Aquaculture. ICLARM Conference Proceedings No. 15. Department of Fisheries, Thailand, and ICLARM, Manila, Philippines, pp. 69–73.

Ofori, J., Abban, E.K., Otoo, E., Wakatsuki, T., 2005. Rice–fish culture: an option for smallholder Sawah rice farmers of the West African lowlands. Ecological Engineering 24, 233–239.

Oo, M.T., Shahabuddin, A.M., Thakur, D.P., Mon, A.A., Yakupitiyage, A., Bart, A.N., et al., 2015. Optimization of phosphorus fertilizer in supplemental feed-fed based Nile tilapia (*Oreochromis niloticus*) ponds. Aquaculture Research 46, 2859–2870.

Perschbacher, P.W., 1995. Algal management in intensive channel catfish production trials. World Aquaculture 26, 65–68.

Pillay, T.V.R., 1990. Aquaculture Principles and Practices. Blackwell Science Ltd, Fishing News Books, Oxford, Edinburgh, London, p. 575.

Pudadera, B.J.J., Corre, K.C., Coniza, E., Taleon, G.A., 1986. Integrated farming of broiler chickens with fish and shrimp in brackishwater ponds. In: Maclean, J.L., Dizon, L.B., Hosillos, L.V. (Eds.), Proceedings of the First Asian Fisheries Forum. Asian Fisheries Society, Manila, Philippines, pp. 141–144.

Rasowo, J., Auma, E.O., 2006. On-farm Trials With Rice-fish Cultivation in the West Kano Rice Irrigation Scheme, 29. NAGA, Kenya, pp. 36–41.

Richard, M., Trottier, C., Verdegem, M.C.J., Hussenot, J.M.E., 2009. Submersion time, depth, substrate type and sampling method as variation sources of marine periphyton. Aquaculture 295, 209–217.

Richard, M., Maurice, J.T., Anginot, A., Paticat, F., Verdegem, M.C.J., Hussenot, J.M.E., 2010. Influence of periphyton substrates and rearing density on *Liza aurata* growth and production in marine nursery ponds. Aquaculture 310, 106–111.

Rothuis, A.J., Nam, C.Q., Richter, C.J.J., Ollevier, F., 1998. Polyculture of silver barb, *Puntius gonionotus* (Bleeker), Nile tilapia, *Oreochromis niloticus* (L.), and common carp, *Cyprinus carpio* L., in Vietnamese ricefields: fish production parameters. Aquaculture Research 29, 661–668.

Sakr, E.M., Shalaby, S.M., Wassef, E.A., El-Sayed, A.-F.M., Moneim, A.I.A., 2015. Evaluation of periphyton as a food source for Nile tilapia (*Oreochromis niloticus*) juveniles fed reduced protein levels in cages. Journal of Applied Aquaculture 27, 50–60.

Sanni, D., Juanich, G., 2006. A feasibility study of rice-fish farming in Western Africa. In: Halwart, M., van Dam, A. (Eds.), Integrated Irrigation and Aquaculture in West Africa- Concept, Practices and Potential, vol. 6. FAO, Rome, pp. 75–78.

Sevilleja, R.C., Cagauan, A.G., Lopez, E.A., Dela Cruz, C.R., van Dam, A.A., 1992. Component technology research in rice-fish systems in the Philippines. In: Dela Cruz, C.R., Lightfoot, C., Costa-Pierce, B.A., Carangal, V.R., Bimbao, M.A.P. (Eds.), Rice-fish Research and Development in Asia. ICLARM Conference Proceedings No. 24, ICLARM, Manila, Philippines, pp. 373–384.

Shevgoor, L., Knud-Hansen, C.F., Edwards, P., 1994. An assessment of the role of buffalo manure for pond culture of tilapia. III. Limiting factors. Aquaculture 126, 107–118.

Shoko, A.P., Limbu, S.M., Mrosso, H.D.J., Mkenda, A.F., Mgaya, Y.D., 2016. Effect of stocking density on growth, production and economic benefits of mixed sex Nile tilapia (*Oreochromis niloticus*) and African sharptooth catfish (*Clarias gariepinus*) in polyculture and monoculture. Aquaculture Research 47, 36–50.

Shrestha, M.K., Lin, C.K., 1996a. Determination of phosphorus saturation level in relation to clay content in formulated pond muds. Aquacultural Engineering 15, 441–459.

Shrestha, M.K., Lin, C.K., 1996b. Phosphorus fertilization strategy in fish ponds based on sediment phosphorus saturation level. Aquaculture 142, 207–219.

Shrestha, M.K., Sharma, R.L., Gharti, K., Diana, J.S., 2011. Polyculture of sahar (*Tor putitora*) with mixed-sex Nile tilapia. Aquaculture 319, 284–289.

Simão, B.R., Brito, L.O., Maia, A.S.C., Miranda, L.C., Azevedo, C.M.D.B., 2013. Stocking densities and feeding strategies in shrimp and tilapia polyculture in tanks. Pesquisa Agropecuária Brasileira 48, 1088–1095.

Sin, A.W., 1980. Integrated fish husbandry systems in Hong Kong, with case studies on duck- fish and goose-fish systems. In: Pullin, R.S.V., Shehadeh, Z.H. (Eds.), Integrated Agriculture-Aquaculture Farming Systems. ICLARM Conference Proceedings No. 4, ICLARM, Manila, Philippines, pp. 113–123.

Soliman, A.K., El-Horbeety, A.A.A., Essa, M.A.R., Kosba, M.A., Kariony, I.A., 2000. Effects of introducing ducks into fish ponds on water quality, natural productivity and fish production together with the economic evaluation of the integrated and non-integrated systems. Aquaculture International 8, 315–326.

Sri-Uam, P., Donnuea, S., Powtongsook, S., Pavasant, P., 2016. Integrated multi-trophic recirculating aquaculture system for Nile tilapia (*Oreochromis niloticus*). Sustainability 8, 592–607.

Tabaro, S.R., Mutanga, O., Rugege, D., Micha, J.-C., 2012a. Rearing rabbits over earthen fish ponds in Rwanda: effects on water and sediment quality, growth, and production of Nile tilapia *Oreochromis niloticus*. Journal of Applied Aquaculture 24, 170–181.

Tabaro, S.R., Mutanga, O., Rugege, D., Micha, J.-C., 2012b. Optimum rabbit density over fish ponds to optimise Nile tilapia production in an integrated rabbit–fish system in Rwanda. African Journal of Aquatic Science 37, 165–174.

Tacon, A.G.J., 1987. The Nutrition and Feeding of Farmed Fish and Shrimp- A Training Manual. 2. Nutrient Source and Composition, p. 129. FAO Field Document. Project GCP/RLA/075/ITA, Field Document NO. 5, Brasilia, Brazil.

Tacon, A.G.J., 1995. Feed formulation and on-farm feed management. In: New, M.B., Tacon, A.G.J., Csavas, I. (Eds.), Farm-made Aquafeeds. FAO Fisheries Technical Paper 343, FAO, Rome, pp. 61–74.

Tahoun, A.-A., Suloma, A., Hammouda, Y., Abo-State, H., El-Haroun, E., 2013. The effect of stocking different ratios of Nile tilapia *Oreochromis niloticus*, striped mullet *Mugil cephalus*, and thinlip grey mullet *Liza ramada* in polyculture ponds on biomass yield, feed efficiency, and production economics. North American Journal of Aquaculture 75, 548–555.

Tendencia, E.A., dela Peña, M.R., Fermin, A.C., Lio-Po, G.C., Choresca Jr., C.H., Inui, Y., 2004. Antibacterial activity of tilapia *Tilapia hornorum* against *Vibrio harveyi*. Aquaculture 232, 145–152.

Tendencia, E.A., dela Peña, M.R., Choresca Jr., C.H., 2005. Efficiency of *Chlorella* sp. and *Tilapia hornorum* in controlling the growth of luminous bacteria in a simulated shrimp culture environment. Aquaculture 249, 55–62.

Thankur, D.P., Yi, Y., Diana, J.S., Lin, C.K., 2004. Effects of fertilization and feeding strategy on water quality, growth performance, nutrient utilization and economic return in Nile tilapia (*Oreochromis niloticus*) ponds. In: Bolivar, R., Mair, G., Fitzsimmons, K. (Eds.), Proceedings of the Sixth International Symposium on Tilapia in Aquaculture. Manila, Philippines, pp. 529–543.

Tian, X., Li, D., Dong, S., Yan, X., Qi, Z., Liu, G., et al., 2001. An experimental study on closed-polyculture of penaeid shrimp with tilapia and constricted tagelus. Aquaculture 202, 57–71.

Tidwell, J.H., Coyle, S., Van Amum, A., Weibel, C., 2000. Production response of freshwater prawn *Macrobrachium rosenbergii* to increasing amounts of artificial substrate in ponds. Journal of the World Aquaculture Society 31, 452–458.

Tidwell, J.H., Bratvold, D., 2005. Utility of added substrates in shrimp culture. In: Azim, M.E., Verdegem, M.C.J., van Dam, A.A., Beveridge, M.C.M. (Eds.), Periphyton: Ecology, Exploitation and Management. CABI Publishing, Wallingford, UK, pp. 247–268.

Tidwell, J.H., Coyle, S.D., Bright, L.A., 2010. Polyculture of Nile Tilapia, *Oreochromis niloticus*, either confined in cages or unconfined in freshwater prawn, *Macrobrachium rosenbergii*, ponds. Journal of the World Aquaculture Society 41, 616–625.

Torres, N.J., Macabale, N.A., Mercado, J.R., 1992. On-farm rice-fish farming systems research in Guimba, Nueva, Philippines. In: Dela Cruz, C.R., Lightfoot, C., Costa-Pierce, B.A., Carangal, V.R., Bimbao, M.A.P. (Eds.), Rice-fish Research and Development in Asia. ICLARM Conference Proceedings No. 24, ICLARM, Manila, Philippines, pp. 295–299.

Uddin, S., Azim, M.E., Wahab, M.A., Verdegem, M.C.J., 2006. The potential of mixed culture of genetically improved farmed tilapia (GIFT, *Oreochromis niloticus*) and freshwater prawn (*Macrobrachium rosenbergii*) in periphyton-based systems. Aquaculture Research 37, 241–247.

Uddin, S., Farzana, A., Fatema, M.K., Azim, M.E., Wahab, M.A., Verdegem, M.C.J., 2007a. Technical evaluation of tilapia (*Oreochromis niloticus*) monoculture and tilapia–prawn (*Macrobrachium rosenbergii*) polyculture in earthen ponds with or without substrates for periphyton development. Aquaculture 269, 232–240.

Uddin, M.S., Rahman, S.M., Azim, M.E., Wahab, M.A., Verdegem, M.C.J., Verreth, J.A.J., 2007b. Effects of stocking density on production and economics of Nile tilapia (*Oreochromis niloticus*) and freshwater prawn (*Macrobrachium rosenbergii*) polyculture in periphyton-based systems. Aquaculture Research 38, 1759–1769.

Uddin, S., Azim, M.E., Wahab, M.A., Verdegem, M.C.J., 2009. Effects of substrate addition and supplemental feeding on plankton composition and production in tilapia (*Oreochromis niloticus*) and water prawn (*Macrobrachium rosenbergii*) polyculture. Aquaculture 297, 99–105.

van Dam, A.A., Beveridge, M.C.M., Azim, M.E., Verdegem, M.C.J., 2002. The potential of fish production based on periphyton. Reviews in Fish Biology and Fisheries 12, 1–31.

van Der Heijden, P.G.M., 2012. Water use at integrated aquaculture-agriculture farms. experiences with limited water resources in Egypt. Global Aquaculture Advocate 4, 28–31.

Veverica, K.L., Bowman, J., Popma, T., 2001. Global experiment: optimization of nitrogen fertilization rate in freshwater tilapia production ponds. In: Gupta, A., McElwee, K., Burke, D., Burright, J., Cummings, X., Egna, H. (Eds.), Eighteenth Annual Technical Report. Pond Dynamics/Aquaculture CRSP. Oregon State University, Corvallis, Oregon, USA, pp. 13–22.

Vromant, N., Rothuis, A.J., Cuc, N.T.T., Ollevier, F., 1998. The effect of fish on the abundance of the rice Caseworm *Nymphula depunctalis* (Guenée) (Lepidoptera: Pyralidae) in direct seeded, concurrent rice-fish fields. Biocontrol Science and Technology 8, 539–546.

Vromant, N., Nam, C.Q., Ollevier, F., 2002. Growth performance and use of natural food by *Oreochromis niloticus* (L.) in polyculture systems with *Barbodes gonionotus* (Bleeker) and *Cyprinus carpio* (L.) in intensively cultivated rice fields. Aquaculture Research 33, 969–978.

Wahab, M.A., Azim, M.E., Ali, M.H., Beveridge, M.C.M., Khan, S., 1999a. The potential of periphyton-based culture of the native major carp calbaush, *Labeo calbasu* (Hamilton). Aquaculture Research 30, 409–419.

Wahab, M.A., Mannan, M.A., Huda, M.A., Azim, M.E., Tollervey, A.G., Beveridge, M.C.M., 1999b. Effect of periphyton grown on bamboo substrates on growth and production of Indian major carp, rohu (*Labeo rohita*). Bangladesh Journal of Fisheries Research 3, 1–10.

Waidbacher, H., Liti, D.M., Fungomeli, M., Mbaluka, R.K., Munguti, J.M., Straif, M., 2006. Influence of pond fertilization and feeding rate on growth performance, economic returns and water quality in a small-scale cage-cum-pond integrated system for production of Nile tilapia (*Oreochromis niloticus* L.). Aquaculture Research 37, 594–600.

Wang, J.-Q., Li, D., Dong, S., Wang, K., Tian, X., 1998. Experimental studies on polyculture in closed shrimp ponds. I. Intensive polyculture of Chinese shrimp *Penaeus chinensis* with tilapia hybrids. Aquaculture 163, 11–27.

Wang, M., Lu, M., 2016. Tilapia polyculture: a global review. Aquaculture Research 47, 2363–2374.

Watanabe, W.O., Losordo, T.M., Fitzsimmons, K., Hanley, F., 2002. Tilapia production systems in the Americas: Technological advances, trends, and challenges. Reviews in Fisheries Science 10, 465–498.

Yakupitiyage, D., 1995. On-farm feed preparation and feeding strategies for carps and tilapias. In: New, M.B., Tacon, A.G.J., Csavas, I. (Eds.), Farm-made Aquafeeds. FAO Fisheries Technical Paper 343, FAO, Rome, pp. 87–100.

Yang, J., Huang, X., 2011. Technology of polyculture of grass carp with tilapia in ponds. Aquaculture 3, 46–48.

Yi, Y., Lin, C.K., 2000. Integrated cage culture in ponds: concepts, practice and perspectives. In: Liao, C.I., Lin, C.K. (Eds.), Proceedings of the First International Symposium on Cage Aquaculture in Asia. Asian Fisheries Society, Quezon City, Philippines, pp. 233–240.

Yi, Y., Lin, C.K., 2001. Effects of biomass of caged Nile tilapia (*Oreochromis niloticus*) and aeration on the growth and yields in an integrated cage-cum-pond system. Aquaculture 195, 253–267.

Yi, Y., Lin, C.K., Diana, J.S., 2003. Hybrid catfish (*Clarias macrocephalus x C. gariepinus*) and Nile tilapia (*Oreochromis niloticus*) culture in an integrated pen-cum-pond system: growth performance and nutrient budget. Aquaculture 217, 395–408.

Yi, Y., Diana, J.S., Lin, C.K., 2004a. Supplemental feeding for red tilapia culture in brackishwater. In: Bolivar, R., Mair, G., Fitzsimmons, K. (Eds.), Proceedings of the Sixth International Symposium on Tilapia in Aquaculture. Manila, Philippines, pp. 451–462.

Yi, Y., Diana, J.S., Shrestha, M.K., Lin, C.K., 2004b. Culture of mixed-sex Nile tilapia with predatory snakehead. In: Bolivar, R., Mair, G., Fitzsimmons, K. (Eds.), Proceedings of the Sixth International Symposium on Tilapia in Aquaculture. Manila, Philippines, pp. 544–557.

Chapter 6

Intensive culture

Chapter outline

6.1 Introduction

Intensive aquaculture is simply the employment of high stocking densities of cultured species, in order to maximize the production with the minimal use of water. Such systems depend exclusively on artificial feeding and water reuse and/or exchange. Intensive systems yield high production, ranging from 100 to >500 t ha^{-1} per year (Muir et al., 2000). However, they require high capital and operating costs as well as high levels of technology and management tools. Therefore, fish farmers should fully consider the following criteria before adopting intensive farming systems:

1. Assurance of free and permanent access to seed supply.
2. Availability of funds needed for construction, maintenance and operation of the system.
3. Availability of technology, management tools and experienced personnel.
4. Awareness of environmental impacts of intensive farming systems and creating the efficient and reliable conditions and mitigation protocols to minimize such impacts.

Tilapia culture has traditionally been relying on extensive and semi-intensive systems in earthen ponds. The expansion of tilapia culture across the world, together with the shortage of freshwater and competition for it with agriculture and other urban activities, has gradually shifted tilapia culture from the traditional semi-intensive systems to the more intensive production systems. These fishes are an ideal candidate for intensive culture due to their ability to tolerate high density and a wide range of environmental conditions, in addition to their high resistance to stress, disease and handling (see Chapter 4 for more details). Tilapia of the genus *Oreochromis*, particularly *Oreochromis niloticus*, *Oreochromis aureus* and *Oreochromis mossambicus* and their hybrids have been reared successfully in intensive systems and therefore have become the preferred cultured species.

The intensive culture of tilapia has been globally expanding, experimentally and/or commercially, in ponds, tanks, raceways, cages, recirculating and aquaponic systems. Water quality (dissolved oxygen (DO), temperature, salinity, ammonia (NH_3), pH, dissolved solid metabolites, etc.), nutrition and feeding, and stocking densities are the

Tilapia Culture. https://doi.org/10.1016/B978-0-12-816541-6.00006-4
Copyright © 2020 Elsevier Inc. All rights reserved.

most important factors which determine the success or failure of intensive culture of tilapia. Water quality requirements of tilapia were addressed in Chapter 4, while nutrition and feeding were covered in Chapter 7. This chapter discusses the intensive culture systems of tilapia, with emphasis on advantages, disadvantages and suitability of each system, in addition to the criteria that lead to successful culture practices.

6.2 Stocking density

Because stocking density is the most important factor affecting intensive fish culture, extensive research has been carried out on the effects of stocking density on tilapia production in different intensive culture systems. Sadly, the available information revealed controversial results (El-Sayed, 2002). This controversy may have been due to the differences in species, sizes, nutrition and feeding, culture systems and water quality. This means that the relationship between stocking density and tilapia growth and survival is a function of a number of biological and physical factors, including the fish life stages, size, sex, social hierarchies and their tolerance to environmental changes, in addition to the configuration and hydrodynamics of culture system (Huang and Chiu, 1997; Muir et al., 2000; El-Sayed, 2002).

The relationship between stocking density and tilapia yield is generally positive (i.e. high fish density leads to high yield) (Watanabe et al., 1990; Siddiqui et al., 1997), while negative correlation usually occurs between stocking density and individual fish growth (Sin and Chiu, 1983; Abou et al., 2007; Azaza et al., 2013; Garcia et al., 2013; Costa et al., 2017). Watanabe et al. (1990) and Huang and Chiu (1997) found also that size variations in Florida red tilapia and tilapia hybrids (*O. niloticus* females × *O. mossambicus* males) increased with increasing stocking density. Size variation may also be related to social hierarchy of the fish. Under crowding conditions, large fish grow bigger and faster and dominate the population, while subordinate individuals grow at much slower rates (El-Sayed and Kawanna, unpublished results; Yousif, 2002). The effects of stocking density (200, 400, 600 and 800 fish m^{-3}) on growth performance and feed utilization of juvenile Nile tilapia (14.9 g) were investigated in a tank-based flow-through system (Azaza et al., 2013). Results indicated that growth rates and net yield were negatively correlated with increased stocking density. Growth heterogeneity, expressed by the inter-individual variations of fish mass, was significantly affected by time, stocking density and their interaction. The difference in growth heterogeneity was positively correlated with stocking density.

Stocking density and feeding frequency have an effect on size hierarchy development (Yousif, 2002). The coefficient of variation of body weights of larval fish fed least frequently (2 times day^{-1}) increased with increasing stocking density (from 0.5 to 2 fish L^{-1}). The two groups which were fed 3 and 4 times day^{-1} showed an inverse relationship with size variation. Size hierarchy in the homogeneous size distributions was observed to re-establish within 2 weeks and increased steadily thereafter, whereas in the nongraded group (mixed group), a steady reduction in size variation was noted with time.

In tilapia culture, it is the fish supply and market demand that determine the price of the produced fish. The farmer should, therefore, carefully define his target consumer, and determine the appropriate stocking density that will produce the size of fish preferred by that consumer. He should also adopt the stocking density which satisfies the maximum production efficiency and producing fish of uniform size. In other words, the farmer should determine whether he wants to produce high yield, but small individual fish (e.g. to be sold in rural areas, at low prices), or he is willing to produce larger individual fish, but lower yield (e.g. for restaurants or export, at high prices).

In addition to the effects of stocking density on tilapia growth and yield, the size at stocking affects tilapia growth and yield. In this regard, McGinty (1986) studied the effects of stocking density on the growth of all-male tilapia. He found that medium-sized group (11–12 cm) gained more weight than small (7–8 cm) or large (15–16 cm) fish groups. The growth of small individuals was depressed due to competition with large- and medium-sized fish, while large fish expended more energy for nest building and egg guarding. More details on the effects of stocking density and stocking sizes on tilapia growth and yield in various culture systems are provided in the following sections.

6.3 Intensive culture in earthen ponds

Pond culture of tilapia is the oldest production system among all systems used for tilapia culture. Semi-intensive culture of tilapia in earthen ponds has been covered in Chapter 5. Despite the widespread expansion of semi-intensive tilapia culture in earthen ponds, little information is available on their intensive culture in these systems. This is probably because tilapia are cultured mostly with other fish species, typically in semi-intensive systems or in integration with other animals and/or plants, especially in Asia, which is the major tilapia producer. In addition, intensive culture of tilapia in earthen ponds is practiced at much smaller scale than other intensive farming systems which are generally adopted.

Intensive tilapia culture in earthen ponds (Fig. 6.1) is affected by a number of factors, including stocking density, species and size, environmental conditions, management strategies and nutrition and feeding. Feeding the fish with complete pelleted feeds and water exchange and/or treatment are also necessary in intensive pond culture. The

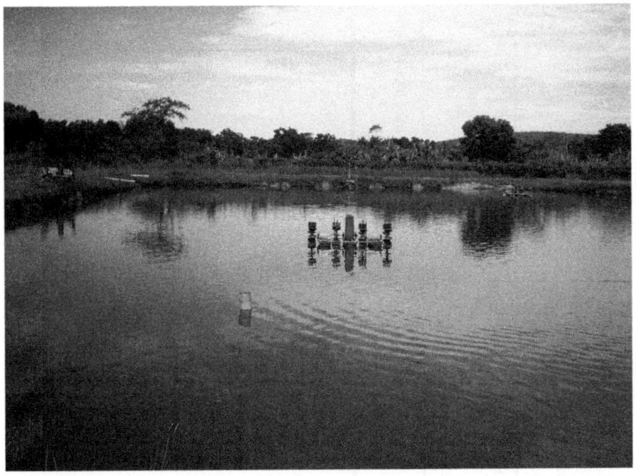

FIGURE 6.1 Intensive culture of tilapia in earthen ponds in Malaysia. *Photograph by A.-F. El-Sayed.*

production of tilapia intensively cultured in earthen ponds in selected countries is summarized in Table 6.1.

6.3.1 Stocking density

As mentioned earlier, tilapia are known to tolerate high stocking density and can withstand extreme crowding conditions. Tilapia have been cultured intensively in earthen ponds in tropics and subtropics for decades. The effects of stocking density on tilapia production in ponds have also been investigated by a number of authors. Sin and Chiu (1983) studied the effects of stocking density and aeration on growth and survival of all-male tilapia hybrids in earthen ponds. The fish were stocked at 30,000, 59,000 and 122,000 fish ha^{-1} in aerated or unaerated ponds in Hong Kong and fed commercial feed (34% crude protein, cp). When the fish were reared in unaerated ponds, the growth was significantly higher at the intermediate density (59,000 fish ha^{-1}) than at the high density (122,000 fish ha^{-1}), while the total yields were 8.4 and 11 t ha^{-1}, at both densities, respectively. Survival and feed utilization efficiency were also better at the higher than the intermediate density. When bigger-size fish (98–112 g) were reared at 30,000 and 111,000 fish ha^{-1}, under continuous aeration for 74 days, average final weights were comparable (192.9 and 214 g $fish^{-1}$ at the low and high density, respectively). The total yield was much higher at the high density (20.5 t ha^{-1}) than at the low density (6.3 t ha^{-1}). Aeration was then essential for good growth and yield at high stocking density, since it increased the yield from 67 to 133 kg ha^{-1} per day.

Intensive culture of tilapia in earthen ponds has been practiced in Israel for many years. Zohar et al. (1984) described the intensive tilapia farming in earthen ponds at high densities with continuous aeration and partial flushing of the pond water. Pruginin et al. (1988) also evaluated the intensive culture of different tilapia hybrids in brackish water ponds in Israel. The Philippines red tilapia showed the best growth rates and fecundity, while Taiwanese fish were the worst. At a density of 30 fish m^{-2} (300,000 ha^{-1}), the yearly production ranged from 80 to 120 t ha^{-1}, with a feed conversion ratio (FCR) ranging from 1.8 to 2.1 and a daily weight gain of 1.3–3.2 g. In association with high summer temperature, both primary production and organic loads increased, and more frequent water replacement was needed. In an intensive tilapia farm in Edku (Behaira Province, Egypt), all-male Nile tilapia fry (about 0.1 g) are generally stocked at a density of 13.3 fish m^{-2} (133,300 fish ha^{-1}). The ponds are aerated with paddle wheels with partial water replacement. The fry are usually fed with extruded feed (32% cp, reduced to 25% cp during fattening stages). After 360 days, the harvest reaches 28.6 t ha^{-1}, with an FCR of 1.4 (Ashour and Ashour, 2013).

6.3.2 Water exchange

The increased summer temperature and photoperiod generally increase both primary production and organic loads in intensive fish ponds. Under such conditions, the level of faeces and other total solids and dissolved metabolites such as ammonia and nitrites in the water will increase. The accumulation of these metabolites has been reported to negatively affect the performance of cultured fish. Therefore, frequent total or partial water exchange and/or aeration will become necessary. The effect of continuous water exchange on the growth of Nile tilapia in earthen ponds (45 m^3) was studied in Brazil (Sipaúba-Tavares et al., 2000). The ponds were subjected to three treatments; no water exchange, no water exchange but provided with aeration at night, or continuous aeration. Water quality (pH, DO, CO_2, NO_2, NH_3, total P and *chlorophyll a*) did not differ among treatments. These results were expected due to the low stocking density (60 fish per pond; 1.3 fish m^{-3}). Fish growth was highest at continuous water exchange, but that system may not be cost-effective, and water limitation may render it inapplicable in many areas.

Water shortage generally dictates the reduction, or even elimination, of water exchange in intensive pond culture systems. In arid areas where freshwater is limited, it would be unwise to replace or exchange culture water. Instead, treatment of this water in such a way that would allow its reuse is a must. Several trials have been conducted on the effects of reducing or eliminating water exchange on the performance of tilapia in intensive pond systems. Chamberlain and Hopkins (1994) reported that water exchange and feed protein level had no impact on the performance of tilapia reared intensively in earthen ponds, if sufficient aeration is provided. The addition of carbon source (wheat

TABLE 6.1 Intensive culture of tilapia in earthen ponds.

Species (country)	Stock data		Growth data			Harvest data		Culture period (days)	Remark	References
	# ha^{-1}	IW	ADG	SGR	FCR	FW	S (%)			
O. n ♂ × *O. m* ♀ (Hong Kong)	59,000	6.6	1.01	2.09	2.4	161.6	88.1	153	690-m^2 ponds, pelleted feed, 34% cp, 59,000 fish ha^{-1} was optimal under unaerated conditions. Aeration improved the growth at high densities.	Sin and Chiu (1983)
	122,000	5.0	0.69	2.00	2.1	112.7	80.3	155		
	30,000	111.7	1.4	0.89	1.7	214.0	100	73		
	111,000	97.7	1.3	0.93	1.8	192.9	96.4	73		
Phil-red	300,000	10–14		3.22		240		160	Brackish water, earthen ponds, lined with PVC, aeration, solids removal. 28% cp. Phl-red, Philippine red; NOR-1 and NOR-2, F1 hybrid of *O. n* × *O. a*; Mos-red, *O. m* red.	Pruginin et al. (1988)
NOR-1	300,000			2.56		190		220		
NOR-2	300,000			2.5		160		220		
Mos-red (Israel)	300,000			1.43		100		220		
O. n (Brazil)	13,333		1.11			314.3	88.7	180	- No water exchange.	Sipaúba-Tavares et al. (2000)
			1.6			423.0	85.5	180	- No water exchange - aeration at night.	
			1.82			474.5	86.7	180	- Continuous aeration.	
O. n (Costa Rica)	15,000	87	1.59	1.15	1,75	210	87	77	Pelleted feed, 34% cp, feeding stopped for 14 days after 50 days, to assess sedimentation and re-suspension rates.	Jiménez-Montealegre et al. (2002)
O. n (Egypt)	133,300	fry (0.1 g)			1.4	270		360		Ashour and Ashour (2013)

Some of the present values were calculated from the original data. *ADG*, average daily gain (g); *FCR*, feed conversion ratio; *FW*, final body weight (g); *IW*, initial body weight (g); *O. a*, *Oreochromis aureus*; *O. m*, *Oreochromis mossambicus*; *O. n*, *Oreochromis niloticus*; *SGR*, specific growth rate.

bran, rice bran (RB), etc.) on water surface, where bacteria can grow and feed on, reduces ammonia accumulation (see Fig. 6.2). Filter feeding fishes such as tilapia and carp can feed on the produced bacteria. By this way, dietary protein can be reduced significantly from 30% to 20%, and the overall cost can be reduced by 50%.

An active sedimentation and re-suspension technique can also be adopted to reduce water exchange in intensive pond culture. This recent development depends on the re-suspension of solid particles from pond sediments into the water column by continuous aeration, mixing, stirring and turbulence because settled particles decomposition on pond bottom can lead to anoxic conditions, while re-suspension favours the aerobic decomposition of the organic matter. The re-suspension of sediments can be an important mechanism of nutrient transfer in the pond and can also help in water purification by increasing the number of nitrifying bacteria in the water column (Milstein et al., 2001a). This system is very suitable for areas facing shortage in water sources, since it is operated with much lower water than in traditional intensive pond systems. In addition, herbivorous and filter feeding fishes (such as tilapia) feed on suspended particles and bacterial bloom. This process leads to additional saving in operational and feed costs.

Avnimelech et al. (1999) described sedimentation and re-suspension systems and the magnitude of sedimentation/re-suspension of particles derived from water column and those from the pond bottom stocked with tilapia and common carp. Milstein et al. (2001b) compared water quality and growth of hybrid tilapia (*O. niloticus* × *O. aureus*) and hybrid sea bass (*Morone saxatilis* × *Morone chrysops*) in conventional intensive ponds with 500% water exchange per day with active

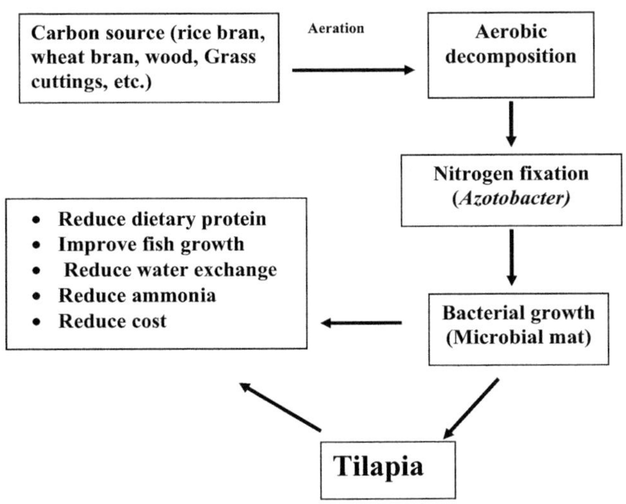

FIGURE 6.2 Production of natural food in tilapia fish ponds. *Reprinted from Aquaculture 179, 149–168, El-Sayed (1999), with permission from Elsevier.*

suspension intensive ponds (with only 8% water exchange per day). They found that bacterial growth and nitrification were higher, while ammonia removal was lower, in active suspension ponds than in classical intensive ponds. Fish growth was similarly good in both systems. This finding confirms the economic advantage of tilapia culture in water-saving active suspension systems, compared to traditional, water-demanding systems.

The rates of sedimentation and suspension can be affected by a number of factors, including fish weight, biomass, primary productivity and carbon: nitrogen (C:N) ratio. Jiménez-Montealegre et al. (2002) measured the rate of sedimentation and suspension of organic carbon and total nitrogen in earthen tilapia ponds, based on nutrient inputs, water quality, fish size and biomass. They found that the rates of total solids sedimentation and suspension were highly correlated with fish weight and biomass, *chlorophyll a*, total suspended solids (TSS), total feed input and Secchi disk visibility.

The C:N ratio plays a significant role in reducing the accumulation of inorganic nitrogen in intensive fish pond. Nitrogen accumulation is controlled by feeding bacteria on carbohydrate source (Fig. 6.2), which results in the uptake of nitrogen from water (Avnimelech, 1999). Thus, adjusting of C:N ratio in fish feed is essential for controlling the change in pond water quality. Chamberlain and Hopkins (1994) suggested that the optimum C:N ratio for bacterial growth is about 15:1. In support, Avnimelech (1999) studied the C:N ratio in tilapia feed, as a control element in aquaculture systems. He found that the addition of carbonaceous substrate in commercial-scale fish ponds reduced inorganic nitrogen and increased bacterial growth that were taken up by tilapia. When a high-protein (30% cp), low-energy diet with a C:N = 11.1:1 was fed at 2% body weight (bw) d^{-1} or a low-protein (20% cp), high-energy diet (C:N = 16.7:1) was fed at 2.6% bw d^{-1}, the low-protein, high-carbohydrate diet has led to the following:

1. Significant reduction in the accumulation of inorganic nitrogen.
2. Increased utilization efficiency of dietary protein.
3. Significant reduction in feed expenditure, feed requirement and feed cost.
4. Better growth rate (2.0 g d^{-1} compared to 1.59 g d^{-1} at 30%) and FCR.

The author (Avnimelech, 1999) suggested that about 20–25 g of carbonaceous materials is needed to convert 1 g of ammonia nitrogen into microbial protein. One advantage of this process is that it is fast and can reduce ammonia to the desired levels within 1–3 days (Avnimelech, 2003). These findings can be very beneficial to intensive tilapia farmers in earthen ponds. These farmers can use cheap carbon and nitrogen sources to partially replace expensive commercial high-protein feeds. The approach of producing single-cell protein(s) in fish ponds should also be encouraged in developing countries where tilapia culture is widely practiced.

6.4 Cage culture

Cage culture of fish has received a considerable attention in recent years as a means of intensive exploitation of water systems, with low capital investment, compared to other traditional intensive farming systems. This system has several attributes that make it an ideal farming system:

1. Relatively low capital investment compared to other intensive culture systems.
2. Ease of observation, management and early detection of stress and disease.
3. Economic treatment of parasites and diseases.
4. Ease of cage movement and relocation.
5. The use of all the available water resources.
6. Ease of fish harvest and low cost of harvesting.
7. Minimum fish handling and reduction of mortality.
8. Optimum use of artificial feed and close observation of fish feeding response.
9. High stocking density, optimum feed utilization and improved growth rates.
10. Reducing pressure on land.
11. Control of reproduction of some species such as tilapia.
12. Can be used for storage and transport of live fish.
13. Easy to control predators and competitors.

Cage culture also has some limitations:

- Risk of theft is high.
- Risk of loss due to cage damage caused by predators or storms.
- High risk of disease outbreaks and difficulty of disease control.
- Low tolerance of fish to poor water quality.
- Complete dependence on high-quality feed.
- Difficult to apply in rough weather.
- Water exchange is essential to remove fish metabolites and maintain good DO inside the cages.
- Rapid fouling of cage frames and nets, which requires continuous cleaning.
- Substantial amounts of feed are lost through cage meshes.
- The accumulation of faeces and metabolites underneath the cage causes negative environmental impacts.

Tilapia cage culture has been practiced experimentally and commercially since the early 1970s (Bardach et al., 1972). Commercial tilapia culture in cages is also expanding at a very fast rate, especially in tropical and subtropical developing countries in Asia, Africa and Latin America (Gibtan et al., 2008; Garcia et al., 2013; Moura et al., 2015; Costa et al., 2017). One of the major advantages of tilapia cage culture is that it can be applied in various water bodies, including rivers, lakes, reservoirs, swamps, ponds, thermal effluents, waste water and seawater (Table 6.2).

6.4.1 Factors affecting cage culture

The success of tilapia cage culture depends on a number of factors, including water quality, water level, tilapia species and strains, stocking density, stocking size, cage size and shape, feed quality and feeding frequency. Some of these factors have already been discussed in the other chapters. Therefore, only cage size and type and stocking density are discussed here.

6.4.1.1 Cage size and type

The sizes of tilapia cages vary considerably according to the farming operations. Breeding cages and fingerling production cages are generally smaller than fattening cages, while experimental cages do not usually exceed few cubic metres. Commercial production cages range from small to medium size (6 to about 100 m^3) (El-Sayed, 2007, 2013; Ofori et al., 2010) to very large size, up to 2000 m^3 (Hecht, 2007). It should be emphasized that the cage size adopted must consider the level of technology available. Large cages appear very suitable for tilapia culture, since they generally result in better growth, reduced feed loss and improved survival even at low levels of DO (Campbell, 1985; McGinty, 1991). Yet, tilapia cage culture is generally practiced in small- to medium-size cages. Different cage types are also used for tilapia culture in different regions of the world. It is very common that locally available materials are used in cage construction, especially in small-scale, rural areas in Africa.

6.4.1.2 Stocking density

Stocking density is another essential factor that influences tilapia performance in cages. The effects of stocking density on growth and survival of tilapia in cages have received considerable attention. A number of studies have been conducted in this regard, and the results have been varying. As expected, increasing fish density may increase total yield, but it will reduce the individual fish growth (Osofero et al., 2009; Asase, 2013; Garcia et al., 2013). Watanabe et al. (1990) found that Florida red tilapia fingerlings reared in sea cages at densities of 500−1000 fish m^{-3} for 30 days had similar growth and feed utilization efficiency. On the other hand, the performance of Nile tilapia reared in floating cages in Thale Noi, Thailand, was significantly affected by stocking density (Chiayvareesajja et al., 1990). The fish were stocked at 20, 76, 200 and 333 individual m^{-3} and fed a weed-based diet, for 3 months. The best

TABLE 6.2 Intensive cage culture of tilapia in some countries.

Species (country)	Stock data		Growth data			Harvest data			Culture period (days)	Remarks	References
	# m^{-3}	IW	ADG	SGR	FCR	FW	Yield ($kg\ m^{-3}$)	S (%)			
Male *O. n* (Egypt)	60–100	5–10			1.2–1.5	300–500	25–40		180–270	25%–30% cp extruded feeds, manual feeding, 600-m^3 floating cages. If overwintered fish (30–50 g) are used, the fish attain 300–500 g in 4–6 months.	El-Sayed (2017)
Male *O. n*, Chitralada strain (Brazil)	250	30.7	1.61	2.15	1.17	150.4	36.9	98.1	74	32% cp feed, 9-m^3 cages suspended in a reservoir. Final body weight was significantly reduced with increasing the density to 450 fish m^{-3}, but biomass was not affected.	Costa et al. (2017)
O. n (Brazil)	133	78	5.73	3.44	0.95	311.1	41.9	96.6	41	6-m^3 cages placed in a hydroelectric reservoir, 42% cp commercial feed.	Garcia et al. (2013)
	333	78	4.11	2.55	1.36	260.2	87.8	96.4	41		
	133	255	6.92	0.81	1.89	809.6	106.2	99.6	118	6-m^3 cages placed in a hydroelectric reservoir, 32% cp feed. At higher density, 25 more days were needed to reach 800 g.	
	150	255	8.8	0.93	1.81	857.5	124.0	98.8	143		
O. n. (Ghana)	50	2.13	1.54	2.75		274.1		77.8	177	8-m^3 cages, 30% cp extruded feed, at 100 and 150 fish m^{-3} growth was significantly lower.	Asase (2013)
Mixed *O. n* (Ghana)	125	25.0	1.72	1.6	2.5	277.5	24.5	77.3	147	30% cp floating extruded feeds, 48-m^3 cages, heavy mortality occurred.	Ofori et al. (2010)
Red tilapia (Chitralada) (Thailand)	158	58.3	3.74		1.44	506.5	57.1	71.2	120	20%–32% cp feeds, 12-m^3 cages, suspended in a river.	Orachunwong et al. (2001)
	100	75	4.43		1.50	606.5	59.2	97.7	120		
	133	88.8	4.26		1.44	600.0	59.6	74.4	120		

Continued

TABLE 6.2 Intensive cage culture of tilapia in some countries.—cont'd

Species (country)	Stock data		Growth data			Harvest data			Culture period (days)	Remarks	References
	# m^{-3}	IW	ADG	SGR	FCR	FW	Yield (kg m^{-3})	S (%)			
O. m × *O. h* (Thailand)	27.5	149	4.03		1.52	769	20.1	95	154	20%–32% cp feed, cages suspended in pond stocked with tilapia fingerlings (2.8 g).	Orachunwong et al. (2001)
	27.2	127	4.26		1.51	736	19.6	98	143		
O. n (Thailand)	20	98.2	0.66		7.80	156.6	3.13	100	90	Bamboo cages, fed pellets containing dry weed, rice bran and FM (4:3:1), 333 fish m^{-3} was best.	Chiayvareesajja et al. (1990)
	67	86.1	0.77		7.50	145.8	9.77	99.7	90		
	200	88.8	0.52		9.90	129.9	25.25	99.6	90		
	333	76.6	0.60		9.60	117.8	38.6	98.5	90		
O. n (GIFT) (Philippines)	20	73.9	0.8–0.9	0.9–1.0	2.8–3.3	156.6–162.6		96–99	90	6-m^3 cage in ponds, fed either commercial feed, farm-made yeast- or compost diets.	Fitzsimmons et al. (1999)
Red tilapia (Mauritius)	61	50.2	1.02	1.13		147.4	9.5	100	95	Seawater cage.	Persand and Bhikajee (1997)
O. s (Kuwait)	200	9.65	1.9	1.9		379.6			193	Seawater cages.	Cruz and Ridha (1991)
O. n (Lesser Antilles)	300	73	3.8	1.49	1.30	616	18.2	97.7	143	36% cp floating pellets, cages suspended in a 2-ha watershed.	Rakocy et al. (2000a)

ADG, average daily gain (g); *FCR*, feed conversion ratio; *FW*, final body weight (g); *IW*, initial body weight (g); *O. n*, *Oreochromis niloticus*; *O. m*, *O. mossambicus*; *O. h Oreochromis hornorum*; *O. s*, *Oreochromis spilurus*; *S*, survival; *SGR*, specific growth rate.

production and profit were obtained at 333 fish m^{-3}, despite that individual growth was better at lower densities. Similarly, the growth of Nile tilapia (78 g) stocked in 6 m^3 cages at 133, 333, 417 and 500 fish m^{-3} in hydroelectric reservoir in Brazil, and fed commercial pelleted feeds (42% cp) for 41 days, was negatively correlated with stocking density (Garcia et al., 2013). Asase (2013) also assessed the effects of stocking density (50, 100 and 150 fish m^{-3}) on growth rates of fingerling Nile tilapia (2.13 g) reared in floating cages (8 m^3) on the Lake Volta, Ghana. The best growth rates were obtained at 50 fish m^{-3}, compared to other densities. However, there was a direct correlation between fish biomass and stocking density.

6.4.2 Cage culture in Asia

Rearing tilapia in cages in Asia has become very popular, especially in Southeast Asian countries such as the People's Republic of China, Philippines, Malaysia, Vietnam, India and Indonesia. Tilapia cage culture in Southeast Asia is spreading, mainly due the favourable weather conditions and availability of suitable water sources. Tilapia culture in cage systems in Southeast Asia has been described by Guerrero (2001). Mozambique tilapia have been the main species cultured in cages in Asia for many years. A big switch to Nile tilapia occurred in recent years, so that Nile tilapia is currently dominating tilapia cage culture and becoming the most favoured species (see Table 6.2).

Cage culture of tilapia has been carried out in lakes and reservoirs in the Philippines since the early 1970s (Guerrero, 2001). The Philippines is currently a pioneer in Asia for Nile tilapia cage culture in lakes and reservoirs (BFAR-PHILMINAQ, 2007). Tilapia culture in floating cages in freshwater environments represents about 32% of total production of farmed tilapia (Romana-Eguia et al., 2013). Both fixed and floating cages of various dimensions are used for tilapia culture in the Philippines. Fixed cages are usually used in shallow water bodies and made of synthetic netting (5 × 5 × 3 m to 15 × 10 × 3 m) and attached to bamboo poles which are staked into the bottom. The cages are properly arranged to allow good water circulation. Floating cages are employed in deep lakes, reservoirs, lagoons and bays and are generally made of bamboo or steel frames and synthetic netting (5 × 5 × 2.5 m to 10 × 10 × 20 m). Tilapia fingerlings (10–20 g) are stocked in floating cages at 15–25, 50–250 and 100–200 fish m^{-3} in extensive, semi-intensive and intensive systems, respectively. The fish are generally fed with supplemental and/or commercial feeds to produce 2.7–7.0, 4–40 and 20–50 kg m^{-3} from these systems, respectively (Romana-Eguia et al., 2013).

Tilapia cage culture is also widely practiced in Indonesia, in rivers, irrigation canals, lakes and reservoirs. Small (8–16 m^3) to medium (100 m^3) cages are generally used in rivers and canals in Java, Sumatra and Kalimantan. The cages are constructed mainly of bamboo or iron bars, with drums, containers or styrofoam as floats. Fish (30–50 g) are stocked at a density of 50–70 m^{-3}. After 3–4 months, 40–50 kg m^{-3} are produced (Nurdjana, 2006). In earlier trials, Hardjamulia and Rukyani (2000) reported that when floating cages (7 × 7 × 2 m) in Jatiluhur Reservoir were stocked with 100–150 kg of Nile tilapia or red tilapia, they produced 626–1200 kg per cage after 60–110 days.

A two-net cage culture system locally known as 'lapis dua' has been developed and applied in reservoirs Saguling, Cirata and Jatiluhur in West Java, Indonesia, since the mid-1990s (Abery et al., 2005; De Silva and Phillips, 2007). Common carp is raised in the inner cage and tilapia in the outer cage. Inner cages are 7 × 7 × 3 m, with bamboo frames, while the depth of the outer cages ranges from 5 to 7 m, depending on the depth of the reservoirs. Cages are generally stocked with fish fingerlings (7–8 cm) at a density of 100 kg each of carp and tilapia. Commercial pelleted feed (26%–28% cp) is provided only for common carp in the inner cage, whereas tilapia in the outer cage are not fed but depend on the fall out of excess feed provided to common carp, and also on available natural foods. Tilapia and carp are harvested at a size of 330–500 and 250 g, respectively.

Cage culture systems were developed in Thailand in the late 1990s and have since expanded in all over the country. Tilapia cage farming has become a popular culture practice in rivers, reservoirs and canals in many parts of Thailand (Fig. 6.3). Most of cage farmers adopt tilapia monoculture, using varieties of red tilapia (*O. niloticus* × *O. mossambicus*) or Nile tilapia. Tilapia cage culture had a significant contribution to total fish production since 2004 (Bhujel, 2013). Generally, cage culture is practiced at small-scale,

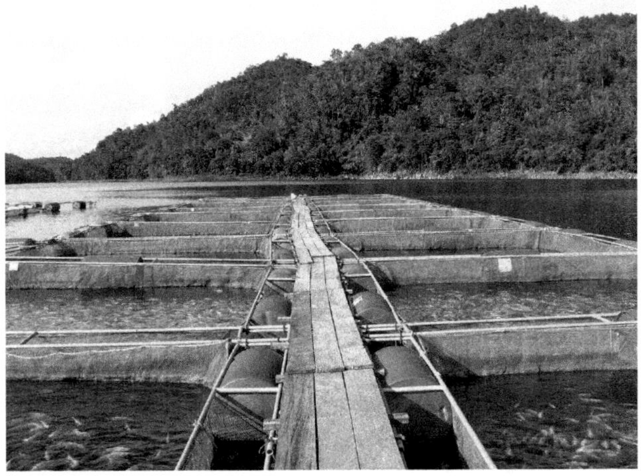

FIGURE 6.3 Red tilapia cage culture in freshwater lakes in Thailand. *Photo provided by Shutterstock.*

artisanal level, mainly in flowing waters, with Chitralada strain being the prime candidate for culture. When 58–89 g fish were stocked in floating cages in Ratchburi River at densities ranging from 100 to 158 fish m^{-3}, and fed commercial diets (20%–32% cp) for 120 days, they attained a final weight of 500–610 g $fish^{-1}$ and a net yield of 57–59.5 kg m^{-3} (Orachunwong et al., 2001). Cages or hapas in ponds, reservoirs and lakes are also used for nursing tilapia seeds. Fry are generally stocked at a density of 500–1000 fry m^{-3}. They are fed with floating pellets or a mixture of RB and fishmeal (2:1), at a daily rate of 5% –10% of body weight or to satiation, 2–4 times a day (Bhujel, 2013).

In Malaysia, cage culture is the second most important aquaculture production system in freshwater environment, only after pond systems (Yusoff, 2015). Intensive cage culture of red tilapia is practiced mainly in rivers, reservoirs and former mining pools (Guerrero, 2001) (Fig. 6.4). Tilapia averaging 700 g are stocked in floating cages measuring 4 × 3 × 2 m, at a density of 2000 fish $cage^{-1}$, for 2 months, then the number is reduced to 600 fish $cage^{-1}$ for another 2 months to reach 1 kg $fish^{-1}$. Modern polyethylene cages are becoming more popular in many freshwater aquaculture operations in Malaysia. The produced fish are exported to Singapore.

In China, tilapia culture is practiced in floating cages (6 × 4 × 3 m) set up in lakes, reservoirs and rivers (Qiuming and Yi, 2004). Juvenile tilapia (>50 g) are stocked at 100–150 fish m^{-3} and fed with artificial feed (28%–35% cp). The fish are harvested after a culture cycle of 120–150 days, at a final weight of 600–800 g and gross yield of 30–60 kg m^{-3}. Dey et al. (2000) suggested that the good performance of tilapia reared at high densities in floating cages in the lakes in China is mainly because these lakes are rich in natural food, which the cultured fish can consume.

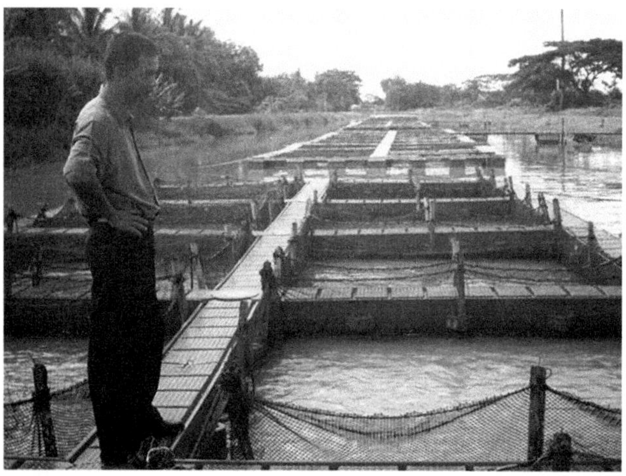

FIGURE 6.4 Tilapia cage culture in flowing rivers in Malaysia. *Photograph by A.-F. El-Sayed.*

Tilapia cage culture in Mekong Delta in Vietnam has been widely expanding during the past few years. Red tilapia are the major cultured tilapia, mainly in wooden floating cages, arrayed in series parallel to the river banks (VASEP, 2016a; Boerlage et al., 2017). Tilapia are farmed mainly for local consumption; however, tilapia export has sharply increased during the past 10 years (VASEP, 2016b). Medium-size cage (10 × 5 × 3.5 m) are generally stocked with tilapia fingerlings (1–10 g) at varying densities; however, the median density is about 175 fish m^{-3}. Fish are fed with pelleted feeds, 2–3 times per day to reach a harvest size ranging from 250 to 500 g in 4–6 months, depending on initial fish size and stocking density. Farmers produce two crops, in average, of red tilapia per cage per year.

Bangladesh is blessed with a plenty of natural freshwater and brackish water resources in the form of lakes, rivers and estuaries, ponds and canals. These water sources can be ideal sites for tilapia cage culture in the country. Trials on tilapia cage culture started in Kaptai Lake in the early 1980s by the Bangladesh Fisheries Development Corporation (BFDC). Since then, progressive development of cage culture has been going on; and this farming system is becoming more popular. A number of private entrepreneurs practice cage culture of GIFT Nile tilapia in the Dhakatia River near Chandpur and Munshiganj region. Fish are stocked at a density of 200–350 fish m^{-3}, to reach 120–190 kg m^{-3} after a culture period of 8–9 months, with an FCR of around 2.0 (Hussain, 2009; Hussain et al., 2013). About 3500 cages are currently in operation in the Dhakatia River and 500 cages along the Meghna River (Baqui and Bhujel, 2011; Hossain et al., 2017).

Cage culture of tilapia in other Asian countries, including India, Taiwan, Singapore, Myanmar and Sri Lanka, is also gaining increasing attention. At this time, very little information is available on tilapia culture in this system in these countries.

6.4.3 Cage culture in Africa

Despite that tilapia cage aquaculture is practiced at different scales in Africa, Egypt remains the most important producer from this system. Over the past two decades, tilapia culture in floating cage has been spreading rapidly throughout the country, especially in the Domiat (Damietta) and Rashid (Rosetta) branches of the Nile River (El-Sayed, 2013). Small-scale (4 × 4 × 2 m) to large-scale (10 × 10 × 6 m) square cages, arranged in groups of arrays, are most common (Fig. 6.5). The cages are made of wooden frames and synthetic netting. Cage floats are made of empty, closed plastic barrels (50 L capacity) fixed underneath the frames of the cages (8–12 floats per 600 m^3 cage). The cages are stocked with tilapia fingerlings (3 to > 50 g) at 60–100 fish m^{-3}. The fish are fed with

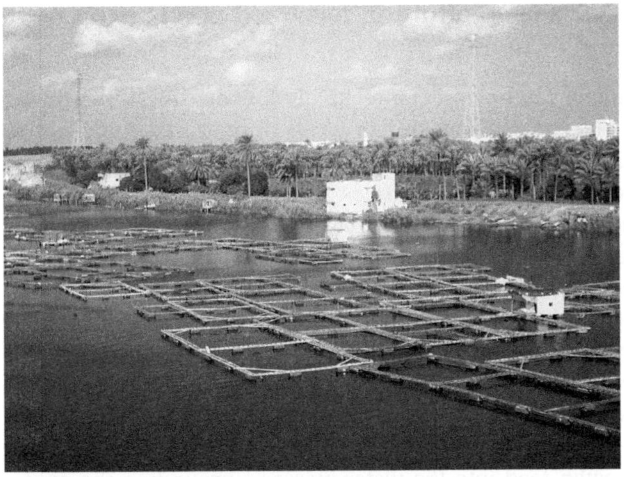

FIGURE 6.5 Arrays of tilapia cages in the Nile River (Rosetta Branch), Egypt. *Photograph by A.-F. El-Sayed.*

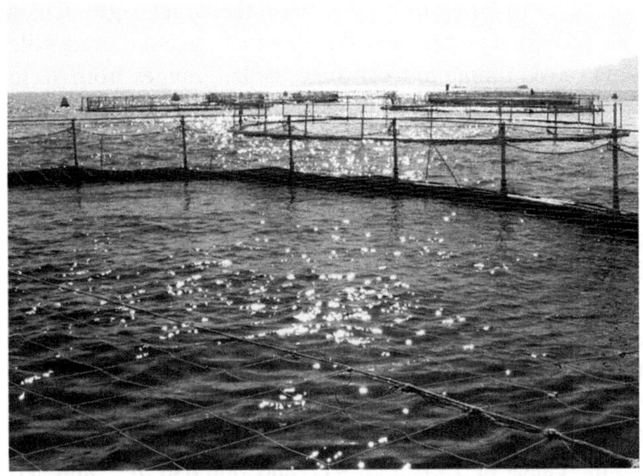

FIGURE 6.6 Large-scale cage culture of tilapia at Lake Harvest Farm, Lake Kariba, Zimbabwe. *Photo provided by R. Brummett.*

commercial extruded (floating) feeds (25%–30% cp), 2 to 3 times per day. The fish reach 300–500 g in 6–9 months, with a total production of 25–40 kg m^{-3} (El-Sayed, 2017).

In the rest of Africa, especially in West sub-Saharan Africa, tilapia cage culture is slowly emerging; with a relatively low contribution to total tilapia production (Jamu, 2001; El-Sayed, 2013). Cage culture is currently practiced in Cote d'Ivoire, Ghana, Kenya, Malawi, Uganda, Zambia and Zimbabwe. Nile tilapia is the only cage-farmed species throughout the region, except in Malawi, where chambo (*Oreochromis shiranus* and *Oreochromis karongae*) are the main species cultured (Blow and Leonard, 2007). Small ($6 \times 4 \times 2$ m) to medium ($6 \times 6 \times 3$ m) cages, made of locally available materials, are generally used in many African countries, particularly in West Africa. Commercial, medium- to large-scale cages (800–1200 m^3) are also used in Ghana (Hecht, 2007). Cages are stocked with tilapia fingerlings (10–30 g) at varying densities, ranging between 63 and 188 fish m^{-3} (Ofori et al., 2009). Both farm-made feeds and commercial feeds (25%–32% cp) are used to feed cage-cultured tilapia. After 5–7 months, the fish can attain a marketable size of 300–500 g.

The largest and most successful commercial farm for cage culture of tilapia (Lake Harvest) is located on Lake Kariba, Zimbabwe (Fig. 6.6). The fish are fed 30%–45% crude protein feeds in the form of sinking and floating pellets and crumbles (Pasipamire, 2009). The production of that farm is some 2000 t yr^{-1}, though the goal is to increase it to 5000 t yr^{-1}. The facility is also provided with a very high standard processing unit. The produced tilapia is exported, either as fresh fillets or frozen, to Europe and the United States (Windmar et al., 2000a). A similar cage farm consisting of 32 cages has been established in Lake Malawi (Malawi), with a target production of 3000 t of chambo (*O. karongae* or *O. shiranus*). Initial stocking density ranges from 65 to 75 fingerlings per m^3 (30 g average weight). Cage-cultured tilapia are generally fed with farm-made or extruded feeds. Feed is dispensed by hand two to three times a day. After a rearing cycle of about 6–9 months, final harvest ranges from 20 to 40 kg m^{-3}.

6.4.4 Cage culture in Latin America and the Caribbean

Tilapia cage culture is rapidly expanding in some Latin American and Caribbean countries, such as Brazil (Lovshin, 2000; Conte et al., 2008; Nunes, 2010; Roriz et al., 2017), Mexico (Fitzsimmons, 2000; Watanabe et al., 2002), Colombia (Popma and Rodriquez, 2000; Watanabe et al., 2002), Honduras, Nicaragua and Cuba (Rojas and Wadsworth, 2007). Specifically, substantial efforts have been directed to research and development of tilapia cage culture in Brazil, compared to other Latin American countries. The culture of Nile tilapia is practiced mainly in floating cages in reservoirs, lakes and rivers and behind hydroelectric power dams all over the country. This system has become the most common aquaculture practice in Brazil; contributing over 40% of total aquaculture production (Roriz et al., 2017). The majority of cages are small scale, ranging from 4 to 20 m^3; however, larger cages (>100 m^3) are also used in some areas. Stocking densities vary considerably, depending on cage size, initial fish size, water quality and operational management. Small cages are generally stocked at 100–300 fish m^{-3}, whereas larger cages are stocked at 25–50 fish m^{-3} (Nunes, 2010; Roriz et al., 2017). Cages are usually constructed with nets made from plastic-coated galvanized steel, stainless steel or synthetic fibres such as polypropylene. Steel nets are more widespread due to their high resistance to predatory fish. Cage frames are made from galvanized steel, stainless steel or high-density polyethylene. The yield ranges from 150 kg m^{-3} per crop in the small cages to 50 kg m^{-3} per crop in the larger cages. Costa et al. (2000) reported that the yield of cage-cultured Nile tilapia or red tilapia in Cear State, Brazil, ranges from 40 to 100 kg m^{-3}. The cage culture of Thai tilapia has resulted in a production of 100–300 kg m^{-3}. Roubach et al. (2003) described a cage-culture system consisting of groups of about 15 cages, each of a size of 4–6 m^3, adopted in the northeast region of Brazil, stocked with juvenile tilapia of 25–30 g to reach 500–650 g in 120 days.

In two consecutive trials, Garcia et al. (2013) determined the appropriate stocking density of Nile tilapia in cages in a hydroelectric reservoir in Brazil and evaluated the effects of size selection on the improvement of fish uniformity. In the initial trial, the fish (78 g) were stocked in 6 m^3 cages at 133, 333, 417 and 500 fish m^{-3} and fed with commercial pelleted feeds (42%) for 41 days. When the fish reached 255 g in average, they were sorted and selected into three sizes and restocked at four densities (133 nonselected, 100, 133 and 150 fish m^{-3}) in order to attain the following harvest yield: 100, 80, 100 and 120 kg m^{-3}, respectively. Commercial feeds (32% cp) were used during this phase. The trial was terminated when the fish reached 800 g. The results revealed that no fish selection was needed when the initial stocking density was reduced from 417 to 133 fish m^{-3}. At this low density, fish growth and feed conversion were better and the time needed to reach harvesting size (800 g) was shorter, leading to a significant reduction in operational cost and an increase in profits. The risk of disease outbreak, fish mortality and deformity were also lower, and DO inside the cages was higher, at low density.

In Mexico, net pens (which use staked sides and rest on the bottom), constructed out of local materials, are commonly utilized by low-income groups or individuals (Fitzsimmons, 2000). More sophisticated, intensive production floating cage are also in use, mainly in irrigation reservoirs. Floating or slow-sinking pelleted feed is generally used for feeding caged fish. Cage culture in Colombia is practiced in large hydroelectric power reservoirs (Popma and Rodriquez, 2000). Cage size ranges from 2.7 to 45 m^3. Sex-reversed tilapia males are commonly stocked at 160–350 fish m^{-3}, at an initial size of about 30 g to reach marketable size of 150–300 g in 6–8 months, using commercial extruded feed (24%–34% cp), yielding 67–116 kg m^{-3}. In Honduras, red tilapia of 5–12 g are cultured in $6 \times 6 \times 2$ m-cages (about 70–80 m^3) suspended in lakes water, and fed pelleted feed (28% cp) (Meyer, 2002). The fish are transferred into cages with increasing netting mesh size according to growth phase until reaching harvest size (450 g).

6.4.5 Cage culture in fertilized ponds and pond effluents

Tilapia can be raised at relatively low densities in fertilized ponds and effluents of fish ponds or industrial sources. The success of this approach depends on fish density, water exchange, fertilization rates and supplemental feeding. As indicated in Chapter 5, tilapia can be raised in fertilized ponds, where dense plankton blooms produce higher fish yield than moderate blooms, especially when small fish were raised. Farming tilapia in earthen ponds in an integrated system has attracted the attention of many researchers in recent years. In these systems, caged fish are usually fed high-protein feed, which results in the accumulation of considerable amounts of metabolic wastes and uneaten feed into the water masses surrounding the cages, and causing water eutrophication and increased organic loads. These wastes can be used as a natural food for filter feeding fish, such as tilapia and carps in integrated systems. The benefits of this type of integration are listed in Chapter 5.

The cage-cum-pond system has been applied with catfish–tilapia (Lin and Diana, 1995; Yi et al., 2003) and tilapia–tilapia (McGinty, 1991; Yi and Lin, 1997, 2001; Yi et al., 1996). McGinty (1991) studied the effects of cage size and the number of noncaged (open-pond) fish on tilapia production in cages suspended in fish ponds. Nile tilapia were stocked in the cages at 250 fish m^{-3} and fed artificial diets. The ponds were stocked with noncaged Nile tilapia fingerlings at a rate of 3000 fish ha^{-1}, or swim-up fry at a rate of 50,000 fry ha^{-1}. The growth of caged fish was increased at the lower number of noncaged fish, and tended to increase with increasing cage size, presumably due to the decrease in feed loss.

In another study, Yi and Lin (1997) investigated the effects of stocking density of noncaged small Nile tilapia on the growth of both caged and noncaged small and large fish in Thailand. Large tilapia were stocked in 4-m^3 net cages at 400 fish $cage^{-1}$, and the cages were suspended in earthen ponds stocked with small tilapia (15–16 g $fish^{-1}$, at two densities; 1.2 or 2 fish m^{-3}). The authors found that stocking densities of noncaged tilapia significantly affected the growth and FCR of both caged and open-pond fish. The growth, FCR and yield of both caged and open-pond fish were better at the low density than at the higher density. The net production of the whole integrated system (caged and noncaged) was significantly higher in the low-density treatment (5.5 t ha^{-1} $crop^{-1}$) than in the high-density treatment (4.5 t ha^{-1} per crop). In addition, large tilapia grew better in integrated system than in open water in the mixed-pond culture system at the same level of stocking densities of small tilapia.

The effects of stocking density of large caged Nile tilapia on the open-pond fish have also been studied (Yi et al., 1996). Large fish (141 g) were stocked at 30, 40, 50, 60 and 70 fish m^{-3} in cages suspended in earthen pond while small Nile tilapia (54 g) were stocked at 2 fish m^{-3} to feed on the wastes of caged fish. The survival of caged tilapia decreased significantly from 91.4% to only 57.2% with increasing stocking density from 30 to 70 fish m^{-3}. The best yield of both caged and open-pond fish was achieved at 50 fish m^{-3}.

The biomass of caged tilapia (i.e. the number of cages per pond) and aeration may also affect the performance of tilapia in integrated cage-cum-pond systems. This hypothesis has been tested by Yi and Lin (2001). The authors stocked Nile tilapia (91–103 g) in one, two, three or four cages suspended in earthen ponds at 50 fish m^{-3}, while fingerlings were stocked in open water at 2 fish m^{-3}. The survival, growth and FCR of caged and noncaged fish were significantly affected by the biomass of caged fish. The average final weight and survival of caged fish decreased with increasing the number of cages. On the other hand, the growth and survival of noncaged fish increased with increasing caged biomass, presumably due the increased feed inputs and wastes from the cages. Aeration of the water increased the growth of only the 4-cage ponds, while the growth of open-pond fish was lower than that in the unaerated ponds, probably due to the increased level of TSS, which resulted in increased aeration-induced mud turbidity and a reduction in primary productivity and natural food supply for the noncaged fish. Water circulation can be an effective solution to water turbidity and will lead to improved DO at night. It will also stimulate phytoplankton production and increase DO through photosynthesis during daytimes (Boyd, 1990).

Walking catfishes are air-breathing fishes that can be grown in ponds at extremely high densities (10 fish m^{-3}), yielding up to 100 t ha^{-1} (Areerat, 1987). These scavenger fishes can be fed with trash fish, chicken offal, slaughterhouse wastes, in addition to pelleted feeds. This generally leads to increased waste production, which in turn, may cause deterioration in water quality and phytoplankton blooms. However, the rich effluents from catfish ponds can be used for tilapia culture in an integrated cage–pond system. Yi et al. (2003) studied the ability of Nile tilapia reared in a semi-intensive system in ponds to utilize the wastes resulting from intensive culture of hybrid catfish (*Clarias macrocephalus* × *Clarias gariepinus*). They found that tilapia yield from catfish-waste system was comparable to that obtained from fertilized ponds. Tilapia recovered considerable amounts of N and P contained in the wastes of intensive catfish culture. The authors suggested that water circulation between catfish pen and tilapia ponds is cost-effective, as it can reduce nutrient contents in pond effluent. Similar results have been reported with walking catfish (*C. macrocephalus*) and catfish hybrids (Lin and Diana, 1995), where the wastes from caged catfish increased phytoplankton productivity in the ponds which supported the growth of Nile tilapia in the same ponds containing the cages. Moreover, tilapia reared in cages feeding on phytoplankton in intensive channel catfish ponds grew reasonably well and improved the water quality in the ponds (Perschbacher, 1995).

In another study, the production and profitability of cage–pond integration of African catfish (*C. gariepinus*) and Nile tilapia with carps was investigated by Mandal et al. (2014). African catfish (3.8 g; 100 fish m^{-3}) and Nile tilapia (48 g; 30 fish m^{-3}) were raised in separate cages in earthen ponds, while carps (silver carp, common carp, bighead carp, rohu, mrigal and grass carp) were stocked in the ponds at 1 fish m^{-2} at 4:2:1.5:1:1:0.5 ratio, respectively. The caged tilapia and catfish were fed on locally made pellet feed (24.1% cp), whereas the ponds were fertilized with diammonium phosphate and urea at a rate of 4.0 kg N and 2.0 kg P ha^{-1} per day for the initial 15 days. The net yield and profitability was significantly higher in the catfish–tilapia–carps integration system (9.4 t ha^{-1} per year) than in the carp polyculture (3.3 t ha^{-1} per year).

Preliminary investigations indicated also that climbing perch (*Anabas testudineus*) may also be cultured with tilapia in integrated cage-cum-pond systems (Phuong et al., 2004). Climbing perch (9 g) were stocked in cages at stocking densities of 50–200 fish m^{-3} and fed pelleted feed (26%–28% cp), while Nile tilapia fingerlings (10 g) were stocked in fertilized earthen ponds at 2 fish m^{-3}. Survival and growth of caged and noncaged fishes were reasonable, despite that FCR of climbing perch was quite high. The best results were achieved at a stocking density of 150 perch m^{-3}.

6.4.6 Tilapia culture in sea cages

The scarcity of freshwater, and the competition for it with other activities such as irrigation, drinking and other urban activities, makes its use for tilapia culture unguaranteed and unsecured. The challenge which faces fish farmers and aquaculture researchers is to use brackish water and seawater, which is available in most of the tropics and subtropics, for tilapia culture. The euryhaline characteristics of tilapia make them an ideal candidate for culture in the saline waters. The tolerance of tilapia to water salinity was discussed in Chapter 4.

Tilapia cage culture in seawater has been tried by a number of researchers, with varying degrees of success, depending on cultured species, size and sex, stocking density cage size and shape and environmental conditions. Watanabe et al. (1990) successfully raised Florida red tilapia in seawater cages in the Bahamas with a survival rate of 84.1%–93.5%. However, the results of that study may not be reliable due to the short duration through which it was carried out (30 days). Persand and Bhikajee (1997) reared red tilapia (*Oreochromis* spp.) in cylindrical seawater cages in Mauritius, for 95 days. The specific growth rate (SGR) (1.13%) and yield (9 kg m^{-3}) were considered low as compared to other similar rearing studies, such as that of Cruz and Ridha (1991) who found that the SGR of *Oreochromis spilurus* grown in sea cages in Kuwait was 1.9%. As mentioned earlier, the difference between both results may have been related to stocking density and species and size, duration of the trials and environmental conditions. Moreover, Al-Ahmed (2002) described the culture of *O. spilurus* in sea cages in Kuwait. Fry are stocked at 600 m^{-3}, while 200 fish m^{-3} are considered optimum for growout phase. In one study, the fish grew from 118 to 323.3 g in 101 days, with a growth rate of 2.03 g d^{-1} and a production of 44 kg m^{-3}. In another study, the fish gained 2.31–3.49 g d^{-1}, with an FCR of 1.47–2.13 and a survival of 95%–97.7%. The main limitation of tilapia culture in sea cages in Kuwait is the decrease in water temperature during winter times (mid-November to mid-April).

Commercial farming of *O. spilurus* in open-sea cages (125 m^3) at a salinity of 37–38‰ has also been carried out in Malta (Agius, 2001), with very promising results. The fish (50 g) were stocked in the cages at the end of June and reached 450–500 g at the end of November (after 5 months), with a mortality rate less than 2%. Once again, as in the case of Kuwait, the main obstacle that limits the expansion of this culture system in Malta is the low water temperature during winter months. It is clear, thus, that rearing certain species of tilapia in seawater cages can be an excellent alternative tilapia culture system, if environmental conditions are favourable.

Currently, there is an ambitious programme for marine aquaculture development in Saudi Arabia, especially in the Red Sea coast. Tilapia (especially *O. spilurus*) is one of the target species selected for this program (Espla, Jeddah, 2019, personal communication). This species grows and spawns normally in full strength sea water (>40%) in Jeddah Fisheries Research Center. Farming trials of *O. spilurus* in sea water in fiberglass tanks are also carried out in a private aquaculture company (Tharawat Seas), with very promising results (Gialamas, Jeddah, 2019, personal communication).

It is clear from the above discussion that tilapia culture in saltwater is highly feasible and could be very profitable. However, more research and development initiatives should be directed to the following areas:

1. Production of more salt-tolerant tilapia strains and hybrids; with emphasis on:
   - gene transfer,
   - genetic studies of intra- and inter-specific variation in salt tolerance,
   - selective breeding to develop salt-tolerant hybrids,
   - more research on hybridization.
2. Optimizing salt tolerance through:
   - optimizing acclimation protocols,
   - adding salt to the diet,
   - better understanding of biochemical pathways and gene networks involved in osmoregulation,
   - understanding environmental adaptation and metabolic connections to osmoregulation. Functional genomics and proteomics can play a significant role in this regard.
3. Improving cold resistance. This can be done through the following approaches:
   - selective breeding,
   - gene transfer,
   - feed manipulation.
4. Improving disease resistance.
5. Re-evaluation of nutrient requirements of tilapia farmed in marine environments.

6.5 Tank and raceway culture

Tank culture of tilapia is becoming more popular, especially in arid and semi-arid areas where freshwater or brackish water is limited. Tanks are generally of smaller size than earthen ponds, and constructed of concrete, fibreglass, wood, metals or any other suitable materials, however, concrete and fibreglass tanks are the most popular. Tanks are generally characterized by smooth internal surfaces to protect the fish from injuries. The following features have been reported to be essential for tank culture of tilapia: (1) tank size and shape, (2) stocking density and size, (3) water exchange and flow rate, and (4) drainage system and sludge removal. The first three factors are discussed in the following sections, while drainage system and sludge removal are explored in Section 6.7.

6.5.1 Tank size and shape

The size and shape of tilapia culture tanks are variable, depending on the culture objectives. Fry and nursery tanks are generally small (<1–3 m^3), while production tanks can reach >30 m^3 (Balarin and Haller, 1983; Martin et al., 2000). In a tilapia farm at Al-Nubaria, near Alexandria, Egypt, the farmer uses 600-m^3 production concrete tanks (20 × 30 × 1 m) with muddy bottom, whereas fish effluents are used to irrigate agricultural crops (El-Sayed, Alexandria, 1998; personal communication).

Tank shape may also affect fish growth and production. Circular tanks have been recommended, since they permit higher water velocities than other tank shapes (Wheaton,

1977), leading to better-conditioned fish. Circular tanks also better distribute the water, are more self-cleaning, use a lower water flow and their construction costs are less than raceways (Balarin and Haller, 1983). However, they create a greater metabolic demand (i.e. a reduction in feed utilization efficiency), presumably due to the continuous movement of the fish.

Rectangular or square tanks (mainly concrete) are also widely used in tilapia culture, as they are easy to construct (Fig. 6.7). However, they have several problems compared with circular tanks. Fish may crowd into tank corners causing oxygen depletion. Small rectangular tanks are also characterized by 'dead spot' and short water circulation, where oxygen depletion may occur, as a result of waste buildup, causing fish stress (Balarin and Haller, 1982). In order to avoid these problems, other tank shapes were adopted. For example, the D-shaped concrete tanks (Fig. 6.8) are successfully used for commercial tilapia production. A large-scale fish farm near Riyadh, Saudi Arabia, uses D-shaped tanks for intensive culture of Nile tilapia (El-Sayed, Riyadh, Saudi Arabia, 1993; personal communication).

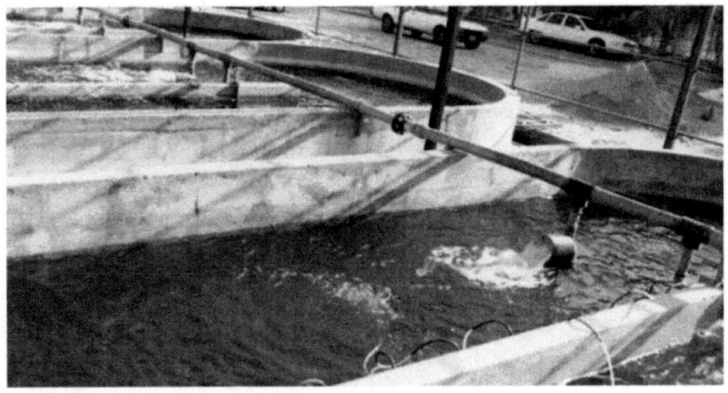

FIGURE 6.8 Intensive culture of Nile tilapia in D-shaped concrete tanks in Saudi Arabia. *Photograph by A.-F. El-Sayed.*

6.5.2 Stocking density and fish size

Stocking density may have a significant effect on final weight and total yield of farmed tilapia raised in tanks and raceways. Maximum density depends on fish size, water flow, aeration and culture systems adopted. Siddiqui et al. (1991a) raised Nile tilapia in concrete tanks using drainage water at a density of 40 fingerlings (4 g) m^{-3}. The fish attained an average final weight of 544 g (21.7 kg m^{-3}) in 415 days. When larger fingerlings (19 g) were used at a density of 64 fish m^{-3}, the fish final weight was 361 g (23.1 kg m^{-3}). When much larger fish (40 g) were stocked at a density of 42.6 m^{-3}, they reached 323 g (13.4 kg m^{-3}) in 164 days (see Table 6.3 for further details). Bailey et al. (2000) found that Nile tilapia stocked at 200 fish m^{-3} in 2-m^3 tanks provided with biofiltration and aeration, and fed a 32% cp diet, attained better daily gain and FCR than fish stocked at 450 m^{-3}. Similar results were obtained with GIFT tilapia (51.1 g) reared in concrete tanks at four densities (8, 17, 25 and 33 fish m^{-3}), under zero culture water exchange, for 30 days (Kpundeh et al., 2013). Growth performance, haematological and serum biochemical indices were all deteriorated with increasing stocking densities at zero water exchange. However, this result might not be reliable, due to the short culture period (only 30 days), the relatively low densities and also because water exchange would be necessary in tank culture system. On the contrary, Watanabe et al. (1993a, 1993b) reported no difference in the growth of Florida red tilapia reared in 23-m^3 flow-through seawater pools at 15, 25 and 35 fish m^{-3}.

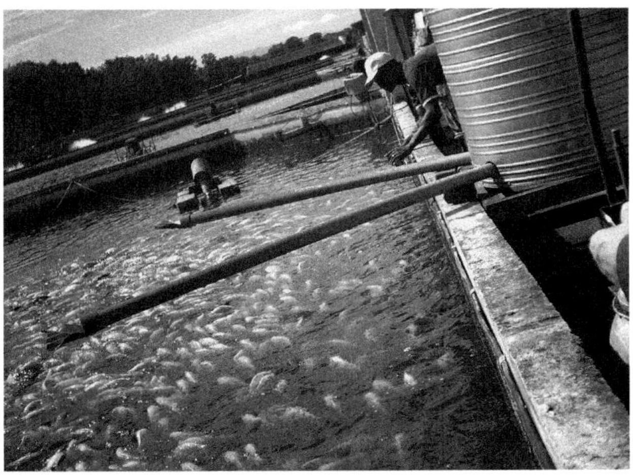

FIGURE 6.7 Intensive culture of red tilapia in rectangular concrete tanks in Malaysia. *Photograph by A.-F. El-Sayed.*

Intensive tank tilapia culture in Egypt is slowly growing, especially in arid and semi-arid areas where freshwater or brackish water is limited (El-Sayed, 2017). Tanks are round or rectangular and of smaller sizes than earthen ponds and constructed mostly of concrete. Circular fibreglass tanks are also gaining popularity. The size and shape of tilapia culture tanks are variable and depend on the culture objectives. Most of the tilapia farmers, using concrete tanks, raise only all-male Nile tilapia (Fig. 6.9). Fish are stocked at densities ranging from 25 to 100 fish m^{-3}, depending on the initial stocking size. Tanks are mostly aerated with air compressors (0.5–1.0 horsepower, depending on tank size and stocking density). Paddle wheels or water spraying over the tank surface are also widely used. Tank water is partially replaced with freshwater when the water quality deteriorates. Some tilapia farmers stock the fish (2–5 g) in tanks in May/June and harvest 200–250 g fish after 5–7 months. Other farmers stock overwintered fingerlings (30–60 g) and harvest 300 to >500 g fish in 6–9 months (El-Sayed, 2013). Total yield of tank-cultured tilapia ranges from 10 to >40 kg m^{-3}

TABLE 6.3 Tank culture of tilapia in selected countries.

Species (country)	Stock data		Growth data			Harvest data			Culture period (days)	Remark	References
	# m^{-3}	IW	SGR	ADG	FCR	FW	Yield (kg m^{-3})	S (%)			
O. n (Saudi Arabia)	40	4	1.18	1.3	2.18	544	21.7		415	Pelleted feed, 34% cp, drainage water, growth stopped during winter months.	Siddiqui et al. (1991a)
O. n (Saudi Arabia)	42.6	40	1.27	1.72	1.96	323	13.4		164	Pelleted feed, 34% cp, drainage water, growth stopped during winter months.	Siddiqui et al. (1991a)
O. n (Saudi Arabia)	64	19	1.7–1.8	0.94–1.06	1.7–2.3	92–104			98	Outdoor concrete tanks, continuous water flow, a rate of 0.5 L min^{-1} kg^{-1} biomass was recommended.	Siddiqui et al. (1991b)
Red tilapia (Malaysia)	159	16.8	1.15–1.63	1.32–1.64	2.49–3.09-	239–292	43.2–51.4	89–93	168	Portable canvas tanks, mixed-feeding strategies, 25% and 35% cp diets. Feeding the fish for 3 days on low-cp diet followed by 3 days on high-cp diet produced the best performance.	Fatan et al. (2005)
O. n (Virgin Islands)	26	71.5	1.17	2.64	1.41	514.4	13.4	99.3	168	6-m^3 circular outdoor tanks, aeration, solids removal twice a day.	Cole et al. (1997)
O. n (Virgin Islands	26	70.4	1.06	2.06	1.51	416.7	10.8	98.9	168	6-m^3 circular outdoor tanks, aeration, no solids removal.	Cole et al. (1997)
O. n (Virgin Islands	200	4.1		0.78	1.22	69.3		92.1	84	32% cp floating pellets, tanks supplied with mircoscreen drum and biological filtration.	Bailey et al. (2000)
	450	4.3		0.60	1.25	55.1		91.9	84		
O. n (Zimbabwe)	46	40	1.11	2.33	1.2–2.0	600	24.0	85	240	30.2% cp commercial feed, 650-m long raceway, water flow 1.7 m^3 s^{-1}.	Windmar et al. (2000b)
O. n (Egypt)	60	52		0.7	2.1	163	9.6	97.8	158	30% cp feed, 150-m^3 circular tanks, aeration, periodic solids removal.	Sadek et al. (1992)
	100	22		0.5	2.3	110	10.3	93.4	175		
	140	15		0.4	2.4	87	11.0	95.0	180		
O. n (Egypt)	25	61.9	0.53–0.66	0.59–0.82		200.1–221.1	4.41–5.39		196	Feeding 25% cp diet at 2% BW day^{-1} was the most cost-effective and affordable feed for farmers	El-Saidy and Gaber (2005)
O. n (Egypt)	34	50	0.97–1.3	1.3–2.55		285–510	9–17		180	250 m^3 concrete tanks, aeration and 3 water exchange rates (5%, 10% and 20% per day). Best growth and harvest obtained at 20% water exchange.	Algazzar et al. (2008)
O. n (Egypt)	40	10–20			1.4–2.8	250–500	20		180	Circular tanks, 30% cp feeds, paddle wheels and water exchange	El-Sayed (personal survey, 2018)
Red tilapia (Thailand)	50	75		0.77	2.25			87.4	70	22% cp diet, circular concrete tanks, solids removal, biological filtration.	Suresh and Lin (1992)
	100	75		0.65	2.57			85.4	70		
	2000	75		0.64	2.61			79.7	70		

ADG, average daily gain (g); *FCR*, feed conversion ratio; *FW*, final body weight (g); *IW*, initial body weight (g); *O. n*, *Oreochromis niloticus*; *S*, survival (%); *SGR*, specific growth rate.

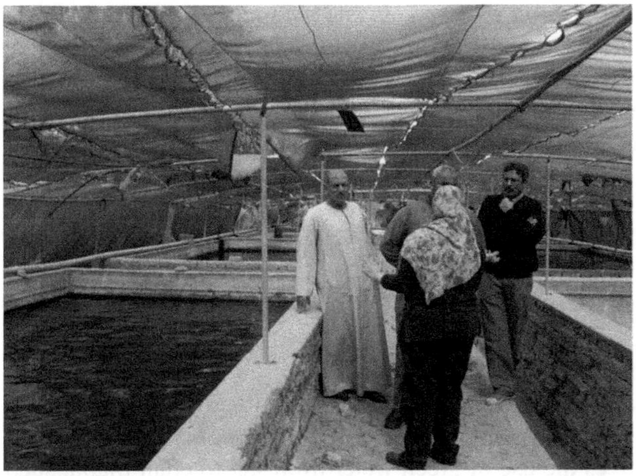

FIGURE 6.9 Intensive culture of Nile tilapia in concrete tanks in Salhia, Sharkia Governorate, Egypt. *Photograph by A.-F. El-Sayed.*

depending on stocking density, water quality, feed and feeding regimes and culture period.

Despite the sophistication and risk of this system, profitability appears quite high compared with other traditional systems. A modern, 4.2-ha concrete tank farm in Salhia, Sharkia Governorate in Egypt, raises monosex tilapia, with very high economic return (El-Sayed, personal survey 2018). Fingerling fish (10–20 g) are stocked in circular tanks (16–18 m diameter; with a volume of 200–250 m^3) at a density of 40 fish m^{-3} and fed with 30% cp floating feed. Paddle wheels and water exchange are adopted for pond management. The water from tilapia tanks is used for irrigating land crops. About 4–5 t per tank (20 kg m^{-3}) are harvested after about 5–7 months, with a final fish weight of 250–500 g per fish.

6.5.3 Water exchange and flow rate

Despite the significant effects that water exchange and flow rate may have on growth and physiological functions of tilapia, little information is available on the subject. Continuous water exchange generally sustains the good quality of culture water, while low or zero water exchange may reduce the quality of the water. In addition, at very high water flow rate, the fish spend substantial amount of dietary energy for continuous swimming, leading to reduced growth and increased mortality (El-Sayed et al., 2005). At low water flow rate, uneaten food, faeces and other fish metabolites may accumulate in fish tanks and adversely affect the water quality. This means that proper water exchange and flow rates should be adopted in order to obtain maximum fish performance.

The effects of water exchange on growth and feed utilization of Nile tilapia reared in outdoor tanks in Saudi Arabia have also been studied (Siddiqui et al., 1991b). Best growth and FCR were achieved at a continuous flow rate of 0.5–1.0 L min^{-1} per kg. Similarly, Balarin and Haller (1983) reported that 100–200 kg m^{-3} per year of tilapia could be produced from commercial tank farms in Kenya, with continuous water flow of 0.5–1.0 L min^{-1} per kg, using commercial balanced feeds. Algazzar et al. (2008) also reported that optimum water exchange rate can make a significant difference in fish production in Wadi Al Natroon Desert, Egypt. The authors stocked Nile tilapia (50 g $fish^{-1}$) in concrete tanks (250 m^3 each) at a density of 34 fish m^{-3}. The tanks were aerated with paddle wheels and subjected to three water exchange rates (5%, 10% and 20% per day). After 6 months, the average fish weights were 285, 410 and 510 g, with a total biomass of 9, 14 and 17 kg m^{-3}, respectively. At 5% exchange rate the tanks required additional aeration through air injection to improve the productivity to reach that of the 10% water exchange rate. Similarly, growth performance, feed efficiency and haematological and serum biochemical parameters of GIFT tilapia juveniles reared in concrete tanks decreased sharply at zero water exchange (Kpundeh et al., 2013).

6.5.4 Raceway culture

Raceway culture system (Fig. 6.10) can be an ideal system for tilapia culture, especially in rural areas where irrigation raceways and canals are available. While rearing tilapia in raceways was reported more than 30 years ago (Balarin and Haller, 1982), studies on the production of tilapia in raceways are also still limited. D'Silva and Maughan (1995) evaluated the effects of stocking density and water quality on red tilapia (*O. mossambicus* × *Oreochromis urolepis*

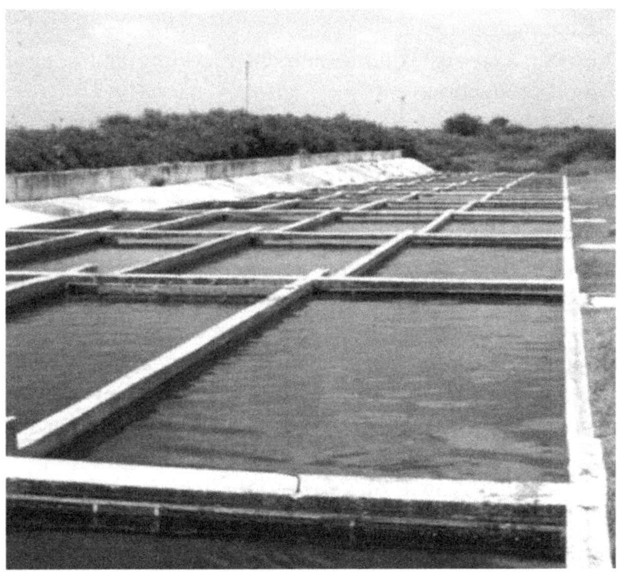

FIGURE 6.10 Intensive culture of tilapia in raceways in Mexico. *Photo provided by K. Fitzsimmons.*

hornorum) reared in pulsed-flow culture systems in irrigation ditches. The fish were stocked at 10, 20, 30, 50 and 70 fish m^{-3}. The results indicated that a 20 fish m^{-3} produced the best marketable yield. Increasing density resulted in increased ammonia concentration and decreased DO levels. Windmar et al. (2000b) described a raceway of 650 m long, divided into five compartments, with a water flow rate of 1.7 $m^3 s^{-1}$ which is used for the production of 480 t of Nile tilapia in Zimbabwe.

6.6 Green water tank culture

Green water tank culture is an intensive culture system where fish wastes and other metabolites are treated in such a way to increase natural primary productivity in culture units. The process involves the oxidation of toxic ammonia (NH_3) and nitrite (NO_2) into relatively nontoxic nitrate (NO_3) through nitrifying bacteria grown on suspended organic matter. The bacteria remove the organic matter from the tanks by using it as food, while the bacteria themselves are used as natural food for filter feeding fishes such as tilapia and carps. However, in green water systems, solid wastes should be removed continuously and both biofiltration and aeration should be provided. Vigorous aeration is necessary to support the suspension of the microbial community, maximize contact between bacteria and waste products and, in turn, increase phytoplankton productivity.

Green water tank culture has many advantages:

1. High system productivity and profitability.
2. Efficient use of water (i.e. minimum or even zero water exchange where only losses due to evaporation and/or solid removal are replaced).
3. The solid waste (sludge) can be used as organic fertilizer.
4. Easy management.
5. Lower feed cost, due to nutrient recycling and natural food production.

Another important advantage of green water system is that it can control the population of pathogenic bacteria in tilapia tanks and reduce their effects. Tendencia and dela Peña (2003) studied the effects of some components of green water system on initial control of luminous bacteria (*Vibrio harveyi*) using tilapia (*Oreochromis hornorum*) and *Chlorella* separately. Tilapia were reared in indoor, circulated tanks at 0, 1 and 3 kg m^{-3}, and the bacteria were inoculated into the tanks at a density of 103 cfu mL^{-1}. The bacteria were not detected in fish tanks 4–6 days after injection. The authors attributed the ability of tilapia to prevent the initial growth of *Vibrio* to the inhibitor properties of lactic acid bacteria (*Enterrococcus durans*) isolated from fish intestine. In addition, Lio-Po et al. (2005) attributed the effectiveness of the green water system to the presence of antiluminous *Vibrio* factors in bacterial, fungal and phytoplankton microbiota and skin mucus of tilapia. When pure *Chlorella* culture was injected with *V. harveyi*, the bacteria were not detected 2–3 days after injection, presumably due to the secretion of antimicrobial compounds from *Chlorella*.

Huervana et al. (2006) found also that green water obtained from tank culture of *O. mossambicus* broodstock has the ability to inhibit luminous vibriosis over a 1-week period. When the green water collected from tilapia tanks was inoculated with *V. harveyi*, the bacteria were not detected. Black tiger shrimp farmers in the Philippines took an advantage of this phenomenon and developed a green water technique as a means of inhibiting bacterial pathogens, especially luminous vibriosis. This technique involves the use of green water from salt-tolerant tilapia such as *O. hornorum* and *O. mossambicus* as rearing water for shrimp culture in ponds. This culture water was able to prevent the onset of luminous vibriosis (Huervana et al., 2006; Lio-Po, 2017).

The viral load of white spot syndrome virus (WSSV), which is the most pathogenic and the longest existing shrimp virus, has also been reported to decrease in the presence of green water (Tendencia et al., 2012). These authors investigated the efficiency of three farming systems against WSSV. Shrimp (*Penaeus monodon*), infected with WSSV by feeding with WSSV-positive shrimp carcass, was tank cultured in green water from tilapia tanks, using *chlorella* as natural food, or with supplementation of molasses to enhance growth of yellow *Vibrio*, while shrimp cultured in seawater served as a control. WSSV was significantly lower in shrimp cultured using green water than in other treatments. However, nitrogenous waste levels were lowest in molasses-added water and highest in green water. These results suggest that the use of green water in combination with the addition of molasses for shrimp culture is highly beneficial for protection against WSSV and improving water quality.

Tilapia culture in green water systems is practiced in Israel (Avnimelech, 1998), the United States (Lutz, 1996) and Virgin Islands (Martin et al., 2000, 2001; Rakocy et al., 2000a, 2000b). Rakocy et al. (2000a, 2000b, 2004) described the green water tank system currently in use in the US Virgin Islands and evaluated its suitability for red tilapia and sex-reversed Nile tilapia culture in a series of studies. Water exchange at 5% d^{-1} did not improve fish survival, growth and yield over a zero water exchange. Sludge removal significantly improved fish performance, but not survival. Weekly application of alum (aluminium sulphate) at 51.5 mg L^{-1} had resulted in a significant increase of Nile tilapia growth and yield. Martin et al. (2000) also reported that Nile tilapia stocked in green water tanks at 26 fish m^{-3} and fed with a 32% cp feed attained biomass of 13.4 kg m^{-3}, an FCR of 1.41 and a survival rate of 99.3%, with an exchange rate of only 0.23% of the tank water per day. Lutz (1996) reported that tilapia production capacity in greenhouse using green water systems in Louisiana is about 250 t yr^{-1}.

6.7 Tilapia culture in recirculating systems

Tilapia have traditionally been cultured in inland-based systems, such as earthen ponds and concrete tanks and, to a lesser extent, raceways. These systems have started to encounter a number of problems that make their long-term sustainability unwarranted. These are:

1. The growing environmental concerns about the effect of the effluents from land-based aquaculture facilities.
2. The limitation and shortage of freshwater supplies together with the competition for it with agricultural, industrial and other urban requirements, especially in arid areas.
3. Increasing land costs, which will limit land use opportunities.
4. Climate changes, which may limit management and production of these systems.
5. Introduction of tilapia into many countries where the environmental conditions are outside their tolerance limits has made the traditional land-based systems unsuitable for tilapia culture in these countries.

Recirculating culture systems 'also known as recycle or closed systems' are an ideal alternative for confronting these difficulties. These systems are characterized by water reuse; i.e. minimal effluent discharge and optimal water conservation. Culture water goes through various treatment processes to restore its quality. These include the removal of solid wastes and suspended metabolites (such as carbon dioxide, ammonia and nitrite), sterilization and aeration. The typical closed system consists of settling tanks (for solids removal), biological and/or mechanical filters (for ammonia removal), ultraviolet (UV) light (for sterilization) and aerators (compressors) or a source of oxygen (Fig. 6.11). A full description of this system has been reviewed by a number of authors (Mires and Anjioni, 1997; Losordo et al., 1999; Muir et al., 2000; van Rijn, 2013; Xiao et al., 2018).

Tilapia culture in recirculating systems is widely spreading in different parts of the world, especially in the areas which face freshwater shortages and/or rough climatic conditions. In southern Israel, commercial culture of tilapia in closed systems is carried out year round in greenhouses, even at low water temperature (19°C) up to 29°C (Muir et al., 2000). At a stocking density of 15 kg m^{-3}, the system produces 25 kg m^{-3} yr^{-1}. Fingerling red tilapia (*O. niloticus* × *O. aureus*) were also grown in indoor tanks or raceway at a density of about 300 fish (40 g) m^{-3} until

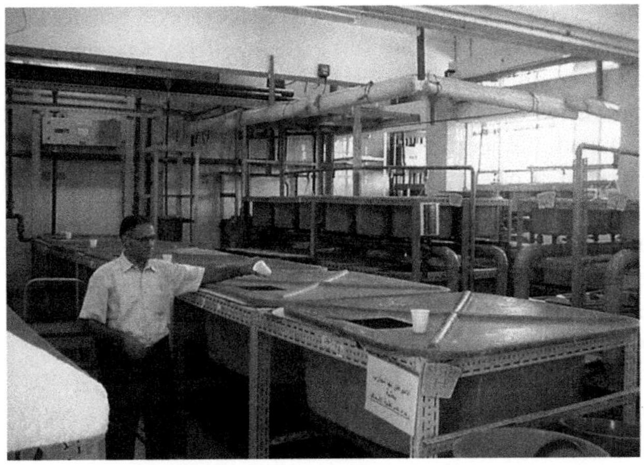

FIGURE 6.11 A recirculating system used for intensive culture of tilapia at the United Arab Emirates University. *Photograph by A.-F. El-Sayed.*

they reached an average weight of 200 g. The density was then reduced to 150 fish m^{-3} during fattening stage to reach 450 g (Muir et al., 2000).

Mires and Amit (1992) described tilapia culture in a closed system known as 'DEKEL System', where water recycles between concrete growout ponds and earthen reservoir serving as a biofilter. This system was able to maintain water quality suitable for tilapia culture. The net yield reached 19.5 kg m^{-2} in 1990. In a later study, Mires and Anjioni (1997) evaluated the technical and economical performance of red tilapia in the DEKEL system and in another closed system supported by a biofilter and pure oxygen supply and referred to as O2BIO. Production in the O2BIO was higher than DEKEL system; however, it was less cost-effective. As a matter of fact, after some technical improvements on DEKET system, the net present value (NPV) > 0 can be obtained after only 2 years, with an internal rate of return (IRR) $= 22\%$ after 4 years. On the contrary, the NPV > 0 of O2BIO can only be reached after 11 years. Only when production reaches 100 kg m^{-2} and the initial investment is reduced from US\$ 600 m^{-2} to US\$ 500 m^{-2}, is an NPV > 0 in O2BIO system obtained, after 6 years. Meanwhile, both systems were not economic due to high production costs and should be improved to produce a positive cash flow.

Tilapia culture in water recycling systems in the United States is also gaining great popularity because their culture in traditional land-based systems is limited due to their tropical nature. Closed systems are currently the most sophisticated, using liquid oxygen, microscreens, fluidized bead biofilters and UV sterilizer. They also have highest stocking densities of any tilapia culture systems (Rosati et al., 1993; Fitzsimmons, 2003). Rosati et al. (1993) determined the carrying capacity and performance of a recirculating system consisting of 18.5 m^3 fibreglass raceway and vertical screen filter when stocked with Nile tilapia under commercial conditions. The fish (15 g) were stocked at 263.2 fish m^{-3}. Final survival was 70%. Oxygen and unionized ammonia became limiting factors when the feed approached 8 and 12 kg day^{-1}. Rosati et al. (1997) further evaluated the performance of Nile tilapia (95% males) reared in a prototype commercial-scale recirculating system. The system consisted of six raceways, with total water capacity of 160 m^3, provided with a rotating drum with screen biofilter, submerged biofilter media and pure oxygen. The fish grew from 15–20 g to 560 g in 6 months. The total yield was 11.33 t $year^{-1}$ (78.8 kg m^{-3} per year).

Tilapia culture in recycle systems has also been reported in other tropical and subtropical regions. Cheong et al. (1987) reported a growth of Taiwanese red tilapia raised in a recycle system, from 0.78 to 438 g in 239 days, with a total production of 49.3–50.2 kg m^{-3}. Watanabe et al. (1997) also described a recycle hatchery system for Florida red tilapia in the Bahamas. In Egypt, tilapia culture in recirculating aquaculture system (RAS) has also been reported to be highly viable and profitable. A pioneering pilot tilapia culture project in RAS in Egypt, funded by the Netherlands government, in an exchange programme, was carried out (Radwan and Leschen, 2011). Monosex Nile tilapia (250 g) was raised in RAS in 24-m^3 concrete tanks (3 × 8 × 1 m), at a density of 93 fish m^{-3}. About 30% of the water volume in the system was replaced daily, in order to clean the system of faeces and other suspended solids. The fish were fed a commercial, 32% cp, extruded feed. After 100 culture days, the average final weight was 450 g, with a production of 41.6 kg m^{-3}. The benefit/cost of this first trial was 1.37. The authors acknowledged that with more modifications and management arrangements, profitability could be increased much further. However, energy cost of the system was relatively high. The appropriate renewable energy sources and technologies need to be developed in order to make RAS sustainable and more economically viable (Table 6.4).

TABLE 6.4 Economic performance of intensive tilapia farming in Egypt.

Costs and returns (US$)	Concrete tanks (Sharkia)[a]	RAS (Kafr El-Shaikh)[b]
Farm size	4.2 ha	140 m^3
Total variable costs (TVC)	19,336	7704
Seeds	545	4333
Feeds	16,364	2327
Protein content (%)	30–35	30–32
Price of feed (US$/t)	684–896	684–704
Fertilizers	Not used	Not used
Labour	727	522
Energy and fuel	700	522
Miscellaneous costs	1000	–
Total fixed costs (TFC)	2680	486
Depreciation	1000	486
Construction depreciation	NA	NA
Equipment depreciation	NA	NA
Land use cost (rental)	1680	NA
Total costs (TC) = TVC + TFC	22,016	8190
Total gross revenue (GR)	32,000	11,230
Net return (NR) = GR − TC	9984	3040
Benefit–cost ratio (BCR) = GR/TC	1.45	1.37

[a] *El-Sayed (2013).*
[b] *Radwan and Leschen (2011).*

The performance of Nile tilapia fingerlings (2 g) has also been evaluated in a hyper-intensive RAS in Mexico. The fish were stocked at 400, 500 and 600 fish m^{-3}, with low water exchange (Gullian-Klanian and Arámburu-Adame, 2013). Fish growth was similar at 400 and 500 fish m^{-3}, with a final weight of 66–67 g after 70 days. At 600 fish m^{-3} the growth was slightly reduced to 60 g $fish^{-1}$.

It should be emphasized here that recirculating system is technically sophisticated and very costly, while tilapia is considered a 'low-priced fish' in many countries. Production of these fishes with high investment in commercial recycle systems may, therefore, be neither cost-effective, nor sustainable in these countries. The message is clear; cost–benefit analyses should be carefully conducted prior to the adoption of tilapia culture in recycle systems in developing countries.

Recirculating systems are characterized by supporting extremely high stocking densities and high net production, compared with other culture systems. However, stocking density has a significant effect on individual fish growth, survival, total production and water quality. A decrease in final individual fish weight and an increase in total yield with increasing stocking density are very commonly observed. Considerable variations in fish size may also occur with increasing fish density in recycle systems (Rosati et al., 1993). Suresh and Lin (1992) evaluated the effects of stocking density on water quality and production of all-male red tilapia juveniles (75 g) stocked in circular tanks at 50, 100 and 200 fish m^{-3} for 70 days. Fish growth, feed efficiency and water quality were inversely correlated with stocking density. However, 100 and 200 fish m^{-3} showed similar performance. Feed digestion and body composition were not affected by stocking density. As mentioned earlier, Bailey et al. (2000) raised Nile tilapia juveniles (4.3 g) in 2-m^3 circular tanks in a recirculating system, at two densities, 200 and 450 fish m^{-3}, for 12 weeks. Fish stocked at 200 fish m^{-3} grew slightly faster than those stocked at 450 fish m^{-3}. The desired survival, uniform size and FCR were not achieved, as a result of using large feed pellets.

6.8 Effluent treatment and management

In recycle systems, as in other culture systems, considerable amounts of fish metabolites, including ammonia, nitrites, organic phosphates, and suspended solids, along with uneaten feed are released into the culture water. These compounds are generally toxic to fish, and have high biological oxygen demand (BOD). If not removed or treated, they may be subject to oxidation, leading to the removal of oxygen from the water, and in turn, producing anaerobic conditions that will stress and/or kill the fish. The magnitude of this problem is much higher in RAS than in flow-through systems, where these compounds can be discharged with effluent water and eliminated through natural processes. Thus, effluent treatment and management become essential for successful aquaculture in recycle systems. Typically, management includes (1) waste settlement and removal; (2) removal of ammonia and nitrites via biofiltration, sterilization and aeration and (3) partial water replacement. In a comprehensive review, van Rijn (2013) described and analyzed solid waste capture and waste water production, treatment and disposal in RAS.

6.8.1 Waste settlement and removal

Solid wastes can be removed through water exchange or backflushing of filters (i.e. mechanical or biofiltration with fixed-film media) (Cole et al., 1997). Waste removal from recirculating systems of tilapia has been reported to improve their performance very significantly. Cole et al. (1997) studied the effects of solid removal (twice a day) on tilapia production and water quality in continuously aerated tanks. The removal of solids significantly increased final fish weight and net yield, but not fish survival, compared to a no-solids-removal system. It also sharply reduced total solids, volatile solids, suspended solids, organic nitrogen, inorganic nitrogen, total phosphorus, chemical oxygen demand (COD) and BOD. However, DO, temperature, NH_4-N and NO_3-N were not significantly affected by solids removal.

Traditional biofiltration, including water exchange, back-flushing, fixed-film media, may be inconvenient to small-scale tilapia farmers in developing countries, mainly due to their (1) occasional failure and (2) high costs, which make them unaffordable for many farmers. Other cheap, locally available biofiltration methods have been tried for solids removal from tilapia culture tanks with great success. For example, the addition of carbon-rich (C-rich) agricultural by-products into fish tanks can be used for solids removal. These C-rich wastes can be combined with nitrogen-rich (N-rich) organic solids discharged from recycle systems to produce marketable compost.

Rice hulls (RH), an abundant by-product of rice polishing in many developing countries, have a good potential as a primary medium for solids removal from RAS (Scott et al., 1998). RH are characterized by (1) a large surface area on which bacteria can grow; (2) oblong shape that facilitates biofilm protection; (3) high availability at no charge; (4) light weight with high porosity and low bulk density and (5) they degrade very slowly because they are composed mainly of silica. Therefore, RH constitute appropriate media which could be used with a three-phase reactor (air, water, and RH) (Greensword, 2017).

A number of studies have evaluated RH as a biocarrier media in RAS. Scott et al. (1998) investigated the use of RH as a primary medium for solids removal from tilapia RAS. These hulls removed 94%, 66% and 63% of settleable solids, TSS and COD, respectively. In another study, the authors evaluated the effects of the direct addition of RH to the culture water on solids removal and found that about 52% of TSS can be removed using this method. Davis et al. (2011) also found that RH have a promising potential for nitrogen oxidation in waste water treatment. Greensword (2017) compared the total ammonia nitrogen (TAN) removal capacities of RH and synthetic plastic media in a three-phase reactor configuration, in ultra-oligotrophic, oligotrophic and lower mesotrophic conditions. He found that RH displayed a TAN conversion rate of 1025 g-N m^{-3}, compared to 1219 g-N m^{-3} displayed by synthetic plastic beads, proving that RH can be a viable biocarrier. These results indicate the high potential of RH in rice-producing developing countries, allowing them to choose for a more affordable integration of modern biofiltration in their aquaculture industries. This type of research is necessary, and should be encouraged, as it indicates that simple, and in the same time efficient, technologies can be used in RAS, in areas where sophisticated technologies are either not available or not affordable.

6.8.2 Removal of ammonia and nitrites

Several methods of ammonia (NH_3) and nitrite (NO_2) removal from culture water are in use, including the biological conversion of ammonia to nitrites and nitrates with nitrifying bacteria in filters or aeration tanks, the adsorption onto ion exchange resins, transfer to the atmosphere by air bubbling through water and chemical reactions with chlorine (Balarin and Haller, 1982). Biological treatment remains the most practical and cost-effective method.

Nitrification is based mainly on biofiltration on fixed media, such as biosedimentation, or biodiscs, or suspended media such as activated sludge.

Different biofiltration types have been described for ammonia removal in recirculating tilapia culture systems. Ridha and Cruz (2001) evaluated the efficiency of two types of biofilter media; polypropylene plastic chips and polyethylene blocks in ammonia removal, water quality and waste accumulation with respect to Nile tilapia reared in a recycle system. No difference in performance efficiency between the two types of media was evident. However, the authors suggested the use of the polypropylene plastic chips because they are cheaper.

Bead filters can be used efficiently for nitrification and clarification of culture water in recirculating culture systems. They can capture solid wastes, stimulate the growth of heterotrophic bacteria and reduce NH_3, NO_2 and O_2 availability for the nitrifying autotrophic bacteria (Lenger and Pfeiffer, 2002). Different types of bead filters are currently in use. Sastry et al. (1999) studied the efficiency of a bubble-washed bead filter in solid capture and biological filtration in a recirculating Nile tilapia culture system at feed loading rates of 16, 24 and 32 kg day^{-1} per m^{-3} of beads. They found that more frequent backflushing improved filter performance and was necessary at higher feeding rates. Five backwashes in 24 h were necessary at the highest feeding load. Similar results have been reported when floating bead filters were used (Lenger and Pfeiffer, 2002). Slow-sand filters have also been widely used for the treatment of effluents within recycle aquaculture systems. These filters are simple, cheap, easy to construct and operate and effectively remove suspended solids. Drennan et al. (1993) evaluated the use of a slow-sand filter for the containment of tilapia eggs and/or fry in a recycle system. The system was very efficient despite the frequent clogging of the bead due to high solids loading.

In some RAS, where ammonia is converted to nitrate, special denitrification reactors, supplied with external or internal carbon sources are used to induce bacterial reduction of nitrate to nitrogen gas under anoxic conditions. A denitrification reactor using internal carbon source was incorporated into Nile tilapia RAS in the Netherlands (Martins et al., 2010). Organic matter is oxidized by reducing NO_3. This RAS reduces water consumption, and NO_3 and organic matter discharge. The performance of a tilapia RAS with and without denitrification was compared for the nutrient utilization efficiency, resource use and waste discharge per kg of fish produced (Eding et al., 2009). The results revealed that the RAS with denitrification requires lower heat, water and bicarbonate; however, its requirement for electricity, oxygen, labour and overall production costs is higher than the conventional RAS. The integration of denitrification has reduced waste discharge by 81% for nitrogen (N), 59% for COD, 61% for total oxygen demand (TOD), 30% for CO_2 and 58% for total dissolved solids.

Aquatic weeds can also remove a considerable portion of solids from RAS. Through competition for light and nutrients in the water, macrophytes usually prevent or, at least, minimize phytoplankton blooming and keep culture water clear. The macrophytes themselves can be used as food for cultured herbivorous fishes such as tilapia and carps. Rakocy and Allison (1981) investigated the efficiency of two floating macrophytes, water hyacinth (*Eichhornia crassipes*) and *Spirodela oligorhiza*, in oxygen uptake from waste water of blue tilapia (*O. aureus*) culture. The fish were stocked in concrete tanks at 16.2, 32.5 and 48.7 fish m^{-3}. Plant populations removed 15.8%, 13.4% and 12% of the waste nitrogen, at the three stocking densities, respectively. Marine algae have also been used for biofiltering waste effluents from closed systems of marine fish and shellfish. *Gracilaria chilensis* (Rhodophyta) was highly efficient in removing soluble nutrients, but had little effect on particulate nutrients, during a separate tank culture of a Chelan fish *Isacia conteptionis*, oyster *Crassostrea gigas* and sea urchin *Loxechinus albus* (Chow et al., 2001). The ammonia from the fish culture and nitrate from the oyster culture were completely removed from the water by the weed.

6.8.3 Water discharge

As discussed earlier, recirculating systems are adopted mainly in areas having limited freshwater sources and rough weather conditions. Economic use of these sources becomes a necessity, and water discharge may not be appropriate. Water recycling and reuse, through post-treatment and/or treatment within the system has been tried for several years as a means of reducing water discharge. Minimizing, or even eliminating, water discharge from tilapia cultured in recycle systems has been investigated with varying degrees of success. Shnel et al. (2002) evaluated the 'zero' discharge from tilapia recirculating system for 331 days in a greenhouse. Neither water nor organic matter was discharged, except for the addition of water to compensate the loss and evaporation. Sludge was also biologically digested, and nitrate was reduced to nitrogen gas. Total tilapia yield was 81.1 kg m^{-3} at a maximum stocking density of 61.8 kg m^{-3}. Inorganic nitrogen concentrations were within acceptable levels for tilapia culture. Water quality remained within the acceptable levels for tilapia throughout the study. Daily average ammonia removal was 0.16 g N m^{-2}, while nitrate removal was most profound in the sedimentation/digestion basin.

About 70% of the phosphorus added with the feed was recovered mostly in the anoxic treatment stage of the system.

6.9 Tilapia production in aquaponic systems

Hydroponic systems are generally the production of plant/vegetable crops in areas smaller than that required under field production; or the production of these vegetables without soils. This practice is done by providing the nutrients that the plant requires with irrigation water. Aquaponics is the integration of hydroponics with aquaculture in a recirculating system, where the wastes and metabolites produced by cultured fish are removed by nitrification and taken up by the plants. The bacteria living in the gravel and in association with the plant roots play a critical role in nutrient removal. Thus, as the aquaculture effluent flows through the aquaculture/hydroponic system, the plants act as a 'biological filter' by removing fish wastes and improving the quality of the culture water. Aquaponic systems have many advantages, including the following:

1. The wastes of one system are used as inputs or fuel for another biological system.
2. The integration of fish and plants increases the diversity and enhances system stability and sustainability.
3. Reducing the volume of waste discharged to the environment and minimizing the negative environmental impacts by water filtration and removing nutrients from water before it leaves the system.
4. Minimizing water exchange and reducing operating costs.
5. The introduction of 'organic products' into the market, which increases farmers' income and supports the local economy.
6. The production of two (or more) food products from one production unit.
7. In arid areas where water is scarce, aquaponics is an appropriate technology that allows food production with re-used water.
8. The system is simple, inexpensive and easy to adopt.

Aquaponics is, therefore, a promising, sustainable food production technology, especially in developing/arid countries, where resources are limited, freshwater is scare and population is increasing.

The site selected for aquaponic system should be stable, protected from winds and floods, exposed to direct sunlight, easily accessible and provided with the necessary utilities. Any aquaponic system should include fish tanks, mechanical and biological filters and plant grows beds (hydroponics). Tank size, shape, colour and material should be carefully chosen. Mechanical filters include sedimentation tanks, radial flow clarifiers, sand or bead filters and baffle filters; however, clarifiers are recommended for small-scale aquaponics. The biological filters are installed between the mechanical filter and the hydroponic containers. They should have a large surface area supplied with sufficient aeration to enhance nitrifying bacterial growth. The media bed (bench bed) hydroponic system, nutrient film technique and deep water culture are the most common hydroponic systems currently in use within aquaponics systems. Full description of aquaponic systems is given by Somerville et al. (2014), Tyson and Simonne (2014) and Nelson (2017).

Tilapia is among the best candidates for aquaponic systems due to their tolerance to high stocking loads and crowding and their resistance to stress, disease, handling and environmental changes. Several studies have considered the production of tilapia in aquaponic systems, with promising results. The Agricultural Experimental Station at the University of Virgin Islands (Fig. 6.12), United States, has a long history of aquaponic research, especially with tilapia production, which started more than three decades ago (Rakocy and Allison, 1981). The production of tilapia in aquaponic systems has also been reported in other geographical regions.

The use of effluents from intensive tank culture of Florida red tilapia for field production of bell peppers had been evaluated (Palada et al., 1999). Water from fish rearing tanks with low (8 fish m^{-3}) and high (16 fish m^{-3}) stocking densities and two daily water exchange rates (0% and 5%) were applied to plots grown with bell peppers 2–3 times weekly. Pepper production from these treatments was compared with that produced through solids (sludge) removed from fish rearing units, cow manure and commercial N fertilizers. Yield from fertigated plots was significantly higher than all other treatments. The yields of pepper from plots fertilized with rearing tank water from two exchange rates were not significantly different from

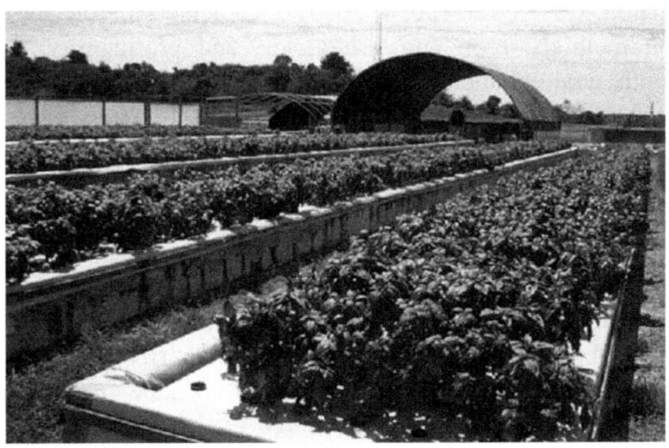

FIGURE 6.12 Tilapia culture in aquaponic system at the University of Virgin Islands. *Photo provided by J. Rakocy and D. Bailey.*

yields produced through inorganic N fertilizer. Tank sludge produced the highest marketable yield. Similarly, Anadu and Barho (2002) compared the production of tomatoes and lettuce grown with blue tilapia in an aquaponic system with those grown in the convention soil. The vegetables grew much faster in aquaponics system, and tomatoes started flowering 2 weeks earlier than soil-grown tomatoes. A prototype tilapia/hydroponic greenhouse recirculating production system for institutional application has been described by Newton et al. (1998) in Blacksburg and Petersburg, Virginia, United States. Tilapia was used as aquaculture species, while vegetables tested included tomatoes and lettuce. The objectives were to produce tilapia crop within 5–6 months and to reuse the effluent water for irrigation and nutrient inputs into the vegetable crops. Rakocy et al. (2001) also described and evaluated an outdoor commercial-scale production of Nile tilapia in an aquaponic system with 13 different types of vegetables.

The production of tilapia and vegetables in aquaponic systems appears very profitable. Rakocy and Bailey (2003) conducted an initial economic analysis of tilapia and lettuce in aquaponics system. The results showed that the return/risk and management for one production unit is US$ 30,874.62 (185,247.73 for 6 units). The authors suggested that break-even prices of tilapia and lettuce could be even lower in other places where production costs (construction costs, electricity, water, labour, etc.) are lower. Producing other vegetables such as okra and herbs (such as basil) in aquaponic systems with tilapia was also profitable (Rakocy and Bailey, 2003). Rakocy et al. (2004) updated the production of tilapia and vegetables in the UVI hydroponic system and compared the yield of okra and basil in this system with conventional field system. The production of these crops was much higher in the aquaponic system. These results clearly justify the adoption of aquaponic systems for fish/vegetable production.

Despite the great potential and expansion of aquaponics, as an important method of food production, only a few studies have considered commercial-scale aquaponics production. Love et al. (2014, 2015) documented the production methods, crop and fish yields, and profitability of commercial aquaponics in the United States and globally, through an online survey. The results revealed that tilapia is the most commonly raised aquatic animals (69% of respondents), followed by ornamental fish (43%), catfish (25%) and other aquatic animals (18%). The most frequently grown plants among commercial producers were leafy green vegetables, herbs, and fruiting crops, including basil (*Ocimum basilicum*, 81% of respondents), salad greens (76%), nonbasil herbs (73%), tomatoes (*Solanum lycopersicum*, 68%), head lettuce (*Lactuca sativa*, 68%), kale (*Brassica oleracea*, 56%), chard (*Beta vulgaris* subspecies *cicla*, 55%), bok choi (*Brassica rapa* subspecies *chinensis*, 51%), peppers (*Capsicum annuum*, 48%) and cucumbers (*Cucumis sativus*, 45%). Among the several factors which were significantly associated with profitability, aquaponics was the respondents' primary source of income.

English (2015) also analyzed the economic feasibility of tilapia, basil and lettuce aquaponics under greenhouse conditions in Arkansas, United States, using the University of the Virgin Islands' Commercial Aquaponics 2 (UVI CA2) system. He found that only lettuce and basil were profitable within the system, while tilapia production resulted in an annual net loss of US$23,020. However, the production of tilapia in combination with hydroponic production achieved net returns of $34,005 for tilapia and lettuce production, $192,733 for tilapia and basil, and $110,579 for tilapia, lettuce and basil. Determined payback period was 1.27 years for tilapia and basil and 2.17 years for tilapia, lettuce and basil. Thus, tilapia and basil production offers lower risk for investors, than tilapia, lettuce and basil. These results suggest that aquaponic food production using the UVI CA2 system could be economically feasible in temperate areas, if the proper crops are selected and the viable markets are available.

Similarly, Kloas et al. (2015) evaluated the use of an aquaponics system to improve sustainability and productivity, and, in the same time, lower environmental emissions. They used innovated aquaponics system for (nearly) emission-free tomato and fish (tilapia) production (ASTAF-PRO) in greenhouses. This double recirculation aquaponic system provided optimum conditions for increasing productivity and preventing adverse interactions between fish and plant units. Tilapia productivity in ASTAF-PRO was similar to that in RAS, while the efficiency of tomato production was similar to conventional hydroponics. This finding indicated that ASTAF-PRO can improve sustainability and productivity, and lower environmental emissions.

Silva et al. (2017) investigated whether biological filters are necessary in aquaponics systems. They evaluated water quality of semi-intensive, small-scale Nile tilapia–pak choi (*Brassica chinensis*) aquaponics system, with and without a bacterial biofilter (BF and NBF) under tropical conditions. At the end of the experiment the individual fresh total weight, dry total weight, edible weight, height and diameter of the pak choi plants were not significantly different between treatments. The yield of food produced was also similar to that reported for pak choi and tilapia grown separately. TAN and nitrite nitrogen (NO_2-N) were higher in the NBF influent than in the BF influent, but they were similar in the effluent of both treatments. These results suggest that the aquaponics plants can act as a biofilter, and that NBF aquaponics system could be used for small-scale farmers in the tropics. The NBF system is also easier to manage and less costly than a BF aquaponics system. In addition, aquaponics system without a biofilter is an ecologically sustainable way of food production for rural communities.

6.10 Biofloc technology

According to National Agricultural Library (NAL) Glossary (United States Department of Agriculture), biofloc technology (BT) is defined as: 'the use of aggregates of bacteria, algae, or protozoa, held together in a matrix along with particulate organic matter for the purpose of improving water quality, waste treatment and disease prevention in intensive aquaculture systems'. In other words, biofloc is a symbiotic process that includes confined aquatic animals, heterotrophic bacteria and other microbial species in the water. Consumption of bioflocs also provides nutritional value to cultured aquatic species. This simply means that BT can be an ideal alternative for sustainable and environmentally friendly aquaculture (Crab et al., 2012). In general, the following benefits can be generated from BT (Hargreaves, 2013):

1. Prevention of the introduction of diseases to fish farms from incoming water.
2. Improvement of biosecurity.
3. Improvement of feed conversion.
4. Improvement of water quality.
5. Improvement of water use efficiency.
6. Increasing land use efficiency.
7. Reduction of sensitivity to light fluctuations.

However, biofloc system may not be as easy as we might think. It is rather technically complicated and more sophisticated than one can imagine. BT may also have some disadvantages (Hargreaves, 2013):

1. Increased energy requirement for vigorous, continuous aeration and mixing.
2. Short response time due to elevated water respiration rates. Thus, monitoring, alarms and emergency power supply are required.
3. Start-up period required.
4. Increased nitrification instability.
5. Alkalinity supplementation required.
6. Increased pollution potential from nitrate accumulation.
7. Inconsistent and seasonal performance for sunlight-exposed systems.

According to Rakocy (2019, personal communication), a typical biofloc system contains a clarifier to remove excess biofloc, alkalinity supplementation tank to reduce the water acidity, heavy aeration, a method for inducing a circular current and denitrification tanks (Figure 6.13). The bioflocs serve as a biofilter in the water column and allow feeding rates much higher than in pond culture. However, high feeding rate leads to high total suspended solids (TSS); which can reach 2000 mg L^{-1} (Rakocy, Virgin Islands, 2019, personal communication). Therefore, introducing a clarifier might be necessary to keep TSS at about 500 mg L^{-1}, which provided good nitrification. Due to the large amount of nitrification in the system, nitrate-nitrogen levels may dramatically increase, reaching up to 700 mg L^{-1}. In this case, denitrification tanks are required to reduce nitrate-nitrogen.

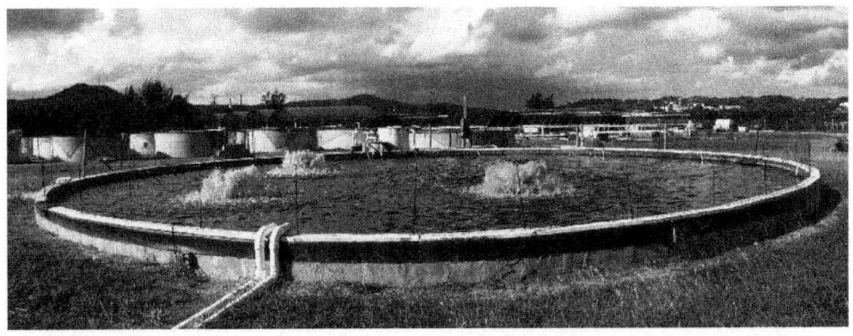

FIGURE 6.13 University of Virgin Islands Biofloc System. *Photo provided by J. Rakocy.*

BT can be applied both in semi-intensive and intensive pond systems and intensive tank and RAS culture systems. In fact, extensive research has been carried out on tilapia culture in biofloc systems under experimental and commercial conditions. Therefore, tilapia is currently among the most common species farmed in biofloc systems. They are able to take up bioflocs as an additional protein source, resulting in a considerable reduction in the cost of production inputs (Crab et al., 2009, 2012).

Avnimelech (2007) reported that tilapia biofloc can contribute to about 50% of their protein requirement. Biofloc also increased Nile tilapia production by 45%, compared to tilapia grown in traditional culture system (Azim and Little, 2008). Growth and survival of tilapia cultured in greenhouse ponds with BT were also excellent, ranging from 80% to 97%, depending on fish size (Crab et al., 2009). Dried and processed bioflocs have been tried as a feed ingredient to replace the conventional protein sources in aquafeed. However, it is unlikely that dried bioflocs could be included in commercial-scale aquafeed manufacturing because only limited quantities are available and also because producing and drying biofloc solids at a commercial scale may not be cost-effective.

The effects of bioflocs on growth, feed digestibility and utilization, and immune response of tilapia have been investigated by a number of researchers. Long et al. (2015) assessed the effects of BT on the growth, digestive enzymes activity, haematology, and immune response of GIFT tilapia, stocked at 3 kg m^{-3}, under light-limited and zero water exchange culture tanks. Glucose was added as a carbon source to the BT treatment to keep a carbon/nitrogen (C/N) ratio of 15/1. BT significantly reduced nitrite and nitrate concentrations compared to the control, BT-free treatment. Fish performance and net yield were also significantly improved in biofloc treatment. In addition, the BT treatment resulted in higher intestine amylase and liver lipase activities, serum glutathione peroxidase and lysozyme activities, while blood parameters were not significantly affected by BT.

The effect of reducing dietary protein level under zero-water exchange systems with or without carbon source, on water quality, growth, immune and antioxidant status of Nile tilapia (48 g) was assessed (Mansour and Esteban, 2017). The fish were fed 20 or 30% cp diet with or without carbon source (wheat milling by-product (WMB) or RB). The highest biofloc volume was obtained when WMB was used as a carbon source. The best growth rates were obtained at 30% cp in the presence of biofloc. However, fish fed 20% cp diet with WMB biofloc attained significantly higher performance than those fed 30% crude protein in clear water. Biofloc treatments significantly improved haematocrit, white blood cells, lymphocytes, plasma proteins, and humoral and cellular immune parameters, and also increased superoxide dismutase and catalase activities.

The growth performance and robustness of Nile tilapia larvae produced from broodstock maintained in a biofloc-based facility was investigated (Ekasari et al., 2015). Molasses (53% C) were added daily into the biofloc system at an estimated C/N ratio of 10/1. The survival rate of the larvae from BT (90%−98%) was much higher than that of the larvae from control group (67%−75%). When the larvae were infected with the pathogenic bacteria (*Streptococcus agalactiae*), these from BT origin showed a significantly higher survival (75%−80%) than the control larvae reared in control, BT-free water (55%). Infection resistance increased upon housing the control larvae in BT water. When the larvae were subjected to salinity stress, the larvae of BT origin showed a higher survival at 1 and 24 h post-salinity stress than for the larvae of control treatment. These results indicate that the use of BT for rearing tilapia broodstock, and larvae can improve the fry quality and production performance.

Biofloc culture environment can also provide appropriate conditions for cyanobacterial productivity, which may affect water quality and fish performance. These microorganisms are associated with cyanotoxins production. Miranda-Baeza et al. (2017) tested this assumption through cyanobacterial (*Oscillatoria* sp.) inoculation in saltwater biofloc system at different levels (0.0, 0.1, 0.5 and 1.0 mg L^{-1}) for 7 weeks. The results indicated that *chlorophyll a* and TSS increased with increasing the concentration of inoculated *Oscillatoria* sp. No significant effects on DO, TAN or NO_2−N were detected. The survival, growth rates and feed efficiency of tilapia hybrid (*O. niloticus* × *O. mossambicus*) reared in saltwater biofloc system were significantly decreased with increasing cyanobacterial concentration.

6.11 Closing remarks

1. The widespread aquaculture of tilapia, especially in areas outside their natural geographical existence together with the shortage of, and competition for, freshwater sources have gradually shifted tilapia culture from traditional semi-intensive to intensive systems.
2. There is an inverse relationship between stocking density and individual fish growth. The farmer should carefully identify his target consumer (i.e. he should decide whether to produce higher yield but smaller fish, or lower yield with larger fish size).
3. Water exchange and/or aeration may be necessary in earthen ponds. The cost-effectiveness of this practice should be carefully investigated taking into account the availability and cost of water, fuel, electricity, etc.
4. Water-saving suspension system may have economic advantages over traditional water-demanding systems in earthen ponds. The re-suspension of sediments can be an important mechanism of nutrient transfer in the pond, and can also serve as water purifier due to the increased number of nitrifying bacteria in the water column.
5. The adjustment of C:N ratio (mainly in fish feeds) is necessary for reducing the accumulation of inorganic nitrogen in intensive tilapia ponds. Proper C:N ratio can reduce ammonia to the desired levels within 1−3 days. A ratio of about 15:1 C:N has been recommended for tilapia. Cheap carbon and nitrogen sources can be used as a partial replacer for expensive commercial high-protein feeds. The approach of producing single-cell protein(s) in fish ponds should also be encouraged in developing countries where tilapia culture is widely practiced.
6. In arid areas where freshwater is limited, water treatment and reuse would be an ideal alternative for intensive tilapia culture.
7. Farming tilapia in cage-cum-pond system appears economic, favourable and successful. However, the farmer must carefully consider the density and size of noncaged and caged species as well as the number of cages (i.e. total biomass). Aeration may also be necessary.
8. Recirculating culture systems are an ideal alternative for tilapia culture. However, these systems are technically sophisticated and very costly, while tilapia is considered a ‘low-priced fish’ in many countries. The production of these fishes with high investment in commercial recycle systems may, therefore, not be sustainable.
9. The addition of carbon-rich agricultural by-products (such as RH) into fish tanks in closed systems can be used for solids removal. This practice can reduce the running costs of the system.
10. Green water tank system is an ideal alternative for tilapia culture, especially in arid areas where freshwater resources are limited.

11. Green water system can control pathogenic bacteria in culture water. Microalgae such as *Chlorella* secrete antimicrobial compounds that inhibit pathogenic bacterial growth. This approach should be further explored.
12. Tilapia production in aquaponic systems can be an efficient and sustainable way of producing tilapia and plant/vegetables, especially in rural, resource-limited areas.
13. Biofloc is a symbiotic process that includes confined aquatic animals, heterotrophic bacteria and other microbial species in the water. Consumption of bioflocs provides nutritional value to cultured aquatic species. Bioflocs can also improve water quality and fish immunity. Therefore, BT can be an ideal alternative for sustainable and environmentally friendly tilapia culture.

References

Abery, N.W., Sukadi, F., Budhiman, A.A., Kartamihardja, E.S., Koeshendrajana, S., Buddhiman, et al., 2005. Fisheries and cage culture of three reservoirs in West Java, Indonesia; a case study of ambitious developments and resulting interactions. Fisheries Management and Ecology 12, 315–330.

Abou, Y., Fiogbe, E.D., Micha, J.C., 2007. Effects of stocking density on growth, yield and profitability of farming Nile tilapia, *Oreochromis niloticus* L., fed *Azolla* diet, in earthen ponds. Aquaculture Research 38, 595–604.

Agius, C., 2001. Commercial culture of *Oreochromis spilurus* in open sea cages. In: Subasinghe, S., Singh, T. (Eds.), Tilapia: Production, Marketing and Technical Developments. Proceedings of the Tilapia 2001 International Technical and Trade Conference on Tilapia. Infofish, Kuala Lumpur, Malaysia, pp. 132–135.

Al-Ahmed, A.A., 2002. Tilapia culture in Kuwait. Global Aquaculture Advocate 5, 31.

Algazzar, M.M., Osman, M.F., Sadek, S., 2008. Effect of water exchange rate on the fish productivity of concrete circulated ponds, Egypt. In: Elghobashy, H., Fitzsimmons, K., Diab, A.S. (Eds.), Proceedings of the Eighth International Symposium on Tilapia in Aquaculture, 12–14 October, 2008, Cairo, Egypt. Central Laboratory Aquaculture Research, Ministry of Agriculture and Land Reclamation, Egypt, pp. 613–615.

Anadu, D.I., Barho, L., 2002. The production of tilapia and vegetables in aquaponics system. In: Proceedings of the Fourth International Conference on Recirculating Aquaculture. US Department of Agriculture, Virginia Polytechnic Institute and State University, Blacksburg, VA, USA, pp. 551–559.

Areerat, S., 1987. *Clarias* culture in Thailand. Aquaculture 63, 355–362.

Asase, A., 2013. Effects of Stocking Density on the Production of Nile tilapia (*Oreochromis niloticus)* in Floating Net Cages on the Volta Lake (M.Phil. degree). University of Ghana, 111 pp.

Ashour, A., Ashour, M., 2013. Successful experience in freshwater fish farming in Egypt. In: Paper Presented at the Third Annual Meeting of Arab Experts and Administrators on "Fisheries Research and Technology Transfer in the Arab Countries", 3–5 December 2013, Cairo, Egypt.

Avnimelech, Y., 1998. Minimal discharge from intensive fish ponds. World Aquaculture 29, 32–37.

Avnimelech, Y., 1999. Carbon/nitrogen ratio as a control element in aquaculture systems. Aquaculture 176, 227–235.

Avnimelech, Y., 2003. Control of microbial activity in aquaculture systems: active suspension ponds. World Aquaculture 34, 19–21.

Avnimelech, Y., 2007. Feeding with microbial flocs by tilapia in minimal discharge bioflocs technology ponds. Aquaculture 264, 140–147.

Avnimelech, Y., Kochva, M., Hargreaves, J.A., 1999. Sedimentation and re-suspension in earthen fish ponds. Journal of the World Aquaculture Society 30, 401–409.

Azaza, M.S., Assad, A., Maghrbi, W., El-Cafsi, M., 2013. The effects of rearing density on growth, size heterogeneity and inter-individual variation of feed intake in monosex male Nile tilapia *Oreochromis niloticus* L. Animal 7, 1865–1874.

Azim, M.E., Little, D.C., 2008. The biofloc technology (BFT) in indoor tanks: water quality, biofloc composition, and growth and welfare of Nile tilapia (*Oreochromis niloticus*). Aquaculture 283, 29–35.

Bailey, D.S., Rakocy, J.E., Martin, J.M., Shultz, M.R., 2000. Intensive production of tilapia fingerlings in a recirculating system. In: Fitzsimmons, K., Filho, J.C. (Eds.), Tilapia Culture in the 21st Century. Proceedings from the Fifth International Symposium on Tilapia Aquaculture. American Tilapia Association and ICLARM, Rio de Janeiro, Brazil, pp. 328–333.

Balarin, J.D., Haller, R.D., 1982. The intensive culture of tilapia in tanks, raceways and cages. In: Muir, J.F., Roberts, R.J. (Eds.), Recent Advances in Aquaculture. Croom Helm, London and Canberra. Westview Press, Boulder Colorado, pp. 267–355.

Balarin, J.D., Haller, R.D., 1983. Commercial tank culture of tilapia. In: Fishelson, L., Yaron, Z. (Eds.), International Symposium on Tilapia in Aquaculture. Tel Aviv University, Tel Aviv, Israel, pp. 473–483.

Baqui, M.A., Bhujel, R.C., 2011. A hands-on training helped proliferation of tilapia culture in Bangladesh. In: Liping, L., Fitzsimmons, K. (Eds.), Better Science, Better Fish, Better Life. Proceedings of the Ninth International Symposium on Tilapia in Aquaculture. AquaFish Collaborative Research Support Program, pp. 311–322.

Bardach, J.E., Ryther, J.H., McLarney, W.O., 1972. Aquaculture: The Farming and Husbandry of Freshwater and Marine Organisms. Wiley Interscience, New York, 868 pp.

BFAR-PHILMINAQ (Bureau of Fisheries and Aquatic Resources), 2007. Managing Aquaculture and Its Impacts: a Guidebook for Local Governments. Bureau of Fisheries and Aquatic Resources (BFAR)-PHILMINAQ Project, Diliman Quezon City, 80 pp.

Bhujel, R.C., 2013. On-farm feed management practices for Nile tilapia (*Oreochromis niloticus*) in Thailand. In: Hasan, M.R., New, M.B. (Eds.), On-Farm Feeding and Feed Management in Aquaculture. FAO Fisheries and Aquaculture Technical Paper No. 583. FAO, Rome, pp. 159–189.

Blow, P., Leonard, S., 2007. A review of cage aquaculture: sub-Saharan Africa. In: Halwart, M., Soto, D., Arthur, J.R. (Eds.), Cage aquaculture – Regional Reviews and Global Overview. FAO Fisheries Technical Paper. No. 498. FAO, Rome, pp. 188–207.

Boerlage, A.S., Dung, T.T., Hoa, T.T., Davidson, J., Stryhn, H., Hammell, K.L., 2017. Production of red tilapia (*Oreochromis* spp.) in floating cages in the Mekong Delta, Vietnam: mortality and health management. Diseases of Aquatic Organisms 124, 131–144.

Boyd, C.E., 1990. Water Quality in Ponds for Aquaculture. Auburn University, Auburn, AL, USA, 482 pp.

Campbell, D., 1985. Large scale cage farming of *Sarotherodon niloticus*. Aquaculture 48, 57–69.

Chamberlain, G.W., Hopkins, J.S., 1994. Reducing water use and feed cost in intensive ponds. World Aquaculture 25, 29–32.

Cheong, L., Chan, F.K., Wong, J., Chou, R., 1987. Observations on the culture of red tilapia (*Oreochromis niloticus* hybrid) in seawater under intensive tank condition using a biodrum. Singapore Journal of Primary Industries 15, 42–56.

Chiayvareesajja, S., Wongwit, C., Tansakul, R., 1990. Cage culture of tilapia (*Oreochromis niloticus*) using aquatic weed-based pellets. In: Hirano, R., Hanyu, I. (Eds.), Proceedings of the Second Asian Fisheries Forum. Asian Fisheries Society, Manila, Philippines, pp. 287–290.

Chow, F., Macchiavello, J., Santa, S.S., Fonck, E., Olivares, J., 2001. Utilization of *Gracilaria chilensis* (Rhodophyta: Gracilariaceae) as a biofilter in the depuration of effluents from tank cultures of fish, oysters and sea urchins. Journal of the World Aquaculture Society 32, 215–220.

Cole, W.M., Rakocy, J.E., Shultz, K.A., Bailey, D.S., 1997. Effects of solids removal on tilapia production and water quality in continuously aerated, outdoor tanks. In: Fitzsimmons, K. (Ed.), Proceedings from the Fourth International Symposium on Tilapia in Aquaculture. Northeast Regional Agriculture Engineering Service, Ithaca, NY, USA, pp. 373–384.

Conte, L., Sonoda, D.Y., Shirota, R., Cyrino, J.E.P., 2008. Productivity and economics of Nile tilapia *Oreochromis niloticus* cage culture in South-East Brazil. Journal of Applied Aquaculture 20, 18–37.

Costa, F.H.F., Sampaio, A.H., Sake-Sampaio, S., Lima, F.M., Matias, J.F.N., Rocha, I.R.C.B., et al., 2000. Tilapia cage culture in reservoirs in Cear State. In: Fitzsimmons, K., Filho, J.C. (Eds.), Tilapia Culture in the 21st Century. Proceedings from the Fifth International Symposium on Tilapia Aquaculture. American Tilapia Association and ICLARM, Rio de Janeiro, Brazil, pp. 393–399.

Costa, Â.A.P., Roubach, R., Dallago, B.S.L., Bueno, G.W., McManus, C., Bernal, F.E.M., 2017. Influence of stocking density on growth performance and welfare of juvenile tilapia (*Oreochromis niloticus*) in cages. Arquivo Brasileiro de Medicina Veterinária e Zootecnia 69, 243–251.

Crab, R., Kochva, M., Verstraete, W., Avnimelech, Y., 2009. Bio-flocs technology application in over-wintering of tilapia. Aquacultural Engineering 40, 105–112.

Crab, R., Defoird, T., Bossier, P., Verstraete, W., 2012. Biofloc technology in aquaculture: beneficial effects and future challenges. Aquaculture 356–357, 351–356.

Cruz, E.M., Ridha, M., 1991. Production of tilapia *Oreochromis spilurus* Gunther stocked at different densities in sea cages. Aquaculture 99, 95–103.

Davis, T.F., Sheffield, R.E., LeBlanc, B.D., Theegala, C., Farlow, J., Hall, S.G., Fall 2011. Rice hulls for wastewater treatment, nitrogen oxidation. Louisiana Agriculture 28–29.

De Silva, S.S., Phillips, M.J., 2007. A review of cage aquaculture: Asia (excluding China). In: Halwart, M., Soto, D., Arthur, J.R. (Eds.), Cage aquaculture – Regional Reviews and Global Overview, FAO Fisheries Technical Paper No. 498. FAO, Rome, pp. 18–48.

Dey, M.M., Bimbao, G.B., Yong, L., Regaspi, P., Kohinoor, A.H.M., Chung, D., et al., 2000. Current status of production and consumption of tilapia in selected Asian countries. Aquaculture Economics and Management 4, 13–31.

Drennan II., D.G., Rahman, M.M., Malone, R.F., 1993. Slow sand filtration technologies for the containment of non-indigenous species in recirculating aquaculture effluents. In: Wang, J.-K. (Ed.), Techniques for Modern Aquaculture. American Society of Agricultural Engineers, St. Joseph, MI, USA, pp. 335–344.

D'Silva, A.M., Maughan, O.E., 1995. Effects of density and water quality on red tilapia (*Oreochromis mossambicus* × *O. urolepis hornorum*) in pulsed-flow culture systems. Journal of Applied Aquaculture 5, 69–76.

Eding, E., Verdegem, M., Martins, C., Schlaman, G., Heinsbroek, L., Laarhoven, B., et al., 2009. Tilapia farming using recirculating aquaculture systems (RAS) - case study in The Netherlands. In: Varadi, L., Bardocz, T., Oberdieck, A. (Eds.), A Handbook for Sustainable Aquaculture: A Product of SustainAqua. Eurofish, Project N°: COLL-CT-2006-030384, pp. 71–95.

Ekasari, J., Rivandi, D.R., Firdausi, A.P., Surawidjaja, E.H., Zairin Jr., M., Bossier, P., et al., 2015. Biofloc technology positively affects Nile tilapia (*Oreochromis niloticus*) larvae performance. Aquaculture 441, 72–77.

El-Saidy, D.M.S.D., Gaber, M.M.A., 2005. Effect of dietary protein levels and feeding rates on growth performance, production traits and body composition of Nile tilapia, *Oreochromis niloticus* (L.) cultured in concrete tanks. Aquaculture Research 36, 163–171.

El-Sayed, A.-F.M., 1999. Alternative dietary protein sources for farmed tilapia spp. Aquaculture 179, 149–168.

El-Sayed, A.-F.M., 2002. Effects of stocking density and feeding levels on growth and feed efficiency of Nile tilapia, *Oreochromis niloticus* (L.) fry. Aquaculture Research 33, 621–626.

El-Sayed, A.-F.M., 2007. Analysis of feeds and fertilizers for sustainable aquaculture development in Egypt. In: Hasan, M.R., Hecht, T., De Silva, S.S., Tacon, A.G.J. (Eds.), Study and Analysis of Feeds and Fertilizers for Sustainable Aquaculture Development. FAO Fisheries Technical Paper No. 497. FAO, Rome, pp. 401–422.

El-Sayed, A.-F.M., 2013. On-farm feed management practices for Nile tilapia *(Oreochromis niloticus)* in Egypt. In: Hasan, M.R., New, M.B. (Eds.), On-farm Feeding and Feed Management in Aquaculture. FAO Fisheries and Aquaculture Technical Paper No. 583. FAO, Rome, pp. 101–129.

El-Sayed, A.-F.M., 2017. Social and economic performance of tilapia farming in Egypt. In: Cai, J., Quagrainie, K.K., Hishamunda, N. (Eds.), Social and Economic Performance of Tilapia Farming in Africa. FAO Fisheries and Aquaculture Circular No. 1130. FAO, Rome, pp. 1–48.

El-Sayed, A.-F.M., Kawanna, M., Mudar, M., 2005. Effects of water flow rates on growth and survival of Nile tilapia fry. World Aquaculture 36, 5–6.

English, L.A., 2015. Economic Feasibility of Aquaponics in Arkansas (M.Sc. thesis). University of Arkansas, Fayetteville, 85 pp.

Fatan, A.A., Hashim, R., Chong, A.S.C., Ali, A., 2005. Enhancement of monosex hybrid red tilapia, *Oreochromis mossambicus* × *O. niloticus* production in portable canvas tanks through mixed-feeding strategies. Journal of Applied Aquaculture 17, 99–111.

Fitzsimmons, K., 2000. Tilapia aquaculture in Mexico. In: Costa-Pierce, B.A., Rakocy, J.E. (Eds.), Tilapia Aquaculture in the Americas, vol. 2. The World Aquaculture Society, Baton Rouge, Louisiana, pp. 171–183.

Fitzsimmons, K., 2003. Tilapia aquaculture in recirculating systems. Aquaculture Magazine 29, 73–76.

Fitzsimmons, K., Circa, A., Jinenez, E.B., Pereda, D., 1999. Development of low-cost supplemental feeds for tilapia in pond and cage culture. In: McElwee, E., Bruke, D., Niles, M., Egna, H. (Eds.), Sixteenth Annual Technical Report. Pond Dynamics/Aquaculture CRSP. Oregon State University, Corvallis, OR, USA, pp. 57–63.

Garcia, F., Romera, D.M., Gozi, K.S., Onaka, E.M., Fonseca, F.S., Schalch, S.H.C., et al., 2013. Stocking density of Nile tilapia in cages placed in a hydroelectric reservoir. Aquaculture 410–411, 51–56.

Gibtan, A., Getahun, A., Mengistou, S., 2008. Effect of stocking density on the growth performance and yield of Nile tilapia [*Oreochromis niloticus* (L., 1758)] in a cage culture system in Lake Kuriftu, Ethiopia. Aquaculture Research 39, 1450–1460.

Greensword, M.A., 2017. Rice Hull Bioreactor for Recirculating Aquaculture (Ph.D. thesis). Louisiana State University, USA.

Guerrero III., R.D., 2001. Tilapia culture in Southeast Asia. In: Subasinghe, S., Singh, T. (Eds.), Tilapia: Production, Marketing and Technical Developments. Proceedings of the Tilapia 2001 International Technical and Trade Conference on Tilapia. Infofish, Kuala Lumpur, Malaysia, pp. 97–103.

Gullian-Klanian, M., Arámburu-Adame, C., 2013. Performance of Nile tilapia *Oreochromis niloticus* fingerlings in a hyper-intensive recirculating aquaculture system with low water exchange. Latin American Journal of Aquatic Research 4, 150–162.

Hardjamulia, I.A., Rukyani, A., 2000. Improved Nile tilapia (GIFT strain) cultured in Indonesia. Naga: The ICLARM Quarterly 23, 38–39.

Hargreaves, J.A., 2013. Biofloc Production Systems for Aquaculture. Southern Regional Aquaculture Center, Publication No. 4503, 12 pp.

Hecht, T., 2007. Review of feeds and fertilizers for sustainable aquaculture development in Sub-Saharan Africa. In: Hasan, M.R., Hecht, T., De Silva, S.S., Tacon, A.G.J. (Eds.), Study and Analysis of Feeds and Fertilizers for Sustainable Aquaculture Development. FAO Fisheries Technical Paper No. 497. FAO, Rome, pp. 77–109.

Hossain, M.,R.A., Rahman, M.A., Akter, S., Hosain, M.E., Niamul Naser, M., 2017. Intervention of tilapia cage culture in the River Dakatia: threaten or blessed to local fish diversity. International Journal of Fisheries and Aquatic Studies 5, 228–232.

Huang, W.-B., Chiu, T.-S., 1997. Effects of stocking density on survival, growth, size variation, and productivity of *Tilapia* fry. Aquaculture Research 28, 165–173.

Huervana, F.H., de la Cruz, J.J.Y., Caipang, C.M.A., 2006. Inhibition of luminous *Vibrio harveyi* by "green water" obtained from tank culture of tilapia, *Oreochromis mossambicus*. Acta Ichthyologica et Piscatoria 36, 17–23.

Hussain, M.G., 2009. A future for tilapia in Bangladesh. AQUA Culture AsiaPacific Magazine 38–40.

Hussain, M.G., Barman, B.K., Karim, M., Keus, E.H.J., 2013. Progress and the future for tilapia farming and seed production in Bangladesh. In: Proceedings of 10th International Symposium on Tilapia in Aquaculture, Jerusalem, Israel, October 6-10, 2013.

Jamu, D., 2001. Tilapia culture in Africa: opportunities and challenges. In: Subasinghe, S., Singh, T. (Eds.), Tilapia: Production, Marketing and Technical Developments. Proceedings of the Tilapia 2001 International Technical and Trade Conference on Tilapia. Infofish, Kuala Lumpur, Malaysia, pp. 105–112.

Jiménez-Montealegre, R., Verdegem, M., Zamora, J.E., Verreth, J., 2002. Organic matter sedimentation and re-suspension in tilapia (*Oreochromis niloticus*) ponds during a production cycle. Aquacultural Engineering 26, 1–12.

Kloas, W., Groß, R., Baganz, D., Graupner, J., Monsees, H., Schmidt, U., et al., 2015. A new concept for aquaponic systems to improve sustainability, increase productivity, and reduce environmental impacts. Aquaculture Environment Interactions 7, 179–192.

Kpundeh, M.D., Xu, P., Yang, H., Qiang, J., He, J., 2013. Stocking densities and chronic zero culture water exchange stress' effects on biological performances, hematological and serum biochemical indices of GIFT tilapia juveniles (*Oreochromis niloticus*). Journal of Aquaculture Research & Development 4 (189), 1–5. https://doi.org/10.4172/2155-9546.1000189.

Lenger, T.A., Pfeiffer, T.J., 2002. Evaluation of supplemental solids removal effects on nitrification rates of floating bead filters. In: Proceedings of the Fourth International Conference on Recirculating Aquaculture. US Department of Agriculture, Virginia Polytechnic Institute and State University, Blacksburg, VA, p. 418.

Lin, C.K., Diana, J., 1995. Co-culture of Nile tilapia (*Oreochromis niloticus*) and hybrid catfish (*Clarias macrocephalus* × *C. gariepinus*) in ponds. Aquatic Living Resources 8, 449–454.

Lio-Po, G.D., 2017. Luminous *Vibrio* and the greenwater culture of the tiger shrimp *Penaeus monodon* with tilapia. In: Perschbacher, P.W., Stickney, R.R. (Eds.), Tilapia in Intensive Co-culture. John Wiley & Sons. Ltd, pp. 81–93.

Lio-Po, G.D., Leaño, E.M., Peñaranda, M.D., Villa-Franco, A.U., Sombito, C.D., Guanzon Jr., N.G., 2005. Anti-luminous *Vibrio* factors associated with the 'green water' grow-out culture of the tiger shrimp *Penaeus monodon*. Aquaculture 250, 1–7.

Long, L., Yang, J., Li, Y., Guan, C., Wu, F., 2015. Effect of biofloc technology on growth, digestive enzyme activity, hematology, and immune response of genetically improved farmed tilapia (*Oreochromis niloticus*). Aquaculture 448, 135–141.

Losordo, T.M., Masser, M.P., Rakocy, J.E., 1999. Recirculating Aquaculture Tank Production Systems: A Review of Component Options. Southern Regional Aquaculture Centre, Publication No. 453, TX, USA, 12 pp.

Love, D.C., Fry, J.P., Genello, L., Hill, E.S., Frederick, J.A., Li, X., et al., 2014. An international survey of aquaponics practitioners. PLoS One 9, e102662. https://doi.org/10.1371/journal.pone.0102662.

Love, D.C., Fry, J.P., Li, X., Hill, E.S., Genello, L., Semmens, K., et al., 2015. Commercial aquaponics production and profitability: findings from an international survey. Aquaculture 435, 67–74.

Lovshin, L.L., 2000. Tilapia culture in Brazil. In: Costa-Pierce, B.A., Rakocy, J.E. (Eds.), Tilapia Aquaculture in the Americas, vol. 2. The World Aquaculture Society, Baton Rouge, LA, pp. 133–140.

Lutz, C.G., 1996. Development of a tank-based tilapia industry in Louisiana. In: Proceedings of the First International Conference on Recirculating Aquaculture. US Department of Agriculture, Virginia Polytechnic Institute and State University, Blacksburg, VA, pp. 1–7.

Mandal, R.B., Jha, D.K., Shrestha, M.K., Pant, J., Rai, S., Pandit, N.P., 2014. Cage-pond integration of African catfish (*Clarias gariepinus*) and Nile tilapia (*Oreochromis niloticus*) with carps. Aquaculture Research 45, 1311–1318.

Mansour, A.T., Esteban, M.Á., 2017. Effects of carbon sources and plant protein levels in a biofloc system on growth performance, and the immune and antioxidant status of Nile tilapia (*Oreochromis niloticus*). Fish & Shellfish Immunology 64, 202–209.

Martin, J.M., Rakocy, J.E., Cole, W.M., 2000. Greenwater tank culture of tilapia. In: Creswell, R.L. (Ed.), Proceedings of the Gulf and Caribbean Fisheries Institute. Gulf and Caribbean Fisheries Institute, c/o

Harbor Branch, Oceanographic Institution, Inc., FL, USA, pp. 330–340. No. 51.

Martin, J.M., Bailey, D.S., Shultz, R.C., Rakocy, J.E., 2001. Effect of three stocking densities on the production of advanced-sized *Oreochromis niloticus* fingerlings in a greenwater tank system. In: Aquaculture 2001- Book of Abstracts. World Aquaculture Society, Baton Rouge, LA, USA, p. 406.

Martins, C.I.M., Eding, E.H., Verdegem, M.C.J., Heinsbroek, L.T.N., Schneider, O., Blancheton, J.P., et al., 2010. New developments in recirculating aquaculture systems in Europe: a perspective on environmental sustainability. Aquacultural Engineering 43, 83–93.

McGinty, A.S., 1986. Effects of size at stocking on competition and growth of all-male tilapia hybrids. Journal of the World Mariculture Society 16, 52–56.

McGinty, A.S., 1991. Tilapia production in cages: effects of cage size and number of noncaged fish. Progressive Fish-Culturist 53, 246–249.

Meyer, D.E., 2002. Tilapia culture in Honduras. Global Aquaculture Advocate 5 (6), 36–37.

Milstein, A., Avnimelech, Y., Zoran, M., Joseph, D., 2001a. Growth performance of hybrid bass and hybrid tilapia in conventional and active suspension intensive ponds. Israeli Journal of Aquaculture/ Bamidgeh 53, 147–157.

Milstein, A., Zoran, M., Kochba, M., Avnimelech, Y., 2001b. Effect of different management practices on water quality of intensive tilapia culture in Israel. Aquaculture International 9, 133–152.

Miranda-Baeza, A., Mariscal-López, M.A., López-Elías, J.A., Rivas-Vega, M.E., Emerenciano, M., Sánchez-Romero, A., et al., 2017. Effect of inoculation of the cyanobacteria *Oscillatoria* sp. on tilapia biofloc culture. Aquaculture Research 48, 4725–4734.

Mires, D., Amit, Y., 1992. Intensive culture of tilapia in quasi-closed water cycled flow-through ponds - the Dekel aquaculture system. Israeli Journal of Aquaculture/Bamidgeh 44, 82–86.

Mires, D., Anjioni, C., 1997. Technical and economic comparative evaluation of two intensive closed water–cycled culture systems for tilapias in Israel. In: Fitzsimmons, K. (Ed.), Proceedings from the Fourth International Symposium on Tilapia in Aquaculture. Northeast Regional Agriculture Engineering Service, Ithaca, NY, USA, pp. 416–425.

Moura, R.S.T., Valenti, W.C., Henry-Silva, G.G., 2015. Sustainability of Nile tilapia net-cage culture in a reservoir in a semi-arid region. Ecological Indicators 66, 574–582.

Muir, J.F., Van Rijn, J., Hargreaves, J., 2000. Production in intensive and recycle systems. In: Beveridge, M.C.M., McAndrew, B.J. (Eds.), Tilapias: Biology and Exploitation. Kluwer Academic Publishers, Dordrecht/Boston/London, pp. 405–445.

Nelson, R.L., 2017. Aquaponics. In: Perschbacher, P.W., Stickney, R.R. (Eds.), Tilapia in Intensive Co-culture. John Wiley & Sons, Ltd, Oxford, UK, pp. 246–260.

Newton, S.H., Mullins, J., Libey, G.S., Kidd, M., 1998. A prototype tilapia/hydroponic greenhouse recirculating production system for institutional application. In: Proceedings of the Second International Conference on Recirculating Aquaculture. US Department of Agriculture, Virginia Polytechnic Institute and State University, Blacksburg, VA, pp. 405–406.

Nunes, A.J.P., 2010. Tilapia cage farm management in Brazil. Global Aquaculture Advocate 12–15.

Nurdjana, M.L., 2006. Indonesian aquaculture development. In: Paper Presented at RCA International Workshop on Innovative Technologies for Eco-Friendly Fish Farm Management and Production of Safe Aquaculture Foods. Bali, December 4–8, 2006.

Ofori, J.K., Dankwa, H.R., Brummett, R., Abban, E.K., 2009. Producing Tilapia in Small Cage in West Africa. WorldFish Center Technical Manual No. 1952. The World Fish Center, Penang, Malaysia, 16 pp.

Ofori, J.K., Abban, E.K., Karikari, A.Y., Brummett, R.E., 2010. Production parameters and economics of small-scale tilapia cage aquaculture in the Volta Lake, Ghana. Journal of Applied Aquaculture 22, 337–351.

Orachunwong, C., Thammasart, S., Lohawatanakul, C., 2001. Recent developments in tilapia feEds. In: Subasinghe, S., Singh, T. (Eds.), Tilapia: Production, Marketing and Technical Developments. Proceedings of the Tilapia 2001 International Technical and Trade Conference on Tilapia. Infofish, Kuala Lumpur, Malaysia, pp. 113–122.

Osofero, S.A., Otubusin, S.O., Daramola, J.A., 2009. Effect of stocking density on tilapia (*Oreochromis niloticus* Linnaeus 1757) growth and survival in bamboo - net cages trial. African Journal of Biotechnology 8, 1322–1325.

Palada, M.C., Cole, W.M., Crossman, S.M.A., 1999. Influence of effluents from intensive aquaculture and sludge on growth and yield of bell peppers. Journal of Sustainable Agriculture 14, 85–103.

Pasipamire, W., 2009. Case Study: Commercial Production of Nile tilapia on Lake Kariba, Zimbabwe. EC FP7 Project, SARNISSA, 22 pp.

Persand, S., Bhikajee, M., 1997. Studies on an experimental fouling resistant mariculture cage for red tilapia in Mauritius. In: Fitzsimmons, K. (Ed.), Proceedings from the Fourth International Symposium on Tilapia in Aquaculture. Northeast Regional Agriculture Engineering Service, Ithaca, NY, USA, pp. 408–415.

Perschbacher, P.W., 1995. Algal management in intensive channel catfish production trials. World Aquaculture 26 (3), 65–68.

Phuong, N.T., Yi, Y., Diana, J.S., Lin, C.K., Bui, T.V., 2004. Integrated cage-cum-pond culture: stocking densities of caged climbing perch in Nile tilapia ponds. In: Bolivar, R., Mair, G., Fitzsimmons, K. (Eds.), Proceedings of the Sixth International Symposium on Tilapia in Aquaculture. Manila, Philippines, pp. 597–598.

Popma, T.J., Rodriquez, F.B., 2000. Tilapia aquaculture in Colombia. In: Costa-Pierce, B.A., Rakocy, J.E. (Eds.), Tilapia Aquaculture in the Americas, vol. 2. The World Aquaculture Society, Baton Rouge, Louisiana, pp. 141–150.

Pruginin, Y., Fishelson, L., Koren, A., 1988. Intensive tilapia farming in brackishwater from an Israeli desert. In: Pullin, R.S.V., Bhukaswan, T., Tonguthai, K., Maclean, J.L. (Eds.), Proceedings of the Second International Symposium on Tilapia in Aquaculture. Conference Proceedings No. 15. Department of Fisheries, Thailand, and ICLARM, Manila, Philippines, pp. 75–81.

Qiuming, L., Yi, Y., 2004. Tilapia culture in China. In: Bolivar, R., Mair, G., Fitzsimmons, K. (Eds.), Proceedings of the Sixth International Symposium on Tilapia in Aquaculture. Manila, Philippines, pp. 18–27.

Radwan, I.A., Leschen, W., 2011. Case Study on Developing Financially Viable Recirculation Aquaculture Systems (RAS) for Tilapia Production in Egypt: Technology Transfer from the Netherlands. EC FP7 Project, SARNISSA, 23 pp.

Rakocy, J.E., Allison, R., 1981. Evaluation of a closed recirculating system for the culture of tilapia and aquatic macrophytes. In: Allen, L.J., Kinney, E.C. (Eds.), Proceedings of the Bio-Engineering Symposium for Fish Culture. American Fisheries Society, Bethesda, MD, pp. 296–307.

Rakocy, J.E., Bailey, D.S., 2003. Initial economic analyses of aquaponic systems. In: Paper Presented at "Beyond Monoculture". Trondheim, Norway, June 6, 2003.

Rakocy, J.E., Bailey, D.S., Martin, J.M., Shultz, R.C., 2000a. Tilapia production systems for the Lesser Antilles and other resource-limited, tropical areas. In: Fitzsimmons, K., Filho, J.C. (Eds.), Tilapia Culture in the 21st Century. Proceedings from the Fifth International Symposium on Tilapia Aquaculture. Rio de Janeiro, Brazil, pp. 651–662.

Rakocy, J.E., Shultz, R.C., Bailey, D.S., 2000b. Commercial aquaponics for the Caribbean. In: Creswell, R.L. (Ed.), Proceedings of the Gulf and Caribbean Fisheries Institute. Gulf and Caribbean Fisheries Institute, c/o Harbor Branch Oceanographic Institution, Inc., No. 51, pp. 353–364.

Rakocy, J.E., Bailey, D.S., Shultz, R.C., Martin, J.M., 2001. Improvements to a commercial-scale aquaponic system and preliminary evaluation of the production of red tilapia *Oreochromis niloticus* and 13 types of vegetables. In: Aquaculture 2001 - Book of Abstracts. World Aquaculture Society, Baton Rouge, LA, USA, p. 544.

Rakocy, J.E., Bailey, D.S., Shultz, R.C., Thoman, E.S., 2004. Update on tilapia and vegetable production in the UVI aquaponic system. In: Bolivar, R., Mair, G., Fitzsimmons, K. (Eds.), Proceedings of the Sixth International Symposium on Tilapia in Aquaculture. Manila, Philippines, pp. 676–690.

Ridha, M.T., Cruz, E.M., 2001. Effect of biofilter media on water quality and biological performance of the Nile tilapia *Oreochromis niloticus* L. reared in a simple recirculating system. Aquacultural Engineering 24, 157–166.

Rojas, A., Wadsworth, S., 2007. A review of cage aquaculture: Latin America and the Caribbean. In: Halwart, M., Soto, D., Arthur, J.R. (Eds.), Cage Aquaculture – Regional Reviews and Global Overview. FAO Fisheries Technical Paper No. 498. FAO, Rome, pp. 70–100.

Romana-Eguia, M.R.R., Larona, M.A., Catacutan, M.R., 2013. On-farm feed management practices for Nile tilapia *(Oreochromis niloticus)* in the Philippines. In: Hasan, M.R., New, M.B. (Eds.), On-farm Feeding and Feed Management in Aquaculture. FAO Fisheries and Aquaculture Technical Paper No. 583. FAO, Rome, pp. 131–158.

Roriz, G.D., Delphino, M.K.D.C., Gardner, I.A., Gonçalves, V.S.P., 2017. Characterization of tilapia farming in net cages at a tropical reservoir in Brazil. Aquaculture Reports 6, 43–48.

Rosati, R., O'Rourke, P.D., Tudor, K., Henry, R.D., 1993. Performance of a raceway and vertical screen filter while growing *Tilapia niloticus* under commercial conditions. In: Wang, J.-K. (Ed.), Techniques for Modern Aquaculture. American Society of Agricultural Engineers, St. Joseph, MI, USA, pp. 303–314.

Rosati, R., O'Rourke, P.D., Foley, P., Tudor, K., 1997. Operation of a prototype commercial-scale recirculating growout system for *Oreochromis niloticus*. In: Fitzsimmons, K. (Ed.), Proceedings from the Fourth International Symposium on Tilapia in Aquaculture. Northeast Regional Agriculture Engineering Service, Ithaca, NY, USA, pp. 330–347.

Roubach, R., Correia, E.S., Zaiden, S., Martino, R.C., Cavalli, R.O., 2003. Aquaculture in Brazil. World Aquaculture 34 (1), 28–34.

Sadek, S., Kallafalah, H., Adell, F., 1992. Tilapia (*Oreochromis niloticus*) biomass yield in commercial farm using circular tanks. Journal of Applied Ichthyology 8, 193–202.

Sastry, B.N., DeLosReyes Jr., A.A., Rusch, K.A., Malone, R.F., 1999. Nitrification performance of a bubble-washed bead filter for combined solids removal and biological filtration in a recirculating aquaculture system. Aquacultural Engineering 19, 105–117.

Scott, J.T., Scott, D.M., Lawson, T.B., 1998. Rice hulls as solids removal media for aquaculture. In: Aquaculture'98 - Book of Abstracts. World Aquaculture Society, Baton Rouge, LA, USA, p. 480.

Shnel, N., Barak, Y., Ezer, T., Dafni, Z., van Rijn, J., 2002. Design and performance of a Zero-discharge tilapia recirculating system. Aquacultural Engineering 26, 191–203.

Siddiqui, A.Q., Howlader, M.S., Adam, A.A., 1991a. Management strategies for intensive culture of Nile tilapia (*Oreochromis niloticus* L.) in tanks using drainage water in Al Hassa region of Saudi Arabia. Arab Gulf Journal of Scientific Research. B, Agricultural and Biological Sciences 9, 149–163.

Siddiqui, A.Q., Howlader, M.S., Adam, A.A., 1991b. Effects of water exchange on *Oreochromis niloticus* (L.) growth and water quality in outdoor concrete tanks. Aquaculture 95, 67–74.

Siddiqui, A.Q., Al-Harbi, A.H., Hafedh, Y.S., 1997. Effects of stocking density on patterns of reproduction and growth of hybrid tilapia in concrete tanks in Saudi Arabia. Asian Fisheries Science 10, 41–49.

Silva, L., Escalante, E., Valdés-Lozano, D., Hernández, M., Gasca-Leyva, E., 2017. Evaluation of a semi-intensive aquaponics system, with and without bacterial biofilter in a tropical location. Sustainability 9, 592–605.

Sin, A.W., Chiu, M.T., 1983. The intensive monoculture of the tilapia hybrid, *Sarotherodon nilotica* (males) × *S. mossambica* (females) in Hong Kong. In: Fishelson, L., Yaron, Z. (Eds.), Proceedings of the International Symposium on Tilapia in Aquaculture. Tel Aviv University, Tel Aviv, Israel, pp. 506–516.

Sipaúba-Tavares, L.H., Yoshida, C.E., de Souza Braga, F.M., 2000. Effects of continuous water exchange on limnology of tilapia (*Oreochromis niloticus*) culture tanks. In: Fitzsimmons, K., Filho, J.C. (Eds.), Tilapia Culture in the 21st Century. Proceedings from the Fifth International Symposium on Tilapia Aquaculture. Rio de Janeiro, Brazil, pp. 279–287.

Somerville, C., Cohen, M., Pantanella, E., Stankus, A., Lovatelli, A., 2014. Small-scale Aquaponic Food Production: Integrated Fish and Plant Farming. FAO Fisheries and Aquaculture Technical Paper No. 589. FAO, Rome, 262 pp.

Suresh, A.V., Lin, C.K., 1992. Effect of stocking density on water quality and production of red tilapia in a recirculated water system. Aquacultural Engineering 11, 1–22.

Tendencia, E.A., dela Peña, M., 2003. Investigations of some components of the green water system which makes it effective in the initial control of luminous bacteria. Aquaculture 218, 115–119.

Tendencia, E.A., Bosma, R.H., Sorio, L.R., 2012. Effect of three innovative culture systems on water quality and whitespot syndrome virus (WSSV) viral load in WSSV-fed *Penaeus monodon* cultured in indoor tanks. Aquaculture 350–353, 169–174.

Tyson, R., Simonne, E., 2014. A Practical Guide for Aquaponics as an Alternative Enterprise. UF/IFAS Extension Service, University of Florida, 100 pp.

van Rijn, J., 2013. Waste treatment in recirculating aquaculture systems. Aquacultural Engineering 53, 49–56.

VASEP (Vietnam Association of Seafood Exporters and Producers), 2016a. An Overview of Vietnam Fishery Sector. VASEP. http://vasep.com.vn/1192/OneContent/tong-quan-nganh.htm.

VASEP (Vietnam Association of Seafood Exporters and Producers), 2016b. Tilapia Exports Set to Shoot Up in Years Ahead. VASEP. http://vietnam.vnanet.vn/english/tilapiaexports-set-to-shoot-up-in-years-ahead-vasep/258011.html.

Watanabe, W.O., Clark, J.H., Dunhkam, J.B., Wicklund, R.I., Olla, B.L., 1990. Culture of Florida red tilapia in marine cages: the effects of stocking and dietary protein on growth. Aquaculture 90, 123–134.

Watanabe, W.O., Ernst, D.H., Chasar, M.P., Wicklund, R.I., Olla, B.L., 1993a. The effects of temperature and salinity on growth and feed utilization of juvenile, sex-reversed male Florida red tilapia cultured in a recirculating system. Aquaculture 112, 309–320.

Watanabe, W.O., Wicklund, R.I., Olla, B.L., 1993b. Saltwater culture of Florida red tilapia: a summary of research at the Caribbean marine research Centre (1985-1991). In: Proceedings of the First International Symposium on Aquaculture: Technology and Investment Opportunities. Ministry of Agriculture and Water, Riyadh, Saudi Arabia, pp. 49–68.

Watanabe, W.O., Wicklund, R.I., Olla, B.L., Head, W.D., 1997. Saltwater culture of the Florida red and other saline tolerant tilapias: a review. In: Costa-Pierce, B.A., Rakocy, J.E. (Eds.), Tilapia Aquaculture in the Americas, vol. 1. World Aquaculture Society, Baton Rouge, LA, pp. 54–141.

Watanabe, W.O., Losordo, T.M., Fitzsimmons, K., Hanley, F., 2002. Tilapia production systems in the Americas: technological advances, trends, and challenges. Reviews in Fisheries Science 10, 465–498.

Wheaton, F.W., 1977. Aquacultural Engineering. John Wiley, New York, 708 pp.

Windmar, M., Jarding, S., Paterson, R., 2000a. Current status of tilapia aquaculture and processing in Zimbabwe. In: Fitzsimmons, K., Filho, J.C. (Eds.), Tilapia Culture in the 21st Century. Proceedings from the Fifth International Symposium on Tilapia Aquaculture. Rio de Janeiro, Brazil, pp. 595–597.

Windmar, M., Jarding, S., Paterson, R., 2000b. Production of 480 tons of tilapia (*Oreochromis niloticus*) at Elanne farm, Zimbabwe. In: Fitzsimmons, K., Filho, J.C. (Eds.), Tilapia Culture in the 21st Century. Proceedings from the Fifth International Symposium on Tilapia Aquaculture. Rio de Janeiro, Brazil, pp. 602–604.

Xiao, R., Wei, Y., An, D., Li, D., Ta, X., Wu, Y., et al., 2018. A review on the research status and development trend of equipment in water treatment processes of recirculating aquaculture systems. Reviews in Aquaculture 1–33.

Yi, Y., Lin, C.K., 1997. Finishing system for large tilapia. In: Fourteenth Annual Technical Report. Pond Dynamics/Aquaculture CRSP, Oregon State University, Corvallis, OR, USA, pp. 146–156.

Yi, Y., Lin, C.K., 2001. Effects of biomass of caged Nile tilapia (*Oreochromis niloticus*) and aeration on the growth and yields in an integrated cage-cum-pond system. Aquaculture 195, 253–267.

Yi, Y., Lin, C.K., Diana, J.S., 1996. Effects of stocking densities on growth of caged adult Nile tilapia (*Oreochromis niloticus*) and on yield of small Nile tilapia in open water in earthen ponds. Aquaculture 146, 205–215.

Yi, Y., Lin, C.K., Diana, J.S., 2003. Hybrid catfish (*Clarias macrocephalus* × *C. gariepinus*) and Nile tilapia (*Oreochromis niloticus*) culture in an integrated pen-cum-pond system: growth performance and nutrient budget. Aquaculture 217, 395–408.

Yousif, O.M., 2002. The effects of stocking density, water exchange rate, feeding frequency and grading on size hierarchy development in juvenile Nile tilapia, *Oreochromis niloticus* L. Emirates Journal of Food and Agriculture 14, 45–53.

Yusoff, A., 2015. Status of resource management and aquaculture in Malaysia. In: Romana-Eguia, M.R.R., Parado-Estepa, F.D., Salayo, N.D., Lebata-Ramos, M.J.H. (Eds.), Proceedings of the International Workshop on Resource Enhancement and Sustainable Aquaculture Practices in Southeast Asia 2014 (RESA). Aquaculture Department, Southeast Asian Fisheries Development Center, Tigbauan, Iloilo, Philippines, pp. 53–65.

Zohar, G., Rappaport, U., Avnimelech, Y., Sarig, S., 1984. Results of the experiments carried out in the Genosar Experimental Station in 1983. Cultivation of Tilapia in high densities and with periodic flushing of the pond water. Bamidgeh 36, 63–69.

Chapter 7

Nutrition and feeding

Chapter outline

7.1 Introduction

Nutrition is the most expensive component in the intensive aquaculture industry, where it represents over 50% of operating costs. Therefore, proper feeding management is a necessary tool for successful tilapia culture practices. A great deal of attention has been paid to aquaculture nutrition in recent years. The challenge that faces tilapia farmers in general, and tilapia nutritionists in developing countries in particular, is the development of commercial, cost-effective tilapia feeds using locally available, cheap and unconventional resources.

Under extensive culture conditions, tilapia depend exclusively on natural food, through fertilization, while both natural foods and supplemental feeds are normally used in semi-intensive farming systems. Tilapia nutrition and feeding in extensive and semi-intensive farming systems are discussed in Chapter 5. The present chapter addresses tilapia nutrition under intensive and super-intensive farming systems. It deals with the requirements of farmed tilapia for the five classes of dietary nutrients, namely protein, lipids, carbohydrates, vitamins and minerals. Consideration is also given to feeding regimes (feeding levels and frequency) and diet form.

7.2 Protein requirements

Proteins are large, complex molecules composed typically of carbon, hydrogen, oxygen and nitrogen, as well as small amounts of sulphur and, sometimes, phosphorus. The principle components of proteins are known as 'amino acids'. Proteins are indispensable for the structure and function of all living organisms.

Protein is the most expensive dietary source in intensive aquaculture. It represents about 50% of total feed costs. Moreover, the dietary protein requirements for maximum performance of fish are generally higher than those of farmed terrestrial animals. Therefore, special attention is paid to the dietary protein requirements of farmed aquatic animals. Determination of dietary protein required for

Tilapia Culture. https://doi.org/10.1016/B978-0-12-816541-6.00007-6
Copyright © 2020 Elsevier Inc. All rights reserved.

optimal performance is also a critical step in developing efficient, sustainable and cost-effective aquafeed formulations.

Protein requirements of tilapia have been extensively studied using dose—response procedures. In this regard, semi-purified test diets containing casein, casein—gelatin mixtures or casein—amino acid mixtures as protein sources or using practical diets in which animal and/or plant ingredients served as dietary protein sources, have been widely used. The utility of the results of many studies are questionable because they were indoor, short-term studies and the outcomes may not be directly applicable in commercial rearing facilities. In addition, casein was traditionally used as a sole dietary protein source in many studies. Casein contains adequate levels of all essential amino acids (EAAs) except arginine. When casein is used as the sole dietary protein source, higher levels would be required to compensate for the arginine deficiency (Teshima et al., 1985a; El-Sayed, 1989). This means that the protein requirements of tilapia would probably have been lower if proper combinations of casein and arginine sources had been used instead of casein alone. Since gelatin is deficient in all EAAs except for arginine, casein/gelatin mixtures are a more suitable protein source in semi-purified tilapia diets. Casein-/gelatin-based diets were found to be utilized more efficiently than casein/amino acid diets (El-Sayed, 1989). It is, therefore, no surprise that the results of protein requirements of tilapia are varying and sometimes contradictory, as shown in Table 7.1.

Protein requirements of tilapia depend, among other things, on fish size or age, protein source, energy content and protein-to-energy (P:E) ratio of the diets. Generally speaking, protein requirement decreases with increasing fish size (Table 7.1). During the larval stages, tilapia (especially Nile tilapia) require about 35%—45% dietary protein for maximum growth performance (El-Sayed and Teshima, 1992). For tilapia juveniles, the protein requirement ranges from 30% to 40%, while adult tilapia require 25%—30% dietary protein for optimum performance (Al Hafedh, 1999; Koch et al., 2017; Liu et al., 2017). On the other hand, tilapia broodstock require 28%—45% dietary protein for optimum reproduction, spawning efficiency, and larval growth and survival, depending on protein source and dietary energy levels (Gunasekera et al., 1996a, 1996b; Siddiqui et al., 1998; El-Sayed et al., 2003; El-Sayed and Kawanna, 2008; de Oliveira et al., 2014; Bombardelli et al., 2017).

7.3 Amino acid requirements

As mentioned earlier, proteins are composed of amino acids, of which about 25 commonly occur in food proteins. These amino acids are divided into two groups:

1. Essential amino acids which cannot be synthesized by living organisms, including fishes, and must be supplied in the diets. These EAAs are arginine (Arg), lysine (Lys), histidine (His), threonine (Thr), valine (Val), leucine (Leu), isoleucine (Iso), methionine (Met), phenylalanine (Phe) and tryptophan (Try).
2. Non-essential amino acids (NEAAs) which can be synthesized by the organism, in the presence of suitable starting materials, including EAAs.

7.3.1 Essential amino acid requirements

Tilapia, like other fishes, require the same 10 EAAs. However, specific EAA requirements of most farmed tilapias, except Nile tilapia (*Oreochromis niloticus*) and, to a lesser extent, Mozambique tilapia (*Oreochromis mossambicus*), have not been determined. Several studies have considered EAA requirements of Nile tilapia and Mozambique tilapia. These requirements are summarized in Table 7.2. The EAA requirements of tilapia vary by species, size, strain, growth stages and amino acid source (e.g. crystalline AA vs. casein/gelatin). It was reported that tilapia fed crystalline EAA-based diets grew at lower rates than those fed casein or casein/gelatin diets (Jackson and Capper, 1982; Teshima et al., 1985a), presumably due to the low pH of the AA-based diets (Wilson et al., 1977). Neutralizing AA-based diets to a pH of 7—7.5 would improve their quality for tilapia (Mazid et al., 1979). Nonetheless, continuous research on amino acid requirements is necessary for formulating efficient, cost-effective and environmentally friendly feeds, using new technologies and tools to understand the complex mechanisms involved in fish growth and feed metabolism.

Commercial tilapia feeds depend mainly on plant protein sources; particularly oilseed plants (e.g. soybean meal (SBM), cottonseed meal (CSM), sunflower seed meal, etc.). These sources are generally deficient in total sulphur amino acids (TSAAs). Therefore, several studies have investigated the requirement, availability, digestibility and metabolism of these amino acids for tilapia. Tilapia requirements for TSAAs can be met by methionine or a methionine—cystine mixture. A methionine:cystine ratio of 50:50 was recommended for the best performance of Nile tilapia (Abdelghany, 2000; Nguyen and Davis, 2009a, 2009b). He et al. (2016) found also that the best survival of juvenile Nile tilapia was obtained at a ratio of 53:47, while methionine digestibility decreased with decreasing methionine:cystine ratios. These authors (He et al., 2017a) evaluated the effect of supplemental L-methionine on growth rates, immune response and antioxidative response of juvenile Nile tilapia (2.3 g). The fish were fed graded levels of methionine (3.2—13.3 g kg^{-1}) at a constant dietary cysteine concentration (0.83 g kg^{-1}). The maximum growth rates were obtained at 9.12 g kg^{-1} dietary methionine. On the other

TABLE 7.1 Protein requirements (%) of cultured tilapia.

Species and life stage	Weight (g)	Protein source	Requirement (%)	References
O. niloticus				
Fry	0.012	FM	45	El-Sayed and Teshima (1992)
	0.51–80	FM	40	Al Hafedh (1999)
	0.56	Casein/gelatin	35	Teshima et al. (1985a)
Fingerlings	1.29	Casein	40	Teshima et al. (1985a)
	2.40	Casein/gelatin	35	Abdelghany (2000)
	3.50	Casein	30	Wang et al. (1985)
GIFT	3.77	FM/casein/SBM/CSM/RSM	35	Kpundeh et al. (2015)
	15.87	FM/SBM/CSM/RSM	35	Liu et al. (2018)
Adults	24	FM/SBM/BM	27.5	Wee and Tuan (1988)
	45–264	FM	30	Al Hafedh (1999)
GIFT males	260.7	FM/casein	29.3	Liu et al. (2017)
	450	SBM/MBM/POM	27.0 (DP)	Koch et al. (2017)
Broodstock		FM/SBM	40	El-Sayed et al. (2003)
		FM	45	Siddiqui et al. (1998)
		Casein/gelatin	35–40	Gunasekera et al. (1996a,b)
	♀ 39.4; ♂ 60.5	FM	40	El-Sayed and Kawanna (2008)
	♀ 95; ♂ 169	FM/SBM	28	Bombardelli et al. (2017)
	764	FM/SBM	38	de Oliveira et al. (2014)
O. mossambicus	Fry	FM	50	Jauncey and Ross (1982)
	0.5–1.0	FM	40	Jauncey (1982)
	6–30	FM	30–35	Jauncey and Ross (1982)
O. aureus	2.50	Casein/albumin	56	Winfree and Stickney (1981)
	7.50	Casein/albumin	34	Winfree and Stickney (1981)
Tilapia zillii	1.40	Casein/gelatin	35	El-Sayed (1987)
O. n × *O. a*	0.60–1.10	FM	32	Shiau and Peng (1993)
	21	SBM	28	Twibell and Brown (1998)
O. n × *O. h*	1.24	–	32	Luquet (1989)
O. m × *O. h*	8.87	–	28	Watanabe et al. (1990)

O. a, Oreochromis aureus; O. h, Oreochromis hornorum; O. m, Oreochromis mossambicus; O. n, Oreochromis niloticus.
BM, blood meal; *CSM*, cottonseed meal; *DP*, digestible protein; *FM*, fish meal; *MBM*, meat and bone meal; *POM*, poultry offal meal; *RSM*, rapeseed meal; *SBM*, soybean meal.

TABLE 7.2 Essential amino acid requirements of Nile tilapia as % of total diet and of total dietary protein (in parenthesis).

Amino acid	Fish wt (g)	Requirement (%)	References
Lysine (Lys)	20.7	0.72	He et al. (2013)
	165	0.52	
	1.44	1.5 (5.41)	Furuya et al. (2012)
	274.9	1.46 (5.8)	Michelato et al. (2016a)
	6.40	- 1.5 (crystalline Lys)	Nguyen and Davis (2016)
		- 1.81 (intact Lys)	
Arginine (Arg)	7.14	1.0 (1% suppl. arginine +1% glutamine)	Pereira et al. (2017)
	6.04	1.82 (6.24)	Yue et al. (2015)
	2.95	1.36 (with 1.53% lysine)	Neu et al. (2016)
		1.18 (4.20)	Santiago and Lovell (1988)
Histidine (His)	4.84	0.82 (3.1)	Michelato et al. (2017)
		0.48	Santiago and Lovell (1988)
Threonine (Thr)		1.05 (3.75)	Santiago and Lovell (1988)
	563.3	1.15	Michelato et al. (2016b)
Valine (Val)		0.78 (2.80)	Santiago and Lovell (1988)
Leucine (Leu)	1.94	1.25 (4.31)	Gan et al. (2016)
		0.95 (3.39)	Santiago and Lovell (1988)
Isoleucine (Iso)		0.87 (3.11)	Santiago and Lovell (1988)
Methionine (Met)		0.75 (2.68)	Santiago and Lovell (1988)
	20.7	0.76	He et al. (2013)
	165	0.55	
	2.3	0.912	He et al. (2017a)
	8.95	- 0.73 at 10.9 MJ kg^{-1} DE - 0.99 at 12.4 MJ kg^{-1} DE	He et al. (2017b)
	1.28	0.81 (in the presence of 0.04% cystine)	Nguyen and Davis (2009b)
Cysteine (Cys)		0.53	Santiago and Lovell (1988)
Phenylalanine (Phe)		1.05 (3.75)	Santiago and Lovell (1988)
Tyrosine (Tyr)		1.79	Santiago and Lovell (1988)
Tryptophan (Try)	38.2	0.29	Zaminhan et al. (2017)
		0.28 (1.00)	Santiago and Lovell (1988)

hand, lower methionine levels were required for maximum plasma complement 4 (C4) content and lysozyme activity (7.50 g kg^{-1}); while maximum C3 content and superoxide dismutase activity were obtained at higher dietary methionine content (9.30 g kg^{-1}).

Since cystine can only be synthesized metabolically from methionine precursor, its presence in the diets is necessary for sparing part of methionine requirement for maximum performance. Therefore, the replacement of cystine for methionine in the diet can minimize methionine levels in practical diets without reducing growth, and in turn, minimize feed cost. Up to 44% of methionine was successfully replaced with cystine in blue tilapia (*Oreochromis aureus*) diets (Liou, 1989). It was also concluded that cystine could replace 47%–49% of TSAA requirement without hampering fish growth performance.

Lysine is another EAA, generally deficient in plant protein sources. Considerable efforts have been paid to dietary lysine requirement of tilapia (Table 7.2). Several studies indicated that lysine requirement of Nile tilapia ranges from 1.4% to 1.5% (Santiago and Lovell, 1988; Furuya et al., 2006, 2012; Michelato et al., 2016a; Nguyen and Davis, 2016). Increasing dietary lysine beyond the required levels may not provide significant additional performance and may even result in reduced growth performance (Furuya et al., 2012). However, the above values are slightly lower than the value reported by NRC (2011) (1.6% for tilapia *Oreochromis* spp.). The requirement of tilapia for phenylalanine (aromatic amino acid) could partially be met by tyrosine (NRC, 1993).

Except the early studies of Jauncey et al. (1983) and Santiago and Lovell (1988), not much attention has been given to other EAA requirements for tilapia. Only a few studies have investigated the requirement of Nile tilapia for arginine (Yue et al., 2015; Neu et al., 2016; Pereira et al., 2017), histidine (Michelato et al., 2017), threonine (Michelato et al., 2016b), leucine (Gan et al., 2016) and tryptophan (Zaminhan et al., 2017) (Table 7.2). These studies demonstrated that the inclusion of these amino acids in the feed resulted in improving growth performance, feed efficiency, immune response and other physiological functions.

7.3.2 Non-essential amino acids

Although NEAAs can be synthesized inside fish body, it has been reported that their dietary supplementation may or may not improve fish performance, physiological functions and immune response, depending on fish species (Gaye-Siessegger et al., 2007). Only a few studies were carried out on the effects of NEAAs on tilapia performance. Mambrini and Kaushik (1994) found that a substitution of 25% of dietary protein by alanine, glutamate or glycine in Nile tilapia diets resulted in 10% reduction in fish growth. A substitution of 50% with a mixture of the three NEAAs resulted in a marked reduction in growth, a lower nitrogen retention and higher nitrogen excretion. Similar results were reported by Gaye-Siessegger et al. (2007), where the utilization of synthetic amino acids by Nile tilapia was poor.

Considerable attention has recently been given to taurine as a feed supplement for farmed fish and shellfish (El-Sayed, 2014). Taurine, or 2-aminoethanesulfonic acid, is an end product of metabolism of sulphur-containing amino acids. It is a neutral β-amino acid, where both the amine group and sulphonic group can be ionized (Jacobsen and Smith, 1968). Despite that taurine is not incorporated into proteins, nor degraded by mammalian tissues (Kuzmina et al., 2010), it is the most abundant free amino acid in animal tissue, accounting for 30%–50% of the entire amino acid pool, depending on the animal species (Jacobsen and Smith, 1968).

Historically, taurine has not been considered as an essential nutrient for fish. However, recent studies indicated that taurine is conditionally essential when these fishes are fed plant protein-based diets deficient in methionine and/or cysteine. The essentiality of taurine for farmed fish depends on fish species and size, natural feeding habits and previous feeding history of the fish (Takagi et al., 2008; Kuzmina et al., 2010; El-Sayed, 2014). Taurine is involved in many physiological functions, including muscular and neural systems development, antioxidation and detoxification, modulation of immune response, calcium transport, retina development, bile acid metabolism, osmotic regulation and endocrine functions (El-Sayed, 2014).

Few recent studies have evaluated the effects of supplemental taurine on growth and reproductive performance of Nile tilapia. Gonçalves et al. (2011) found that supplemental taurine is essential for optimum performance of Nile tilapia (*O. niloticus*) larvae. Similar results were reported by Al-Feky et al. (2016a). Nile tilapia larvae fed with SBM-based diets supplemented with exogenous dietary taurine showed significantly better growth, survival and feed efficiency than those given taurine-free diets. About 9.7 g kg^{-1} dietary taurine was required for optimum performance. Al-Feky et al. (2016b) found also that spawning performances, including spawning frequencies, total number of spawnings per tank, number of spawnings per female and absolute fecundity, were all significantly improved with increasing dietary taurine up to 0.8%. Eggs produced from broodstock fed 8.3 g kg^{-1} taurine exhibited significantly higher hatchability and required shorter time for hatching and yolk-sac absorption and also resulted in higher larval weight than at other dietary taurine levels. These findings demonstrated the inability of Nile tilapia to synthesize taurine and suggest that exogenous taurine is essential for optimum growth and reproductive performance of these fish. The interactions between dietary taurine and methionine in Nile tilapia fed plant protein-based diet have also been demonstrated by Michelato et al. (2018). Fish fed diets supplemented with methionine, taurine or a mixture of both exhibited similar growth performance. This indicates that dietary taurine supplementation has a sparing effect on the methionine requirement of Nile tilapia.

7.4 Protein sources

Since purified and semi-purified protein sources are not recommended for tilapia under commercial culture conditions, other conventional and unconventional, locally available dietary protein sources should be sought. Research has evaluated many such sources for different species of tilapia, with varying results. It is appropriate to highlight these protein sources for tilapia, with emphasis on the sources that have economic potential and are locally available, especially in developing countries (see El-Sayed, 1999 for more details). The suggested inclusion levels of these sources in diets of different tilapia species and sizes are given in Table 7.3.

A wide variety of unconventional protein sources, including animal proteins, plant proteins, single-cell proteins (SCPs) and industrial and agricultural wastes have been evaluated with respect for their utility in farmed tilapia feeds. Some sources proved cost-effective, while others were not. The following evaluation of alternative protein sources will provide farmers and nutritionists with information on the advantages and disadvantages of such feed ingredients as well as their proper inclusion levels in tilapia feeds.

7.4.1 Animal protein sources

7.4.1.1 Fish meal

Fish meal (FM) has been traditionally used as the main protein source in the aquafeed industry, due to its high protein content and balanced EAA profile. FM is also an excellent source of essential fatty acids (EFAs), digestible energy, minerals and vitamins. The increased demand for FM, coupled with a significant shortage in global FM production, has created sharp competition for its use by the animal feed industry. As a result, FM has become the most expensive protein commodity in animal and aquaculture feeds in recent years (El-Sayed, 1998, 1999). Many developing countries have realized that, in the long run, they will be unable to afford FM as a major protein source in aquafeed. Many attempts have been made to partially or totally replace FM with less expensive, locally available protein sources.

7.4.1.2 Fishery by-products

Despite the fact that large amounts of fishery by-products and by-catch are produced annually in the world, little attention has been paid to the commercial use of these by-products for tilapia. The exception is fish silage (FS) and shrimp meals, where several studies have considered their use as an FM replacer in tilapia feeds. The results indicated that between 30% and 75% FS can be successfully incorporated in tilapia feed, depending on fish species and size, silage source and diet composition (Fagbenro, 1994; Fagbenro et al., 1994). Wassef et al. (2003) found also that growout Nile tilapia (28.6 g) responded better to FS than fry or fingerlings. They also reported that 50% FS was most cost-effective, while about 75% was required when FS + SBM (1:1) were used. Similar results were reported by Madage et al. (2015), where up to 50% of dietary FM can be replaced with tilapia silage in test diets for red tilapia hybrids (*O. mossambicus* × *O. niloticus* × *O. aureus*). It is evident that FS has a potential as a protein source for tilapia.

On the other hand, the quality of FS is affected by the fermentation and/or silaging methods. For example, diets containing formic acid-preserved FS reduced growth performance of tilapia, presumably due to acidity of the diet and a high proportion of free amino acids in the FS. It has been suggested that acidity reduces diet acceptance and affects protease activity in fish guts (Hardy et al., 1983), while free amino acids may depress fish appetite (Wilson et al., 1984). Shrimp meal has also been successfully used as a protein source for tilapia. Nile tilapia utilized shrimp head meal at up to 60% of the diet without adverse effects on their performance (Nwanna and Daramola, 2000). Moreover, Mansour (1998) and El-Sayed (1998) reported that shrimp meal can replace FM in red tilapia (*O. niloticus* × *Oreochromis hornorum*) and Nile tilapia diets, at 50% and 100%, respectively, without significant retardation in weight gain and feed efficiency.

Abdelghany (2003) evaluated gambusia (*Gambusia affinis*) fish meal (GFM) as a replacement for herring FM protein in diets for red tilapia (*O. niloticus* × *O. mossambicus*). The growth of fish fed GFM at up 50% substitution level was not different from that of herring FM-based diet. Partial or complete substitution of GFM for FM did not affect feed utilization efficiency and digestibility of protein, dry matter and gross energy of the diets. Economic analysis showed that the best cost-effective results were achieved at 50% substitution level. Goddard et al. (2008) found also that fisheries by-catch and waste-processing meals could totally replace FM (commercial anchovy meal) in practical diets for Nile tilapia.

7.4.1.3 Terrestrial animal by-products

Terrestrial animal by-products including poultry by-product meal (PBM), blood meal (BM), hydrolysed feather meal (HFM) and meat and bone meal (MBM) have been widely used as protein sources for tilapia, due to their high protein content and good EAA profiles. However, they may be deficient in one or more of the EAA. The most limiting

TABLE 7.3 Tested and recommended levels of different protein sources for tilapia.

Source (specification)	Levels tested (%)	Requirement (%)	Species (weight, g)	References
Animal sources				
Gambusia meal	0–100	50	*Oreochromis niloticus* × *Oreochromis mossambicus*	Abdelghany (2003)
Shrimp meal	100	100	*Oreochromis niloticus* (20)	El-Sayed (1998)
Shrimp meal	100	100	Red tilapia (9)	Mansour (1998)
Shrimp head waste	0–60	60	*O. niloticus* (1.4)	Nwanna and Daramola (2000)
FS	0–75	50	Red tilapia (2.1)	Madage et al. (2015)
FS + SBM or MBM, PBM or HFM (1:1)	0–75	50–75	*O. niloticus* (8)	Fagbenro (1994), Fagbenro et al. (1994)
PBM + Met + Lys + Thr	0–100	50	*O. n* (0.88)	Aydin and Gümüş (2013)
MBM + Met	40–50	50	*O. niloticus* (11 mg)	Tacon et al. (1983)
MBM	100	100	*O. niloticus* (20)	El-Sayed (1998)
MBM	100	100	Red tilapia (9)	Mansour (1998)
MBM + BM (2:3)	0–100	100	*O. mossambicus* (1)	Davies et al. (1989)
BM	0–100	100	*O. mossambicus* (1)	Davies et al. (1989)
BM	100	<100	*O. niloticus* (20)	El-Sayed (1998)
BM	100	<100	Red tilapia (9)	Mansour (1998)
HFM	0–100	66	*O. niloticus* (0.01)	Bishop et al. (1995)
HFM ± EAA	10–50	30	*O. niloticus* (4–5)	Tacon et al. (1983)
Animal by-products	0–100	100	*O. niloticus* (0.1)	Rodriguez-Serna et al. (1996)
Chicken offal silage	0–20	20	*O. niloticus* (10.8)	Belal et al. (1995)
Black soldier fly	0–100	75	*O. niloticus (3)*	Muin et al. (2017)
Housefly maggot meal	0–100	100	*O. niloticus (2)*	Ogunji et al. (2008)
Housefly maggot meal	0–100	75	*O. niloticus (69)*	Wang et al. (2017)
Super worm meal	0–100	50	*O. niloticus (5.7)*	Jabir et al. (2012)
Oilseed plants				
SBM ± Met	75	75	*O. niloticus* (0.8)	Tacon et al. (1983)
SBM	0–100	75	*O. mossambicus* (50)	Jackson et al. (1982)

Continued

TABLE 7.3 Tested and recommended levels of different protein sources for tilapia.—cont'd

Source (specification)	Levels tested (%)	Requirement (%)	Species (weight, g)	References
SBM ± Met	0–100	67	Hybrids (4.47)	Shiau et al. (1989)
Soy protein concentrate	0–100	100	*O. niloticus* (3.2)	Abdelghany (1997)
SBM + EAA + DCP+oil	0–100	100	Hybrids (84)	Viola et al. (1988)
SBM + DCP + oil	0–100	100	Hybrids (169)	Viola et al. (1988)
SB flour + PMM (75:25)	25–75	25	*O. niloticus* (7)	Sadiku and Jauncey (1995)
CSM ± Lys	100	100	*O. niloticus* (20)	El-Sayed (1990)
CSM	0–100	50	*O. mossambicus* (12)	Jackson et al. (1982)
CSM	0–100	80	*Tilapia zillii* (1.5)	El-Sayed (1987)
Sesame seed meal	0–75	25	*T. zillii* (2.4)	El-Sayed (1987)
Groundnut cake	0–100	25	*O. mossambicus* (30)	Jackson et al. (1982)
Rapeseed meal	0–75	75	*O. mossambicus* (13)	Jackson et al. (1982)
Copra meal	0–50	25–50	*O. mossambicus* (31)	Jackson et al. (1982)
Defatted cocoa cake	100	100	*Tilapia guineensis* (52)	Fagbenro (1988)
Palm kernel cake	0–100	60	*O. niloticus* (2.5)	Omoregie and Ogbemudia (1993)
Palm kernel cake	20–50	50	*O. mossambicus* (8.4)	Lim et al. (2001)
Macadamia press cake	0–100	50	*O. niloticus* (7.5–12)	Balogun and Fagbenro (1995)
Macadamia press cake	100	100	*T. guineensis* (NA)	Fagbenro (1993)
Sunflower meal	0–50	20	*Tilapia rendalli* (0.93)	Olvera-Novoa et al. (2002)
Aquatic plants				
Spirulina	0–100	40	*O. mossambicus* (0.3)	Olvera-Novoa et al. (1998)
Azolla pinnata	8–42	42	*O. niloticus* (0.011)	Santiago et al. (1988)
A. pinnata	0–100	<25	*O. niloticus* (4–40)	El-Sayed (1992)
Hydrodictyon	0–100	20	*O. niloticus* (1)	Appler (1985)
Hydrodictyon	0–100	20	*T. zillii* (1)	Appler (1985)
Eleocharis ochrostachys	20–40	20–30	*O. niloticus* (7)	Klinnavee et al. (1990)
Potamogeton	25–50	25	*O. niloticus* (14.5)	Essa (1997)

Duckweed	0–100	50–100	*Tilapia* sp. (NA)	Skillicorn et al. (1993)
Duckweed (*Lemna*)	0–50	50	*O. niloticus* (14.5)	Essa (1997)
Duckweed (*Spirodela*)	0–100	30	*O. niloticus* (13.9)	Fasakin et al. (1999)
Grain legumes				
Leucaena leaf meal	0–50	<25	*O. mossambicus* (50)	Jackson et al. (1982)
Cassava leaf meal	20–100	<100	*O. niloticus* (14–15)	Ng and Wee (1989)
Jack bean meal (cooked in distilled water)	20–30	20	*O. niloticus* (7.6)	Fagbenro et al. (2004)
Jack bean meal (cooked in trona solution)	20–30	30	*O. niloticus* (7.6)	Fagbenro et al. (2004)
Alfalfa LPC	15–55	35	*O. mossambicus* (0.3)	Olvera-Novoa et al. (1990)
Cowpea LPC	0–50	20–30	*O. niloticus* (0.16)	Olvera-Novoa et al. (1997)
Corn gluten feed + SBM	100	100	*O. niloticus* (30)	Wu et al. (1995)
Corn gluten + SBM	100	100	*O. niloticus* (30)	Wu et al. (1995)
Corn coproducts	0–100	50	Hybrids (21)	Twibell and Brown (1998)
Coffee pulp	0–39	13–26	*Oreochromis aureus* (4–10)	Ulla Rojas and Weerd (1997)
Toasted lima bean + Met	20–80	40–80	*O. niloticus* (5)	Adeparusi and Olute (2000)
LE-DDGS	0–50	30	Hybrid (6)	Chatvijitkul et al. (2016)
LE-DDGS + Lys + 2% fat	0–50	50	Hybrid (2.2)	

Levels tested are a substitution of standard dietary protein (mainly FM), SBM or whole diet. Recommended levels are based on biological and/or economic evaluation.
BM, blood meal; *CSM*, cottonseed meal; *DCP*, dicalcium phosphate; *FM*, fish meal; *HFM*, hydrolysed feather meal; *LE-DDGS*, lipid-extracted distillers dried grains with solubles; *LPC*, leaf protein concentrate; *MBM*, meat and bone meal; *Met*, methionine; *NA*, not available; *PBM*, poultry by-product meal; *PMM*, poultry meat meal; *SB*, soybean; *SBM*, soybean meal.

EAAs in these by-products are lysine (in PBM, HFM), isoleucine (BM) and methionine (MBM, BM, HFM) (Tacon and Jackson, 1985). If these by-products are included in feeds at the proper ratios, the EAA deficiencies can be overcome and the quality of such diets is likely to improve (Tacon et al., 1983; Davies et al., 1989). Tacon et al. (1983) found that hexane-extracted MBM or MBM:BM (4:1) supplemented with methionine successfully replaced up to 50% of FM protein in Nile tilapia fry diets. Similarly, up to 50% of FM protein can be replaced by PBM protein with Lys, Met and Thr supplementation in diets for Nile tilapia fry without adverse effects on growth performance, feed utilization and body composition (Aydin and Gümüş, 2013). Furthermore, Davies et al. (1989) found that optimum MBM/BM ratios could replace up to 75% of FM in diets fed to *O. mossambicus* fry. They also found that diets containing MBM or high MBM/BM ratios (3:1 and 2:3) were superior to FM even at a 100% substitution level. Cost-benefit analyses indicated that these sources can be used as single dietary protein sources for Nile tilapia (El-Sayed, 1998). On the contrary, BM and HFM are not efficiently utilized by tilapia due to low digestibility and poor EAA profiles (Viola and Zohar, 1984; Davies et al., 1989; Bishop et al., 1995). Thompson et al. (2012) also reported that diets containing high levels of SBM, but free of PBM, cannot be well utilized by Nile tilapia fry even with methionine and lysine supplementation. A diet containing a relatively high SBM level (46%), combined with PBM (22%), without amino acid supplementation, resulted in higher growth rates than the SBM-based diets. The authors suggested that practical, well-balanced diets for juvenile Nile tilapia can be achieved without FM and amino acid supplementation, when SBM and PBM were included at 20% each.

Terrestrial animal by-product silage has been successfully used as a protein source for tilapia. Belal et al. (1995) fed *O. niloticus* fingerlings (10.8 g) test diets containing 0%–20% chicken offal silage (COS), made from chicken viscera, as a replacement of FM. They found that the growth and body composition of fish fed COS up to 20% level were similar to that of fish fed an FM-based diet. High inclusion levels of COS should be tested in order to determine the proper inclusion level.

7.4.1.4 Insect and worm meals

Insect-based proteins have recently been recognized as an efficient and cheap alternative to FM and soybean in aquaculture feeds. The nutritional values of insects such as housefly (*Musca domestica*), black soldier fly (BSF) (*Hermetia illucens*), blowfly (*Chrysomya megacephala*) and mealworm beetle (*Tenebrio molitor*) are reasonably good. They contain high protein (up to > 55%) and lipid (up to 35%) levels (Sing et al., 2014; Muin et al., 2017; Wang et al., 2017). However, the nutritional value of these insects highly varies, depending on insect species, harvested stage, production substrate and processing methods. These insects have been evaluated as alternative protein sources in tilapia diets with promising results (Ogunji et al., 2008; Sing et al., 2014; Muin et al., 2017; Wang et al., 2017).

A number of studies have considered the use of housefly (*M. domestica*) maggot meal (MM) as a potential protein source for farmed tilapia. Earlier studies indicated that up to 100% of the FM can be replaced with MM (Ogunji et al., 2008) and blowfly (*C. megacephala*) MM (Sing et al., 2014) in practical diets for Nile tilapia fingerlings without affecting fish performance. More recently, Wang et al. (2017) assessed housefly MM as a replacer of FM protein in practical feeds for Nile tilapia, at 0%, 25%, 50%, 75% and 100% substitution levels. There was no significant difference in feed intake and apparent digestibility coefficient between the treatments. Replacing up to 75% of FM protein with MM did not have an impact on the growth performance, feed utilization and survival, whereas the complete replacement of FM caused significant retardation in fish performance and survival. Increasing substitute levels were accompanied with the declining concentrations of nitrite nitrogen and total phosphorus (TP) in the water. This study suggested that at 50% substitution level, MM can serve as a renewable, cost-effective, and environmentally superior alternative protein source for Nile tilapia.

The BSF is a non-pest tropical insect, with a huge potential as a protein source in animal feed industry. The BSF larvae can grow very quickly, with a growout cycle taking about 2 weeks to reach a weight of 0.25 g per larva (Maquart et al., 2018). They can also feed on a wide range of substrates, including manures and food wastes. The larvae contain 28%–48% crude protein, with an excellent amino acid profile and 12%–42% lipid, depending on the substrate on which they were produced (Newton et al., 1977; Maquart et al., 2018). This high nutritional value makes BSF an ideal FM replacer in commercial fish feed. However, the use of BSF as a feed ingredient for tilapia has been controversial. Earlier studies of Bondari and Sheppard (1987) indicated that blue tilapia fed chopped or whole BSF larvae resulted in depressed fish growth compared to commercial diet. The author referred the poor performance to the use of fresh larvae, which reduced the dry matter and protein intake, and also because they contain high chitin content, an almost indigestible sugar. On the other hand, opposite results were reported by Devic et al. (2018) who assessed the incorporation of BSF larvae meal (BSFM) into Nile tilapia (5.7 g) test diet at 0.0%, 3.0%, 5.0% and 8.0%, as a partial substitute of FM and SBM. They found that growth performance, feed utilization efficiency and whole body composition were not adversely affected by BSFM inclusion level. However, BSFM replacement levels were relatively low (0%–8%); it would have been more logic and meaningful if a wider substitution range had been tested.

The nutritional value of yellow mealworm (*T. molitor*) (TM) was evaluated as an FM substitute for Nile tilapia (Sánchez-Muros et al., 2016). Dietary protein from FM was replaced by 50% protein from SBM or TM; or 75% of FM protein was replaced with SBM (50%) and TM (25%). The results indicated that an inclusion of TM up to 50% substitution did not affect feed intake, protein digestibility and muscle amino acid composition. However, TM inclusion at both levels reduced growth rates and affected the muscle fatty acid profile. These results suggest that TM cannot be used at high inclusion levels, presumably due to their high chitin content and the toxins that they may contain.

Rapatsa and Moyo (2017) investigated mopane worm (*Imbrasia belina*) meal as a protein source in the diet of Mozambique tilapia (*O. mossambicus*). The worm meal replaced FM at 10%, 20%, 40% and 60% levels. Growth rates, feed efficiency, digestive enzyme activities and profit index increased with increasing mopane worm inclusion levels. This result suggests that mopane worm meal may be a good candidate for the replacement of FM in Mozambique tilapia diets. Also, Jabir et al. (2012) found that up to 50% of dietary FM in Nile tilapia diet can be replaced by super worm (*Zophobas morio*) meal (SWM). Additional SWM resulted in significant retardation in fish performance.

7.4.2 Plant protein sources

7.4.2.1 Oilseed plants

7.4.2.1.1 Soybean meal

Among plant protein sources, SBM contains the highest protein content and has the best EAA profile. However, SBM is deficient in sulphur-containing amino acids (Met, Lys, Cys) and contains endogenous antinutrients, including protease (trypsin) inhibitor, phytohaemagglutinin and antivitamins. Some of the factors can be destroyed or inactivated during thermal processing (El-Sayed et al., 2000).

SBM can be used as a total or partial protein source for farmed tilapia, depending on fish species and size, dietary protein level, SBM source and processing methods, and culture systems employed. For example, it was found that prepressed, solvent-extracted SBM, with or without Met supplementation, successfully replaced up to 75% of FM in the diet of Nile tilapia fry (Tacon et al., 1983), *O. mossambicus* (Jackson et al., 1982) and 67% in the case of tilapia hybrids (Shiau et al., 1989). In the meantime, supplementing SBM with the deficient EAA did not improve fish growth, and therefore was proven unnecessary (Teshima and Kanazawa, 1988).

The utilization of SBM in tilapia feeds may be limited by dietary minerals (phosphorus in this case), rather than the deficient EAA. It was reported that the noninclusion of the deficient EAA to SBM-based diet did not result in any growth retardation, while SBM supplemented with 3% dicalcium phosphate (DCP) and oil completely replaced FM without any adverse effects on fish growth (Viola et al., 1986, 1988). The nonnecessity of EAA supplementation has also been reported with other oilseed plants (El-Sayed, 1987, 1990).

It should be realized that the quality of SBM (and other plant protein sources) for tilapia depends on the processing methods. For example, Wassef et al. (1988) found that the germination and defattening of SBM reduced the activity of protease inhibitors. Heating SBM also destroys the antinutritional factors and helps rupture the cellulose membrane surrounding the cell and releases the cell contents making them more available. Boiling of full-fat SBM at 100°C for 1 h also improves its quality and reduces trypsin inhibitor activity for Nile tilapia. However, El-Sayed et al. (2000) found that full-fat SBM contained traces of protease inhibitors even after thermal treatment (at 200°C for 10 min) or soaking for 3 days, leading to an increase in trypsin secretion (to compensate for the reduced activity) in Nile tilapia.

7.4.2.1.2 Cottonseed meal/cake

CSM is one of the most available plant protein sources in tropical and subtropical regions. It is also one of the best protein candidates for tilapia in developing countries, due to its high availability, relatively low price, good protein content (26%–54%, depending on processing methods) and amino acid profile. However, it contains relatively low levels of Cys, Lys and Met in addition to its high content of gossypol (a phenolic antinutrient) that may limit the use of CSM in tilapia feeds. Results on the use of CSM and CSC (cottonseed cake) indicated that replacement of more traditional protein sources at between 50% and 100% can be effective in tilapia feed, depending on CSM source, processing methods and fish species and size (see Table 7.3).

7.4.2.1.3 Other oilseed by-products

Other oilseed by-products, including groundnut, sunflower, rapeseeds, sesame seeds, copra, macadamia, cocoa cake and palm kernel, may have a good potential as protein sources for tilapia. However, few studies have been conducted to evaluate these ingredients, with varying, and sometimes contradictory results. For example, Jackson et al. (1982) found that rapeseed meal could effectively replace up to 75% of FM protein in *O. mossambicus* diets, without significant retardation in fish performance. On the contrary, Davies et al. (1990) found that only 15% rapeseed meal could effectively replace FM/SBM in *O. mossambicus* diets, while higher levels resulted in poor growth and feed efficiency due to the high content of glucosinolate (antinutrient) in rapeseed. Similar results were reported with respect to the use of macadamia press cake as a protein source for tilapia. Agbo et al. (2011) found that groundnut (*Arachis hypogaea* L.) cake and groundnut husk protein could replace at least 50% and 20% of FM protein, respectively, in the diet of Nile tilapia fingerlings without any adverse effects on growth, feed efficiency, body composition and nutrient digestibility.

Sesame seeds are deficient in Lys and zinc. The supplementation of either Lys or zinc significantly improved the growth and survival of *Tilapia zillii*, in addition to the disappearance of the disease symptoms (El-Sayed, 1987). Therefore, Lys or zinc may meet the requirement of one another, supporting the argument that certain minerals rather than EAA deficiency may be the limiting factor in sesame seeds.

7.4.2.1.4 Effects of phytase supplementation

Many plant protein sources contain high levels of phytic acid, which binds with divalent minerals such as Ca, P, Zn, Mn, Mg and Fe to form water-insoluble salts, rendering the minerals unavailable. When these plants are used as the primary source of protein in a tilapia feed, higher supplementary mineral levels may be required, particularly if the culture water is deficient in one or more of the required minerals. The inclusion of bacterial phytase in tilapia diets can be effective in reducing phytic acid activity and improving the utilization of plant protein sources. Phytase may also reduce the effect of antinutritional factors, protect amino acids from degradation and decrease leaching of water soluble components (Riche et al., 2001).

Many studies indicated that the addition of phytase into tilapia diets has improved growth rates, digestibility and utilization of dietary protein phosphorous (Riche et al., 2001; Liebert and Portz, 2005; Rachmawati et al., 2018; Li et al., 2019). These studies demonstrated that about 500–1000 phytase units kg^{-1} feed are required for optimum performance, depending on dietary plant protein/animal protein ratios and mineral contents of the diets. In addition, phytase supplementation to Nile tilapia fed low dietary phosphorus improved immune response and reduced the pathological lesions of liver, spleen, stomach and intestines (Abo Norag et al., 2018).

On the contrary, Hu et al. (2016) found that supplemental microbial phytase did not improve growth rates and feed conversion ratio of hybrid tilapia (*O. niloticus* ♀ × *O. aureus* ♂). Moreover, microbial phytase stimulated intestinal inflammation and stress status, as indicated by the upregulation of intestinal expressions of the cytokine genes (tnf-α and tgf-β) and hsp70. This particular study indicates that dietary microbial phytase may lead to mixed effects on farmed tilapia, suggesting that phytases should be carefully selected as aquafeed additives and those that may induce intestinal inflammation should be avoided.

7.4.2.2 Aquatic plants

Several studies have been conducted on the use of aquatic plants in tilapia feeds. Among these plants, the duckweed (family: Lemnaceae) is the most promising. Fresh duckweed is an excellent food source for tilapia, as it contains about 35%–45% crude protein with good amino acid and mineral profiles. It can be easily cultivated, and it grows at a tremendous rate to yield 10–50 dry mt ha^{-1} yr^{-1}, depending on cultivation environment (Leng et al., 1995). Duckweed can be used as a single food source for farmed tilapia. A study in Bangladesh (Skillicorn et al., 1993) indicated that when duckweed was used as a single nutritional input for tilapia in earthen ponds, fish production reached 7.5 mt ha^{-1} yr^{-1}. Furthermore, with better pond management and stocking density, the annual production per ha can reach 10 mt or more. Dry duckweed is also a good protein and energy alternative for tilapia. It can replace up to 50% of the commercial feed without adverse effects on fish performance (Essa, 1997). Fasakin et al. (1999) found also that replacing FM with up to 30% sun-dried duckweed supported the growth of Nile tilapia and was cost-effective. Up to 25% fermented duckweed was also successfully included in the diets of Nile tilapia fingerlings (Velásquez et al., 2015).

The use of *Azolla*, a freshwater fern that has a symbiotic relationship with nitrogen fixing cyanobacteria *Anabaena azollae*, as a fresh or dried feed ingredient for farmed tilapia has also been investigated, with controversial results. El-Sayed (1992) evaluated *Azolla pinnata* as an FM replacer for Nile tilapia fingerlings and adults at 0%–100% substitution levels. Fish fed with *A. pinnata* showed extremely poor performance even at the lowest inclusion level (25%). Similar results were reported on *O. niloticus* (Almazan et al., 1986) and *Tilapia rendalli* fed *Azolla microphylla* (Micha et al., 1988). It seems from these studies that the acceptability of *Azolla* to tilapia is poor.

In contrast, between 30% and 42% of FM-based diets fed to Nile tilapia has been successfully replaced by *Azolla* meal without negatively affecting fish performance (Santiago et al., 1988; Naegel, 1997). When Nile tilapia fingerlings (16.2 g) were fed *Azolla filiculoides* as a main dietary component at 30%, 35% and 40%, no significant differences were found in fish performance, production and net profit among all diets (Abou et al., 2007a). In another 90-day study, Abou et al. (2007b) found that up to 20% of FM can be replaced with dry *A. filiculoides* in diets fed to juvenile Nile tilapia males (15 g) reared in earthen ponds, without any significant adverse effects on growth performance and feed utilization. In addition, Azolla-based diets resulted in considerable economic return compared to FM-based diet.

Other aquatic plants, including *Hydrodictyon reticulatum*, coontail (*Ceratophyllum demersum*), chuut-nuu (*Eleocharis ochrostachys*) and *Potamogeton gramineous* can be used as a partial replacement of protein or carbohydrate for different tilapia species. However, these sources should be carefully looked at, since some other aquatic plants such as *Elodea trifoliate* and *Myriophyllum spicatum* have been reported to reduce tilapia performance. In addition, when dry *C. demersum* and *Potamogeton amplifolius* were incorporated in Nile tilapia diets at 13%, 26% and 38% (33%, 66% and 100% of wheat bran), they resulted in a significant reduction in fish performance (Balkhasher, 2012). Growth rates and feed utilization of fish fed fermented *P. amplifolius* at 13% and 26% inclusion level were not significantly different ($P > .05$) from fish fed the control diet. At 38% inclusion level, fish performance was significantly reduced. On the other hand, fermented *C. demersum* produced extremely poor performance at all inclusion levels.

Marine algae also have a high potential as a source of protein and n-3 EFAs, or as feed additives. However, only a few studies have considered marine algae as feed ingredients in tilapia feeds. Azaza et al. (2008) demonstrated that up to 20% of SBM can be replaced by ulva meal (*Ulva rigida*) in practical Nile tilapia diets without any detrimental effects on fish performance. It was also found that 50% of corn gluten could be replaced by spirulina meal (*Spirulina platensis*) in Nile tilapia larval diets (Hussein et al., 2013). Nile tilapia were also fed diets containing 20%−60% red algae (*Gracilaria arcuata*) as a replacement of FM (Younis et al., 2018). Fish growth performance was significantly reduced with algal supplementation; however, feed efficiency did not differ between fish fed the control diet and those fed 20% *Gracilaria*. The authors concluded that up to 20% red algae, *G. arcuata,* could be incorporated, as a FM replacer, in Nile tilapia diets.

7.4.2.3 Grain legumes

Many leguminous or cereal plants and by-products can be used as partial protein sources for tilapia. Among these, leucaena leaf meal (LLM, 30% crude protein), brewery wastes, corn products (corn gluten, corn distiller's grain, corn co-products, corn gluten feed), cassava leaf meal (CLM), green gram legume, lima bean and leaf protein concentrates are of prime importance. However, most of leguminous or cereal plants are deficient in certain EAA (e.g. Arg, Thr, Iso, His and Met are deficient in LLM) and may contain antinutrients, such as mimosine (a toxic nonprotein amino acid) found in LLM (Lim and Dominy, 1991). Therefore, proper processing of these sources (heating, soaking, cooking, etc.) may improve their quality for tilapia. Osman et al. (1996) reported that cooked or sun-dried LLM produced better performance of Nile tilapia than did sodium hydroxide-treated or rumen liquor-incubated LLM.

Other legume seeds have been tested as protein sources for tilapia. Ng and Wee (1989) found that the performance of Nile tilapia fed CLM was reduced with increasing CLM levels in the diets. However, fish growth was significantly improved when CLM was supplemented with 0.1% Met. Similarly, when the green gram legume (*Phaseolus aureus*) was fed to Nile tilapia fry at different dietary protein levels, the best growth rates were observed at 25% substitution level (De Silva and Gunasekera, 1989). Fagbenro et al. (2004) found that jack bean (*Canavalia ensiformis*) can be a useful partial substitute for FM in tilapia feed. Up to 20% of SBM protein was provided by jack bean seeds cooked in distilled water, whereas cooking in trona solution increased the inclusion level to 30%.

El-Sayed et al. (2016) evaluated the use of guar meal (GM) as a protein source for Nile tilapia fingerlings (20 g) at different substitution levels (0%−100%). The results indicated that fish performance was excellent at all GM inclusion levels, but fish performance and feed efficiency were significantly retarded with increasing dietary GM up to 20% level. However, the cost−benefit analysis of the test diets indicated that GM-based diets, even at 100% substitution, were economically better than the control, SBM-based diet. These results suggest that GM can totally replace SBM in Nile tilapia feeds. In an earlier study, Al Hafedh and Siddiqui (1998) reported that guar seeds could successfully replace up to 50% of FM in the diets of Nile tilapia, without adverse effects on growth and feed utilization.

Distiller's dried grains with solubles (DDGS) are a dried by-product resulting from the fermentation of dry-milled grains to ethanol. DDGS has attracted the attention as an alternative dietary protein in tilapia diets due to its low price (compared to conventional sources) and good protein (wheat: 38.7%−45.7% and corn: 28%−33%) and amino acid contents (Coyle et al., 2004; Lim et al., 2007, 2011a; Schaeffer et al., 2009). Therefore, DDGS can replace FM in tilapia diets at different levels, depending on diets composition, DDGS source, fish species and size and culture conditions. Coyle et al. (2004) reported that an FM-free diet containing 30% DDGS, 26% MBM and BM and 16% SBM provided good growth in hybrid tilapia (*O. niloticus* × *O. aureus*). Lim et al. (2007) found also that corn DDGS supplemented with exogenous lysine can be included in juvenile Nile tilapia diet at 40% level, without affecting their growth performance and body composition. Similarly, Chatvijitkul et al. (2016) found that up to 30% lipid-extracted distillers dried grains with solubles (LE-DDGS) could be used as a substitute for SBM in practical diets for hybrid tilapia (*O. niloticus* × *O. aureus*) without reducing fish growth. With lysine and lipid supplementation, as much as 50% LE-DDGS can be successfully included in hybrid tilapia diets.

As mentioned earlier, most of the mentioned plant sources may contain high levels of phytic acid, which binds with divalent minerals such as Ca, P, Zn, Mn, Mg, and Fe to form water-insoluble salts, which reduce the bioavailability of these minerals. When these plants are used as a primary source of protein in a tilapia feed, higher supplementary mineral levels may be required, particularly if the culture water is deficient in one or more of the required minerals.

7.4.3 Single-cell proteins

SCPs are a group of microorganisms including unicellular algae, fungi, bacteria, cyanobacteria and yeast. The use of SCP for tilapia in semi-intensive and intensive farming systems has attracted attention in recent years. SCP production is a simple, cheap and effective way of producing natural fish food. For example, if a carbon source (such as wheat bran, rice bran and cellulose) is sprayed on the surface of pond water with continuous aeration, at the optimum carbon:nitrogen ratio (15:1), bacterial growth will increase (Chamberlain and Hopkins, 1994). The bacteria consume the carbon source as energy and reduce ammonia concentration through nitrification, while the fish feed on the bacteria (see Fig. 6.2, Chapter 6). In such cases, cheap carbon and nitrogen sources can partially replace expensive commercial protein sources in tilapia feeds. More attention should be given to the production of SCP in fish ponds in developing countries where tilapia culture is widely practiced.

Biofloc technology can be an excellent source of SCP for semi-intensive and intensive tilapia farming. Biofloc is 'aggregates of bacteria, algae, or protozoa, held together in a matrix along with particulate organic matter'. These microorganisms are an ideal SCP source for farmed tilapia, especially in intensive tank systems. The use of biofloc technology in tilapia culture is covered in details in Chapter 6.

7.5 Economic evaluation of protein sources

Most of the protein sources used in tilapia feeds have been evaluated from biological and nutritional points of view. Economic evaluation of such feed inputs for tilapia has not been given enough attention. Only a few studies have demonstrated that despite the fact that many of these feed inputs produced lower biological performance than standard proteins (mainly FM), cost–benefit analyses indicated that they were economically better. For example, economic evaluation of CSM (El-Sayed, 1990), corn gluten feed and meal (Wu et al., 1995), and animal by-product meal (Rodriguez-Serna et al., 1996; El-Sayed, 1998) as protein sources for Nile tilapia; brewery waste (Oduro-Boateng and Bart-Plange, 1988) for *Tilapia busumana* and cocoa cake (Fagbenro, 1988) for *Tilapia guineensis* indicated that profit indices of these protein sources were better than for FM-based feeds. The authors suggested the use of these sources as total FM replacers for tilapia. As mentioned above, El-Sayed et al. (2016) evaluated GM as a protein source for Nile tilapia. Growth performance and feed efficiency were significantly reduced with increasing dietary GM up to 20% level. However, economic analysis indicated that GM was economically superior to SBM, even at 100% substitution. However, more work is needed to economically evaluate the other unconventional protein sources that are commonly used in tilapia feeds.

7.6 Measurement of dietary energy

Dietary energy content is generally expressed in three different ways: gross (total) energy (GE), digestible energy (DE) and metabolic energy (ME). Theoretically, ME is preferred to GE and DE, since it accounts for energy loss from protein metabolism, and in turn, provides a more precise estimate of the energy used for growth. But the determination of ME is difficult because of the problems associated with collecting fish metabolites. It is also suspected that ME offers little advantage over DE since energy losses via gills and urine are small. Therefore, it may be more appropriate to use DE as a measurement of dietary energy because it can be easily determined. The digestibility coefficients of a number of ingredients commonly used in tilapia feeds have been determined (Table 7.4). It is more appropriate to use the values reported for tilapia than ME or DE values reported for other fish species. If DE is not available, GE is likely to be the only useful alternative.

Another major problem associated with the determination of dietary energy requirements of tilapia is the interchangeable and inconsistent use of terminology. Many authors have used ME and DE values interchangeably and used varying energy values for the same ingredient under the same terminology. In addition, energy values reported for other fish species have been widely used in the preparation of tilapia diets (see El-Sayed and Teshima, 1991 for details).

7.7 Dietary lipid requirements

Tilapia, like other vertebrates, require dietary lipids for the following physiological functions:

1. A source of EFAs supply.
2. Energy production and protein sparing.

TABLE 7.4 Protein and (organic matter) digestibility (%) by tilapia of some feed ingredients commonly used in feed manufacturing.

Ingredient	1a (*O. n*)	2a (*O. a* × *O. n*)	3a (*O. n*)	4b (*O. n*)	5a (*O. n*)	6a (*O. n*)	7c (*O. n*)	8c (*O. n* × *O. a*)
Animal sources								
Fish meal	92.2		72 (58)	92	94			90.2 (89.2)
Sardine						87 (80)		
Tuna						82		
Anchovy						94	90.(86)	
Meat and bone meal	92.2							
Poultry offal meal				74 (59)		74 (59)		87.2 (79.2)
Shrimp meal		74		87				
Silkworm pupa meal	91.1							
Plant sources								
Azolla				75				
Brewers grains		63	62 (42)			63 (30)		
Cooked cassava meal						74		
Casein				97				
Copra meal				56	81	81		
Corn grains (raw)						83 (76)		75.1 (61.4)
Corn grains (cooked)						90		
Corn gluten meal	90.7			97				96.5 (83.4)
Cottonseed meal		90	31 (−24)			90		
Cottonseed cake					90			
Groundnut meal			79 (72)					
Palm kernel meal			−26 (−89)					
Rapeseed meal								85 (57.3)
Soybean meal	90.9	91		93	93	91 (57)	93	96.2 (84.5)
Sunflower seed meal								99.2 (65.5)
Sunflower seed cake							86–89 (42)	
Wheat germ meal	95.5							
Wheat middlings						76 (58)		
Wheat bran							75 (30)	83.6 (38.8)

1: Watanabe et al. (1996), 2: Degani et al. (1997), 3: Luquet (1989), 4: Lorico-Querijero and Chiu (1989), 5: Moreau (1996), 6: Hanley (2000), 7: Maina et al. (2002), 8: Sklan et al. (2004). a = % protein and (organic matter) digestibility; b = true digestibility; c = apparent digestibility.
O. a, Oreochromis aureus; O. n, Oreochromis niloticus.

TABLE 7.5 Lipid requirements of tilapia.

Tilapia species (and size in g)	Levels tested (% of diet)	Requirements (% of diet)	References
Tilapia zillii (1.85)	1.7–15	15.0	El-Sayed and Garling (1988)
Oreochromis niloticus (0.9–1.6)	3–19	15.0	Teshima et al. (1985b)
Oreochromis aureus	0–10	10.0	Stickney and Wurts (1986)
O. aureus × *O. niloticus*		12.0	Jauncey and Ross (1982)
Oreochromis mossambicus × *O. niloticus* (1.2)	6–24	18.0	De Silva et al. (1991)
O. niloticus × *O. aureus* (1.34)	0–20	12.0	Chou and Shiau (1996)
O. mossambicus × *O. aureus* (67)	3.72–11.45	3.6	Fitzsimmons et al. (1997)
O. niloticus (GIFT) (2.6)	1.73–16.55	9.34	Wang et al. (2011)
O. niloticus (34.5)	3–9	>3 (6–9)	Hooley et al. (2014)
Adult *O. niloticus* (GIFT) (220)	3.3–12.4	7.54	Tian et al. (2015)
O. aureus × *O. niloticus* (8)	3.9–7.7	6.0	Ma et al. (2016)
O. niloticus larvae (0.042)	1.2–18.4	8.56	Qiang et al. (2017)

3. Normal growth and development.
4. Carrying and assisting in the absorption of fat-soluble vitamins.
5. Structure and maintenance of cell membrane integrity and flexibility.
6. Precursors of steroid hormones.
7. Improving the texture and flavour of the diet and fatty acid composition of the fish.

Tilapia are known to utilize dietary lipids very efficiently. Dietary lipids may spare more protein for growth than do carbohydrates (Teshima et al., 1985b; El-Sayed and Garling, 1988). Dietary lipid requirement of tilapia is varying considerably, depending on dietary protein and energy contents, lipid source, pellets form, fish species and developmental stage and water quality. Generally speaking, early studies revealed higher lipid requirement (10%–18%) than the recent studies (6%–9%) (Table 7.5). Jauncey (2000) reported that the protein content in diets of tilapia hybrids (*O. niloticus* × *O. aureus*) could be reduced from 40% to 30% by increasing the dietary lipid level to 12%, with a decrease of P:E ratio from 100.0 to 83.3 mg protein $kcal^{-1}$ DE, but beyond 12% level growth rates decreased. Similar dietary lipid level was also reported on the same hybrid (Chou and Shiau, 1996). De Silva et al. (1991) reported that tilapia hybrids (*O. mossambicus* × *O. niloticus*) require 18% dietary lipid for optimum performance. Fingerling *T. zillii* also required 15% dietary lipids for maximal growth and feed utilization.

On the other hand, much lower lipid levels (6%–9%) were suggested by many, more recent, studies (Lim et al., 2009; Hooley et al., 2014; Tian et al., 2015; Ma et al., 2016; Qiang et al., 2017). These values are close to the lipid levels which are currently used in commercial tilapia feeds worldwide. Increasing dietary lipid beyond these levels may increase tissue and whole-body lipid levels (Tian et al., 2015). This may also increase feed prices due to the continuous increase in the prices of fish oil (FO) and plant oils.

When Nile tilapia larvae (0.042 g) were fed diets containing varying lipid levels, the best growth and feed efficiency were obtained at 8.56% level (Qiang et al., 2017). Even at 3.6% dietary lipid the growth of *O. mossambicus* × *O. aureus* hybrids was similar to fish fed 6% or 8% lipid, as long as dietary energy value was balanced with suitable carbohydrates (Fitzsimmons et al., 1997). Ma et al. (2016) studied the effects of extruded and pelleted diets with differing lipid levels (3.9%–7.7%) on growth rates, nutrient retention and serum biochemical indices of tilapia hybrid (*O. aureus* × *O. niloticus*). They found that extruded diets were better utilized than pelleted diets. The optimum dietary lipid level for best performance was 6.0% in both the pelleted and extruded diets.

7.7.1 Lipid sources

Plant oils, including oilseed plant oils (soybean oil (SBO), sunflower oil, cottonseed oil, linseed oil, sesame oil, etc.)

and vegetable oils (VOs) have been widely used as dietary lipid sources for farmed tilapia. Animal fats such as beef tallow, lard oil and animal by-product fat have also been tested and showed controversial results. Yildirim-Aksoy et al. (2007) found also that the performance of Nile tilapia fingerlings fed semi-purified diets supplemented with 7% of corn oil (CO), menhaden FO or linseed oil (LSO) was similar. Fish fed beef tallow (BT) showed much lower growth rates and nutrient utilization. A combination of FO + CO + BT or LSO + CO + BT produced superior growth to other groups.

Ng and Wang (2011) evaluated the effects of dietary lipid source on the reproductive performance of Nile tilapia broodfish. The fish were fed isonitrogenous (35% protein) and isolipidic (10%) with added FO, FO and crude palm oil (CPO) (FO + CPO; 1:1), CPO or linseed oil (LSO) as lipid sources. The best reproductive performance (time at first spawning number of eggs per fish, inter-spawning intervals, spawning frequency and egg hatchability) was obtained in fish fed the CPO-containing diets. The authors concluded that CPO can be used as a cost-effective lipid source in broodstock diets to increase tilapia fry production. Alongside the same line, Ng et al. (2013) assessed the effects of VOs on the growth, tissue fatty acid composition and oxidative stability of red hybrid tilapia. The fish were fed diets containing FO, FO + CPO; 1:1, LSO + CPO; 1:1, CPO or SBO. Growth rates and feed efficiency were not significantly different among diets. Moreover, SBO and CPO diets enhanced the resistance of tilapia tissues to lipid peroxidation; but they led to a significant reduction in EPA, DHA and n-3/n-6 ratios in the fillets. However, the authors suggested using an FO-based finishing diet for improving DHA, EPA and n-3/n-6 ratio in fish flesh.

VO, including canola oil (rich in monoenes), perilla oil (rich in n-3 polyunsaturated fatty acids, PUFA), sunflower oil (rich in n-6 PUFA) and refined, bleached, deodorized palmolein (rich in saturates) were evaluated by Teoh and Ng (2016) as a total replacement of FO in the diets of tilapia hybrid (*Oreochromis* sp.) (8.9 g). With the exception of sunflower oil, total FO replacement by other VOs did not significantly reduce fish growth performance. However, dietary VO significantly affected the fatty acid composition of tilapia fillet and whole body. Tilapia fed the VO diets which do not contain long-chain polyunsaturated fatty acids (PUFA) longer than C18 recorded high amounts of n-6 and n-3 LC-PUFA in their body lipids. This result suggests that VO-based diets can trigger $\Delta5$ and $\Delta6$ fatty acid desaturase activities. Similar results were reported on Nile tilapia fingerlings (9 g) fed diets containing SBO, rapeseed oil (RSO), linseed oil (LSO) and pork lard (PL) as a total replacement of FO (Peng et al., 2016). The replacement of FO with RSO, LSO or PL did not affect growth or feed utilization; only SBO exhibited lower specific growth rate and feed utilization efficiency. FO, LSO and RSO resulted in the lowest hepatosomatic index (HSI), hepatopancreas lipid content, hepatopancreas malondialdehyde contents, lipoprotein lipase and malate dehydrogenase activities in fish liver. Fish fed FO or LSO showed higher aspartate transaminase and alanine transaminase activities in liver and higher total antioxidant capacity, superoxide dismutase and alkaline phosphatase (ALP) activities in serum; however, the values of these parameters were lower in fish fed PL compared to other groups. This study showed that alternative lipid sources (except SBO), especially linseed oil, could be used successfully in tilapia diets.

7.7.2 Essential fatty acid requirements

It is known that coldwater fishes and marine fishes require n-3 polyunsaturated fatty acids (n-3 PUFA), while freshwater fishes inhabiting warmwater environments tend to require n-6 PUFA. This may suggest that tilapia would utilize plant oils (rich in n-6 fatty acids) more efficiently than FOs (rich in n-3 fatty acids). However, information on fatty acid requirements of tilapia has been contradictory. Several studies indicated that tilapia require n-6 EFA rather than n-3 EFA (Stickney et al., 1982; Stickney and McGeachin, 1983). The growth of Nile tilapia fed on a fish oil-containing diet (rich in n-3 EFA) was significantly reduced as compared with one containing SBO or corn oil (rich in n-6 EFA) (Takeuchi et al., 1983). Similar results were reported on Nile tilapia broodstock, where fish fed with fish oil-containing diets had significantly poor reproductive performance compared to those fed SBO diets (Santiago and Reyes, 1993). Li et al. (2013) found also that despite both linoleic acid (LA; 18:2n-6) and linolenic acid (LNA; 18:3n-3) are dietary essential for growth of hybrid tilapia (*O. niloticus* × *O. aureus*), dietary LA alone, at a level of 1.14%, can meet the EFA requirement of juvenile fish.

On the other hand, many other studies indicated that tilapia may require both n-3 EFA and n-6 EFA. Stickney and McGeachin (1983) found that 10% SBO or 10% FO produced similar growth of blue tilapia. Furthermore, Chou and Shiau (1999) found that both n-3 and n-6 highly unsaturated fatty acids (HUFA) are required for maximum performance of tilapia hybrids (*O. niloticus* × *O. aureus*). El-Sayed et al. (2005) found that Nile tilapia broodstock reared in brackish water required n-3 HUFA for optimum spawning performance, while the reproductive performance of fish reared in freshwater was not affected by dietary lipid source. Chen et al. (2013) quantified the optimum requirement of dietary LNA for Nile tilapia fingerlings (2.1 g). The fish were fed diets containing similar lipid level but varying in LNA content (0.0%–2.04%). The results showed that the optimum requirement of dietary LNA for juvenile tilapia is 0.45%–0.64%. Increasing dietary LNA levels resulted in increased LNA and 22:6n-3 contents, but decreased 20:4n-6 and 20:5n-3 levels in fish tissues. These findings are in agreement with the results of Chou and Shiau (1999) and Chou et al. (2001) who suggested that hybrid tilapia may require both n-6 and n-3 FAs in their diets. It is evident that the requirements of tilapias for EFA are species specific, and more work is needed to quantify the EFA requirements of different tilapias under different culture systems and different water environments. The prices, availability and affordability of oil sources should also be considered when deciding which fatty acid source will be used. It might be more cost-effective to use one lipid source, which produces lower performance than using another, more growth promoting, but much more expensive source.

7.8 Carbohydrate utilization

Carbohydrates are the cheapest sources of dietary energy for humans, fish and domestic animals. Carbohydrates are also the most available food source in the world. Tilapias are mainly herbivorous and are expected to utilize dietary carbohydrates more efficiently than carnivorous fishes. Tilapia can efficiently utilize as much as 35%–40% digestible carbohydrate (Anderson et al., 1984; El-Sayed and Garling, 1988; Qiang et al., 2014). In addition, increasing dietary carbohydrate results in the sparing of dietary protein for growth. Wang et al. (2017) reported the enhancement of protein-sparing effect of starch on Nile tilapia growth when dietary protein was low. However, excessive dietary carbohydrates may lead to negative impacts on fish performance and physiological functions, presumably due to the imbalance of the ratio between protein and energy contents. Increasing dietary carbohydrate (dextrin) inclusion in the diets of adult Nile tilapia to 50% resulted in a significant retardation in fish growth and feed conversion ratio (FCR) (Boonanuntanasarn et al., 2018).

Traditionally, wheat bran, corn and rice bran have been used as the major dietary carbohydrate sources for tilapia. A number of other unconventional sources have been evaluated for different tilapia species. El-Sayed (1991) found that up to 20% sugarcane bagasse could be included in *T. zillii* diets without significant retardation in fish growth and feed digestibility. However, Nile tilapia fed sugarcane bagasse diets exhibited poor performance. Cacao husks successfully replaced wheat bran, wheat flour or rice bran in tilapia feeds at up to 20% inclusion level (Pouomogne et al., 1997). Barley seeds replaced up to 30% of dietary corn in Nile tilapia diets without adverse effects on fish performance (Belal, 1999). El-Sayed (2003) studied the use of fresh and fermented water hyacinth by Nile tilapia fingerlings as a supplement of wheat bran at 20% and 40% levels (10% and 20% of the diet). He found that at 10% level, fermented and fresh water hyacinth produced similar performance to the control diet. At the level of 20% of the diet, fermented water hyacinth was better utilized than fresh water hyacinth.

Carbohydrate utilization by tilapia is affected by a number of factors, including carbohydrate source, other dietary ingredients, fish species and size and feeding frequency. Tilapia have been reported to utilize complex sugars (starch) more efficiently than disaccharides and monosaccharides (Anderson et al., 1984; Shiau and Chen, 1993; Shiau and Lin, 1993). In support, it was found that lipogenic enzyme activities in tilapia liver were higher in fish fed starch diets than in fish fed a glucose diet (Lin and Shiau, 1995), indicating that these activities are adaptive to dietary carbohydrate source. On the contrary, a study by Qiang et al. (2014) indicated that high dietary glucose levels (40%) were utilized well as an energy source by GIFT juveniles. Liver lipogenic enzyme activities were higher in glucose-fed fish than in those fed wheat starch.

The carbohydrate-to-lipid (CHO:L) ratio is an important factor affecting the carbohydrate utilization and ligogenic enzyme activities. El-Sayed and Garling (1988) fed *T. zillii* test diets with varying CHO (12%–41%) and lipid (1.7%–14.8%) with CHO:L ranging from 0.8 to 24.1. The performances of fish fed diets with CHO:L ratios ranging from 0.8 to 8.8 were not significantly different. A diet with higher CHO:L (24.1) produced significantly lower performance, presumably due to an EFA deficiency in the diet. Similar results were found in fingerling Nile tilapia fed diets differing in carbohydrate (18%–40%) and lipid (8.1%–19.5%) with a CH:L ratio of 0.9–4.95 (Ali and Al-Asgah, 2001). The best performance was obtained at a CHO:L ratio of 3.3 (about 35% CHO and 10.6% lipids). Further increase in CHO:L ratio resulted in a significant decrease in fish growth and nutrient utilization. The HSI increased with a decrease in the CHO:L ratio and was the highest with a CHO:L ratio of 0.94 and lowest with a CHO:L ratio of 4.95.

The requirement of niacin, which is a precursor of certain coenzymes needed for carbohydrate metabolism, is affected by dietary protein source (Shiau and Suen, 1992). In addition, dietary chromium chloride or chromic oxide was found to improve glucose (but not starch) utilization by tilapia (Shiau and Lin, 1993; Shiau and Liang, 1995). The quality of dietary carbohydrates for tilapia is influenced by their fibre content. Shiau et al. (1988) found that increasing dietary carboxymethylcellulose (CMC) depressed stomach emptying, carbohydrate digestion and absorption, fish growth and feed conversion efficiency. The inclusion of 10% guar gum, carrageenan, CMC and cellulose in tilapia diets resulted in significant decrease in fish performance. Moreover, as low as 2% dietary chitin or chitosan depressed tilapia growth (Shiau and Yu, 1999).

Carbohydrate utilization by tilapia is also affected by daily feeding frequency. Tung and Shiau (1991) and

Shiau and Lei (1999) have demonstrated that increasing feeding frequency (from 2 to 6 times day^{-1}, or continuous feeding) improved carbohydrate utilization, growth rates and protein sparing. Fish size also affects carbohydrate utilization. When two sizes of tilapia (0.46 and 4.55 g) were fed glucose or starch, larger fish utilized glucose more efficiently than smaller fish, while starch was utilized equally by both sizes (Tung and Shiau, 1993).

Carbohydrates may contain amylase inhibitors, or other antinutrients that reduce their utilization by fishes. El-Sayed et al. (2000) found that wheat bran contains protease inhibitor, the activity of which may negatively affect food digestibility. Processing of dietary carbohydrates may, therefore, improve their quality for tilapia. In this regards, El-Sayed (1991) found that cooking sugarcane bagasse slightly improved its utilization by *T. zillii*. As noted above, El-Sayed (2003) found that fermented water hyacinth was better utilized than fresh water hyacinth when incorporated in Nile tilapia diets at 20% levels, while at 10% inclusion level both fermented and fresh hyacinth were utilized equally.

7.9 Vitamin requirements

Vitamins are organic compounds that are generally required in small quantities in animal diets. They act as cofactors or substrates in normal metabolic reactions. Vitamins are subdivided into water-soluble (macrovitamins, based on the levels required) and fat-soluble groups. Vitamin deficiency may result in nutrition-related diseases, poor growth or increase susceptibility to infections.

Vitamin supplementation is not necessary for tilapia in semi-intensive farming systems, while in intensive systems, supplemental dietary vitamins may be necessary. However, it is difficult to accurately determine the vitamin requirement of tilapia in intensive systems because they consume significant amounts of vitamins along with the natural food they consume from culture water. The vitamin requirements of these fishes have not been sufficiently studied. The species that has been relatively studied in detail is hybrid tilapia (*O. niloticus* × *O. aureus*), while limited information is available on vitamin requirements of other tilapia species. However, a number of recent studies have tackled the vitamin requirements of Nile tilapia.

The requirements of tilapia for fat-soluble vitamins have not been well investigated, except vitamin A. A number of studies have recently been carried out on the effects of vitamin A supplementation on growth rates, feed efficiency, haematology and immune response of Nile tilapia. Guimarães et al. (2014) found that vitamin A is essential for Nile tilapia. Fingerling Nile tilapia were fed diets supplemented with different levels of vitamin A (0, 2500, 5000, 10,000 and 20,000 IU kg^{-1} diet). Fish fed a vitamin A-free diet suffered from lower growth, poor feed efficiency ratio, haemorrhages, operculum deformity, fin erosion, darker body colouration, lethargy and lower haematological parameters compared to vitamin A-fed groups. Vitamin A supplementation at 3910 IU kg^{-1} was sufficient to prevent these deficiency signs. In addition, supplemental vitamin A enhanced serum protein, lysozyme activity and superoxide anion production. Nonetheless, serum total immunoglobulin and spontaneous complement activity and resistance of Nile tilapia to *Streptococcus iniae* infection challenge were not affected by dietary vitamin A. Growth retardation and clinical problems were also recorded in Nile tilapia fed vitamin A-free diet; and 5400 IU of retinol kg^{-1} diet was recommended to alleviate these symptoms and sustain normal growth (Campeche et al., 2009). Similar results were also reported by Guimarães et al. (2016) where 1.2 mg retinol kg^{-1} diet was required to prevent deficiency signs and promote proper growth and health status of these fish.

Vitamin E (DL-α-tocopheryl acetate) was also found essential for normal performance of tilapia. When GIFT tilapia were fed test diets supplemented with 0, 40, 200 and 1000 mg kg^{-1} vitamin E, fish fed the vitamin E-free diet showed significantly lower growth, feed efficiency and survival rate than those fed vitamin E-supplemented diets (Wu et al., 2017). Fish fed vitamin E-free diet also had significantly poorer cohesiveness, resilience and chewiness than other groups. At least 40 mg vitamin E kg^{-1} diet was suggested to improve growth performance, fillet quality and antioxidant capacity, whereas about 573.8–582.3 and 655–752.5 mg kg^{-1} were required for optimum fillet texture and serum antioxidant capacity. Similar results were reported in hybrid tilapia, *O. niloticus* × *O. aureus* (Huang et al., 2003).

Since vitamins C and E are antioxidants, they are among the most important nutrients that influence the immune system. They provide cellular defence against reactive oxygen species which damage biological membranes. The interactive effects of vitamins C and E on growth, immunity and resistance of Nile tilapia to *S. iniae* challenge were evaluated (Lim et al., 2010). The fish were fed diets supplemented with vitamin C (0, 100 and 2000 mg kg^{-1}) and E (0, 50 and 500 mg kg^{-1}). About 23 mg kg^{-1} vitamin E (found in the basal diet) was sufficient for promoting growth and feed efficiency, but 50 mg kg^{-1} was required to enhance fish survival. Vitamin E concentrations in the diets did not affect vitamin C concentration in the liver, but increasing dietary vitamin C increased liver vitamin E. Vitamin C-free diet significantly lowered red blood cells (RBCs) and haemoglobin and increased corpuscular volume. Total immunoglobulin was higher, while lysozyme activity was lower, in fish fed 2000 mg kg^{-1} vitamin C diets. Vitamin E at 500 mg kg^{-1} diet significantly decreased alternative complement activity. On the other hand, vitamin C did not affect fish mortality following *S. iniae* challenge, while supplemental vitamin E significantly improved fish survival.

Few studies were also carried out on the effects of vitamin C (ascorbic acid or its salts) on growth, feed efficiency of young and adult Nile tilapia and on their reproductive performance. The results indicated that dietary vitamin C requirement of tilapia varies considerably, depending on the forms of vitamin C used, other dietary components, fish species, strains and size and culture conditions (see Table 7.6). Huang et al. (2016) fed GIFT Nile tilapia (70 g) with diets containing 23.8–339.0 mg kg^{-1} vitamin C (L-ascorbyl-2-polyphosphate). They found that increasing dietary vitamin C level up to 41.9 mg kg^{-1} increased growth rate of tilapia, beyond which no further improvement occurred in fish growth. Dietary vitamin C also had significant effects on enzyme activities of serum ALP, aspartate aminotransferase and alanine aminotransferase, and also on serum albumin and total protein content. The authors concluded that vitamin C requirement for optimum growth of GIFT tilapia is 45.0 mg kg^{-1} diet. In another study, vitamin C requirement of adult (220 g) GIFT tilapia was investigated in cages (Wu et al., 2015). The fish were fed semi-purified diets containing 10.22 (control) to 382.54 mg kg^{-1} vitamin C. The results revealed that vitamin C requirement of adult GIFT was 53.05, 180.53 and 185.86 mg kg^{-1}, based on weight gain, hepatic and muscle vitamin C contents, respectively.

The reproductive efficiency and egg and larvae quality of Nile tilapia broodstock (70 g for female and 153 g for male) fed different levels of vitamin C (ascorbyl monophosphate) (0.0–942 mg kg^{-1} diet) were also investigated by Sarmento et al. (2018). The results indicated that broodfish require much higher vitamin C than other growth stages. The highest gonadosomatic index, total and relative fecundity and larval measurements were found at 599 mg vitamin C kg^{-1} diet. Hatching rate and egg and larvae production per female were directly related to vitamin C levels. Haematocrit, erythrocytes, leukocytes, total plasma protein values and larval survival were lowest in females fed a vitamin C-free diet and improved with vitamin C supplementation. The resistance to air exposure by newly hatched larvae was greatest for those individuals from females receiving the 942 mg vitamin C kg^{-1} diet, intermediate with the 599 mg and lowest with the 0 mg vitamin C kg^{-1} diet. The authors concluded that dietary supplementation of 599 vitamin C kg^{-1} is required for optimizing reproductive parameters, blood variables and eggs and larval quality of Nile tilapia.

Few other studies assessed the requirement of Nile tilapia for thiamin (vitamin B_1), niacin (vitamin B_3) and pyridoxine (vitamin B_6). Lim et al. (2011b) found that 3.5 mg kg^{-1} dietary thiamin is required for optimum growth, feed efficiency, survival, prevention of neurological symptoms, and maintaining normal levels of RBC count, haematocrit (Ht), serum pyruvate, and proximate body composition of Nile tilapia. Higher niacin levels were required by GIFT tilapia (87 g), where a minimum of 20.4 mg kg^{-1} dietary niacin was required for maximal growth, and 84.6 mg kg^{-1} for the highest liver niacin level (Jiang et al., 2014). The effect of dietary pyridoxine supplementation on the growth performance of fingerling Nile tilapia (8.4 g) and the haematological response under heat stress was assessed (Teixeira et al., 2012). When the fish were fed a pyridoxine-free diet, they showed the lowest weight gain and protein retention. They required 10 mg pyridoxine (pyridoxal HCl) kg^{-1} diet for the normal growth, health maintenance and reduction of heat stress.

The following can be observed from Table 7.6:

- Niacin requirement is affected by dietary carbohydrates. Tilapia fed simple sugars (glucose) required lower niacin levels than fish fed polysaccharides (dextrin).
- Because ascorbic acid is unstable, and loses its activity during processing and storage, more stable forms of ascorbic acids should be used. L-ascorbyl-2-sulphate (C2S), L-ascorbyl-2-monophosphate-magnesium (C2MP-Mg) and L-ascorbyl-2-monophosphate-sodium (C2MP-Na) could be used.
- Vitamin E requirement increases with increasing dietary lipid level.
- The requirement of vitamin K for tilapia has not been determined.

It has been reported that tilapia may not require certain vitamins, since the fish are able to synthesize them. Lovell and Limsuwan (1982) and Sugita et al. (1990) found that dietary supplementation of vitamin B_{12} is not required by tilapia. They suggested that these fishes can synthesize that vitamin in their digestive tracts by intestinal microorganisms. However, further studies are needed to verify these suggestions.

7.10 Mineral requirements

Minerals are inorganic elements that are required by animals to maintain many of their metabolic functions. These functions can be summarized as follows (Jauncey, 1998):

- Structure of hard skeletons such as bones and teeth.
- Osmoregulation.
- Structure of soft tissues.
- Nerve impulse and transmission and muscle contraction.
- Body acid-base equilibrium and regulation of the pH of the blood and other fluids.
- Cofactors in metabolism, catalysts and enzyme activators.
- Minerals serve as components of many enzymes, vitamins, hormones and respiratory pigments.

Little information is available on the mineral requirements of tilapia, and therefore, their response to

TABLE 7.6 Vitamin requirements and deficiency symptoms of tilapia.

Vitamin	Fish species	Requirement (mg kg^{-1})	Deficiency symptoms	References
Niacin (B_3)	*O. n* (GIFT)	20.4		Jiang et al. (2014)
	O. n × *O. a*	26 (fed glucose)	Haemorrhage, deformed snout, gill and skin oedema, fin and mouth lesion	Shiau and Suen (1992)
		121 (fed dextrin)		
Biotin (B_7)	*O. n* × *O. a*	0.06		Shiau and Chin (1999)
Choline	*O. n* × *O. a*	1000		Shiau and Lo (2000)
Pantothenic acid (B_5)	*O. a*	10	Low growth, haemorrhage, anaemia, sluggishness, high mortality, hyperplasia of epithelial cells of gill lamellae	Soliman and Wilson (1992a)
Thiamin (B_1)	*O. m* × *O. n*	2.5 (seawater, 32‰)	Low growth and feed efficiency, low haematocrit	Lim and Leamaster (1991)
	O. n	3.5	Neurological disorders, anorexia, reduced growth and feed efficiency, low RBC count and haematocrit and increased mortality	Lim et al. (2011b)
Riboflavin (B_2)	*O. a*	6	Anorexia, low growth, high mortality, fin erosion, loss of body colour, cataract, dwarfism	Soliman and Wilson (1992b)
	O. m × *O. n*	5 (seawater, 32‰)		Lim et al. (1993)
Pyridoxine (B_6)	*O. n* × *O. a*	1.7–9.5 (28% cp)	Low growth, high mortality, abnormal neurological signs, anorexia, convulsions, caudal fin erosion, mouth lesion	Shiau and Hsieh (1997)
		15–16.5 (36% cp)		
	O. n	10		Teixeira et al. (2012)
Vitamin C	*O. n*	599 (C2MP) (for optimum reproductive performance)		Sarmento et al. (2018)
	O. n (GIFT) adult	• 53.05 (C2S) (for optimum growth) • 186 (C2S) (for optimum hepatic Vitamin C content) • 180.53 (C2S) (for optimum muscle Vitamin C content)		Wu et al. (2015)
	O. n (GIFT)	• 45 (C2S) (for optimum growth) • 115 (C2S) (for optimum hepatic Vitamin C content) • 119 (C2S) (for optimum muscle Vitamin C content)		Huang et al. (2016)
	O. n	420 (ascorbic acid)		Soliman et al. (1994)
	O. a	50 (ascorbic acid)		Stickney et al. (1984)
	O. n × *O. a*	79 (ascorbic acid)		Shiau and Jan (1992)

Continued

TABLE 7.6 Vitamin requirements and deficiency symptoms of tilapia.—cont'd

Vitamin	Fish species	Requirement (mg kg^{-1})	Deficiency symptoms	References
	O. n × *O. a*	41–48 (C2S)		Shiau and Hsu (1995)
	O. n × *O. a*	37–42 (C2MP-Mg)		Shiau and Hsu (1995)
	O. n × *O. a*	63.4 (C2MP-Na)		Shiau and Hsu (1995)
	O. s	11–200 (C2S)		Al-Amoudi et al. (1992)
D	*O. n* × *O. a*	374.8 IU		Shiau and Hwang (1993)
E	*O. a*	10 (at 3% lipid)	Low growth and FCR, skin haemorrhage, muscle dystrophy, impaired erythropoiesis, ceroid in liver and spleen, abnormal skin colouration	Roem et al. (1990)
		25 (at 6% lipid)		
	O. n	50–100 (5% lipid)		Satoh et al. (1987)
		500 (10%–15% lipid)		
	O. n	40 (for growth); 573.8–582.3 (for fillet texture)		Wu et al. (2017)
	O. n × *O. a*	42–44 (5% lipid)		Shiau and Shiau (2001)
		60–66 (12% lipid)		
A	*O. n*	5000 IU	Low growth, restless, abnormal movement, blindness, exophthalmia, haemorrhage, pot belly syndrome, reduced mucus secretion, high mortality	Saleh et al. (1995)
	O. n	3505–3545 IU	Low growth, haemorrhages around the snout areas, decrease of appetite	Guimarães et al. (2014)
	O. n	1.2	Resting and abnormal swimming, exophthalmia, haemorrhages on skin and at the base of fins, serous fluids in abdominal cavity, neutropenia, reduction in RBC count and haematocrit and haemoglobin levels and high mortality	Guimarães et al. (2016)
Inositol	*O. n* × *O. a*	400		Shiau and Su (2005)

O. a., *Oreochromis aureus*; *O. m*, *Oreochromis mossambicus*; *O. n*, *Oreochromis niloticus*; *O. s*, *Oreochromis spilurus*.
C2MP-Mg, L-Ascorbyl-2-monophosphate-magnesium; *C2MP-Na*, L-Ascorbyl-2-monophosphate-sodium; *C2S*, L-Ascorbyl-2-sulphate.

TABLE 7.7 Mineral requirements of tilapia.

Mineral	Species	Requirement (mg kg^{-1})	References
Calcium	*Oreochromis aureus*	7000	Robinson et al. (1987)
	Oreochromis niloticus	3500	Shiau and Tseng (2007)
Phosphorus	*O. niloticus*	<9000	Watanabe et al. (1980)
	O. niloticus	4600	Haylor et al. (1988)
	O. niloticus	6120–8910	Schamber et al. (2014)
	O. niloticus (GIFT)	8600	Yao et al. (2014)
	O. niloticus × *O. aureus*	7000	Viola et al. (1986)
	O. niloticus × *O. aureus*	9500–10,000	Zhang et al. (2015)
	O. aureus	5000	Robinson et al. (1987)
Potassium	*O. niloticus* × *O. aureus*	2100–3300	Shiau and Hsieh (2001)
Magnesium	*O. aureus*	500	Reigh et al. (1991)
	O. niloticus	600–800	Dabrowska et al. (1989)
	O. niloticus	200.0 (in FW); 25.0 (in SW)	Lin et al. (2013)
Zinc	*O. niloticus*	30.0	Eid and Ghonim (1994)
	O. niloticus	79.0	do Carmo e Sá et al. (2004)
	O. aureus	20.0	McClain and Gatlin (1988)
	O. niloticus × *O. aureus*	105.0–115.0[a]	Li and Huang (2016)
	O. niloticus	37.2 and 52.1[b]	Huang et al. (2015)
Manganese	*O. niloticus*	12.0	Watanabe et al. (1988)
	O. niloticus × *O. aureus*	7.0	Lin et al. (2008)
Iron	*O. niloticus*	60.0	Kleemann et al. (2003)
Chromium	*O. niloticus* × *O. aureus*	139.6	Shiau and Shy (1998)
Copper	*O. niloticus* × *O. aureus*	4.0	Shiaut and Ning (2003)
	O. niloticus	6.0	Damasceno et al. (2016)
	O. niloticus	17.0	Tang et al. (2017)
Selenium	*O. niloticus*	>1.0–<2.0 (Se-Met)	Lee et al. (2016)

[a]*Fish were fed on a soybean meal-based diet containing 15.5 g kg^{-1} phytic acid.*
[b]*37.2 based on weight gain and 52.1 based on bone Zn content.*

dietary minerals is not fully understood. The requirements of tilapia for 10 minerals, namely, calcium, phosphorus, magnesium, zinc, manganese, potassium, iron, copper, selenium and chromium, have been studied (Table 7.7). Nonetheless, phosphorus (P) and zinc (Zn) have received much more attention than other minerals. The mineral requirements of tilapia depend on fish species and size, mineral source and mineral contents of both culture water and fish feed.

Extensive research has been conducted on phosphorus requirements of different tilapias. The availability of dietary phosphorus to tilapia depends on phosphorus source (monobasic vs. dibasic form) and fish species and size. Available phosphorus (AP) provides more reliable value of the P requirement than total phosphorus (TP) (Antony Jesu Prabhu et al., 2013) because about 67% of the TP in plant feedstuffs is present as phytate-P, which is not available to fish (Sugiura et al., 2004). It was found that P in FM was more available than that in plant sources such as soybean, sorghum and wheat. The P availability in plant-based diets can be significantly increased following pretreatment with microbial phytase (Cao et al., 2008). These authors fed Nile tilapia with plant protein diets pretreated with phytase (1000 U kg^{-1}) and supplemented with graded levels of mono calcium phosphate at 0%–2.5% of the diet. Diets pretreated with phytase provided better growth and feed efficiency than nontreated groups. Apparent digestibility coefficient of P was also significantly improved by phytase pretreatment. Supplemental P was reduced by 50% when the diets were pretreated with phytase, without adversely affecting fish performance.

Viola et al. (1986) found that about 0.7% dietary phosphorus was sufficient for optimum growth of large male tilapia hybrids, while small fish required about 1% phosphorus. The best growth and bone mineralization of *O. aureus* fed casein-based diets was obtained at 0.7% dietary calcium and 0.5% phosphorus (Robinson et al., 1987). Schamber et al. (2014) found that large Nile tilapia (145 g) require at least 6100 mg kg^{-1} dietary AP for optimal growth performance, body composition and bone mineralization. The minimum dietary requirement of AP for maintaining optimal growth of smaller GIFT tilapia (46 g) reared in freshwater was 8600 mg kg^{-1} (Yao et al., 2014).

Significant attention has also been given to zinc (Zn) requirement of tilapia. The requirement may depend on tilapia species and size, Zn source and basal diets composition. Early studies showed that the Zn requirement for maximum growth of *O. aureus* was 20 mg kg^{-1} (McClain and Gatlin, 1988), whereas *O. niloticus* require 30 mg kg^{-1} (Eid and Ghonim, 1994). Huang et al. (2015) found also that the dietary Zn requirement for optimal growth of adult Nile tilapia (167 g) was 37.2 mg kg^{-1}, while maximum bone Zn content was obtained at 52.1 mg Zn kg^{-1} diet.

On the other hand, higher Zn requirement values were reported by a number of authors. do Carmo e Sá et al. (2004) found that Nile tilapia juveniles (13.3 g) fed plant-based diets containing different levels of $ZnSO_4$-H_2O (0–400 mg kg^{-1}) require 44.50 mg kg^{-1} Zn for optimum weight gain and 79.51 mg kg^{-1} for best body Zn concentration. The authors concluded that the optimum supplemental zinc in vegetable-based diets to juvenile Nile tilapia is 79.51 mg kg^{-1} diet. Much higher Zn requirement for Nile tilapia was reported by Li and Huang (2016) who evaluated the effect of dietary Zn levels (31–227 mg kg^{-1}) on growth, enzyme activity and body trace elements of hybrid tilapia (*O. niloticus* × *O. aureus*) fingerlings (2.9 g). They found that dietary Zn requirement of fish fed on a SBM-based diet containing 15.5 mg kg^{-1} phytic acid is 105–115 mg kg^{-1}, which is about 100 mg kg^{-1} higher than the reported requirement for these fish when fed on a phytate-free diet.

Zinc source may also affect tilapia growth and nutrient utilization. In this regard, Zhao et al. (2011) compared the effects of varying levels (0–60 mg kg^{-1} diet) of zinc sulphate ($ZnSO_4$) or zinc methionine (ZnMet) at two carbohydrate levels (35 or 40%) on growth and carbohydrate utilization of hybrid tilapia (*O. niloticus* × *O. aureus*) (3 g). Fish fed with a diet supplemented with 60 mg Zn from either $ZnSO_4$ or ZnMet had better growth rate and protein efficiency ratio than those fed with lower Zn levels. The enzymes involved in carbohydrate metabolism were also significantly affected by Zn levels and sources. The glucose 6-phosphate dehydrogenase (G6P-DH) in fish fed with the 20 mg ZnMet kg^{-1} diet and the pyruvate kinase (PK) levels in fish fed with 20 mg kg^{-1} $ZnSO_4$ and 30 mg kg^{-1} ZnMet diet were higher than those in fish fed with the 40% carbohydrate diet. This result suggests that supplemental dietary zinc from both ZnMet and $ZnSO_4$ significantly affects the growth performance and carbohydrate utilization of hybrid tilapia.

The requirement of tilapia for other minerals was not well investigated. Only a few studies were carried out on the effects of potassium, manganese, magnesium, selenium and copper on growth, feed utilization and physiological functions of tilapia. Potassium requirement of tilapia hybrids (*O. niloticus* × *O. aureus)* is 0.02–0.03 g kg^{-1} (Shiau and Hsieh, 2001). Watanabe et al. (1988) recommended 3–4 mg kg^{-1} copper for Nile tilapia. Ishak and Dollar (1968) found that *O. mossambicus* reared in water containing 25 ppm manganese (Mn) and fed diets supplemented with 2.8 mg kg^{-1} manganese suffered from poor growth, high morality, anorexia and loss of equilibrium. Supplementing the diets with up to 35 mg kg^{-1} manganese did not improve fish performance. Adding manganese to the water helped the fish overcome some of the deficiency signs, while adding manganese to both the water and the diet resulted in the best performance. On the other hand, Watanabe et al. (1988) reported that 12 mg kg^{-1} Mn were recommended for Nile tilapia. On the other hand, Lin et al. (2008) found that growth rate, feed efficiency and survival of juvenile tilapia hybrid (*O. niloticus* × *O. aureus*) were not affected by dietary Mn. However, hepatic, bone and muscle Mn concentrations were increased with increasing Mn supplementation. Hepatic manganese superoxide dismutase (Mn SOD) activity was also higher in fish fed diets with 5.9–33.4 mg manganese kg^{-1} diet than that in fish fed the control diet. The authors suggested that 7 mg Mn kg^{-1} diet is adequate for juvenile tilapia hybrids.

From 0.59 to 0.77 g kg^{-1} magnesium (Mg) was required for optimum growth of Nile tilapia (Dabrowska et al., 1989), while 0.5 g kg^{-1} was needed for *O. aureus* (Reigh et al., 1991). Mg and protein requirements of tilapia are significantly affected by one another. Dabrowska et al. (1989) fed Nile tilapia diets containing two protein levels (24% and 44%) and 4 Mg levels (0.07. 0.68, 1.0 and 3.2 g kg^{-1}). They found that Mg-deficient or Mg-excessive diets resulted in poor growth, feed utilization efficiency, while about 0.59–0.77 g kg^{-1} Mg was adequate for optimum performance. At the low protein level, increasing Mg to 3.2 g kg^{-1} resulted in poor performance, while at the higher protein level, increasing dietary Mg had only a slight negative effect on fish growth. At the high protein level, fish fed a Mg-deficient diet absorbed Mg from culture water at a higher rate than those reared on the low-protein diet. In addition, fish fed a low protein–high Mg diet exhibited a decrease in blood haematocrit and haemoglobin contents, accompanied by sluggishness in fish movement.

Lin et al. (2013) quantified the dietary Mg requirement for hybrid tilapia (*O. niloticus* × *O. aureus*) reared in freshwater and seawater environments. A semi-purified basal diet containing 25–570 mg Mg kg^{-1} diet was fed to fingerling tilapia (0.88 g) reared either in the freshwater or seawater (32 ppt) environment. Tilapia reared in freshwater attained the highest weight gain at $\geq$150 mg kg^{-1} supplemental Mg. Plasma alkaline phosphatase (ALP) activity was highest in fish fed diets with 230 and 300 mg Mg kg^{-1}. The concentration of Mg in whole body, scale, muscle and plasma increased with increasing dietary Mg up to 230 mg kg^{-1} and levelled off with further increase in dietary Mg. In the seawater environment, growth rate, plasma ALP activity, whole body, scale, muscle and plasma Mg levels were not significantly affected by dietary Mg. This study concluded that optimum dietary Mg requirement for tilapia reared in freshwater is about 200 mg kg^{-1} diet, whereas about 25 mg Mg kg^{-1} is required for tilapia reared in seawater.

Selenium (Se) requirement of juvenile Nile tilapia (1.85 g) was assessed using selenomethionine as a source of Se at different levels (0.3–14.7 mg kg^{-1} diet) (Lee et al., 2016). The highest growth rate and feed efficiency were obtained in fish fed 2.06 mg Se kg^{-1}. The survival rate of fish fed 6.31 and 14.7 mg Se kg^{-1} was significantly lower than those of fish fed lower Se levels, whereas lysozyme activity of fish fed 0.30 mg Se kg^{-1} was significantly lower than those of fish fed other Se concentrations. Myeloperoxidase (MPO) and SOD activities increased with increasing Se levels up to 6.31 mg kg^{-1} and declined afterwards. This study indicated that the minimum Se requirement for optimum performance of Nile tilapia is 1.06 mg kg^{-1} diet. These results also suggested that optimum dietary Se requirement of juvenile Nile tilapia is >1.06 but <2.06 mg kg^{-1}, whereas between 6.31 and 14.7 mg kg^{-1} diet could induce Se toxicity.

Copper (Cu) is an important element for organism and functions as a cofactor in various redox enzymes. Cu deficiency can cause growth retardation, low feed efficiency and various diseases (Tang et al., 2017). However, high Cu levels may induce toxic effects and reduce fish performance and nutrient utilization, therefore Cu requirement should be carefully assessed. A couple of studies have considered the Cu requirement of tilapia. Tang et al. (2017) evaluated the effects of dietary Cu on growth rates, antioxidant and immune activity in fingerling hybrid tilapia (*O. niloticus* × *O. aureus*) (0.7 g) fed diets containing graded levels of Cu (1–129 mg kg^{-1}). They found that 17 mg kg^{-1} of dietary Cu improved the growth rate, survival, condition factor and feed conversion ratio. Dietary Cu also increased the activity of SOD and lysozyme and reduced the activity of glutathione (GSH), alanine aminotransferase and aspartate aminotransferase. At high dietary CU (>65 mg kg^{-1}), fish growth, feed utilization efficiency and survival were decreased. Similarly, Nile tilapia (8 g) were fed diets supplemented with Cu (0, 4.0, 6.0, 8.0, 1000 and 1500 mg kg^{-1}) (Damasceno et al., 2016). Cu supplementation at 0–8 mg kg^{-1} diet did not change growth rate and liver Cu concentrations; however, at 6 mg Cu kg^{-1} growth rate was slightly better. At 1000 and 1500 mg Cu kg^{-1}, growth performance, plasma protein, RBC, haematocrit (Htc) and haemoglobin concentration (Hb) were impaired. However, it should be mentioned that dietary Cu requirement in these studies is much higher than that previously reported by Shiaut and Ning (2003) who reported that juvenile tilapia hybrids require only 4 mg Cu kg^{-1} diet.

Iron source has a significant effect on iron requirement of tilapia. Shiau and Su (2003) found that ferric citrate ($FeC_6H_5O_7$-H_2O) was half as effective as ferrous sulphate ($FeSO_4$-$7H_2O$) in meeting the iron requirement of juvenile tilapia, *O. niloticus* × *O. aureus*. Fish fed diets supplemented with $FeC_6H_5O_7$ as a source of iron required 150–160 mg Fe kg^{-1} diet for optimum performance. When dietary $FeSO_4$ was used, the requirement was reduced by about 50% (85 mg Fe kg^{-1}).

7.11 Feeding regimes and practices

7.11.1 Feeding levels

Accurate determination of daily ration in fish farms is of prime necessity for best farm management. Overfeeding (Fig. 7.1) will result in waste of feed and money, in addition to the environmental impacts it might cause. Underfeeding, on the other hand, will lead to reduced growth performance and total harvest. Nonetheless, feeding regimes are still one of the most disputable areas in tilapia nutrition and feeding. Some researchers suggested that daily feed be provided to the fish as a percentage of fish body weight, while others recommend the ad libitum (or satiation) regimes for best growth and feed utilization. When ad libitum feeding is practiced, feed should be available all the times (e.g. through automatic or demand feeders), while in satiation regime, the fish are fed as much as they can consume. Regardless of this dispute, the feeding regime of farmed tilapia is not fully understood. Varying results have been reported regarding feeding levels, amounts and frequency of different tilapia. For example, optimum growth of Nile tilapia was obtained at a frequency of four times per day when the fish were fed ad libitum (De Silva et al., 1986). When the fish were fed a restricted ration

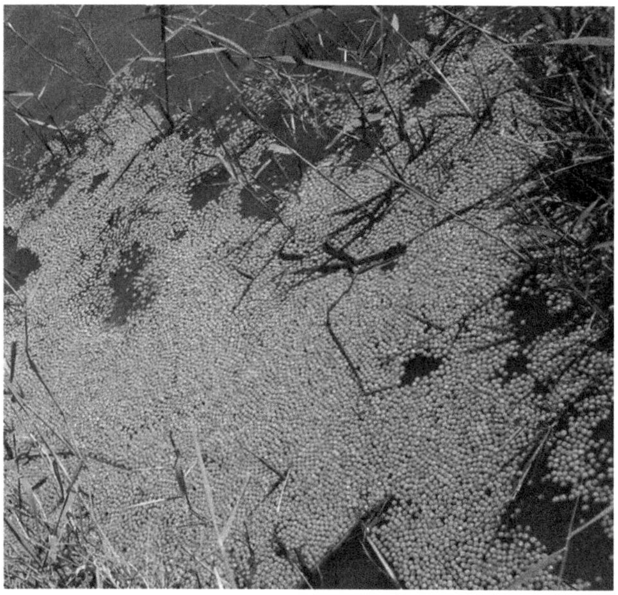

FIGURE 7.1 Overfeeding tilapia pond. Winds moved unconsumed feed to shallow, grass areas, where it could not be easily accessed by the fish, causing economic and environmental losses. *Photograph by A.-F. El-Sayed.*

of 3% of their body weight (BW) day^{-1}, the best performance was achieved at one or two feedings per day. These results suggested that restricted feeding regime was better than ad libitum which may result in feed waste. However, Nile tilapia hybrids (*Oreochromis urolepis hornorum* × *O. mossambicus*) reared in marine cages showed maximum growth at feeding rates near satiation (Clark et al., 1990). A feeding rate of 6% BW d^{-1} and a feeding frequency of two meals per day was suggested for optimum growth of GIFT during the fry phase (0.85 g) (Huang et al., 2015).

In an interesting study, Chowdhury et al. (2013) developed a bioenergetics-based factorial model to determine feed requirement and waste output of tilapia produced under commercial conditions, using data collected from 64 published studies. The authors analyzed body chemical composition, basal metabolism, energy budget and body phosphorus composition of tilapia fed different diets reported in these studies. Three realistic production scenarios were adopted. The scenario 1 depicted a commercial diet used in a validation trial, with high protein (40%, 32% and 28%) and energy (17.8, 16.7 and 16.3 MJ GE kg^{-1}) levels for nursery, pre-growout and growout stages, respectively. The diets in the other two scenarios contained progressively lower crude protein and gross energy levels than those in scenario 1 (Table 7.8). Feeding rates were estimated at these three scenarios of variable digestible protein and energy levels. Estimated feeding rates ranged from 8.4% to 11.5% for nursery fish (1 g), reduced to 0.8%–1.2% for the largest size (800 g) (see Table 7.8).

It is clear from this study that feeding rates decrease at higher dietary protein and energy levels, and increase with decreasing the concentration of these nutrients. One may ask which scenario is economically better for tilapia farmers. The answer is not that easy because other factors may also affect the feeding levels, such as diet form, pellet size, feeding frequency, fish density, water quality, etc. Therefore, the decision should be taken by the farmer himself, based on the preset objectives, targeted outputs, prevailing farming conditions and careful cost–benefit analyses of each scenario.

7.11.2 Feeding frequency

Because tilapia have small stomachs and are characterized with continuous feeding behaviour, more frequent feeding would be appropriate for them. Meanwhile, feeding levels and frequency of tilapia decrease with increasing fish size. During larval stages, the fishes require a daily ration of about 20%–30% of their body weight, divided into 6-8 feedings. Fish fingerlings require 3%–4% of body weight, dispensed three to four times daily. It has been indicated that increasing feeding levels above fish requirements may reduce feed digestibility and utilization efficiency (Meyer-Burgdorff et al., 1989).

A feeding trial was conducted to evaluate the appropriate feeding frequency for cage-cultured red tilapia (*O. mossambicus* × *O. hornorum*) in Thailand (Orachunwong et al., 2001). Fish were stocked in floating cages suspended in earthen ponds and fed a commercial tilapia feed (25% cp) ad libitum 2, 3, and 4 times daily. Feeding 3–4 times day^{-1} has resulted in better growth and FCR than twice a day. Dividing the daily ration of tilapia reared in cages into 3-4 feedings would probably reduce feed loss compared to once or twice a day. Similarly, feeding juvenile Nile tilapia (34.4 g), to apparent satiation, two to three times per day resulted in the best growth and feed efficiency (Riche et al., 2004). Thongprajukaew et al. (2017) also reported that the best performance of sex-reversed Nile tilapia (11.8 g) was obtained at two meals per day (0600 and 1800 h). However, smaller tilapia may require more frequent feeding to satisfy their nutrient requirement. For example, the optimum feeding frequency of juvenile Nile tilapia (1.0–5.8 g) was four times daily (Daudpota et al., 2016). On the contrary, a feeding frequency of 2 meals d^{-1} (6% BW d^{-1}) was suggested for optimum growth of GIFT during the fry phase (0.85 g) (Huang et al., 2015).

7.11.3 Feeding methods

Feeding methods (hand-feeding, blower feeding, automatic feeders or demand feeders) may affect tilapia performance. Hand-feeding is recommended in small-scale tilapia farms because it allows the feeder to regulate the amount of feed

TABLE 7.8 General daily feeding rates (% of body weight) based on the digestible energy requirement of tilapia reared at 27–30°C growing from 1 to 800 g for feeds in three feed composition scenarios.

		Feed requirement (% BW d^{-1})		
Production stage	**Fish mean weight (g)**	**Scenario 1 (validation trial)[a]**	**Scenario 2[b]**	**Scenario 3[c]**
Nursery	1	8.4	11.0	13.4
	10	4.0	6.1	6.3
	25	3.0	4.5	4.7
Pre-growout	50	3.6	5.5	5.7
	100	2.4	3.7	3.8
	200	1.6	2.5	2.6
Growout	300	1.5	2.3	2.4
	400	1.2	1.9	1.9
	500	1.0	1.6	1.7
	600	0.9	1.4	1.5
	700	0.8	1.3	1.3
	800	0.8	1.2	1.2
Feed conversion ratio		1.24	1.27	1.32

[a]*The diet contains 40%, 32% and 28% cp and 17.8, 16.7 and 16.3 MJ GE kg^{-1}, for nursery, pre-growout and growout stages, respectively.*
[b]*The diet contains 38%, 30% and 26% cp and 17.3, 16.3 and 15.8 MJ GE kg^{-1}, for nursery, pre-growout and growout stages, respectively.*
[c]*The diet contains 35%, 28% and 24% cp and 16.6, 15.8 and 15.3 MJ GE kg^{-1}, for nursery, pre-growout and growout stages, respectively.*
From: Chowdhury et al. (2013). Aquaculture 410–411, 138–147.

required, prevent overfeeding and observe fish behaviour and feeding activity. However, automatic feeders, feed blowers and demand feeders are usually used with large commercial farms (Figs. 7.2 and 7.3). Hargreaves et al. (1986) found no difference in the performance of *O. aureus* fed by automatic feeders and those fed fixed rations. They recommended that automatic feeders be used because they reduced 88%–94% of the labour requirement. Rakocy et al. (2000) also recommended demand feeders for tilapia reared in cages suspended in watershed ponds. Similarly, demand feeders provide excellent growth and feed conversion of tilapia reared in marine cages, in addition to reducing labour. Endo et al. (2002) found that self-fed Nile tilapia had significantly lower blood cortisol, higher phagocytic activity of their macrophages, higher antibody production and higher number of blood lymphocytes. The authors suggested that self-feeding reduced fish stress and improved their immune response.

7.11.4 Diet form

Farmed tilapia are known to accept a wide range of diet forms. The acceptance is affected by fish size, stocking density, culture system and natural food availability. For example, Nile tilapia fingerlings and juveniles reared in floating cages responded better to mashed than pelleted feed, while large fish grew better on pelleted diet (Guerrero, 1980). In addition, when the fish were fed moist or dry pellets in cages, moist feed was utilized slightly better than dry feed; however, the leaching rate was higher in moist than in dry feeds. Meanwhile, the growth of Nile tilapia fry fed pellet crumbles and unpelleted diets was not different (Santiago et al., 1987). Tilapia can also consume both floating and sinking pellets very efficiently. Allison et al. (1979) found also that sinking pellets were better utilized by blue tilapia than unpelleted feed.

Generally speaking, floating pellets may be more preferable to sinking pellets due to the following attributes:

- Complete starch gelatinization;
- Better digestibility and stability;
- Better FCR;
- Removal of antinutritional factors during heat treatment; and
- Fish feeding can be observed, and feeding levels can be controlled.

However, extruded feeds are more expensive than compressed feeds due to the higher production costs. Also, extrusion technology and skilled personnel may not always be available.

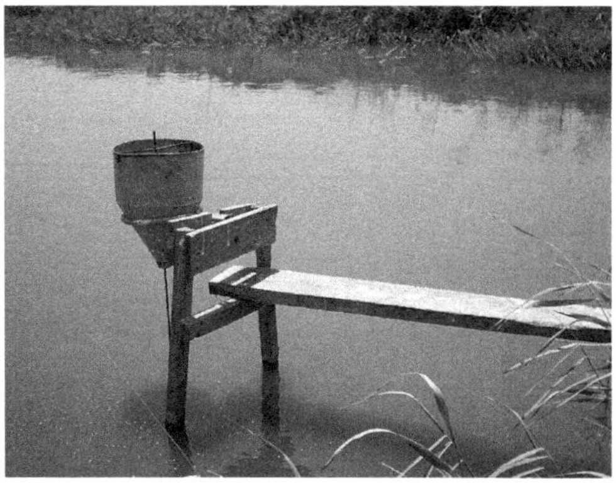

FIGURE 7.2 Demand feeders in earthen tilapia ponds in Egypt. *Photograph by A.-F. El-Sayed.*

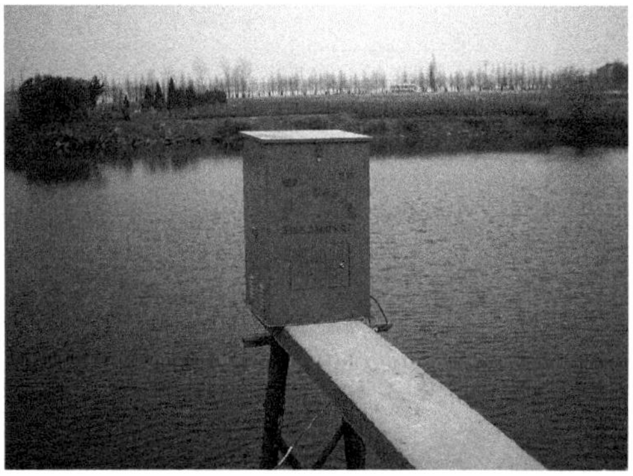

FIGURE 7.3 Automatic feeder in tilapia ponds in China. *Photograph by A.-F. El-Sayed.*

7.11.5 Feed colour

Feed colour may affect tilapia performance, particularly in intensive farming systems. El-Sayed (2004) evaluated the effects of feed colour on the growth and survival of Nile tilapia fingerlings reared in indoor, recirculating system. The fish were fed four test diets with different colours, red, light green, dark blue and yellow, in addition to a commercial, light-brown diet. Fish fed dark-coloured diets (red and dark blue) had better performance than those fed light-coloured diets (green and yellow). The red diet produced the best growth rate while the yellow diet resulted in the poorest performance. El-Sayed et al. (2013) further elaborated the effects of feed colour on the performance of Nile tilapia fry (0.01 g) and fingerling (5.3 g). The fish were fed test diets with six different colours (dark blue, dark green, red, dark brown, yellow and light brown). The best growth rates, feed efficiency, survival and body protein were achieved in larvae fed on dark-coloured diets (dark blue and dark green), while light-coloured diets (yellow and light brown) produced lower performance. In case of fingerlings, fish performance, survival and body composition were not significantly affected by feed colours. These results suggest that Nile tilapia larvae are visual feeders, and they prefer dark-coloured diets to light-coloured diets, while fingerling fish showed no preference to diet colours.

7.12 Closing remarks

1. With the exception of Nile tilapia and Mozambique tilapia, the EAA requirements of farmed tilapias are not known. Some NEAAs (such as taurine) may be conditionally essential and therefore should be given more attention.
2. A wide variety of unconventional dietary protein sources have been tested for tilapias. Most of these sources could partially or totally replace standard protein sources (mainly FM) in tilapia feeds.
3. Insect and worm meals have recently been recognized as an efficient and cheap alternative to FM and soybean in aquaculture feeds. Commercial production of insect meal is still a challenge, due to the undeveloped technology and high production costs.
4. The digestibility by tilapia of a number of feed ingredients that are commonly used in tilapia feed has been determined. DE could be used to calculate the energy contents of practical tilapia feed if these ingredients are used. If DE is not available, GE should be used instead of using DE or ME values reported for other fish species.
5. Extensive work should be conducted on the utilization of unconventional carbohydrate sources by tilapia, especially in developing countries, where these sources are available at low prices.
6. Earlier studies revealed high lipid requirements for farmed tilapia (10%−18%), while a significant reduction in lipid requirements has recently been achieved. Currently, commercial tilapia feeds contain 6%−9% lipids.
7. Despite the fact that tilapia require n-6 EFA, n-3 EFA may also be required, especially when the fish are reared in brackish water.
8. The requirements of tilapia for fat-soluble vitamins have not been well investigated; except for vitamin A, and, to a lesser extent, vitamin E. On the other hand, water-soluble vitamins have been relatively well covered, especially vitamin C.
9. The requirements of 10 minerals, namely, calcium, phosphorus, magnesium, zinc, manganese, potassium, iron, copper, selenium and chromium, have been studied for tilapia. Dietary phosphorus and zinc have received much more attention than other minerals. Determination of the dietary mineral requirements of tilapia should consider the relationship between dietary protein and energy and essential minerals.

10. The feeding regime (level, amount, frequency) of cultured tilapias is influenced by several factors, including fish species, size and age, diet form (pellets, crumbles, mash, dry, moist, floating, sinking) and culture system. These factors should be fully considered for best on-farm feed and feeding management for tilapia.
11. Feed colour may affect the growth and feed utilization of tilapia. Nile tilapia are visual feeders during their larval stages, preferring dark-coloured diets to light-coloured diets. Other nonvisual stimulators may be more important for food detection during fingerling and adult stages. More work is needed to support this argument.

References

Abdelghany, A.E., 1997. Optimum ratio between anchovy fish meal and soy protein concentrate in formulated diets for Nile tilapia (*Oreochromis niloticus* L.). In: Fitzimmons, K. (Ed.), Proceedings from the Fourth International Symposium on Tilapia in Aquaculture. Northeast Regional Agriculture Engineering Service, Ithaca, NY, USA, pp. 31–39.

Abdelghany, A.E., 2000. Replacement value of cystine for methionine in semi-purified diets supplemented with free amino acids for the Nile tilapia *Oreochromis niloticus* L. fry. In: Fitzsimmons, K., Filho, J.C. (Eds.), Tilapia Culture in the 21st Century. Proceedings from the Fifth International Symposium on Tilapia Aquaculture. Rio de Janeiro, Brazil, pp. 109–119.

Abdelghany, A.E., 2003. Partial and complete replacement of fish meal with gambusia meal in diets for red tilapia '*Oreochromis niloticus* × *O. mossambicus*'. Aquaculture Nutrition 9, 145–154.

Abo Norag, M.A., El-Shenawy, A.M., Fadl, S.E., Abdo, W.S., Gad, D.M., Rashed, M.A., 2018. Effect of phytase enzyme on growth performance, serum biochemical alteration, immune response and gene expression in Nile tilapia. Fish & Shellfish Immunology 80, 97–108.

Abou, Y., Fiogbé, E.D., Micha, J.-C., 2007a. Effects of stocking density on growth, yield and profitability of farming Nile tilapia, *Oreochromis niloticus* L., fed *Azolla* diet, in earthen ponds. Aquaculture Research 38, 595–604.

Abou, Y., Fiogbé, E.D., Micha, J.-C., 2007b. A preliminary assessment of growth and production of Nile tilapia, *Oreochromis niloticus* L., fed *Azolla*-based-diets in earthen ponds. Journal of Applied Aquaculture 19, 55–69.

Adeparusi, E.O., Olute, B.W., 2000. Effects of methionine-supplemented toasted lima bean (*Phaseolus lunatus*) diets on growth of *Oreochromis niloticus*. In: Fitzsimmons, K., Filho, J.C. (Eds.), Tilapia Culture in the 21st Century. Proceedings from the Fifth International Symposium on Tilapia Aquaculture. American Tilapia Association and ICLARM, Rio de Janeiro, Brazil, pp. 125–130.

Agbo, N.W., Adjei-Boateng, D., Jauncey, K., 2011. The potential of groundnut (*Arachis hypogaea* L.) by-products as alternative protein sources in the diet of Nile tilapia (*Oreochromis niloticus*). Journal of Applied Aquaculture 23, 367–378.

Al Hafedh, Y.S., Siddiqui, A.Q., 1998. Evaluation of guar seed as a protein source in Nile tilapia, *Oreochromis niloticus* (L.) practical diets. Aquaculture Research 29, 703–708.

Al Hafedh, Y.S., 1999. Effects of dietary protein on growth and body composition of Nile tilapia, *Oreochromis niloticus* L. Aquaculture Research 30, 385–393.

Al-Amoudi, M.M., El-Nakkadi, A.M.N., El-Nouman, B.M., 1992. Evaluation of optimum dietary requirement of vitamin C for the growth of *Oreochromis spilurus* fingerlings in water from the Red Sea. Aquaculture 105, 165–173.

Al-Feky, S.S.A., El-Sayed, A.-F.M., Ezzat, A.A., 2016a. Dietary taurine enhances growth and feed utilization in larval Nile tilapia (*Oreochromis niloticus*) fed soybean meal-based diets. Aquaculture Nutrition 22, 457–464.

Al-Feky, S.S.A., El-Sayed, A.-F.M., Ezzat, A.A., 2016b. Dietary taurine improves reproductive performance of Nile tilapia (*Oreochromis niloticus*) broodstock. Aquaculture Nutrition 22, 392–399.

Ali, A., Al-Asgah, N.A., 2001. Effect of feeding different carbohydrate to lipid ratios on the growth performance and body composition of Nile tilapia (*Oreochromis niloticus*). fingerlings. Animal Research 50, 91–100.

Allison, R., Smitherman, R.O., Gabrero, J., 1979. Effects of high density culture and form of feed on reproduction and yield of *Tilapia aurea*. In: Pillay, T.V.R., Dill, W.A. (Eds.), Advances in Aquaculture. Fishing News Books Ltd, Farnham, UK, pp. 168–170.

Almazan, G.J., Pullin, R.S.V., Angeles, A.F., Manalo, T.A., Agbayani, R.A., Trono, M.T.B., 1986. *Azolla pinnata* as a dietary component for Nile tilapia *Oreochromis niloticus*. In: Maclean, J.L., Dizon, L.B., Hosillos, L.V. (Eds.), Proceedings of the First Asian Fisheries Forum. Asian Fisheries Society, Manila, Philippines, pp. 523–528.

Anderson, J., Jackson, A.J., Matty, A.J., Capper, B.S., 1984. Effects of dietary carbohydrate and fibre on the tilapia *Oreochromis niloticus* (Linn.). Aquaculture 37, 303–314.

Antony Jesu Prabhu, P., Schrama, J.W., Kaushik, S.J., 2013. Quantifying dietary phosphorus requirement of fish – a meta-analytic approach. Aquacutlure Nutrition 19, 233–249.

Appler, H.N., 1985. Evaluation of *Hydrodictyon reticulatum* as a protein source in feeds for *Oreochromis* (*Tilapia*) *niloticus* and *Tilapia zillii*. Journal of Fish Biology 27, 327–334.

Aydin, B., Gümüş, E., 2013. Replacement of fishmeal by poultry by-product meal, supplemented with lysine, methionine, and threonine, in diets for fry of Nile tilapia (*Oreochromis niloticus*). Israeli Journal of Aquaculture – Bamidgeh 65, 885–892.

Azaza, M.S., Mensi, F., Ksouri, J., Dhraief, M.N., Brini, B., Abdelmouleh, A., et al., 2008. Growth of Nile tilapia (*Oreochromis niloticus* L.) fed with diets containing graded levels of green algae ulva meal (*Ulva rigida*) reared in geothermal waters of southern Tunisia. Journal of Applied Ichthyology 24, 202–207.

Balkhasher, A.A.S., 2012. The Use of Some Freshwater Macrophytes as Feed Ingredients for Nile Tilapia (*Oreochromis niloticus*) (M.Sc. thesis). Alexandria University, Egypt.

Balogun, A.M., Fagbenro, O.A., 1995. Use of macadamia presscake as a protein feedstuff in practical diets for tilapia, *Oreochromis niloticus* (L.). Aquaculture Research 26, 371–377.

Belal, I.E.H., Al-Owaifeir, A., Al-Dosari, M., 1995. Replacing fish meal with chicken offal silage in commercial *Oreochromis niloticus* (L.). feed. Aquaculture Research 26, 855–858.

Belal, I.E.H., 1999. Replacing dietary corn with barley seeds in Nile tilapia, *Oreochromis niloticus* (L.), feed. Aquaculture Research 30, 265–269.

Bishop, C.D., Angus, R.A., Watts, A., 1995. The use of feather meal as a replacement for fishmeal in the diet of *Oreochromis niloticus* fry. Bioresource Technology 54, 291–295.

Bombardelli, R.A., dos Reis Goes, E.S., de Negreiros Sousa, S.M., Syperreck, M.A., Goes, M.D., de Oliveira Pedreira, A.C., et al., 2017. Growth and reproduction of female Nile tilapia fed diets containing different levels of protein and energy. Aquaculture 479, 817–823.

Bondari, K., Sheppard, D.C., 1987. Soldier fly, *Hermetia illucens* L., larvae as feed for channel catfish, *Ictalurus punctatus* (Rafinesque), and blue tilapia, *Oreochromis aureus* (Steindachner). Aquaculture and Fisheries Management 18, 209–220.

Boonanuntanasarn, S., Kumkhong, S., Yoohat, K., Plagnes-Juan, E., Burel, C., Marandel, L., et al., 2018. Molecular responses of Nile tilapia (*Oreochromis niloticus*) to different levels of dietary carbohydrates. Aquaculture 482, 117–123.

Campeche, D.F.B., Catharino, R.R., Godoy, H.T., Cyrino, J.E.P., 2009. Vitamin A in diets for nile tilapia. Scientia Agricola 66, 751–756.

Cao, L., Yang, Y., Wang, W.M., Yakupitiyage, A., Yuan, D.R., Diana, J.S., 2008. Effects of pretreatment with microbial phytase on phosphorous utilization and growth performance of Nile tilapia (*Oreochromis niloticus*). Aquaculture Nutrition 14, 99–109.

Chamberlain, G.W., Hopkins, J.S., 1994. Reducing water use and feed cost in intensive ponds. World Aquaculture 25 (3), 29–32.

Chatvijitkul, S., Davis, D.A., Lim, C.E., 2016. Lipid extracted distillers dried grains with solubles (LE-DDGS) as a partial replacement for soybean meal in hybrid tilapia (*Oreochromis niloticus* × *O. aureus*) diets. Aquaculture 459, 131–136.

Chen, C., Sun, B., Li, X., Li, P., Guan, W., Bi, Y., et al., 2013. N-3 essential fatty acids in Nile tilapia, *Oreochromis niloticus*: quantification of optimum requirement of dietary linolenic acid in juvenile fish. Aquaculture 416–417, 99–104.

Chou, B.S., Shiau, S.Y., 1996. Optimal dietary lipid level for growth of juvenile hybrid tilapia, *Oreochromis niloticus* × *Oreochromis aureus*. Aquaculture 143, 185–195.

Chou, B.S., Shiau, S.-Y., 1999. Both n-6 and n-3 fatty acids are required for maximum growth of juvenile hybrid tilapia, *Oreochromis niloticus* × *Oreochromis aureus*. North American Journal of Aquaculture 61, 13–20.

Chou, B.S., Shiau, S.Y., Hung, S.S.O., 2001. Effect of dietary cod liver oil on growth and fatty acids of juvenile hybrid tilapia. North American Journal of Aquaculture 63, 277–284.

Chowdhury, M.A.K., Siddiqui, S., Hua, K., Bureau, D.P., 2013. Bioenergetics-based factorial model to determine feed requirement and waste output of tilapia produced under commercial conditions. Aquaculture 410–411, 138–147.

Clark, J.H., Watanabe, W.O., Ernst, D.H., 1990. Effect of feeding rate on growth and diet conversion of Florida red tilapia reared in floating marine cages. Journal of the World Aquaculture Society 21, 16–24.

Coyle, S.D., Mengel, G.J., Tidwell, J.H., Webster, C.D., 2004. Evaluation of growth, feed utilization and economics of hybrid tilapia, *Oreochromis niloticus* × *Oreochromis aureus,* fed diets containing different protein sources in combination with distillers dried grains with solubles. Aquaculture Research 35, 365–370.

Dabrowska, H., Meyer-Burgdorff, K., Gunther, K.D., 1989. Interaction between dietary protein and magnesium level in tilapia (*Oreochromis niloticus*). Aquaculture 76, 277–291.

Damasceno, F.M., Fleuri, L.F., Sartori, M.M.P., Amorim, R.L., Pezzato, L.E., da Silva, R.L., et al., 2016. Effect of dietary inorganic copper on growth performance and hematological profile of Nile tilapia subjected to heat-induced stress. Aquaculture 454, 257–264.

Daudpota, A.M., Abbas, G., Kalhoro, I.B., Shah, S.S.A., Kalhoro, H., Hafeez-Ur-Rehman, M., et al., 2016. Effect of feeding frequency on growth performance, feed utilization and body composition of juvenile Nile tilapia, *Oreochromis niloticus* (L.) reared in low salinity water. Pakistan Journal of Zoology 48, 171–177.

Davies, S.J., Williamson, J., Robinson, M., Bateson, R.I., 1989. Practical inclusion levels of common animal by-products in complete diets for tilapia (*Oreochromis mossambicus*, Peters). In: Proceedings of the Third International Symposium on Feeding and Nutrition of Fish. Tuba, Japan, pp. 325–332.

Davies, S.J., McConnell, S., Bateson, R.I., 1990. Potential of rapeseed meal as an alternative protein source in complete diets for tilapia (*Oreochromis mossambicus,* Peters). Aquaculture 87, 145–154.

de Oliveira, M.M., Ribeiro, T., Orlando, T.M., de Oliveira, D.G., Drumond, M.M., de Freitas, R.T., Rosa, P.V., 2014. Effects crude protein levels on female Nile tilapia (*Oreochromis niloticus*) reproductive performance parameters. Animal Reproduction Science 150, 62–69.

De Silva, S.S., Gunasekera, R.M., Keembiyahetty, C., 1986. Optimum ration and feeding frequency in *Oreochromis niloticus* young. In: Mclean, J.L., Dizon, L.B., Hosillos, L.V. (Eds.), Proceedings of the First Asian Fisheries Forum. Asian Fisheries Society, Manila, Philippines, pp. 559–564.

De Silva, S.S., Gunasekera, R.M., 1989. Effect of dietary protein level and amount of plant ingredient (*Phaseolus aureus*) incorporated into the diets on consumption, growth performance and carcass composition in *Oreochromis niloticus* fry. Aquaculture 80, 121–133.

De Silva, S.S., Gunasekera, R.M., Shim, K.F., 1991. Interactions of varying protein and lipid levels in young red tilapia: evidence of protein sparing. Aquaculture 95, 305–318.

Degani, G., Viola, S., Yehuda, Y., 1997. Apparent digestibility of protein and carbohydrate in feed ingredients for adult tilapia (*Oreochromis aureus* × *O. niloticus*). Israeli Journal of Aquaculture – Bamidgeh 49, 115–123.

Devic, E., Leschen, W., Murray, F., Little, D.C., 2018. Growth performance, feed utilization and body composition of advanced nursing Nile tilapia (*Oreochromis niloticus*) fed diets containing Black Soldier Fly (*Hermetia illucens*) larvae meal. Aquaculture Nutrition 24, 416–423.

do Carmo e Sá, M.V.C., Pezzato, L.E., Ferreira Lima, M.M.B., de Magalhães Padilha, P., 2004. Optimum zinc supplementation level in Nile tilapia *Oreochromis niloticus* juveniles diets. Aquaculture 238, 385–401.

Eid, A.E., Ghonim, S., 1994. Dietary zinc requirement of fingerling *Oreochromis niloticus*. Aquaculture 119, 259–264.

El-Sayed, A.-F.M., 1987. Protein and Energy Requirements of Tilapia zillii (Ph.D. thesis). Michigan State University, East Lansing, MI, USA.

El-Sayed, A.-F.M., Garling Jr., D.L., 1988. Carbohydrate-to-lipid ratio in diets for *Tilapia zillii* fingerlings. Aquaculture 73, 157–163.

El-Sayed, A.-F.M., 1989. Evaluation of semipurified test diets for *Tilapia zilli* fingerlings. Journal of the World Aquaculture Society 20, 240–244.

El-Sayed, A.-F.M., 1990. Long-term evaluation of cotton seed meal as a protein source for Nile tilapia, *Oreochromis niloticus*. Aquaculture 84, 315–320.

El-Sayed, A.-F.M., 1991. Evaluation of sugarcane bagasse as a feed ingredient for the tilapias *Oreochromis niloticus* and *Tilapia zillii*. Asian Fisheries Science 4, 53–60.

El-Sayed, A.-F.M., Teshima, S., 1991. Tilapia nutrition in aquaculture. Reviews in Aquatic Sciences 5, 247–265.

El-Sayed, A.-F.M., 1992. Effects of substituting fish meal with *Azolla pinnata* in practical diets for fingerling and adult Nile tilapia *Oreochromis niloticus* L. Aquaculture and Fisheries Management 23, 167–173.

El-Sayed, A.-F.M., Teshima, S., 1992. Protein and energy requirement of Nile tilapia, *Oreochromis niloticus*, fry. Aquaculture 103, 55–63.

El-Sayed, A.-F.M., 1998. Total replacement of fishmeal with animal protein sources in Nile tilapia, *Oreochromis niloticus* (L.), feeds. Aquaculture Research 29, 275–280.

El-Sayed, A.-F.M., 1999. Alternative dietary protein sources for farmed tilapia spp. Aquaculture 179, 149–168.

El-Sayed, A.-F.M., Moyano, F.J., Martinez, I., 2000. Assessment of the effect of plant inhibitors on digestive protease of Nile tilapia using *in vitro* assays. Aquaculture International 8, 403–415.

El-Sayed, A.-F.M., 2003. Effects of fermentation methods on the nutritive value of water hyacinth for Nile tilapia, *Oreochromis niloticus* (L.) fingerlings. Aquaculture 218, 471–478.

El-Sayed, A.-F.M., Mansour, C.R., Ezzat, A.A., 2003. Effects of dietary protein levels on spawning performance of Nile tilapia (*Oreochromis niloticus*) broodstock reared at different water salinities. Aquaculture 220, 619–632.

El-Sayed, A.-F.M., 2004. Feed colour affects growth, feed utilization of Nile tilapia. Global Aquaculture Advocate 7 (2), 76.

El-Sayed, A.-F.M., Mansour, C.R., Ezzat, A.A., 2005. Effects of dietary lipid source on spawning performance of Nile tilapia (*Oreochromis niloticus*) broodstock reared at different water salinities. Aquaculture 248, 187–196.

El-Sayed, A.-F.M., Kawanna, M., 2008. Effects of dietary protein and energy levels on spawning performance of Nile tilapia (*Oreochromis niloticus*) broodstock in a recycling system. Aquaculture 280, 179–184.

El-Sayed, A.F.M., El-Ghobashy, A.E., El-Mezayen, M.M., 2013. Effect of feed colour on growth and feed utilization of Nile tilapia (*Oreochromis niloticus* L.) larvae and fingerlings. Aquaculture Nutrition 19, 870–876.

El-Sayed, A.-F.M., 2014. Is dietary taurine supplementation beneficial for farmed fish and shrimp? a comprehensive review. Reviews in Aquaculture 6, 241–255.

El-Sayed, A.-F.M., Abo-State, H., Tahoun, A.-A., 2016. Evaluation of guar meal as a dietary protein source for Nile tilapia (*Oreochromis niloticus*) reared in hapa-in-pond system. Journal of Fisheries and Aquatic Science 11, 317–322.

Endo, M., Kumahara, C., Yoshida, T., Tabata, M., 2002. Reduced stress and increased immune responses in Nile tilapia kept under self-feeding conditions. Fisheries Science 68, 253–257.

Essa, M.A., 1997. Utilization of some aquatic plants in diets for Nile tilapia, *Oreochromis niloticus*, fingerlings. Egyptian Journal of Aquatic Biology and Fisheries 1, 19–34.

Fagbenro, O.A., 1988. Evaluation of defatted cocoa cake as a direct feed in the monosex culture of *Tilapia guineensis* (Pisces: Cichlidae). Aquaculture 73, 201–206.

Fagbenro, O.A., 1993. Observations on macadamia presscake as supplemental feed for monosex *Tilapia guineensis* (Pisces: Cichlidae). Journal of Aquaculture in the Tropics 7, 91–94.

Fagbenro, O.A., 1994. Dried fermented fish silage in diets for *Oreochromis niloticus*. Israeli Journal of Aquaculture – Bamidgeh 46, 140–147.

Fagbenro, O.A., Jauncey, K., Haylor, G., 1994. Nutritive value of diets containing dried lactic acid-fermented fish silage and soybean meal for juvenile *Oreochromis niloticus* and *Clarias gariepinus*. Aquatic Living Resources 7, 79–85.

Fagbenro, O.A., Adeparusi, E.O., Jimoh, W.A., 2004. Nutrient quality of detoxified jackbean (*Canavalia ensiformis* L. DC) seeds coked in distilled water or trona solution and evaluation of the meal as a substitute for soybean meal in practical diets for Nile tilapia. In: Bolivar, R., Mair, G., Fitzsimmons, K. (Eds.), Proceedings of the Sixth International Symposium on Tilapia in Aquaculture. Manila, Philippines, pp. 289–300.

Fasakin, E.A., Balogun, A.M., Fasuru, B.E., 1999. Use of duckweed, *Spirodela polyrrhiza* L. Schleiden, as a protein feedstuff in practical diets for tilapia, *Oreochromis niloticus* L. Aquaculture Research 30, 313–318.

Fitzsimmons, K., Dickenson, G., Brand, C., Davis, J., 1997. Effect of reducing dietary lipid levels on growth and body composition of hybrid tilapia in an intensive recirculating-water system. Progressive Fish-Culturist 59, 293–296.

Furuya, W.M., Santos, V.G., Silva, L.C.R., Furuya, V.R.B., Sakaguti, E.S., 2006. Digestible lysine requirements of Nile tilapia juveniles. Revista Brasileira de Zootecnia 35, 937–942.

Furuya, W.M., Graciano, T.S., Vidal, L.V.O., Xavier, T.O., Gongora, L.D., Righetti, J.S., et al., 2012. Digestible lysine requirement of Nile tilapia fingerlings fed arginine-to- lysine balanced diets. Revista Brasileira de Zootecnia 41, 485–490.

Gan, L., Zhou, L.L., Li, X.X., Yue, Y.R., 2016. Dietary leucine requirement of juvenile nile tilapia, *Oreochromis niloticus*. Aquaculture Nutrition 22, 1040–1046.

Gaye-Siessegger, J., Focken, U., Abel, H., Becker, K., 2007. Influence of dietary non-essential amino acid profile on growth performance and amino acid metabolism of Nile tilapia, *Oreochromis niloticus* (L.). Comparative Biochemistry and Physiology 146, 71–77.

Goddard, S., Al-Shagaa, G., Ali, A., 2008. Fisheries by-catch and processing waste meals as ingredients in diets for Nile tilapia, *Oreochromis niloticus*. Aquaculture Research 39, 518–525.

Gonçalves, G.S., Ribeiro, M.J.P., Vidotti, R.M., Sussel, F.R., 2011. Taurine Supplementation in Diets for Nile tilapia (*Oreochromis niloticus*). World Aquaculture 2011, Natal, Brazil, 6–10 June, 2011. Abstract # 639. World Aquaculture Society.

Guerrero III., R.D., 1980. Studies on the feeding of *Tilapia nilotica* in floating cages. Aquaculture 20, 169–175.

Guimarães, I.G., Lim, C., Yildirim-Aksoy, M., Li, M.H., Klesius, P.H., 2014. Effects of dietary levels of vitamin A on growth, hematology, immune response and resistance of Nile tilapia (*Oreochromis niloticus*) to *Streptococcus iniae*. Animal Feed Science and Technology 188, 126–136.

Guimarães, I.G., Pezzato, L.E., Santos, V.G., Orsi, R.O., Barros, M.M., 2016. Vitamin A affects haematology, growth and immune response of Nile tilapia (*Oreochromis niloticus*, L.), but has no protective effect against bacterial challenge or cold-induced stress. Aquaculture Research 47, 2004–2018.

Gunasekera, R.M., Shim, K.F., Lam, T.J., 1996a. Effect of dietary protein level on spawning performance and amino acid composition of eggs of Nile tilapia, *Oreochromis niloticus* (L.). Aquaculture 146, 121–134.

Gunasekera, R.M., Shim, K.F., Lam, T.J., 1996b. Influence of protein content of broodstock diets on larval quality and performance in Nile tilapia, *Oreochromis niloticus* (L.). Aquaculture 146, 245–259.

Hanley, F., 2000. Digestibility coefficients of feed ingredients for tilapia. In: Fitzsimmons, K., Filho, J.C. (Eds.), Tilapia Culture in the 21st Century. Proceedings from the Fifth International Symposium on Tilapia Aquaculture. American Tilapia Association and ICLARM, Rio de Janeiro, Brazil, pp. 163–172.

Hardy, R.W., Shearer, K.D., Stone, F.E., Weig, D.H., 1983. Fish silage in aquaculture diets. Journal of the World Mariculture Society 14, 695–703.

Hargreaves, J.A., Rakocy, J.E., Nair, A., 1986. An evaluation of fixed and demand feeding regimes for cage culture of *Oreochromis aureus*. In: Mclean, J.L., Dizon, L.B., Hosillos, L.V. (Eds.), The First Asian Fisheries Forum. Asian Fisheries Society, Manila, Philippines, pp. 335–340.

Haylor, G.S., Beveridge, M.C.M., Jauncey, K., 1988. Phosphorous nutrition of juvenile *Oreochromis niloticus*. In: Pullin, R.S.V., Bhukaswan, T., Tonguthai, K., Maclean, J.L. (Eds.), Proceedings of the Second International Symposium on Tilapia in Aquaculture. ICLARM Conference Proceedings No. 15. Department of Fisheries, Bangkok, Thailand, and ICLARM, Manila, Philippines, pp. 341–345.

He, J.Y., Titan, L.X., Lemme, A., Gao, W., Yang, H.J., Niu, J., et al., 2013. Methionine and lysine requirements for maintenance and efficiency of utilization for growth of two sizes of tilapia *(Oreochromis niloticus)*. Aquaculture Nutrition 19, 629–640.

He, J.Y., Han, B., Tian, L.-X., Yang, H.-J., Zeng, S.-L., Liu, Y.-J., 2016. The sparing effect of cystine on methionine at a constant TSAA level in practical diets of juvenile Nile tilapia *Oreochromis niloticus*. Aquaculture Research 47, 2031–2039.

He, J.Y., Long, W.Q., Han, B., Tian, L.X., Yang, H.J., Zeng, S.L., et al., 2017a. Effect of dietary L-methionine concentrations on growth performance, serum immune and antioxidative responses of juvenile Nile tilapia, *Oreochromis niloticus*. Aquaculture Research 48, 665–674.

He, J.Y., Tian, L.X., Lemme, A., Figueiredo-Silva, C., Gao, W., Yang, H.J., et al., 2017b. The effect of dietary methionine concentrations on growth performance of juvenile Nile tilapia *(Oreochromis niloticus)* fed diets with two different digestible energy levels. Aquaculture Nutrition 23, 76–89.

Hooley, C.G., Barrows, F.T., Paterson, J., Sealey, W.M., 2014. Examination of the effects of dietary protein and lipid levels on growth and stress tolerance of juvenile tilapia, *Oreochromis niloticus*. Journal of the World Aquaculture Society 45, 115–126.

Hu, J., Ran, C., He, S., Cao, Y., Yao, B., Ye, Y., et al., 2016. Dietary microbial phytase exerts mixed effects on the gut health of tilapia: a possible reason for the null effect on growth promotion. British Journal of Nutrition 115, 1958–1966.

Huang, C.H., Chang, R.J., Huang, S.L., Chen, W., 2003. Dietary vitamin E supplementation affects tissue lipid peroxidation of hybrid tilapia, *Oreochromis niloticus* × *O. aureus*. Comparative Biochemistry and Physiology B 134, 265–270.

Huang, F., Jiang, M., Wen, H., Wu, F., Liu, W., Tian, J., et al., 2015. Dietary zinc requirement of adult Nile tilapia (*Oreochromis niloticus*) fed semi-purified diets, and effects on tissue mineral composition and antioxidant responses. Aquaculture 439, 53–59.

Huang, F., Jiang, M., Wen, H., Wu, F., Liu, W., Tian, J., et al., 2016. Dietary vitamin C requirement of genetically improved farmed tilapia, *Oreochromis niloticus*. Aquaculture Research 47, 689–697.

Huang, Q., Huang, K., Ma, Y., Qin, X., Wen, Y., Sun, L., et al., 2015. Feeding frequency and rate effects on growth and physiology of juvenile genetically improved farmed Nile tilapia. North American Journal of Aquaculture 77, 503–512.

Hussein, E.E.-S., Dabrowski, K., El-Saidy, D.M.S.D., Lee, B.-J., 2013. Enhancing the growth of Nile tilapia larvae/juveniles by replacing plant (gluten) protein with algae protein. Aquaculture Research 44, 937–949.

Ishak, M., Dollar, A.M., 1968. Studies on Manganese uptake in *Tilapia mossambica* and *Salmo gairdneri*. 1. Growth and survival of *Tilapia mossambica* in response to manganese. Hydrobiologia 31, 572–584.

Jabir, M.D.A.R., Razak, S.A., Vikineswary, S., 2012. Nutritive potential and utilization of super worm (*Zophobas morio*) meal in the diet of Nile tilapia (*Oreochromis niloticus*) juvenile. African Journal of Biotechnology 11, 6592–6598.

Jackson, A.J., Capper, B.S., 1982. Investigations into the requirements of tilapia *Sarotherodon mossambicus,* for dietary methionine, lysine and arginine in semi-synthetic diets. Aquaculture 20, 289–297.

Jackson, A.J., Capper, B.S., Matty, A.J., 1982. Evaluation of some plant proteins in complete diets for the tilapia, *Sarotherodon mossambicus*. Aquaculture 27, 97–109.

Jacobsen, J.G., Smith, L.H., 1968. Biochemistry and physiology of taurine and taurine derivatives. Physiological Reviews 48, 424–511.

Jauncey, K., 1982. The effects of varying dietary protein level on the growth, food conversion, protein utilization and body composition of juvenile tilapias (*Sarotherodon mossambicus*). Aquaculture 27, 43–54.

Jauncey, K., Ross, B., 1982. A Guide to Tilapia Feeds and Feeding. University of Stirling, Scotland, 111 pp.

Jauncey, K., Tacon, A.G.J., Jackson, A.J., 1983. The quantitative essential amino acid requirements of *Oreochromis (Sarotherodon). mossambicus*. In: Fishelson, L., Yaron, Z. (Eds.), Proceedings of the International Symposium on Tilapia in Aquaculture. Tel-Aviv University, Israel, pp. 328–337.

Jauncey, K., 1998. Tilapia Feeds and Feeding. Pisces Press Ltd, Stirling, Scotland, 241 pp.

Jauncey, K., 2000. Nutrient requirements. In: Beveridge, M.C.M., McAndrews, B.J. (Eds.), Tilapias: Biology and Exploitation. Kluwer Academic Publishers, London, UK, pp. 325–327.

Jiang, M., Huang, F., Wen, H., Yang, C., Wu, F., Liu, W., et al., 2014. Dietary niacin requirement of GIFT tilapia, *Oreochromis niloticus*, reared in freshwater. Journal of the World Aquaculture Society 45, 333–341.

Kleemann, G.K., Barros, M.M., Pezzato, L.E., Sampaio, F.G., Ferrari, J.C., Valle, J.B., et al., 2003. Iron Requirement for Nile tilapia *Oreochromis niloticus*. In: World Aquaculture 2003 - Book of Abstracts, vol. 1. World Aquaculture Society, Baton Rouge, LA, USA, p. 82.

Klinnavee, S., Tansakul, R., Promkuntong, W., 1990. Growth of Nile tilapia (*Oreochromis niloticus)* fed with aquatic plant mixtures. In: Hirano, R., Hanyu, I. (Eds.), The Second Asian Fisheries Forum. Asian Fisheries Society, Manila, Philippines, pp. 283–286.

Koch, J.F.A., Barros, M.M., Teixeira, C.P., Carvalho, P.L.P.F., Fernandes Junior, A.C., Cintra, F.T., et al., 2017. Protein-to-energy ratio of 21.43 g MJ^{-1} improves growth performance of Nile tilapia at the final rearing stage under commercially intensive rearing conditions. Aquaculture Nutrition 23, 560–570.

Kpundeh, M.D., Qiang, J., He, J., Yang, H., Xu, P., 2015. Effects of dietary protein levels on growth performance and haemato-immunological parameters of juvenile genetically improved farmed tilapia (GIFT), *Oreochromis niloticus*. Aquaculture International 23, 1189–1201.

Kuzmina, V.V., Gavrovskaya, L.K., Ryzhova, O.V., 2010. Taurine. Effect on exotrophia and metabolism in mammals and fish. Journal of Evolutionary Biochemistry and Physiology 46, 19–27.

Lee, S., Nambi, R.W., Won, S., Katya, K., Bai, S.C., 2016. Dietary selenium requirement and toxicity levels in juvenile Nile tilapia, *Oreochromis niloticus*. Aquaculture 464, 153–158.

Leng, R.A., Stanbolie, J.H., Bell, R., 1995. Duckweed- a potential high-protein feed resource for domestic animals and fish. Livestock Research for Rural Development 7 (1), 11 p. http://www.cipav.org.co/lrrd/lrrd7/1/3.htm.

Li, M.-R., Huang, C.-H., 2016. Effect of dietary zinc level on growth, enzyme activity and body trace elements of hybrid tilapia, *Oreochromis niloticus* × *O. aureus*, fed soya bean meal-based diets. Aquaculture Nutrition 22, 1320–1327.

Li, E., Lim, C., Klesius, P.H., Welker, T.L., 2013. Growth, body fatty acid composition, immune response, and resistance to *Streptococcus iniae* of hybrid tilapia, *Oreochromis niloticus* × *Oreochromis aureus*, fed diets containing various levels of linoleic and linolenic acids. Journal of the World Aquaculture Society 44, 42–55.

Li, X.-Q., Zhang, X.-Q., Chowdhury, M.A.K., Zhang, Y., Leng, X.-J., 2019. Dietary phytase and protease improved growth and nutrient utilization in tilapia (*Oreochromis niloticus* × *Oreochromis aureus*) fed low phosphorus and fishmeal-free diets. Aquaculture Nutrition 25, 46–55.

Liebert, F., Portz, L., 2005. Nutrient utilization of Nile tilapia *Oreochromis niloticus* fed plant-based low phosphorus diets supplemented with graded levels of different sources of microbial phytase. Aquaculture 248, 111–119.

Lim, C., Dominy, W.G., 1991. Utilization of plant proteins by warmwater fish. In: Akiyama, D.M., Tan, R.K.H. (Eds.), Proceedings of Aquaculture Feed Processing and Nutrition Workshop. American Soybean Association, Singapore, pp. 163–172.

Lim, C., Leamaster, B., 1991. Thiamine requirements of red hybrid tilapia grown in seawater. Journal of the World Aquaculture Society 22, 36A.

Lim, C., Leamaster, B., Brock, J.A., 1993. Riboflavin requirements of fingerling red tilapia grown in seawater. Journal of the World Aquaculture Society 24, 451–458.

Lim, H.-A., Ng, W.-K., Lim, S.-L., Ibrahim, C.O., 2001. Contamination of palm kernel meal with Aspergillus flavus affects its nutritive value in pelleted feeds for tilapia, *Oreochromis mossambicus*. Aquaculture Research 32, 895–905.

Lim, C., Garcia, J.C., Yildirim-Aksoy, M., Klesius, P.H., Shoemaker, C.A., Evans, J.J., 2007. Growth response and resistance to *Streptococcus iniae* of Nile tilapia, *Oreochromis niloticus*, fed diets containing distillers dried grains with solubles. Journal of the World Aquaculture Society 38, 231–237.

Lim, C., Yildirim-Aksoy, M., Li, M.H., Welker, T.L., Klesius, P.H., 2009. Influence of dietary levels of lipid and vitamin E on growth and resistance of Nile tilapia to *Streptococcus iniae* challenge. Aquaculture 298, 76–82.

Lim, C., Yildirim-Aksoy, M., Welker, T., Klesius, P.H., 2010. Growth performance, immune response, and resistance to *Streptococcus iniae* of Nile tilapia, *Oreochromis niloticus*, fed diets containing various levels of vitamins C and E. Journal of the World Aquaculture Society 41, 35–48.

Lim, C., Li, E., Klesius, P.H., 2011a. Distiller's dried grains with solubles as an alternative protein source in diets of tilapia. Reviews in Aquaculture 3, 172–178.

Lim, C., Yildirim-Aksoy, M., Barros, M.M., Klesius, P., 2011b. Thiamin requirement of nile tilapia, *Oreochromis niloticus*. Journal of the World Aquaculture Society 42, 824–833.

Lin, J.H., Shiau, S.Y., 1995. Hepatic enzyme adaptation to different dietary carbohydrates in juvenile tilapia *Oreochromis niloticus* × *O. aureus*. Fish Physiology and Biochemistry 14, 165–170.

Lin, Y.-H., Lin, S.-M., Shiau, S.-Y., 2008. Dietary manganese requirements of juvenile tilapia, *Oreochromis niloticus* × *O. aureus*. Aquaculture 284, 207–210.

Lin, Y.-H., Ku, C.-Y., Shiau, S.-Y., 2013. Estimation of dietary magnesium requirements of juvenile tilapia, *Oreochromis niloticus* × *Oreochromis aureus*, reared in freshwater and seawater. Aquaculture 380–383, 47–51.

Liou, C.H., 1989. Lysine and Sulfur Amino Acid Requirements of Juvenile Blue Tilapia (*Oreochromis aureus*) (Ph.D. thesis). Texas A & M University, College Station, TX, USA, 101 pp.

Liu, W., Jiang, M., Wu, J.-P., Wu, F., Tian, J., Yang, C.-G., et al., 2017. Dietary protein level affects the growth performance of large male genetically improved farmed tilapia, *Oreochromis niloticus*, reared in fertilized freshwater cages. Journal of the World Aquaculture Society 48, 718–728.

Liu, W., Wen, H., Luo, Z., 2018. Effect of dietary protein levels and feeding rates on the growth and health status of juvenile genetically improved farmed tilapia (*Oreochromis niloticus*). Aquaculture International 26, 153–167.

Lorico-Querijero, B., Chiu, Y.N., 1989. Protein digestibility studies on *Oreochromis niloticus* using chromic oxide indicator. Asian Fisheries Science 2, 177–191.

Lovell, R.T., Limsuwan, T., 1982. Intestinal synthesis and dietary nonessentiality of vitamin B_{12} for *Tilapia nilotica*. Transactions of the American Fisheries Society 11, 485–490.

Luquet, P., 1989. Practical considerations on the protein nutrition and feeding of tilapia. Aquatic Living Resources 2, 99–104.

Ma, F., Li, X.Q., Li, B.A., Leng, X.J., 2016. Effects of extruded and pelleted diets with differing lipid levels on growth, nutrient retention and serum biochemical indices of tilapia (*Oreochromis aureus* × *Tilapia nilotica*). Aquaculture Nutrition 22, 61–71.

Madage, S.S.K., Medis, W.U.D., Sultanbawa, Y., 2015. Fish silage as replacement of fishmeal in red tilapia feeds. Journal of Applied Aquaculture 27, 95–106.

Maina, J.G., Beames, R.M., Higgs, D., Mbugua, P.N., Iwama, G., Kisia, M., 2002. Digestibility and feeding value of some feed ingredients fed to tilapia *Oreochromis niloticus* (L.). Aquaculture Research 33, 853–862.

Mambrini, M., Kaushik, S.J., 1994. Partial replacement of dietary protein nitrogen with dispensable amino acids in diets of Nile tilapia, *Oreochromis niloticus*. Comparative Biochemistry and Physiology A 109, 469–477.

Mansour, C.R., 1998. Nutrient Requirements of Red Tilapia Fingerlings (M.Sc. thesis). Alexandria University, Alexandria, Egypt.

Maquart, P.O., Murray, F., Leschen, W., Netwon, R., Little, D., September 2018. Black soldier fly- A future for tilapia feed? International Aquafeed 20–22.

Mazid, A.M., Tanaka, Y., Katayama, T., Rahman, A.M., Simpson, K.L., Chichester, C.O., 1979. Growth response of *Tilapia zillii* fingerlings fed isocaloric diets with variable protein levels. Aquaculture 18, 115–122.

McClain, W.R., Gatlin, D.M., 1988. Dietary zinc requirement of *Oreochromis aureus* and effects of dietary calcium and phytate on zinc bioavailability. Journal of the World Aquaculture Society 19, 103–108.

Meyer-Burgdorff, K., Osman, M.F., Gunther, K.D., 1989. Energy metabolism in *Oreochromis niloticus*. Aquaculture 79, 283–291.

Micha, J.-C., Antoine, T., Wery, P., Van Hove, C., 1988. Growth, ingestion capacity, comparative appetency and biochemical composition of *Oreochromis niloticus* and *Tilapia rendalli* fed with *Azolla*. In: Pullin, R.S.V., Bhukaswan, T., Tonguthai, K., Maclean, J.L. (Eds.), Proceedings of the Second International Symposium on Tilapia in Aquaculture. ICLARM Proceedings No. 15. Department of Fisheries, Thailand, and ICLARM, Manila, Philippines, pp. 347–355.

Michelato, M., de Oliveira Vidal, L.V., Xavier, T.O., de Moura, L.B., de Almeida, F.L.A., Pedrosa, V.B., et al., 2016a. Dietary lysine requirement to enhance muscle development and fillet yield of finishing Nile tilapia. Aquaculture 457, 124–130.

Michelato, M., Vidal, L.V.O., Xavier, T.O., Graciano, T.S., De Moura, L.B., Furuya, V.R.B., et al., 2016b. Dietary threonine requirement to optimize protein retention and fillet production of fast-growing Nile tilapia. Aquaculture Nutrition 22, 759–766.

Michelato, M., Zaminhan, M., Boscolo, W.R., Nogaroto, V., Vicari, M., Artoni, R.F., et al., 2017. Dietary histidine requirement of Nile tilapia juveniles based on growth performance, expression of muscle-growth-related genes and haematological responses. Aquaculture 467, 63–70.

Michelato, M., Furuya, W.M., Gatlin, D.M., 2018. Metabolic responses of Nile tilapia *Oreochromis niloticus* to methionine and taurine supplementation. Aquaculture 485, 66–72.

Moreau, Y., 1996. Measurement of the apparent digestibility coefficients for *Oreochromis niloticus* of agro-industrial by-products available in Cote d'Ivoire. In: Pullin, R.S.V., Lazard, J., Legendre, M., Amon Kottias, J.B., Pauly, D. (Eds.), Proceedings of the Third International Symposium on Tilapia in Aquaculture. ICLARM Conference Proceedings No. 41. ICLARM, Penang, Malaysia, pp. 204–210.

Muin, H., Taufek, N.M., Kamarudin, M.S., Razak, S.A., 2017. Growth performance, feed utilization and body composition of Nile tilapia, *Oreochromis niloticus* (Linnaeus, 1758) fed with different levels of black soldier fly, *Hermetia illucens* (Linnaeus, 1758) maggot meal diet. Iranian Journal of Fisheries Sciences 16, 567–577.

Naegel, L.C.A., 1997. *Azolla* meal as a supplemental feed ingredient for tilapias. In: Fitzsimmons, K. (Ed.), Proceedings from the Fourth International Symposium on Tilapia in Aquaculture. Northeast Regional Agriculture Engineering Service, Ithaca, NY, USA, pp. 20–30.

Neu, D., Boscolo, W., Zaminhan, M., Almeida, F., Sary, C., Furuya, W., 2016. Growth performance, biochemical responses, and skeletal muscle development of juvenile Nile tilapia, *Oreochromis niloticus*, fed with increasing levels of arginine. Journal of the World Aquaculture Society 47, 248–259.

Newton, G., Booram, C., Barker, R., Hale, O., 1977. Dried larvae meal as a supplement for swine. Journal of Animal Science 44, 395–400.

Ng, W.K., Wee, K.L., 1989. The nutritive value of cassava leaf meal in pelleted feed for Nile tilapia. Aquaculture 83, 45–58.

Ng, W.-K., Wang, Y., 2011. Inclusion of crude palm oil in the broodstock diets of female Nile tilapia, *Oreochromis niloticus*, resulted in enhanced reproductive performance compared to broodfish fed diets with added fish oil or linseed oil. Aquaculture 314, 122–131.

Ng, W.-K., Chong, C.-Y., Wang, Y., Romano, N., 2013. Effects of dietary fish and vegetable oils on the growth, tissue fatty acid composition, oxidative stability and vitamin E content of red hybrid tilapia and efficacy of using fish oil finishing diets. Aquaculture 372–375, 97–110.

Nguyen, T.N., Davis, D.A., 2009a. Methionine requirement in practical diets for juvenile Nile tilapia, *Oreochromis niloticus*. Journal of the World Aquaculture Society 40, 410–416.

Nguyen, T.N., Davis, D.A., 2009b. Re-evaluation of total sulphur amino acid requirement and determination of replacement value of cystine for methionine in semi-purified diets of juvenile Nile tilapia,*Oreochromis niloticus*. Aquaculture Nutrition 15, 247–253.

Nguyen, L., Davis, D.A., 2016. Comparison of crystalline lysine and intact lysine used as a supplement in practical diets of channel catfish (*Ictalurus punctatus*) and Nile tilapia (*Oreochromis niloticus*). Aquaculture 464, 331–339.

NRC (National Research Council), 1993. Nutrient Requirements of Fish. National Academy of Science, Washington, DC, USA, 141 pp.

NRC (National Research Council), 2011. Nutrient Requirements of Fish and Shrimp. National Academy of Science, Washington, DC, USA, 392 pp.

Nwanna, L.C., Daramola, J.A., 2000. Harnessing of shrimp head waste in Nigeria for low cost production of tilapia, *Oreochromis niloticus* (L.). In: Fitzsimmons, K., Fhlho, J.C. (Eds.), Tilapia Aquaculture in the 21st Century. Proceedings from the Fifth International Symposium on Tilapia in Aquaculture. Rio De Janeiro, Brazil, pp. 174–178.

Oduro-Boateng, F., Bart-Plange, A., 1988. Pito brewery waste as an alternative protein source to fishmeal in feeds for *Tilapia busumana*. In: Pullin, R.S.V., Bhukaswan, T., Tonguthai, K., Maclean, J.L. (Eds.), The Second International Symposium on Tilapia in Aquaculture. ICLARM Conference Proceedings No. 15. Department of Fisheries, Thailand, and ICLARM, Manila, Philippines, pp. 357–360.

Ogunji, J.O., Kloas, W., Wirth, M., Schulz, C., Rennert, B., 2008. Housefly maggot meal (magmeal) as a protein source for *Oreochromis niloticus* (Linn.). Asian Fisheries Science 21, 319–331.

Olvera-Novoa, M.A., Campos, G.S., Sabido, G.M., Martínez-Palacios, C.A., 1990. The use of alfalfa leaf protein concentrate as a protein source in diets for tilapia (*Oreochromis mossambicus*). Aquaculture 90, 291–302.

Olvera-Novoa, M.A., Pereira-Pacheco, F., Olvira-castillo, L., Perez-Flores, V., Navarro, L., Samano, J.C., 1997. Cowpea (*Vigna unguiculata*) protein concentrate as replacement for fish meal in diets for tilapia (*Oreochromis niloticus*) fry. Aquaculture 158, 107–116.

Olvera-Novoa, M.A., Domínguez-Cen, L.J., Olvira-Castillo, L., Martínez-Palacios, C.A., 1998. Effect of the use of the microalgae *Spirulina maxima* as fish meal replacement in diets for tilapia, *Oreochromis mossambicus* (Peters), fry. Aquaculture Research 29, 709–715.

Olvera-Novoa, M.A., Olvira-Castillo, L., Martínez-Palacios, C.A., 2002. Sunflower seed meal as a protein source in diets for *Tilapia rendalli* (Boulanger, 1896) fingerlings. Aquaculture Research 33, 223–229.

Omoregie, E., Ogbemudia, F.I., 1993. Effects of substituting fish meal with palm kernel meal on growth and food utilization of the Nile tilapia, *Oreochromis niloticus*. Israeli Journal of Aquaculture – Bamidgeh 45, 113–119.

Orachunwong, C., Thammasart, S., Lohawatanakul, C., 2001. Recent developments in tilapia feeds. In: Subasinghe, S., Singh, T. (Eds.), Tilapia: Production, Marketing and Technical Developments. Proceedings of the Tilapia 2001 International Technical and Trade Conference on Tilapia. Infofish, Kuala Lumpur, Malaysia, pp. 113–122.

Osman, M.F., Omar, E., Nour, A.M., 1996. The use of leucaena leaf meal in feeding Nile tilapia. Aquaculture International 4, 9–18.

Peng, X., Li, F., Lin, S., Chen, Y., 2016. Effects of total replacement of fish oil on growth performance, lipid metabolism and antioxidant capacity in tilapia *(Oreochromis niloticus)*. Aquaculture International 24, 145–156.

Pereira, R.T., Rosa, P.V., Gatlin, D.M., 2017. Glutamine and arginine in diets for Nile tilapia: effects on growth, innate immune responses, plasma amino acid profiles and whole-body composition. Aquaculture 473, 135–144.

Pouomogne, V., Gabriel, T., Pouemegne, J.-B., 1997. A preliminary evaluation of cacoa husks in practical diets for juvenile Nile tilapia (*Oreochromis niloticus*). Aquaculture 156, 215–223.

Qiang, J., Yang, H., He, J., Wang, H., Zhu, Z.X., Xu, P., 2014. Comparative study of the effects of two high-carbohydrate diets on growth and hepatic carbohydrate metabolic enzyme responses in juvenile GIFT tilapia (*Oreochromis niloticus*). Turkish Journal of Fisheries and Aquatic Sciences 14, 515–525.

Qiang, J., He, J., Yang, H., Sun, Y.-L., Tao, Y.-F., Xu, P., et al., 2017. Dietary lipid requirements of larval genetically improved farmed tilapia, *Oreochromis niloticus* (L.), and effects on growth performance, expression of digestive enzyme genes, and immune response. Aquaculture Research 48, 2827–2840.

Rachmawati, D., Samidjan, I., Elfitasari, T., 2018. Effect of the phytase enzyme addition in the artificial feed on digestibility of feed, feed conversion ratio and growth of GIFT tilapia saline fish (*Oreochromis niloticus*). Nursery Stadia I. In: Third International Conference on Tropical and Coastal Region Eco Development 2017. IOP Conference Series: Earth and Environmental Science, vol. 116, p. 012009.

Rakocy, J.E., Bailey, D.S., Martin, J.M., Shultz, R.C., 2000. Tilapia production systems for the Lesser Antilles and other resource-limited, tropical areas. In: Fitzsimmons, K., Filho, J.C. (Eds.), Tilapia Culture in the 21st Century. Proceedings from the Fifth International Symposium on Tilapia Aquaculture. Rio de Janeiro, Brazil, pp. 651–662.

Rapatsa, M.M., Moyo, N.A.G., 2017. Evaluation of *Imbrasia belina* meal as a fishmeal substitute in *Oreochromis mossambicus* diets: growth performance, histological analysis and enzyme activity. Aquaculture Reports 5, 18–26.

Reigh, R.C., Robinson, E.D., Brown, P.B., 1991. Effect of dietary magnesium on growth and tissue magnesium content of blue tilapia (*Oreochromis aureus*). Journal of the World Aquaculture Society 22, 192–200.

Riche, M., Trottier, N.L., Ku, P.K., Garling, D.L., 2001. Apparent digestibility of crude protein and apparent availability of individual amino acids in tilapia (*Oreochromis niloticus*). fed phytase pretreated soybean meal diets. Fish Physiology and Biochemistry 25, 181–194.

Riche, M., Oetker, M., David, I.H., Smith, T., Garling, D.L., 2004. Effect of feeding frequency on consumption, growth, and efficiency in juvenile tilapia (*Oreochromis niloticus*). Israeli Journal of Aquaculture – Bamidgeh 56, 247–255.

Robinson, E.H., LaBomascus, D., Brown, P.B., Linton, T.L., 1987. Dietary calcium and phosphorus requirements of *Oreochromis aureus* reared in calcium-free water. Aquaculture 64, 267–276.

Rodriguez-Serna, M., Olvera-Novoa, M.A., Carmona-Osalde, C., 1996. Nutritional value of animal by-product meal in practical diets for Nile tilapia *Oreochromis niloticus* (L.). fry. Aquaculture Research 27, 67–73.

Roem, A.J., Kohler, C.C., Stickney, R.R., 1990. Vitamin E requirements of the blue tilapia *Oreochromis aureus* (Steindachner) in relation to dietary lipid levels. Aquaculture 87, 155–164.

Sadiku, S.O.E., Jauncey, K., 1995. Soybean flour-poultry meat meal blends as dietary protein source in practical diets of *Oreochromis niloticus* and *Clarias gariepinus*. Asian Fisheries Science 8, 159–168.

Saleh, G., Eleraky, W., Gropp, J.M., 1995. A short note on the effects of vitamin A hypervitaminosis and hypovitaminosis on health and growth of tilapia (*Oreochromis niloticus*). Journal of Applied Ichthyology 11, 382–385.

Sánchez-Muros, M.J., De Haro, C., Sanz, A., Trenzado, C.E., Villareces, S., Barroso, F.G., 2016. Nutritional evaluation of *Tenebrio molitor* meal as fish meal substitute for tilapia (*Oreochromis niloticus*) diet. Aquaculture Nutrition 22, 943–955.

Santiago, C.B., Aldaba, M.B., Reyes, O.S., 1987. Influence of feeding rate and diet form on growth and survival of Nile tilapia (*Oreochromis niloticus*) fry. Aquaculture 64, 277–282.

Santiago, C.B., Lovell, R.T., 1988. Amino acid requirements for growth of Nile tilapia. Journal of Nutrition 118, 1540–1546.

Santiago, C.B., Aldaba, M.B., Reyes, O.S., Laron, M.A., 1988. Response of Nile tilapia (*Oreochromis niloticus*). fry to diets containing *Azolla* meal. In: Pullin, R.S.V., Bhukaswan, T., Tonguthai, K., Maclean, J.L. (Eds.), Proceedings of the Second International Symposium on Tilapia in Aquaculture. ICLARM Proceedings No. 15. Department of Fisheries, Thailand, and ICLARM, Manila, Philippines, pp. 377–382.

Santiago, C.B., Reyes, O.S., 1993. Effects of dietary lipid source on reproductive performance and tissue lipid levels of Nile tilapia *Oreochromis niloticus* (L.). broodstock. Journal of Applied Ichthyology 9, 33–40.

Sarmento, N.L.A.F., Martins, E.F.F., Costa, D.C., Mattioli, C.C., da Costa Julio, G.S., Figueiredo, L.G., et al., 2018. Reproductive efficiency and egg and larvae quality of Nile tilapia fed different levels of vitamin C. Aquaculture 482, 96–102.

Satoh, S.T., Takeuchi, T., Watanabe, T., 1987. Requirement of tilapia for alpha tocopherol. Nippon Suisan Gakkaishi 53, 119–124.

Schaeffer, T.W., Brown, M.L., Rosentrater, K.A., 2009. Performance characteristics of Nile tilapia (*Oreochromis niloticus*) fed diets containing graded levels of fuel-based distiller's dried grains with solubles. Journal of Aquaculture Feed Science and Nutrition 1, 78–83.

Schamber, C.R., Boscolo, W.R., Natali, M.R.M., Michelato, M., Furuya, V.R.B., Furuya, W.M., 2014. Growth performance and bone mineralization of large Nile tilapia (*Oreochromis niloticus*) fed graded levels of available phosphorus. Aquaculture International 22, 1711–1721.

Shiau, S.-Y., Yu, H.L., Hwa, S., Chen, S.Y., Hsu, S.I., 1988. The influence of carboxymethyl cellulose on growth, digestion, gastric emptying time and body composition of tilapia. Aquaculture 70, 345–354.

Shiau, S.-Y., Kwok, C.C., Huang, J.Y., Chen, C.M., Lee, S.L., 1989. Replacement of fish meal with soybean meal in male tilapia

(*Oreochromis niloticus* × *O. aureus*) fingerling diet at a suboptimal protein level. Journal of the World Aquaculture Society 20, 230–235.

Shiau, S.-Y., Jan, F.L., 1992. Dietary ascorbic acid requirement of juvenile tilapia, *Oreochromis niloticus* × *O. aureus*. Nippon Suisan Gakkaishi 58, 671–675.

Shiau, S.Y., Suen, G.S., 1992. Estimation of the niacin requirements for tilapia fed diets containing glucose or dextrin. Journal of Nutrition 122, 2030–2036.

Shiau, S.-Y., Chen, M.J., 1993. Carbohydrate utilization by tilapia (*Oreochromis niloticus* × *O. aureus*) as influenced by different chromium sources. Journal of Nutrition 123, 1747–1753.

Shiau, S.-Y., Hwang, J.Y., 1993. Vitamin D requirement of juvenile hybrid tilapia, *Oreochromis niloticus* × *O. aureus*. Nippon Suisan Gakkaishi 59, 553–558.

Shiau, S.-Y., Lin, S.F., 1993. Effects of supplemental dietary chromium and vanadium on the utilization of different carbohydrates in tilapia, *Oreochromis niloticus* × *O. aureus*. Aquaculture 110, 321–330.

Shiau, S.-Y., Peng, C.Y., 1993. Protein sparing effect by carbohydrates in diets for tilapia. *Oreochromis niloticus* × *O. aureus*, Aquaculture 117, 327–334.

Shiau, S.-Y., Hsu, T.S., 1995. L-Ascorbyl-2-sulfate has equal antiscorbutic activity as L-ascorbyl-2-monophosphate for tilapia, *Oreochromis niloticus* × *O. aureus*. Aquaculture 133, 147–157.

Shiau, S.-Y., Liang, H.S., 1995. Carbohydrate utilization and digestibility by tilapia, *Oreochromis niloticus* × *O. aureus,* are affected by chromic oxide inclusion in the diet. Journal of Nutrition 125, 976–982.

Shiau, S.-Y., Hsieh, H.L., 1997. Vitamin B_6 requirements of tilapia, *Oreochromis niloticus* × *O. aureus* fed two dietary protein concentrations. Fisheries Science 63, 1002–1007.

Shiau, S.-Y., Shy, S.M., 1998. Dietary chromic oxide inclusion level required to maximize glucose utilization in hybrid tilapia *Oreochromis niloticus* × *O. aureus*. Aquaculture 161, 355–362.

Shiau, S.-Y., Chin, Y.H., 1999. Estimation of dietary biotin requirement of juvenile hybrid tilapia, *Oreochromis niloticus* × *O. aureus*. Aquaculture 170, 71–78.

Shiau, S.-Y., Lei, M.S., 1999. Feeding strategy does affect carbohydrate utilization by hybrid tilapia, *Oreochromis niloticus* × *O. aureus*. Fisheries Science 65, 553–557.

Shiau, S.-Y., Yu, Y.P., 1999. Dietary supplementation of chitin and chitosan depresses growth in tilapia, *Oreochromis niloticus* × *O. aureus*. Aquaculture 179, 439–446.

Shiau, S.-Y., Lo, P.S., 2000. Dietary choline requirements of juvenile hybrid tilapia, *Oreochromis niloticus* × *O. aureus*. Journal of Nutrition 130, 100–103.

Shiau, S.-Y., Hsieh, J.F., 2001. Quantifying the dietary potassium requirement of juvenile hybrid tilapia, *Oreochromis niloticus* × *O. aureus*. British Journal of Nutrition 85, 213–218.

Shiau, S.-Y., Shiau, L.F., 2001. Reevaluation of the vitamin E requirement of juvenile tilapia, *Oreochromis niloticus* × *O. aureus*. Animal Science 72, 529–534.

Shiaut, S.Y., Ning, Y.C., 2003. Estimation of dietary copper requirements of juvenile tilapia, *Oreochromis niloticus* × *O. aureus*. Animal Science 77, 287–292.

Shiau, S.Y., Su, L.-W., 2003. Ferric citrate is half as effective as ferrous sulfate in meeting the iron requirement of juvenile tilapia, *Oreochromis niloticus* × *O. aureus*. Journal of Nutrition 133, 483–488.

Shiau, S.-Y., Su, S.-L., 2005. Juvenile tilapia (*Oreochromis niloticus* × *O. aureus*) requires dietary myo-inositol for maximal growth. Aquaculture 243, 273–277.

Shiau, S.-Y., Tseng, H.-C., 2007. Dietary calcium requirements of juvenile tilapia, *Oreochromis niloticus* × *O. aureus*, reared in fresh water. Aquaculture Nutrition 13, 298–303.

Siddiqui, A.Q., Al Hafedh, Y.S., Ali, S.A., 1998. Effect of dietary protein level on the reproductive performance of Nile tilapia, *Oreochromis niloticus* (L.). Aquaculture Research 29, 349–358.

Sing, K., Kamarudin, M., Wilson, J., Azirun, M., 2014. Evaluation of blowfly (*Chrysomya megacephala*) maggot meal as an effective, sustainable replacement for fishmeal in the diet of farmed juvenile red tilapia (*Oreochromis* sp.). Pakistan Veterinary Journal 34, 288–292.

Skillicorn, P., Spira, W., Journey, W., 1993. Duckweed Aquaculture: A New Aquatic Farming System for Developing Countries. The World Bank, Washington, D.C., 76 pp.

Sklan, D., Prag, T., Lupatsch, I., 2004. Apparent digestibility coefficients of feed ingredients and their prediction in diets for tilapia *Oreochromis niloticus* × *Oreochromis aureus* (Teleostei, Cichlidae). Aquaculture Research 35, 358–364.

Soliman, A.K., Wilson, R.P., 1992a. Water-soluble vitamin requirements of tilapia. 1. Pantothenic acid requirement of blue tilapia, *Oreochromis aureus*. Aquaculture 104, 121–126.

Soliman, A.K., Wilson, R.P., 1992b. Water-soluble vitamin requirements of tilapia. 2. Riboflavin requirement of blue tilapia, *Oreochromis aureus*. Aquaculture 104, 309–314.

Soliman, A.K., Jauncey, K., Roberts, R.J., 1994. Water-soluble vitamin requirements of tilapia: ascorbic acid (vitamin C) requirement of Nile tilapia, *Oreochromis niloticus*. Aquaculture and Fisheries Management 25, 269–278.

Stickney, R.R., McGeachin, R.B., Robinson, E.H., Arnold, G., Suter, L., 1982. Growth of *Tilapia aurea* as a function of degree of dietary lipid saturation. Proceedings of the Annual Conference of Southeastern Association of Fish and Wildlife Agencies 36, 172–181.

Stickney, R.R., McGeachin, R.B., 1983. Effects of dietary lipid quality on growth and food conversion of tilapia. Proceedings of the Annual Conference Southeastern Association of Fish and Wildlife Agencies 37, 352–357.

Stickney, R.R., McGeachin, R.B., Lewis, D.H., Marks, J., Sis, R.F., Robinson, E.H., et al., 1984. Response of *Tilapia aurea* to dietary vitamin C. Journal of the World Mariculture Society 15, 179–185.

Stickney, R.R., Wurts, W.A., 1986. Growth response of blue tilapia to selected levels of dietary menhaden and catfish oils. Progressive Fish-Culturist 48, 107–109.

Sugita, H., Miyajima, C., Deguchi, Y., 1990. The vitamin B_{12}- producing ability of intestinal bacteria isolated from tilapia and channel catfish. Nippon Suisan Gakkaishi 56, 701.

Sugiura, S.H., Hardy, R.W., Roberts, R.J., 2004. The pathology of phosphorus deficiency in fish-a review. Journal of Fish Diseases 27, 255–265.

Tacon, A.G.J., Jauncey, K., Falaye, A., Pantah, M., MacGowen, I., Stafford, E., 1983. The use of meat and bone meal, hydrolyzed feather meal and soybean meal in practical fry and fingerling diets for *Oreochromis niloticus*. In: Fishelson, L., Yaron, Z. (Eds.), Proceedings of the International Symposium on Tilapia in Aquaculture. Tel-Aviv University, Israel, pp. 356–365.

Tacon, A.G.J., Jackson, A.J., 1985. Utilization of conventional and unconventional protein sources in practical fish feeds. In: Cowey, C.B.,

Mackie, A.M., Bell, J.G. (Eds.), Nutrition and Feeding in Fish. Academic Press, London, pp. 119–145.

Takagi, S., Murata, H., Goto, T., Endo, M., Yamashita, H., Ukawa, M., 2008. Taurine is an essential nutrient for yellowtail *Seriola quinqueradiata* fed non-fish meal diets based on soy protein concentrate. Aquaculture 280, 198–205.

Takeuchi, T., Satoch, S., Watanabe, T., 1983. Requirement of *Tilapia nilotica* for essential fatty acids. Nippon Suisan Gakkaishi 49, 1127–1134.

Tang, L., Huang, K., Xie, J., Yu, D., Sun, L., Huang, Q., et al., 2017. Dietary copper affects antioxidant and immune activity in hybrid tilapia (*Oreochromis niloticus* × *Oreochromis aureus*). Aquaculture Nutrition 23, 1003–1015.

Teixeira, C.P., Barros, M.M., Pezzato, L.E., Fernandes Jr., A.C., Koch, J.F.A., Padovani, C.R., 2012. Growth performance of Nile tilapia, *Oreochromis niloticus*, fed diets containing levels of pyridoxine and haematological response under heat stress. Aquaculture Research 43, 1081–1088.

Teoh, C.-Y., Ng, W.-K., 2016. The implications of substituting dietary fish oil with vegetable oils on the growth performance, fillet fatty acid profile and modulation of the fatty acid elongase, desaturase and oxidation activities of red hybrid tilapia, *Oreochromis* sp. Aquaculture 465, 311–322.

Teshima, S., Kanazawa, A., Uchiyama, Y., 1985a. Optimum protein levels in casein-gelatin diets for *Tilapia nilotica* fingerlings. Memoirs of the Faculty of Fisheries, Kagoshima University 34, 45–52.

Teshima, S., Kanazawa, A., Uchiyama, Y., 1985b. Effects of dietary protein, lipid and digestible carbohydrate levels on the weight gain, feed conversion efficiency and protein efficiency ratio of *Tilapia nilotica*. Memoirs of the Kagoshima University, Research Centre for the South Pacific 6, 56–71.

Teshima, S., Kanazawa, A., 1988. Nutritive value of methionine-enriched soy plastein for *Oreochromis niloticus* fry. In: Pullin, R.S.V., Bhukaswan, T., Tonguthai, K., Maclean, J.L. (Eds.), Proceedings of the Second International Symposium on Tilapia in Aquaculture. ICLARM Conference Proceedings No. 15. Department of Fisheries, Thailand, and ICLARM, Manila, Philippines, pp. 393–399.

Thompson, K.R., Velasquez, A., Patterson, J.T., Metts, L.S., Webster, C.D., Brady, Y.J., et al., 2012. Evaluation of plant and animal protein sources as partial or total replacement of fish meal in diets for Nile tilapia fry and juvenile stages. North American Journal of Aquaculture 74, 365–375.

Thongprajukaew, K., Kovitvadhi, S., Kovitvadhi, U., Preprame, P., 2017. Effects of feeding frequency on growth performance and digestive enzyme activity of sex-reversed Nile tilapia, *Oreochromis niloticus* (Linnaeus, 1758). Agriculture and Natural Resources 51, 292–298.

Tian, J., Wu, F., Yang, C.G., Jiang, M., Liu, W., Wen, H., 2015. Dietary lipid levels impact lipoprotein lipase, hormone-sensitive lipase, and fatty acid synthetase gene expression in three tissues of adult GIFT strain of Nile tilapia, *Oreochromis niloticus*. Fish Physiology and Biochemistry 41, 1–18.

Tung, P.H., Shiau, S.-Y., 1991. Effect of meal frequency on growth performance of hybrid tilapia, *Oreochromis niloticus* × *O. aureus*, fed different carbohydrate diets. Aquaculture 92, 343–350.

Tung, P.H., Shiau, S.-Y., 1993. Carbohydrate utilization versus body size in tilapia, *Oreochromis niloticus* × *O. aureus*. Comparative Biochemistry and Physiology 104A, 585–588.

Twibell, R.G., Brown, P.B., 1998. Optimal dietary protein concentration for hybrid tilapia *(Oreochromis niloticus* × *Oreochromis aureus)* fed all-plant diets. Journal of the World Aquaculture Society 29, 9–16.

Ulla Rojas, J.B., Weerd, H.V., 1997. The growth and feed utilization of *Oreochromis aureus* fingerlings fed diets with various coffee pulp levels. In: Fitzsimmons, K. (Ed.), Proceedings from the Fourth International Symposium on Tilapia in Aquaculture. Northeast Regional Agriculture Engineering Service, Ithaca, New York, USA, pp. 40–49.

Velásquez, Y.C., Kijora, C., Wuertz, S., Schulz, C., 2015. Effect of fermented aquatic macrophytes supplementation on growth performance, feed efficiency and digestibility of Nile tilapia (*Oreochromis niloticus*) juveniles fed low fishmeal diets. Livestock Research for Rural Development 27 (9), 1–8.

Viola, S., Zohar, G., 1984. Nutrition studies with market size hybrids of tilapia (*Oreochromis*). in intensive culture. Bamidgeh 36, 3–15.

Viola, S., Zohar, G., Arieli, Y., 1986. Phosphorus requirements and its availability from different sources for intensive pond culture species in Israel. Part 1. Tilapia. Bamidgeh 38, 3–12.

Viola, S., Arieli, Y., Zohar, G., 1988. Animal-protein-free feeds for hybrid tilapia (*Oreochromis niloticus* × *O. aureus*) in intensive culture. Aquaculture 75, 115–125.

Wang, A.M., Han, G.M., Feng, G.N., Yang, W.P., Guo, J.H., Wang, T., et al., 2011. Effects of dietary lipid levels on growth performance, nutrient digestibility and blood biochemical indices of GIFT tilapia (*Oreochromis niloticus*). Acta Hydrobiologica Sinica 35, 80–87.

Wang, K., Takeuchi, T., Watanabe, T., 1985. Effect of dietary protein levels on growth of *Tilapia nilotica*. Bulletin of the Japanese Society of Scientific FIsheries 51, 133–140.

Wang, L., Li, J., Jin, J.N., Zhu, F., Roffeis, M., Zhang, X.Z., 2017. A comprehensive evaluation of replacing fishmeal with housefly (*Musca domestica*) maggot meal in the diet of Nile tilapia (*Oreochromis niloticus*): growth performance, flesh quality, innate immunity and water environment. Aquaculture Nutrition 23, 983–993.

Wang, X.-X., Chen, M.-y., Wang, K., Ye, J.-d., 2017. Growth and metabolic responses in Nile tilapia (*Oreochromis niloticus*) subjected to varied starch and protein levels of diets. Italian Journal of Animal Science 16, 308–316.

Wassef, E.A., Plammer, G., Poxton, M., 1988. Protease digestion of the meals of ungerminated and germinated soybeans. Journal of Food Science and Agriculture 44, 201–214.

Wassef, E.A., Sweilam, M.A., Attalah, R.F., 2003. The use of fermented fish silage as a replacement for fish meal in Nile tilapia (*Oreochromis niloticus*) diets. Egyptian Journal of Nutrition and Feeds 6, 357–370.

Watanabe, T., Takeuchi, T., Murakami, A., Ogino, C., 1980. The availability to *Tilapia nilotica* of phosphorus in white fish meal. Bulletin of the Japanese Society of Scientific FIsheries 46, 897–899.

Watanabe, T., Satoh, S., Takeuchi, T., 1988. Availability of minerals in fish meal to fish. Asian Fisheries Science 1, 175–195.

Watanabe, T., Takeuchi, T., Satoh, S., Kiron, V., 1996. Digestible crude protein contents in various feedstuffs determined with four freshwater fish species. Fisheries Science 62, 278–282.

Watanabe, W.O., Clark, J.H., Dunhkam, J.B., Wicklund, R.I., Olla, B.L., 1990. Culture of Florida red tilapia in marine cages: the effects of stocking and dietary protein on growth. Aquaculture 90, 123–134.

Wee, K.L., Tuan, N.A., 1988. Effects of dietary protein level on growth and reproduction of Nile tilapia (*Oreochromis niloticus*). In: Pullin, R.S.V., Bhukaswan, T., Tonguthai, K., Maclean, J.L. (Eds.), Proceedings of the Second International Symposium on Tilapia in

Aquaculture. ICLARM Conference Proceedings No. 15. Department of Fisheries, Thailand and ICLARM, Manila, Philippines, pp. 401–410.

Wilson, R.P., Harding, D.E., Garling Jr., D.L., 1977. The effect of dietary pH on amino acid utilization and the lysine requirement of fingerling channel catfish. Journal of Nutrition 107, 166–170.

Wilson, R.P., Freeman, D.W., Poe, E.W., 1984. Three types of catfish offal meals for channel catfish fingerlings. Progressive Fish-Culturist 46, 126–132.

Winfree, R.A., Stickney, R.R., 1981. Effects of dietary protein and energy on growth, feed conversion efficiency and body composition of *Tilapia aurea*. Journal of Nutrition 111, 1001–1012.

Wu, F., Huang, F., Wen, H., Jiang, M., Liu, W., Tian, J., et al., 2015. Vitamin C requirement of adult genetically improved farmed tilapia, *Oreochromis niloticus*. Aquaculture International 23, 1203–1215.

Wu, F., Jiang, M., Wen, H., Liu, W., Tian, J., Yang, C.G., et al., 2017. Dietary vitamin E effects on growth, fillet textural parameters, and antioxidant capacity of genetically improved farmed tilapia (GIFT), *Oreochromis niloticus*. Aquaculture International 25, 991–1003.

Wu, Y.V., Rosati, R.R., Sessa, D., Brown, P.B., 1995. Utilization of corn gluten feed by Nile tilapia. Progressive Fish-Culturist 57, 305–309.

Yao, Y.F., Jiang, M., Wen, H., Wu, F., Liu, W., Tian, J., et al., 2014. Dietary phosphorus requirement of GIFT strain of Nile tilapia *Oreochromis niloticus* reared in freshwater. Aquaculture Nutrition 20, 273–280.

Yildirim-Aksoy, M., Lim, C., Davis, D.A., Shelby, R., Klesius, P.H., 2007. Influence of dietary lipid sources on the growth performance, immune response and resistance of Nile tilapia, *Oreochromis niloticus*, to *Streptococcus iniae* challenge. Journal of Applied Aquaculture 19, 29–49.

Younis, E.M., Al-Quffail, A.S., Al-Asgah, N.A., Abdel-Warith, A.A., Al-Hafedh, Y.S., 2018. Effect of dietary fish meal replacement by red algae, *Gracilaria arcuata*, on growth performance and body composition of Nile tilapia *Oreochromis niloticus*. Saudi Journal of Biological Sciences 25, 198–203.

Yue, Y., Zou, Z., Zhu, J., Li, D., Xiao, W., Han, J., et al., 2015. Effects of dietary arginine on growth performance, feed utilization, haematological parameters and non-specific immune responses of juvenile Nile tilapia (*Oreochromis niloticus* L.). Aquaculture Research 46, 1801–1809.

Zaminhan, M., Boscolo, W.R., Neu, D.H., Feiden, A., Furuya, V.R.B., Furuya, W.M., 2017. Dietary tryptophan requirements of juvenile Nile tilapia fed corn-soybean meal-based diets. Animal Feed Science and Technology 227, 62–67.

Zhang, Y.-F., Yue, Y.-R., Tian, L.-X., Liu, Y.-J., Wang, A.-L., Yang, H.-J., et al., 2015. Dietary phosphorus requirements of juvenile hybrid tilapia (*Oreochromis niloticus*♀ × *O. aureus*♂) fed fishmeal-free practical diets. Israeli Journal of Aquaculture – Bamidgeh 67, 1179–1191.

Zhao, H.X., Cao, J.M., Liu, X.H., Zhu, X., Chen, S.C., Lan, H.B., et al., 2011. Effect of supplemental dietary zinc sources on the growth and carbohydrate utilization of tilapia Smith 1840, *Oreochromis niloticus* × *Oreochromis aureus*. Aquaculture Nutrition 17, 64–72.

Further reading

Abdel-Ghany, H.M., El-Sayed, A.-F.M., Ezzat, A.A., Essa, M.A., Helal, A.M., 2019. Dietary lipid sources affect cold tolerance of Nile tilapia *(Oreochromis niloticus)*. Journal of Thermal Biology 79, 50–55.

Green, B.W., Rawles, S.D., Schrader, K.K., Gaylord, T.G., McEntire, M.E., 2019. Effects of dietary protein content on hybrid tilapia (*Oreochromis aureus* × *O. niloticus*) performance, common microbial off-flavor compounds, and water quality dynamics in an outdoor biofloc technology production system. Aquaculture 503, 571–582.

Hassaan, M.S., El-Sayed, A.I.M., Soltan, M.A., Iraqi, M.M., Goda, A.M., Davies, S.J., et al., 2019. Partial dietary fish meal replacement with cotton seed meal and supplementation with exogenous protease alters growth, feed performance, hematological indices and associated gene expression markers (GH, IGF-I) for Nile tilapia. *Oreochromis niloticus*, Aquaculture 503, 282–292.

Kabir, K.A., Schrama, J.W., Verreth, J.A.J., Phillips, M.J., Verdegem, M.C.J., 2019. Effect of dietary protein to energy ratio on performance of nile tilapia and food web enhancement in semi-intensive pond aquaculture. Aquaculture 499, 235–242.

Li, E., Lim, C., Cai, C., Klesius, P.H., 2011. Growth response and resistance to *Streptococcus iniae* of Nile tilapia, *Oreochromis niloticus*, fed diets containing different levels of wheat distiller's dried grains with solubles with or without lysine supplementation. Animal Feed Science and Technology 170, 246–255.

Li, X.-Q., Zhang, X.-Q., Kabir Chowdhury, M.A., Zhang, Y., Leng, X.-J., 2019. Dietary phytase and protease improved growth and nutrient utilization in tilapia (*Oreochromis niloticus* × *Oreochromis aureus*) fed low phosphorus and fishmeal-free diets. Aquaculture Nutrition 25, 46–55.

Mufatto, L.M., Nobrega, R.O., Menoyo, D., Fracalossi, D.M., 2019. Dietary ratios of n-3/n-6 fatty acids do not affect growth of Nile tilapia at optimal temperatures (28°C) nor at temperatures that simulate the onset of winter (22°C). Aquaculture Nutrition 25, 646–661.

Chapter 8

Reproduction and seed production

Chapter outline

8.1 Introduction

As mentioned in Chapter 1, tilapia culture is expanding at an extremely high rate. The more tilapia culture is expanded, the more it becomes vital to produce sufficient amounts of seeds to meet the increasing demand of tilapia farmers. The current status of tilapia culture in many countries suggests that there is a gap between seed supplies and farmers' demand. Tilapia seed producers are also usually faced with a number of constraints that limit the management of mass seed production (Little et al., 1993; Bhujel, 2000). These include early maturation of tilapia, which may lead to overcrowding and fish stunting, low fecundity, successive reproductive cycles and asynchronous spawning. Despite tilapia seeds being easily produced in captivity, poor broodstock and hatchery management can result in reduced growth rates of produced seeds. In many cases, produced seeds suffer from poor quality, low survival, deformation, genetic pollution and lack of traceability (Mohan, 2007).

Generally speaking, the major weaknesses and threats of tilapia seed production are as follows:

- Poor quality broodstock;
- Insufficient quality seed supply, particularly in Africa;
- Poor seed production facilities and infrastructures;
- High hatchery operating costs (feeds, chemicals, electricity, fuel, etc.);
- Poor hatchery management;
- Unregulated imported seed;
- Poor seed dissemination and marketing strategies;

Tilapia Culture. https://doi.org/10.1016/B978-0-12-816541-6.00008-8
Copyright © 2020 Elsevier Inc. All rights reserved.

- Poor standardization and certification systems;
- Poor governance and legislation and
- Increased chances of disease transfer.

Therefore, understanding the value chain of tilapia reproduction and seed production is essential for sustainable, cost-effective and high-quality tilapia seed production. In other words, facing the above weaknesses and gabs is necessary for optimizing hatchery operation and maximizing tilapia culture outputs.

This chapter addresses the major issues of tilapia reproduction, including modes of reproduction, broodstock management, hatchery management, environmental factors and larval rearing. It is hoped that such discussion will clarify the so many problems associated with tilapia seed production and improve our understanding of tilapia reproduction and seed production.

8.2 Modes of reproduction

Tilapia are currently divided into two main generic groups according to their modes of reproduction:

1. 'Substrate spawners' (guarders), which include the fishes belonging to the genus *Tilapia* (e.g. *Tilapia zillii*, *T. rendalli*) (Coward and Bromage, 2000). For substrate spawners, both males and females build and defend the nest and protect the fertilized eggs and hatched larvae until they become independent of their parents. The courtship in these fishes lasts for several days (Coward and Bromage, 2000).
2. 'Mouthbrooders', where fertilized eggs are incubated into the parents' buccal cavities (Fig. 8.1). This group is further divided into two genera:
   (a) *Oreochromis* (maternal mouthbrooders), including *Oreochromis niloticus*, *O. aureus*, *O. mossambicus*, where only females brood the eggs in their mouths.
   (b) *Sarotherodon* (biparental mouthbrooders) (e.g. *Sarotherodon galilaeus*), where both males and females brood and defend the fertilized eggs and hatched fry, and paternal mouthbrooders (e.g. *S. melanotheron*) where only males brood the eggs (Turner and Robinson, 2000). Courtship in these fishes lasts for several hours to several days (Rana, 1990a; Coward and Bromage, 2000).

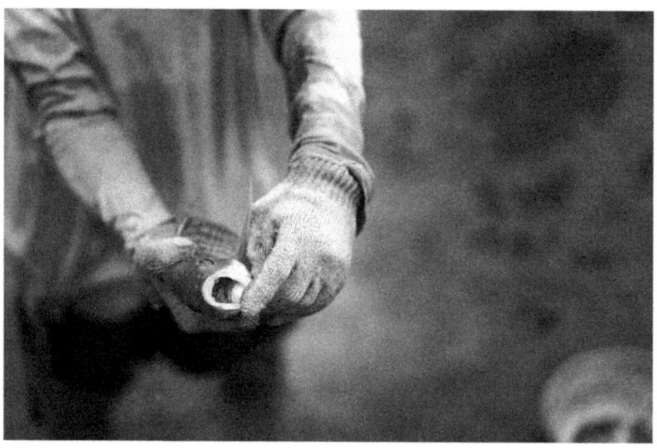

FIGURE 8.1 Eggs are being released from mouthbrooding Nile tilapia female. *Photo provided by Shutterstock.*

The majority of cultured tilapia belong to the maternal mouthbrooding *Oreochromis* genus, where Nile tilapia alone represented 70.2% of global production of farmed tilapia in 2017 (FAO, 2019). The reproduction mode of this species is quite interesting. Breeding starts with building and defending the spawning territory by the males, followed by courtship between resident male and visiting female which lasts for only few hours (Rana, 1990a) after which egg releasing and fertilization occurs. Nile tilapia female repeatedly releases a string of about 20–50 eggs, then the male passes right over the eggs, with his genital papilla pressing against the bottom of the nest or tank bottom, and release a cloud of milky milt. The female returns immediately and picks the fertilized eggs into her mouth.

Studies have shown that Nile tilapia egg fertilization also occurs inside the female's mouth (not outside). Mansour (2001) observed that Nile tilapia female releases the eggs on the bottom of the aquarium and immediately collects them into her mouth before fertilization. Then, the male comes closer with his genital papilla near the female's mouth and starts releasing his milky milt, where the female starts sucking it into the mouth. This process usually lasts for about 4–6 min, after which the female leaves the spawning area. Similar observations have been reported by Myers and Hershberger (1991) and Goncalves-de-Freitas and Nishida (1998). This phenomenon has also been recorded in another tilapia, *O. macrochir* (Fryer and Iles, 1972).

Another strange and interesting phenomenon of Nile tilapia reproduction is the 'sneaking' behaviour of subordinate males. Goncalves-de-Freitas and Nishida (1998) found that the dominant male establishes a territory, constructs nests and attracts the female. However, in a number of cases the authors observed that a subordinate male sneaks between the spawning couple after egg delivery and starts releasing milt near the female's mouth and close to the released eggs. The female then sucks the milt and picks up the eggs into her mouth. The authors suggested that these two mating tactics (territorial and sneaking) could be a part of an evolutionary stable strategy. Sneaking behaviour has also been reported in another mouthbrooding cichlid species, *Pseudosimochromis curvifrons* (Kuwamura, 1987).

From the foregoing discussion, it is clear that fertilization of the eggs of some tilapia species (e.g. *O. niloticus* and *O. macrochir*) occurs inside and/or outside the females' mouth. It is not known 'when' and 'why' these fish prefer either method. Also, the question concerning why only some subordinate males display sneaking behaviour remains to be answered.

8.3 Age and size at first maturity

The age and size at first maturity of tilapia vary considerably between species, and even within strains of same species (Macintosh and Little, 1995; Bhujel, 2000). Under favourable natural conditions, Nile tilapia reach their sexual maturity at a size of 20–30 cm (150–250 g) (Lowe-Mcconnell, 1958; Trewavas, 1983). However, tilapia may mature at small sizes in many parts of the world; a phenomenon indicating that these fishes are under stressful environmental conditions and/or overexploitation (Duponchelle and Panfili, 1998; Duponchelle and Legendre, 2000).

In a natural habitat, age and size at first maturity of tilapia are affected by environmental conditions (Lowe-Mcconnell, 1982), geographical barriers (Faunce, 2000), overfishing (Ojuok et al., 2007), food supply (Santiago et al., 1985; Siddiqui et al., 1997; El-Sayed et al., 2003) and water body area (Duponchelle and Panfili, 1998). Duponchelle and Panfili (1998) found that age and size at maturity of Nile tilapia collected from large and small water bodies were positively correlated with the reservoir area. They also found that the range of variation in age at first maturity between populations was much higher than that of size at maturity. The authors suggested that these variations may have been related to the differences in environmental variables (phenotypic plasticity) rather than the genetic differences.

Under aquaculture conditions, tilapia generally mature at smaller sizes than in natural environments. De Graaf et al. (1999) and El-Sayed et al. (2003) found that farmed Nile tilapia reach their first maturation at about 30 g. Generally speaking, the size at first maturation of Nile tilapia females under aquaculture conditions ranges from 30 to 50 g, as has been reported by Siraj et al. (1983), Lester et al. (1988), De Silva and Radampola (1990) and Mansour (2001). This size is considerably small compared with a size of 150–250 g (20–30 cm) at which these fish mature under favourable natural conditions (Lowe-Mcconnell, 1958; Gwahaba, 1973).

Feed quantity and quality and feeding regimes also affect size at first maturity and productivity of tilapia broodfish. Many authors found that the mean weight of Nile tilapia at first spawning tended to increase with increasing dietary protein level (De Silva and Radampola, 1990; El-Sayed et al., 2003).

8.4 Fecundity and egg characteristics

Fecundity can be defined in various ways, including the following:

1. Potential fecundity: the number of mature eggs in female's ovary immediately before spawning (Payne and Collinson, 1983). This definition assumes that all ripening oocytes are ovulated and only few eggs are retained in the ovary after spawning (Coward and Bromage, 2000). This definition, however, may not fit with multiple-spawning fishes such as tilapia, as it underestimates their fecundities (Wootton, 1979).
2. Fecundity can also be defined as the number of fry produced by tilapia female throughout its lifetime (Lowe-McConnell, 1955). This definition may not also be appropriate for tilapia under aquaculture conditions because broodstocks are used only for a relatively short time during their optimum reproduction period (Rana, 1990a). It was suggested, therefore, that the definition of fecundity should be restricted to 'the number of fry produced per year' (Mires, 1982). This modified definition takes into account (1) the effects of environmental factors, (2) the underestimation of reproductive potential because the number of fry is often less than the number of eggs released and (3) that the correlation between the number of eggs and number of fry released may be weak.

Tilapia are characterized by low fecundity and relatively large egg size (Lowe-McConnell, 1959; Peters, 1983; Duponchelle et al., 1997). For example, Nile tilapia produce from <100 to >3000 eggs per spawn, with egg size ranging from <2 to 7.9 mm (De Graaf et al., 1999). On the other hand, substrate spawners produce much higher numbers of smaller eggs (1–1.5 mm) than mouthbrooding tilapia (Wohlfarth and Hulata, 1983; Coward and Bromage, 1999). The fecundity and egg sizes of various tilapias reared under different environmental and culture conditions are summarized in Table 8.1.

In most tilapias, fecundity varies considerably among fishes of the same species, and even among females of similar sizes, especially in large fish classes (Coward and Bromage, 1999). In addition, fecundity and egg size are directly related to fish size, length or age, but with high variability (Rana, 1986; Little, 1989; Ridha and Cruz, 1989). Little (1989) found that small Nile tilapia broodfish produced many more eggs, with shorter spawning intervals, than large fish, over a period of 105–116 days. However, larger females usually produce more eggs per clutch than smaller females. On the other hand, eggs per spawn were found to correlate with maternal age, but not with body weight (Getinet, 2008). Eggs per spawn of females of 4, 9, 16 and 24 months, increased by twofold between 4- and

TABLE 8.1 Optimum fecundity of different tilapias at different sex ratios and stocking rates.

Species	Culture system	Fish weight (g) Male	Fish weight (g) Female	♂:♀ ratio	Stocking density m^{-3}	Eggs female^{-1} (average)	Remark	Reference
Oreochromis niloticus	Glass aquaria		42–75	1:3	28	305–753 (507) spawn^{-1}	Fed 40% cp in fresh water	El-Sayed et al. (2003)
	Closed	162–211	112–177	1:3	4	3165 kg^{-1} mo^{-1} (678)	Fed 45% cp	Ridha and Cruz (1999)
	Closed	117–177	92–160	1:3	20	50.9 kg^{-1} d^{-1}	Photoperiod of 2500 lux, for 18 h	Ridha and Cruz (2000)
	Concrete tanks	439	206	1:3	1.67	39.1 g^{-1} (1328)	Fed 45% cp	Siddiqui et al. (1998)
O. niloticus × *O. aureus*	Concrete, outdoor tanks	226	189–294	1:2	2	18.8 kg^{-1} d^{-1}	Fed 34% cp	Siddiqui and Harbi (1997)
	Concrete, outdoor tanks	226	294–437	1:3	2	25.3 kg^{-1} d^{-1}	Fed 34% cp	Siddiqui and Harbi (1997)
Tilapia zillii	Glass aquaria		29–419	1:2		461–11,640 (4.9–84.3 g^{-1})		Coward and Bromage (1999)

24-month-old females. Percent fertilization and hatchability decreased with age of females. The author concluded that optimum age range for reproducible production of good quality eggs is 6–18 months. It was also found that large eggs contain more yolk and lead to larger fry with better growth and higher resistance to starvation and severe environmental conditions (Rana and Macintosh, 1988). The direct correlation between fish size and fecundity was not found in *T. zillii* (Coward and Bromage, 1999), *T. tholloni* and *S. melanotheron* (Peters, 1983).

One may ask whether it is better to use small broodfish which could collectively yield more eggs per culture unit, or larger fish with higher individual egg production, but at longer intervals. The decision should be taken by hatchery managers, based on the preset objectives and targeted outputs.

8.5 Broodstock management

The achievement of maximum sustainable seed production of tilapia depends, to a large extent, on broodstock management. Information on broodstock selection, nutrition, fecundity, stocking density, sex ratio and environmental conditions is crucial for maximizing hatchery production efficiency. It is of paramount importance to highlight these parameters.

8.5.1 Broodstock selection

Maintaining pure, high-quality broodstock is probably the core of successful seed production. The selection of proper broodfish will certainly have subsequent effects on the quantity and quality of produced offspring. Husbandry of broodstock during gonads development and maturation is also essential for quality seed production. The following measures/characteristics should be considered in broodstock selection:

1. Broodfish should be genetically pure, and fishes from unknown or questionable origins must be avoided.
2. Broodfish should not be too small because small fish are less fecund and less efficient at egg incubation and fry protection (Rana, 1986).
3. Broodfish should not be too old, and must not have spawned several times, because fecundity decreases with maternal age and successive spawnings (Rana, 1986). Increased spawning frequency may also result in poor quality seed.
4. Broodfish should be in good shape and free of deformities and injuries.
5. Inferior and unwanted tilapia must be prevented from entering broodstock ponds; therefore, incoming water should be filtered continuously.

8.5.2 Stocking density and sex ratio

Maintaining the correct stocking density and sex ratio of farmed tilapia will certainly improve hatchery efficiency and mass production of tilapia seeds. Suboptimal broodstock density will result in low seed production (Mires, 1982). Also, high broodfish density often reduces seed production (Bevis, 1994), presumably due to aggression and fighting between males leading to reduction in courtship, egg fertilization and incubation (Behrends and Smitherman, 1983; Ridha and Cruz, 1999). Guerrero (1982) reported also that tilapia mucus contains a substance that may cause autoallergic responses and inhibit reproduction at high broodstock densities. Similarly, the percentage of spawning females of *O. niloticus* × *O. hornorum* hybrids was inversely correlated with broodfish stocking density, due to chemical or behavioural factors (Lovshin, 1982).

Several stocking densities have been suggested for optimum seed production of tilapia, depending on tilapia species, broodstock size and condition, culture systems and water quality. Therefore, it is no surprise that varying, and sometimes controversial, results have been reported on the relationship between stocking density of broodstock and seed production. Hughes and Behrends (1983) suggested that 5 fish m^{-2} be adopted for optimum seed production of Nile tilapia in suspended net enclosures. On the other hand, only 29% of Nile tilapia females reared in hapas in ponds in Thailand spawned at 10 fish m^{-2}, compared to 39% and 42% at 5 and 2.5 m^{-2} (Bevis, 1994). In the meantime, Little (1992) found that six fish m^{-2} was most optimum for Nile tilapia reared in hapas suspended in fertilized ponds. Meanwhile, Ridha and Cruz (1999) found that 4 fish m^{-2} had better seed production and spawning synchrony than at 8 and 12 fish m^{-2}. Table 8.1 summarizes the sex ratios and stocking densities suggested for optimum seed production of different tilapias.

Extensive work has been carried out on sex ratios of tilapia broodstock because suboptimal ratio leads to reduction in seed production, waste of resources and unnecessary increase in running costs. Therefore, different sex ratios have been adopted for different tilapias, with varying results. The male:female ratio ranges from 1:5 in ponds and 1:10 in tanks and hapas (Little and Hulata, 2000). A ratio of 1:<3 appears optimum, and is suggested, especially when synchronized spawning is required. Hughes and Behrends (1983) found that in Nile tilapia, a male:female ratio of 1:2 produced more seed than 1:3 ratio. Conversely, a male: female ratio of 1:2.5 and 1:3 produced more eggs than 1:1.5 and 1:2 in Nile tilapia (Akar, 2012). Mires (1982) reported also that 3:1 and 2:1 sex ratios in tilapia hybrids were more productive than 1:1 and 1:2 ratios, presumably due to the effects of 'male pressure' or the increase in spawning frequency of individual females. Nevertheless, it is uncommon to stock more males than females in spawning units, as this may lead to male aggression and fighting and cause severe harm to the females.

It is clear that no single sex ratio can be adopted for optimum reproduction efficiency of tilapia. It is the hatchery operator's job to decide the most appropriate sex ratio, taking into account the tilapia species, size and age, culture system and hatchery conditions. The optimum sex ratio may also be affected by the broodstock density. Broussard et al. (1983) found that increasing broodstock density, at a fixed male:female sex ratio of 1:3 had a negative effect on fry production of Nile tilapia reared in ponds. The authors referred that effect to the increasing competition between territorial males and/or constraints imposed by feed availability.

8.5.3 Spawning intervals

As stated earlier, one of the main characteristics of tilapia is their early maturity and asynchronous and successive spawning. They can spawn several times a year, if suitable ambient environmental and culture conditions are attained. In these multiple-spawning fishes, females' ovaries contain oocytes of different developmental stages. Coward and Bromage (1998) found that up to 20% of immediately postspawned *T. zillii* ovary was occupied by unspawned mature eggs. Residual eggs that progress into atresia have also been reported in postspawned *O. niloticus* ovaries (Peters, 1983). Immediately after spawning, the tilapia ovary regenerates very rapidly and previtellogenic stages are recruited into vitellogenic and late vitellogenic stages in as short as 1 week (Coward and Bromage, 1998, 2000).

As a result of different gonadal developmental stages in tilapia, spawning intervals are expected to vary considerably among species, and even within the same species. These intervals are influenced by fish size, age, stocking density, sex ratio, nutrition status, culture conditions and environmental factors. For example, Siraj et al. (1983) found that first- and second-year classes of Nile tilapia spawned at short intervals (7–12 days), while third-year class fish spawned at longer intervals (10–20 days). Getinet (2008) also reported that the age of tilapia females affects their spawning intervals. Nile tilapia females of the same age ensured consistent egg diameter, protein and lipid contents, fertilization and hatchability at a cost of altering fecundity and spawning interval. Temperature also influences the interspawning interval (Msiska and Costa-Pierce, 1997).

Many studies have also indicated that the removal of eggs and fry from females' mouths accelerates vitellogenesis and shortens the intervals between successive spawnings (Lovshin and Ibrahim, 1988; Tacon et al., 1996; Baroiller et al., 1997). Mair et al. (1993) found that the interspawning interval of Nile tilapia was 37.5% shorter when eggs were removed from females' mouths at 4-day intervals, as compared to females allowed to incubate their eggs naturally. Similarly, Baroiller et al. (1997) found that interspawning interval of incubating Nile tilapia females was 27 days compared to only 15 days in nonincubating groups. In addition, the removal of Nile tilapia eggs and fry from the mouths of females increases seed production (Little et al., 1993; Macintosh and Little, 1995). Macintosh and Little (1995) reported that removing eggs and fry of Nile tilapia at 5- and 10-day intervals has resulted in a significant increase in seed production kg^{-1} female day^{-1}, compared to seeds produced from natural incubation. A 5-day cycle of seed removal from females' mouths is a common practice in commercial tilapia hatcheries in Thailand (Bhujel, 2000). On the other hand, parental care may suppress the reproductive potential of tilapia (Lee, 1979). Therefore, longer interspawning intervals were reported in females naturally incubating their eggs. This has been attributed mainly to feed deprivation during brooding time, which usually leads to the delay of subsequent oogenesis (Lee, 1979; Tacon et al., 1996).

8.5.4 Broodstock exchange

Exchange of tilapia male and female broodfish, after a period of conditioning, could be an effective tool for improving seed production, spawning synchrony and spawning frequency. Conditioning is the separation of males and females in different conditioning units, at high densities, for a period of rest between spawnings (Bhujel, 2000). During this period, the fish must be provided with good quality feed and appropriate feeding regimes (Bhujel, 2000). Conditioning of tilapia broodstock has been a common practice in some Asian countries for many years.

Partial or total exchange of Nile tilapia females with resting females at 5–10-day intervals significantly improved seed and fry production (Macintosh and Little, 1995; Little et al., 2000). Costa-Pierce and Hadikusumah (1995) found that the best seed production was achieved at a rotation of 10–16 days. Seed production was negatively correlated with initial broodstock density and initial female body weight, but positively correlated with dietary protein level. Meanwhile, Lovshin and Ibrahim (1988) found that exchanging Nile tilapia male and female broodfish after 21 days of conditioning resulted in 16% increase in egg and fry production over a 105 day-spawning experiment, compared to nonexchange or female only exchange. Similar results have been reported by Little et al. (1993), where conditioned males and females produced more eggs and fry and spawned more frequently than nonconditioning or employing only conditioned females.

It should be emphasized that more frequent disturbance and exchange of broodfish or conditioning for long periods may lead to negative effects on reproduction efficiency. Little et al. (1993) found that conditioning of Nile tilapia females for 20 days caused 18% reduction in seed production, possibly due to the reabsorption of ripe eggs in the ovary, which occurs after about a week, if the females do not spawn, as reported by Peters (1983). The quality of fish sperms may also decline with resting for long time, due to continuous production and release of spermatozoa into the lumen of the testes, leading to negative effects on the sperm quality (Purdom, 1995). Based on these results, it is suggested that relatively short periods of resting (about 5–15 days) appear optimal for tilapia broodfish.

The positive effects of conditioning on reproduction efficiency of tilapia have been related to the higher activity of rested males in courtship, compared to nonrested males (Bhujel, 2000). Fertilization capacity of tilapia sperms may also be affected by resting conditions. Rana (1986) found that the fertilizing capacity of Nile tilapia sperms sharply decreased from about 90% to only 20% with increasing mating frequency, presumably due to the production of immature spermatozoa. Replacing old breeders with yearling breeders may also improve spawning efficiency. Smith et al. (1991) found that first-year class Florida red tilapia breeders produced more eggs and fry than year class two. The authors suggested that old breeders be replaced by younger yearling breeders.

8.6 Broodstock nutrition

Spawning performance and seed production of tilapia are directly related to broodstock nutrition (Watanabe et al., 1985; Bhujel et al., 2001; El-Sayed and Kawanna, 2008; El-Sayed et al., 2003, 2005a,b). Despite eggs being able to absorb some nutrients directly from water, egg yolk remains the major source of nutrition for embryonic development in fish. Exogenous nutrition of broodfish provides the essential nutrients required for gonadal development of females and the performance of produced seeds (Santiago et al., 1983; Gunasekera et al., 1997). Therefore, inadequate food supply for fish broodstock will lead to poor reproductive performance and seed production (Gunasekera et al., 1996a, 1996b; Gunasekera and Lam, 1997; Bhujel, 2000).

8.6.1 Protein requirements

Protein requirements of tilapia broodstock depend on species and size, dietary protein and energy sources, and rearing systems. Several studies have investigated the protein requirements of Nile tilapia broodstock, while little attention has been paid to other tilapia species. Most of these studies indicated that the size at first spawning, fecundity, spawning frequency and egg hatchability increased with increasing dietary protein level. Generally speaking, these fish require about 30%–45% dietary protein for optimum reproductive performance and seed production (Santiago et al., 1985; De Silva and Radampola, 1990; Gunasekera et al., 1995, 1996a; Siddiqui et al., 1998; Bhujel et al., 2001; El-Sayed et al., 2003; El-Sayed and Kawanna, 2008; de Oliveira et al., 2014). On the other hand, Cissé (1988) found that fecundity and spawning frequencies of *S. melanotheron* were not significantly affected by dietary protein levels. The protein requirements of tilapia broodstock are summarized in Table 8.2. More studies are needed to investigate the effects of dietary protein on reproductive output of other tilapia broodstocks.

The ratio between dietary protein and energy (P:E ratio) in fish feeds is crucially important for (1) ensuring the adequate use of energy and spare protein for anabolic processes, (2) avoiding restricting nutrient consumption due to high energy levels and (3) preventing the accumulation of excessive fats, which would adversely affect the health of reproducing fish (El-Sayed and Kawanna, 2008; Oliva-Teles, 2012). Nonetheless, the P:E ratio for tilapia broodstock is not well studied. Only a few studies have investigated the effects of P:E ratio in broodstock diets on their spawning performance, with varying, and sometimes contradictory, results. For example, El-Sayed and Kawanna (2008) fed Nile tilapia females diets containing 30%, 35% and 40% cp and 14.6, 16.7 and 18.8 MJ GE kg^{-1}. Spawning performances, including total number of spawnings per tank, number of spawnings per female, absolute fecundity and average number of eggs per spawn were all significantly lower at 30% cp than at higher protein levels. At all protein levels, increasing dietary energy from 14.6 to 18.8 MJ GE kg^{-1} resulted in a significant decrease in fish fecundity. At all energy levels, egg hatchability increased with increasing dietary protein levels. Regardless of dietary energy, eggs produced from broodstock fed 30% and 35% cp exhibited significantly lower hatchability and needed less time for hatching and yolk-sac absorption, and resulted in lower larval length than those fed a 40% protein diet. These results suggest that a diet containing 40% dietary protein and about 16.7 MJ GE kg^{-1} should be adopted for the best spawning performance of Nile tilapia broodstock reared in a recycling system.

On the contrary, Bombardelli et al. (2017) suggested that Nile tilapia females fed diets containing lower protein and energy levels produce a greater number of eggs per gram of body weight than those given higher levels. These authors fed female Nile tilapia with diets containing 28%, 34% and 40% digestible protein (DP), and 11.72, 14.23 and 16.74 MJ kg^{-1} digestible energy (DE). The absolute fecundity of females was not affected by dietary treatments, whereas the relative fecundity was inversely correlated to DE. This result suggests that the females fed diets with the lowest protein and energy levels used their body reserves in the reproductive process, ensuring egg production at the cost of somatic growth. The authors recommended the use of a diet containing 28% DP and 16.74 MJ kg^{-1} DE for Nile tilapia broodstock.

Dietary taurine was found to improve reproductive performance of Nile tilapia broodstock. Al-Feky et al. (2016) reported that 8 g kg^{-1} supplemental taurine

TABLE 8.2 Protein requirements (%) of Nile tilapia broodstock.

Range tested (%)	Requirement (%)	Culture system	Remarks	Reference
20–50	35	Closed	Isocaloric diets	Wee and Tuan (1988)
20–35	30	Closed		De Silva and Radampola (1990)
20 and 40	40	Outdoor tanks	Only two protein levels tested, natural food may have affected the results	Santiago et al. (1985)
10–35	35	Tanks	Isocaloric diets	Gunasekera et al. (1996a)
25–45	45			Siddiqui et al. (1998)
15.5, 25 and 30	30	Hapas in fertilized ponds	15.5%, 25% and 30% cp refer to herbivorous diet, large and small catfish pellets, respectively	Bhujel et al. (2001)
25–40	40	Glass aquaria	Isocaloric diets	El-Sayed et al. (2003)
25–45	40	Closed system	At 400 kcal GE 100 g^{-1}	El-Sayed and Kawanna (2008)
32–40	38	Masonry tanks	Continuous water flow	de Oliveira et al. (2014)
28–40 DP	28 DP	Hapa pens	At 16.74 MJ DE kg^{-1}	Bombardelli et al. (2017)

maximized spawning performances, including spawning frequencies, number of spawnings per female and absolute fecundity. Eggs produced from broodstock fed 8 g kg^{-1} taurine also exhibited higher hatchability and needed shorter time for hatching and yolk-sac absorption, as well as resulted in higher larval growth than other dietary taurine levels.

8.6.2 Lipid requirements

The quality and quantity of dietary lipids have been shown to significantly affect the reproduction of tilapia. A number of studies have considered the effects of dietary lipid source on the reproductive performance and tissue lipids of tilapia, with controversial results. Santiago and Reyes (1993) fed Nile tilapia broodstock diets containing different oil sources (cod liver oil, corn oil, soybean oil, coconut oil, or a mixture of cod liver oil and corn oil (1:1)) for 24 weeks. They found that fish fed the cod liver oil (rich in n-3 HUFA) had the best somatic growth, the highest level of lipid in the liver and muscle, but the poorest reproductive performance, while soybean oil (rich in n-6 FA) resulted in the highest overall reproductive performance. However, the results of Santiago and Reyes (1993) may be questionable, due to a number of reasons. First, the initial stocking sizes of males and females were very large (ranged from 95 to 128 g for males and 90–124 g for females). These fish may have spawned a number of times before stocking, which in turn may have affected their fecundity and spawning efficiency. Second, the energy content of the diets was very low (2.8 kcal g^{-1}, using the DE values of channel catfish). These energy values may have not been sufficient to meet both somatic and reproductive performances of the fish. Third, the male:female ratio adopted (1:1) may have led to male aggression and fighting, causing severe harm to the females, whereas the recommended sex ratio under aquarium conditions is 1:3 (or 1:>3) (Little and Hulata, 2000).

Contradictory results have been reported by El-Sayed et al. (2005a) who studied the effect of dietary lipid source and water salinity on spawning performance of Nile tilapia broodstock and growth of their larvae. The fish were fed diets with three different soybean oil:cod liver oil (SBO:CLO) ratios (5:0, 2:3 and 0:5) at three water salinities (0, 7 and 14‰) for 165 days. At 0‰, the size at first maturation, spawning intervals egg hatchability, days to hatch, yolk sac absorption time and larval weight were not significantly affected by dietary oil source, while the inclusion of fish oil (FO) in the diets increased the absolute fecundity and number of eggs per spawn at each salinity. At 7 and 14‰, fish fed CLO or CLO/SBO mix spawned at shorter intervals, and more frequently than those fed SBO. In addition, eggs produced from broodstock fed SBO at 7 and 14‰ needed more time for hatching and yolk-sac absorption and resulted in poorer larval weight than those fed CLO or CLO/SBO mix. This result indicates that either n-6 or n-3 fatty acids could meet the requirement of Nile tilapia broodfish reared at 0‰. At that salinity, fish fed n-3 essential fatty acids (EFAs) may also have sufficient ability to elongate and desaturate *18:2*n-6 into long chain FA, as reported by Kanazawa et al. (1980) and El-Sayed and Garling (1988). This result also reveals that Nile tilapia broodfish reared in brackish water (7 and 14‰) require a source of dietary n-3 HUFA for optimum spawning performance, while plant oil (SBO) may meet the requirements of broodfish reared in fresh water (0‰). Again, more work is needed to verify the relationship between dietary lipid levels and fatty acids and spawning performance of different tilapia species reared under different culture conditions.

Other oil sources, such as palm oil, may be used as an alternative, cost-effective dietary lipid source for tilapia broodstock. This assumption was tested by Ng and Wang (2011) who fed GIFT tilapia broodstock diets containing FO, FO and crude palm oil (CPO) (FO + CPO; 1:1), CPO or linseed oil (LSO) as lipid sources. CPO, either solely or in combination with FO, resulted in improved reproductive performance, compared to FO or LSO. First spawning occurred much earlier in fish fed CPO diet than at other oil sources. CPO-based diets also produced higher fecundity, higher spawning frequency (at shorter interspawning interval) and higher hatchability. The authors suggested that the inclusion of CPO in tilapia broodstock diets can be cost-effective for increasing tilapia seed production. Similar results were also obtained by Hajizadeh and Shinn (2016) who found that palm oil can replace FO in diets fed to Nile tilapia broodstock. Fish fed PO-based diets had better fecundity, spawning intervals and eggs and larval quality than those fed the control diet.

8.6.3 Vitamins and minerals requirements

Very little attention has been paid to vitamin requirements of tilapia broodstock, despite their positive effects on the reproductive performance of farmed fish. Soliman et al. (1986) found that supplementation of ascorbic acid at 1250 mg kg^{-1} dry diet of *O. mossambicus* significantly improved egg hatchability and the condition and survival rate of their fry. Similarly, when Nile tilapia broodstock were fed diets with graded levels of vitamin C (ascorbyl monophosphate), the best reproductive performance, blood variables and eggs and larvae quality were achieved at 599 mg vitamin C kg^{-1} diet (Sarmento et al., 2018).

It has also been found that vitamin E deficiency in Nile tilapia feed causes lack of sexual colouration (light skin colour) and reduces reproductive activity (Schimittou, 1993). Nascimento et al. (2014) assessed the effects of graded levels of vitamin E (200, 300, 400 and 500 mg kg^{-1}) on spawning activity of Nile tilapia broodstock. Vitamin E supplementation positively affected fish fecundity, spawning frequency, hatching rate and larval production and survival. About 400 mg vitamin E kg^{-1} feed was sufficient to support the best reproductive performance. The effects of dietary vitamin C (L-ascorbic acid), vitamin E and selenium, at concentrations of 120, 34 and 0.2 mg kg^{-1} diet, respectively, either solely or combined, on the reproductive performance of Nile tilapia were also investigated (El-Gamal et al., 2007). GSI, egg size, fecundity, spawning rate, hatching rate and larval survival were all significantly higher in the group fed with the combination of vitamins E and C and selenium than in other groups.

Despite the essentiality of minerals for fish growth and general metabolism, studies on the effects dietary mineral supplementation on reproductive performance of tilapia are almost lacking. Only Carvalho et al. (2018) found that available phosphorus significantly affects spawning frequency, absolute and relative fecundity, interspawning intervals and egg hatchability of Nile tilapia females. The best reproductive performance was achieved at 6.6 g phosphorus kg^{-1} diet. It is evident, therefore, that extensive work is urgently needed on quantitative lipid requirements, energy requirements, protein sparing effects by dietary lipids or carbohydrates and vitamins and mineral requirements of tilapia broodstock under different culture systems.

8.6.4 Feeding management

8.6.4.1 Feeding levels

Feeding management of tilapia broodstock can significantly affect reproductive performance, hatchery efficiency and profitability. Since mouthbrooding tilapia incubate the eggs and fry in their mouths and do not eat during incubation periods, it is unwise to feed them at abundant and constant rates (Miranova, 1977; Bhujel, 2000). Instead, a higher feeding rate immediately after seed harvesting, followed by a lower feeding rate and/or no feeding (if broodfish are raised in a green-water system), might be more economic and more efficient in terms of reproductive performance (Bhujel, 2000). In support, Miranova (1977) found that the egg production of *O. mossambicus* was higher with restricted food (25%–50% of the satiation ration) than with abundant food, despite the fact that abundant feeding resulted in better growth of females than restricted feeding. This result suggested that the reproduction of tilapia is stimulated by a decrease in the food ration. Similarly, Coward and Bromage (1999) studied the effects of high and low rations on the growth and reproductive performance of *T. zillii* for 550 days. They found that fish maintained upon the higher ration were significantly larger than fish fed a reduced ration. Also, high rations produced a higher mean total fecundity than low ration, though the mean egg diameter and gonadosomatic index remained unchanged. When adjusting spawning data to a common maternal fish size, using a one-factor analysis of covariance (ANCOVA), the authors did not detect significant differences between the two ration levels in terms of mean total fecundity and egg diameter. Furthermore, the ovaries of fish fed the low ration possessed high ratios of early and late perinucleolar oocytes and fewer late-vitellogenic/maturing oocytes than the ovaries of fish fed the higher ration. The authors suggested that, under prolonged food restriction, the female *T. zillii* sacrifices somatic growth for maintaining reproductive efficiency.

In addition to the above findings, Siddiqui et al. (1997) found that the fecundity of hybrid tilapia (*O. niloticus* × *O. aureus*) fed at 0.5%, 1%, 2% and 3% body weight a day^{-1} increased with increasing feeding rate. However, fecundity g^{-1} female was higher at lower feeding levels (0.5% and 1%) than at higher feeding levels (2% and 3%). Egg size, hatchability, fry length and weight were not affected by feeding levels. It is clear thus while food restriction leads to growth retardation and reduction in total fecundity, it tends to increase spawning frequency, total number of eggs over a discrete period and the amount of energy allocated to egg production.

It is suggested that when the demand for seed is low, broodstock should be stunted, by stocking them at higher densities under restricted feeding regimes, to minimize seed production. When market demand for seed increases, stunted broodfish are restocked at the required densities and fed at higher feeding rates, in order to compensate for early growth retardation and produce more seed compared to the normal broodfish. This assumption was tested by Bhujel et al. (2007), who assessed the reproductive performance of prestunted and normal Nile tilapia broodfish at varying feeding rates (1%, 2% and 3% BW d^{-1}). Results showed that stunted broodfish required a feeding rate of 3% (or higher) for optimum seed output, while 2% feeding was sufficient for normal broodfish.

8.6.4.2 Feeding frequency

Feeding frequency is another important factor affecting fish reproduction. A number of studies have investigated the effects of feeding frequency and schedules on spawning performance and seed output of tilapia. Ungsethaphan (1995) found that *O. niloticus* fed twice day^{-1} at low feeding rates (0.5% and 1.0% of body weight) produced more seed, compared to those fed once a day. When feeding level was increased to 1.5% of body mass day^{-1} seed production was decreased. As tilapia are continuous grazers in nature, feeding them at shorter intervals may lead to better seed production (Bhujel, 2000). However, feeding more than twice a day may not be cost-effective due to labour intensity. Feeding tilapia broodstock with high energy diets at low feeding rates might also be better than feeding larger amounts of low energy diet.

The effect of scheduled use of high-protein and low-protein diets on growth and fry production of Nile tilapia broodstock have been investigated (Santiago and Laron, 2002). The fish were fed a high-protein diet (HP, 40% cp) or a low-protein diet (LP, 25% cp) or HP for 1–3 days followed by LP for 1–4 days for 54 weeks. Fry production was not significantly affected by the feeding schedule for broodstock. However, cost/benefit analyses indicated that feeding broodstock on 1HP-1LP and 3HP-2LP feeding schedules gave the highest spawning and economic performance. This finding indicates that feed quality, feeding schedules and feed costs should be considered for achieving optimum reproductive performance. It also gives fish farmers and managers an option in the management of feeding their tilapia broodstocks.

8.7 Environmental factors

Environmental factors play a main role in releasing the genetic potential (Duponchelle et al., 1997) and seed production in tilapia (Little et al., 1994; Bhujel et al., 2001). Therefore, good water quality and other environmental conditions should be maintained for successful and sustainable reproductive activity and seed production of these fishes. In this regard, the following environmental parameters are of prime importance.

8.7.1 Dissolved oxygen

As indicated in Chapter 4, tilapias can survive at low levels of dissolved oxygen (DO) due to their ability to utilize atmospheric oxygen (Chervinski, 1982; Popma and Lovshin, 1996). However, the effects of DO on reproductive and spawning activities of tilapia have not been well studied. The available information indicates that low DO (<0.5 mg L^{-1}), generally occurring in the early morning in outdoor fish ponds, has negative impacts on the ovarian growth, courtship, seed production and quality and the ability of tilapia females to mouthbrood eggs and fry (Bevis, 1994; Little and Hulata, 2000). Low DO also causes a reduction in feed intake, behavioural and morphological changes (melanin pigments in the skin) (Bhujel, 2000). These stressful conditions have been reported to cause disease incidence, inhibit reproduction and spawning activities, cause oocyte atresia and decrease fecundity and hatchability (Schimittou, 1993).

8.7.2 Temperature

Tilapias are eurythermal fishes that can tolerate a wide range of temperatures ranging from 8 to >40°C (Philippart and Ruwet, 1982). Most tilapia species were reported to reproduce successfully at about 22°C (Popma and Lovshin, 1996; El-Naggar et al., 2000). This was not the case in *O. mossambicus*, where no spawning occurred at 22°C, while increasing water temperature from 25 to 31°C significantly increased their seed production (Miranova, 1977). Tilapia reproduction generally slows at 21–24°C, while the optimum temperature for reproduction ranges from 25 to 30°C (Rothbard, 1979; Popma and Lovshin, 1996). At temperatures higher than 35°C, reproductive performance has been found to be very poor (Bevis, 1994; Little et al., 1997). Spawning units should therefore be designed and constructed in such a way to meet severe climatic conditions. Increasing temperature through passive daytime heating and conservation of warmer water overnight can improve hatchery efficiency (Little and Hulata, 2000). Concrete tanks built in greenhouses (Fig. 8.2) can be an ideal design for this system. Greenhouse tanks enable tilapia to spawn all year round, especially in temperate zones where temperature sharply drops during winter months (I. Radwan, Kafr El-Shaikh, Egypt, 2005; personal communication). This will also help tilapia farmers nurse the fry during winter time and stock them in fattening ponds at much bigger sizes than the size they generally use under natural conditions. Wind breaks and deep hapas in ponds have been successfully used to reduce the effects of cold weather in Vietnam and Thailand (Cao, 1998; Dan and Little, 2000). Reducing the effects of hot weather through shading and deepening fish ponds have also been successful (El-Sayed et al., 1996; Bhujel, 1999).

An interaction between endocrine control of reproduction and temperature has been implied. Cornish et al. (1997) found that the secretion of luteinizing-like hormone (LH-like H) and follicle stimulating-like hormone (FSH-like H) was related to increasing water temperature leading to increasing spawning efficiency of *O. mossambicus*.

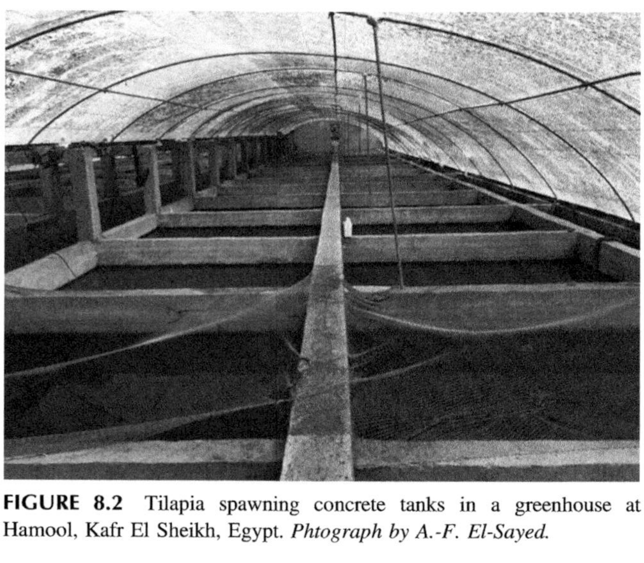

FIGURE 8.2 Tilapia spawning concrete tanks in a greenhouse at Hamool, Kafr El Sheikh, Egypt. *Phtograph by A.-F. El-Sayed.*

8.7.3 Salinity

Salinity is another important parameter for tilapia reproduction, since these fishes are salinity-tolerant. A great deal of attention has been paid to the culture of tilapia in brackish water and seawater, due to the shortage of, and competition for, fresh water in many parts of the world. This means that there is a great scope for tilapia culture in coastal areas using either salinity-acclimated seed produced from freshwater hatcheries or establishing the hatcheries in brackish water by diluting the seawater with fresh water (Suresh and Lin, 1992).

The effects of salinity on tilapia reproduction have been studied by a number of authors, with varying, and sometimes controversial results, depending on tilapia species and strains. For example, Wardoyo (1991) studied the effects of different salinity levels (0, 10, 15, 20 and 25‰) and acclimation regimes (direct and gradual exposures) on survivals, weight gains and reproductive performance of three strains of Nile tilapia (Egypt, Ghana and Ivory Coast) and red tilapia hybrid (Red tilapia). He found that spawning success and eggs hatchability of Egypt and Ghana strains and red tilapia were reduced with increasing water salinity, but were not affected by strains or acclimation regimes. On the other hand, fecundity (eggs g^{-1} per female) was not affected by salinity levels or strains. Meanwhile, hatchability rates were higher for late eggs (>3 days) than for early eggs (<3 days). Hatchability of early eggs was also higher at 10 and 15‰ than at 0 and 20‰.

Corre (1981) reported also that Nile tilapia spawned at 14‰, while no spawning occurred at 28‰. Similar observations were reported by Watanabe (1985) and Fineman-Kalio (1988) who found that these fish reproduce successfully at salinities ranging from 13.5 to 29‰ and cease reproduction at salinities higher than 30‰, despite 95% of females being gravid. However, Watanabe and Kuo (1985) reported that the same species can reproduce at salinities ranging from fresh water to 32‰, but extremely poor egg hatchability was obtained in full-strength seawater. Hatchability was similar for eggs spawned in fresh water, 10 and 15‰, and was considerably lower than at 5‰. On the other hand, Mozambique tilapia (*O. mossambicus*) is more salinity-tolerant than other tilapias and can reproduce at water salinity ranging from 10 to 49‰ (Chervinski, 1982). Furthermore, their reproduction efficiency is better in brackish water than in fresh water. Uchida and King (1962) found that seed production of *O. mossambicus* was approximately three times higher in brackish water (8.9−15.2‰) than in fresh water.

The effect of salinity on the reproduction of blue tilapia *(O. aureus)* was also evident. Available information indicated that nest building did not occur in fish reared in seawater, and in turn, gonadosomatic index dropped, causing nonoccurrence of reproduction (Chervinski and Yashouv, 1971; Chervinski and Zorn, 1974). Al-Ahmad et al. (1988) found that fecundity, egg hatching success and fry survival of *O. spilurus* was twice in groundwater (4‰) compared to seawater (40‰). Ernst et al. (1991) found that seed production of Florida red tilapia breeders was significantly greater at low salinity (5‰) than in brackish water (18‰) and the proportion of brooding females and number of seed per clutch were greater at 5‰ than at 18‰. In another study, Liao and Chang (1983) noted that breeding behaviour of Taiwanese red tilapia was inhibited in brackish water and seawater compared to fresh water.

It is obvious that salinity-tolerant tilapia species, strains and hybrids tend to reproduce more efficiently at low and moderate salinities than at high salinities. The failure of tilapia to reproduce at high salinities could be attributed to the resorption of the eggs, as a result of the osmotic stress (Chervinski and Yashouv, 1971). High salinities were also found to suppress the aggression of dominant tilapia males (Watanabe et al., 1988). To overcome this aggression, male broodfish may be kept in saline water during times of low seed demand.

8.7.4 Photoperiod and light intensity

Photoperiod plays a significant role in fish growth, metabolism and reproduction through melatonin secretion (key hormone engaged in regulating endogenous rhythms) (Boeuf and Le Bail, 1999; Bromage et al., 2001). Fishes are also characterized by photoreceptor cells in both the eye and pineal organ (Boeuf and Le Bail, 1999). The receptivity of fish to light depends on fish species and developmental stages (Barlow et al., 1995). The effects of light intensity and photoperiod on fish growth, body pigmentation, locomotor activity rhythms, sexual maturation and reproduction of several fish species have been studied (Silva-Garcia, 1996; Boeuf and Le Bail, 1999; Purchase et al., 2000; Trippel and Neil, 2002).

In nature, tilapia show some degrees of sensitivity to light intensity and photoperiod (Lowe-McConnell, 1959). The reproductive activity of some cichlids living in clear waters was found to be modulated by lunar cycle. Okorie (1973) found that advanced gonadal maturation of Nile tilapia in Lake Victoria was higher during full moon than at new moon. Similar effects of lunar periodicity on breeding activity of *T. mariae* have been reported (Schwank, 1987). It was also assumed that moonlight enhances the effectiveness of parental care (Schwank, 1987). Baroiller et al. (1997) found that the peak of spawning activity of Nile tilapia reared in outdoor tanks for 20 months occurred when water temperature and photoperiod were at their peaks (about 27°C and 16 h, respectively).

Various tilapia species spawn at certain times of the day, at a favourable temperature and photoperiod. This behaviour suggests nychthermal cyclicity (daytime spawning and nighttime rest) in these fishes. The effect of nychthermal periodicity on tilapia breeding is evident. About 99% of Nile tilapia reared in aquaria at a 12L:12D photoperiod cycle spawned during the afternoon of light periods, with 84% spawned between 14.00 and 16.00 h (Baroiller et al., 1997).

Despite the effects that light intensity and photoperiod may have on reproductive performance of tilapia, very few studies have considered these effects under culture conditions. Most of these studies suggested that about 12–14.5 h photoperiod be adopted for optimum spawning activity. Rothbard and Pruginin (1975) recommended also a 12–14 h light phase, at a temperature of 25–29°C, for the induction of natural interspecific spawning between *O. niloticus* and *O. aureus*. Similarly, Ridha et al. (1998) found that *O. spilurus* breeders reared under longer photoperiods exhibited higher fecundity. However, that result is questionable since only two photoperiods were used (13 and 14 h). Furthermore, Ridha and Cruz (2000) found that the best seed production and spawning performance of Nile tilapia were achieved at a light intensity of 2500 lux and a photoperiod of 18 h day^{-1}. Increasing photoperiod during winter using artificial light has led to the production of red tilapia fry all year round (Galman et al., 1988). On the other hand, the use of accelerated artificial light (600-W) for 14.5 h day^{-1} at 27–30 C did not affect seed production of Florida red tilapia (Smith et al., 1991). It appears, therefore, that the response of tilapia to photoperiods is species-specific.

On the contrary, Campos-Mendoza et al. (2004) found that Nile tilapia reared under long daylength (18L:6D) exhibited higher fecundity, and lower interspawning intervals, compared with fish reared at shorter light hours. It is clear, therefore, that more work is needed to resolve this dispute and determine the photoperiod required for optimum spawning performance of farmed tilapia.

In order to elucidate this discrepancy, Biswas et al. (2005) evaluated photoperiod manipulation to control reproduction and, in turn, overcome the problem of overcrowding in Nile tilapia. Fish broodstock were exposed to 6L:6D, 12L:12D and 14L:10D. Reproductive parameters, including fecundity, gamete quality and offspring viability, were evaluated. Steroid levels (estradiol-17β, E_2; testosterone, T) were analyzed on days one and three post spawning and at 3-day intervals afterwards. The authors found that females exposed to 12L:12D and 14L:10D spawned successfully throughout the study, while the spawning of fish exposed to 6L:6D was arrested after three to four spawning cycles, with a significant decrease in plasma levels of E_2. These findings suggest that photoperiod manipulation can be used as a useful and safe tool for controlling excessive reproduction of farmed tilapia.

Similarly, El-Sayed and Kawanna (2007) found that the fecundity, spawning frequency and interspawning intervals were significantly better in Nile tilapia reared at 12L:12D than at 18L:6D and 6L:18D cycles. Broodstock exposed to long photoperiods (18L:6D and 24L:0D) had the lowest spawning performance, but exhibited the highest biomass and best growth rates, compared to fish subjected to intermediate photoperiod (12L:12D). Fish that spawned more frequently (at 12L:12D) exhibited lower average weights, presumably due to the use of substantial amount of dietary energy for gonads development and spawning activity, rather than for somatic growth. These fish depend on their energy reserve, as they fast during egg and fry brooding. It is obvious from these studies that adopting a photoperiod similar to natural photoperiods (about 12L:12D) will result in better seed production.

8.7.5 Water level and exchange

Water level has been reported to affect reproduction efficiency of tilapia in nature (Noakes and Balon, 1982; Philippart and Ruwet, 1982). Noakes and Balon (1982) found that a high water level increased the reproductive activity of tilapia females, resulting in smaller males being recruited into the breeding population. Partial water change at frequent intervals may also improve seed output and spawning synchrony (Bhujel, 2000). Guerrero (1982) suggested that tilapia mucus contains a hormone-like substance that inhibits reproduction, especially at high densities. Regular exchange of pond water may remove this substance and improve reproduction efficiency. Water exchange also improves DO and flushes out harmful substances, such as undigested food, faeces and other metabolites, such as ammonia, nitrite and nitrates (Mires, 1982). It is no surprise, therefore, that seed output from ponds filled with new water is higher than from ponds with water used for long periods (Bhujel, 2000). This suggests that pond water should be frequently changed.

8.7.6 Interactive effects of environmental factors

The effects of a single factor on fish growth and reproduction is generally disadvantageous because it does not consider the possible interactive effects with other factors. If interaction between effective factors occurs, the adoption of a one-factor-at-a-time design will likely lead to poor results; thus, understanding the significant interaction will be more meaningful. A number of studies investigated the combined effects of different factors on growth performance and reproductive output of tilapia. Watanabe et al. (1993) and Likongwe et al. (1996) reported an occurrence of synergistic effect between temperature and salinity upon the growth and survival in tilapia. The combined effects of temperature (20–34 °C), salinity (0–18‰) and pH (5–10) on egg fertilization and hatchability of GIFT tilapia were also investigated (Hui et al., 2014). The results showed significant interactive effects of the three factors on fertilization and hatching. The maximum fertilization and hatching rates occurred at 27.3°C/9.2‰/7.4 temperature/salinity/pH combination.

In a similar approach, the effects of feeding levels (1 or 4% BW day^{-1}), stocking densities (3 or 10 females m^{-2}) and water-flow rates (3.6 or 21 L min^{-1}) on the fecundity, spawning frequency and egg quality of Nile tilapia were investigated by Tsadik and Bart (2007). Under both feeding levels, higher relative fecundity was observed at lower stocking density (3 female m^{-2}) and water-flow rate (3.6 L min^{-1}) than in other treatments. High feeding level (4% BW day^{-1}) increased somatic growth and number of eggs spawn^{-1}, but did not affect relative fecundity. Higher stocking density (10 female m^{-2}) significantly lowered eggs spawn^{-1}, while higher water-flow rate (21 L min^{-1}) increased growth rate but lowered relative fecundity (eggs kg^{-1} per day). The authors concluded that lower feeding level (1% BW day^{-1}), lower stocking density (3 female m^{-2}) and lower water flow rate (3.6 L min^{-1}) could be adopted as a management strategy for improving tilapia seed production.

8.8 Production of monosex tilapia

Mixed-sex culture of tilapia has been a common practice in many countries for decades. However, extensive attention has been given to monosex culture of tilapia during the past 2 decades. Monosex tilapia may have many attributes that make them an excellent candidate for aquaculture. Among these are the following:

- High growth rates and feed utilization efficiency.
- High tolerance to severe environmental conditions including temperature, salinity, low DO, etc.
- Higher energy conservation.
- Reduced aggressiveness.
- Greater uniformity of size at harvest.
- Better flesh quality and appearance.
- High resistance to stress and diseases.
- Role in controlling overreproduction.

The following methods have been used for production of monosex tilapia: (1) manual sorting; (2) hormonal sex reversal; (3) interspecific hybridization; (4) androgenesis and gynogenesis; (5) triploidy and (6) transgenesis. The first three methods are discussed here, while androgenesis and gynogenesis, triploidy and transgenesis are addressed in Chapter 13 (Recent Technological Innovations).

8.8.1 Manual sexing

Manual sexing of tilapia fingerlings was widely used in the past (Hickling, 1963). It is an easy technique, but it is extremely laborious, is stressful for the fish and often leads to inaccurate results due to the presence of females as a result of human error (Penman and McAndrew, 2000). Therefore, this method is rarely used. The technique of manual sorting is based on assessing the number of openings in the urinogenital papillae: the male has a single urinogenital opening, while the female has two separate openings. The accuracy of this method ranges from 80% to 90% (Penman and McAndrew, 2000). Accuracy also increases with increasing fish size.

8.8.2 Hormonal sex reversal

Hormonal sex reversal has been extensively used for sex determination and producing monosex fish for aquaculture purposes. Steroid hormones or hormone analogues as well as nonsteroid compounds (Table 8.3) are commonly used for producing monosex tilapia. The hormones are generally incorporated into larval feeds and administered to undifferentiated larvae at their very early larval stages (preferably at first feeding) for sufficient time to enable sex reversal. The use of hormones has been under increasing public criticism due to their possible health and environmental impacts. As a result, the use of hormones for sex reversal of tilapia is either licensed (in the United States) or banned (in Europe) (Penman and McAndrew, 2000).

TABLE 8.3 Steroid hormones, hormone analogues and nonsteroid compounds used for producing monosex tilapia.

Hormone (compound)	Abbreviation
17α-methyldihydrotestosterone	MDHT
17α-methyltestosterone	MT
17α-ethynyltestosterone	ET
17α-methyl-5-androstan-3-17β-diol	
Androstenedione	AN
17β-oestradiol	E2
17α-ethynyloestradiol	EE
Fadrozole (Aromatase inhibitor)	F
Trenbolone acetate	TBA
11β-hydroxyandrostenedione	11β-OHA4
Aromatase inhibitor	AI
Diethylstilbestrol	DES
Tamoxifen	
Acriflavine	

8.9 All-male production

8.9.1 Oral-hormone administration

Many steroid hormones, steroid analogues, or nonsteroid compounds have been widely used in male sex reversal of various tilapia species. The percentage of sex-reversed males depends mainly on the type of hormones, dose, timing and duration of administration, fish species, and size/age of larvae, as indicated in Table 8.4. Available data indicate that 17α-methyltestosterone (MT) hormone is the

TABLE 8.4 Production of male tilapia using natural and synthetic steroids (full names of the hormones are given in Table 8.3).

Species	Hormone	Route	Optimum dose	Timing	Duration (days)	% males	Remarks	Reference
O. n	F	Food	200–500	7 dph	30	92.5–96	Genetically females	Kwon et al. (2000)
	F	Food	75–100	Fry	30	100		Afonso et al. (2001)
	ET	Food	60	Fry	25–28	91–99.4		Vera-Cruz and Mair (1994)
	MT	Food	30	Fry	21	99		Guerrero and Guerrero (1988)
	MT	Food	60	10.4 mm	14–28	82–92		Smith and Phelps (1997)
	TBA	Immersion	250 μg L^{-1}	10 dpf	2 h	98–100	Exposed to ultrasound for 2 h	Bart (2002)
	AN	Immersion	100–250 μg L^{-1}	10 dpf	2 h	92	Exposed to ultrasound for 2 h	Bart (2002)
	MT	Immersion	50 μg L^{-1}	10 dpf	2 h	98	Exposed to ultrasound for 2 h	Bart (2002)
	MDHT	Immersion	250 μg L^{-1}	10 dpf	2 h	98–100	Exposed to ultrasound for 2 h	Bart (2002)
	MT	Food	60	10 dpf	10-30 dpf	92		Gale et al. (1999)
	MT	Immersion	500 μg L^{-1}	10 and 13 dpf	3 h	87		Gale et al. (1999)
	MDHT	Immersion	500 μg L^{-1}	10 and 13 dpf	3 h	83–100		Gale et al. (1999)
	MDHT	Immersion	1800 μg L^{-1}	14 dph	4 h	100	Single immersion	Wassermann and Afonso (2003)
	MT	Immersion	1800 μg L^{-1}	10 and 14 dph	4 h	98.3	Two immersions	Wassermann and Afonso (2003)
	ET	Immersion	1800 μg L^{-1}	14 dph	4 h	86.7	Two immersions	Wassermann and Afonso (2003)

Continued

TABLE 8.4 **Production of male tilapia using natural and synthetic steroids (full names of the hormones are given in Table 8.3).—cont'd**

Species	Hormone	Route	Optimum dose	Timing	Duration (days)	% males	Remarks	Reference
O. m	MDHT	Immersion	5–10 μg L^{-1}	10 dph	10 d	100		Varadaraj and Pandian (1987)
	MT	Food	30	9–11 mm	18	98		Guerrero (1975)
	ET	Food	60	9–11 mm	18	100		Guerrero (1975)
O. a	MT	Immersion	0.6 ppm	9–11 mm	35	62.3		Torrans et al. (1988)
	MT	Food	50	9 mm	42	100		Hines and Watts (1995)
	ET	Food	60	Fry	25–28	83–97		Mélard and Ducarme (1993), Mélard et al. (1995)
	TBA	Food	25	9.1 mm	28	98.3		Galvez et al. (1996)
O. s	MT	Food	70	Fry	38	90		Ridha and Lone (1990)
	MT	Immersion	2.5 ppm	Yolk-sac fry	4 days	100	In BW, later fed MT at 50 mg kg^{-1} feed	Lone and Ridha (1993)
Red tilapia	11β-OHA4	Food	50	10 dpf	28	99.1		Desprez et al. (2003)
O. n × *O. a*	Tamoxifen	Food	100	9 mm	42	100		Hines and Watts (1995)
O. n × *O. a*	ET	Food	60	Fry	25–28	96–100		Rothbard et al. (1983)

Oral doses are in mg kg^{-1} feed. *O. a* = *O. aureus*; *O. m* = *O. mossambicus*; *O. n* = *O. niloticus*; *O. s* = *O. spilurus*.

most common and successful hormone used for tilapia sex reversal (Guerrero and Guerrero, 1988; Ridha and Lone, 1990; Lone and Ridha, 1993; Penman and McAndrew, 2000; Beardmore et al., 2001). The doses of steroid hormones tested for sex reversal of tilapia ranged from <30 to 100 mg kg^{-1} food, provided to the fish for <15–>60 days. However, the best results have been reported at a dose of 30–60 mg kg^{-1} administered for about 25–30 days (Guerrero and Guerrero, 1988; Vera-Cruz and Mair, 1994; Green et al., 1997). Guerrero (1975) found that the administration of 30 mg 17α-ethynyltestosterone (ET) kg^{-1} feed for 18 days produced 98% males in *O. mossambicus*, while 60 mg kg^{-1} produced 100% males. MT produced 98% and 85% males at 30 and 60 mg kg^{-1}. Excessive doses of hormones may therefore reduce the percentage of sex-reversed fish, increase fish mortality and cause sterility or paradoxical sex reversal (Green et al., 1997; Beardmore et al., 2001).

8.9.2 Effects of phytoestrogens on sex reversal

Phytoestrogens, which are plant-derived substances with estrogenic activity, may affect reproductive development and sex differentiation in fish. They may either have the same effects as estrogen or block estrogen's effects (Bennetau-Pelissero et al., 2001; Green and Kelly, 2009), depending on the ratio of phytoestrogens to endogenous estrogens, aromatase activity, animal species and reproductive status, length of the exposure and method of administration (Tsai et al., 2000; Trant et al., 2001; Andersen et al., 2003).

Soybean (SB), which is widely used as a major protein source for farmed fish, contains high levels of phytoestrogens; mainly genistein and daidzein. Therefore, the use of SB in broodstock diets may affect reproductive development and sex differentiation in fish, due to the presence of these phytoestrogens. This assumption has been tested on Nile tilapia by El-Sayed et al. (2012) in two consecutive experiments. The first experiment investigated the sex ratio of newly hatched Nile tilapia larvae (0.01 g) fed SB-based diet, without or with supplementation of 17α-MT at 60 mg kg^{-1} diet, for 28 days. The control, soybean meal (SBM)-based diet produced significantly higher percentage of females (77%) than the FM-based diet (52%). The addition of MT to SBM resulted in a significant reduction in percentage of females (31%); however, this percentage was significantly higher than that produced by FM-based diet treated with MT (only 3% females). The second experiment investigated the effects of different concentrations (0, 10, 20 and 30 mg kg^{-1}) of pure, crystalline genistein and daidzein (the major phytoestrogens contained in SB) on sex reversal of Nile tilapia larvae fed on an FM-based diet treated with MT. The control, hormone-free diet produced almost equal ratio of females and males (0.96:1). The addition of MT significantly increased the percentage of males, while daidzein and genistein reduced this percentage, especially at high concentration (30 mg kg^{-1}). These results clearly demonstrated that phytoestrogen contents of SBM have estrogenic effects on Nile tilapia larvae. Therefore, SB meal and other plant protein sources containing high levels of phytoestrogens should be avoided as protein sources for Nile tilapia larvae during sex reversal treatments.

8.9.3 The use of nonsteroidal alternatives

The use of hormones for sex reversal has been under increasing public criticism due to their potential health and environmental impacts. Therefore, recent studies have considered the use of nonsteroidal compounds to manipulate sex inversion. Nonsteroidal compounds may exhibit antagonistic or agonistic effects to sex steroids that are generally involved in sexual differentiation in fishes. When tilapia hybrids (*O. niloticus* × *O. aureus*) were fed tamoxifen-treated diets, a 100% male was produced at a dose of 100 mg kg^{-1} feed (Hines and Watts, 1995). When acriflavine was used, 89% and 85% males were produced at 15 and 50 mg kg^{-1} diet.

Tribulus terrestris is an annual herb, belonging to family Zygophyllaceae, widely distributed around the world, and well adapted to grow in dry climate. *T. terrestris* is known to elevate the testosterone levels in mammals (Gauthaman et al., 2002). Omitoyin et al. (2013) evaluated *T. terrestris* extract as a natural sex-reversal agent in Nile tilapia larvae. Newly hatched larvae were fed test diets containing 0.0, 1.0, 1.5, 2.0 and 2.5 g of *T. terrestris* extract kg^{-1} diet, in addition to another diet containing 50 mg MT kg^{-1}. Percentage of males increased with increasing *T. terrestris* extract to reach its maximum value of 85.7% at 2.5 g kg^{-1}.

Pulse-Electric Field Inductions have been tried to induce male sex reversal in Nile tilapia fertilized eggs (Bunthawin et al., 2015). The eggs (two to three days post fertilization) were induced in square-wave electric fields of 0.25–87.50 kV m^{-1}. Verification of sex reversal of treated eggs was carried out with autopsies of 2-month-old sex-reversed fry using the acetocarmine stain method. The results indicated that the optimal conditions for sex reversal were three square wave pulses of 87.50 kV m^{-1} electric fields. This technique resulted in 89% sex reversal, with less than 25% egg mortality.

8.9.4 Immersion techniques

Oral administration of hormones for sex reversal of tilapia is generally safe and successful; however, hormone traces from uneaten food and metabolites are often of a major environmental concern. Immersing fish fry in hormone solution for short periods of time has attracted the attention as a successful alternative tool to overcome this problem. One of the major advantages of the immersion technique is the substantial decrease in treatment period and the reduction of possible effects of the hormones on the workers (Gale et al., 1999). This technique is also characterized by minimal intervention, which is usually reduced to the time when the fish is most sensitive to the treatments. In spite of these attributes, the use of immersion technique for masculinization of tilapia has not been developed for practical and commercial use.

The percentage of sex-reversed males produced by immersion technique ranges from <60% to 100%, depending on fish species, type and dose of hormone and immersion period (Table 8.4). Varadaraj and Pandian (1987) found that the immersion of *O. mossambicus* in 5 or 10 μg L^{-1} of 17α-methyl-5-androsten-3-17β-diol for 10 days post hatch (dph) caused 100% masculinization. Similar results were reported with *O. spilurus* immersed in MT (2.5 mg L^{-1}) for 4 days in brackish water, followed by oral administration of the hormone at 50 mg kg^{-1} for 35 days (Lone and Ridha, 1993). The exposure of Nile tilapia fry to 500 μg L^{-1} 17α-methyldihydrotestosterone (MDHT) for 3 h on days 10 and 13 post fertilization (dpf) also resulted in 83%–100% males (Gale et al., 1999), while low concentration of MDHT and MT (100 μg L^{-1}) caused lower male percentage. Afonso and Leboute (2003) also investigated masculinizing potency of ET, MT and MDHT applied to Nile tilapia larvae at 14 dph, in two consecutive trials. In the first trial, the fish were subjected to a single 4-h immersion dose at concentrations ranging from 200 to 1800 μg L^{-1}. In the second trial, the fish were immersed in these androgens at 1800 μg L^{-1} for 4 h either as a single immersion at 14 days or double immersions at 10 and 14 dph. The authors found that when different concentrations were applied, the best male proportion was achieved at 1800 μg L^{-1}, but none of the treatments produced 100% male (86%–90%). The results of the second trial confirmed that of the first trial. However, two immersions slightly improved male proportion, especially in MT-treated group, where the male proportion increased from 92% to 98%, but decreased male percentage in MDHT group to 94% compared to 100% at one immersion.

The exposure of fish larvae to ultrasound is believed to increase the transport of hormone from the water into fish body, leading to higher masculinization rate (Bart, 2002). Bart (2002) studied the effects ultrasound exposure time (1 and 2 h) on sex reversal of Nile tilapia using four different hormones (androstenedione (AN), MDHT, MT and trenbolone acetate; (TBA)). He found that subjecting the fry (10 dpf) to ultrasound for 2 h resulted in a significant increase in male percentage, compared to 1-h exposure. In addition, TBA (250 μg L^{-1}) produced 98%–100% males and was not significantly different from 100 μg L^{-1}. Lower percentage of males was produced with MDHT treatment (90.5%).

The immersion of tilapia eggs, instead of fry, has recently emerged as an effective tool of inducing sex reversal. When fertilized eggs are immersed in the hormone solution, the hormone is absorbed through passive diffusion across the lipid membrane of the egg. One major advantage of this technique is the substantial reduction in the amount of hormone used, since little amounts of water are generally used for egg incubation compared to the amounts used in larval holding units. As yet, little information is available on sex reversal of tilapia using immersion technique. A few studies have been reported in this regard. Anon (2002; cited in Cagauan et al., 2004) reported that the immersion of 2-d old Nile tilapia eggs in MT at 500 μg L^{-1}, for 24h has resulted in 88% males. Cagauan et al. (2004) also evaluated sex reversal of Nile tilapia in the Philippines, by immersing fertilized eggs (3–4 d old) in different concentrations of MT (0, 200, 400, 600 and 800 μg L^{-1}) for 24, 48, 72 and 96 h. The highest male proportion of 91% was obtained at 800 μg L^{-1} for 96 h. However, the results of this study are questionable. At 72 and 96 h, it is very likely that some of the eggs (which were already 3–4 d old) have hatched into sac fry. It is possible therefore that, at long immersion times (72 and 96 h), the authors may have immersed sac fry rather than eggs. Further investigations are therefore urgently needed to improve the immersion technique in order to increase the percentage of sex-reversed tilapia to 100% or close to 100%.

Oestrogen biosynthesis is mediated by the steroidogenic enzyme cytochrome P450 aromatase, which converts androgens to estrogens (Afonso et al., 2001). Therefore, nonsteroidal aromatase inhibitors (AIs) have been shown to alter the sex of several animals including tilapia. Afonso et al. (2001) fed Nile tilapia larvae with diets containing 0, 50, 75 and 100 mg kg^{-1} of the AI fadrozole for 15 and 30 days, starting 9 days after hatching. Regardless of the feeding period, the proportion of males was significantly higher in the treated groups, but 100% males were produced at the high doses (75 and 100 mg kg^{-1}) for 30 days. These results were confirmed by Kwon et al. (2002) who found that treating XX Nile tilapia female fry with AI at 28 or 36°C resulted in 99%–100% males. In addition, Sun et al. (2014) reported reversal of differentiated ovaries into functional testis in Nile tilapia by long-term feeding with a diet containing AI (fadrozole), at a concentration of 200 μg g^{-1} diet. Fish with longer sex differentiation needed longer treatment time for successful sex reversal. Spermatogonia were transformed from oogonia or germline stem cell-like cells distributed in germinal epithelium. The morphological and histological characteristics of sex-reversed gonads were more similar to testis, whereas their gene expression profiles remained closer to the female fish. The transdifferentiation was driven by suppression of female pathway genes and activation of male pathway genes.

8.10 All-female production

8.10.1 Hormonal sex reversal

In many fish species, females grow at higher rates, and attain larger sizes, than males. Males may also mature before females reaching marketable size, leading to dispersion of sizes and reduction in production. The production of all-female fish is an effective way of solving the problems and controlling reproduction of cultured tilapia. Therefore, the interest in producing all-female population, for aquaculture purposes, has increased. As for males, several natural or synthetic steroids, mainly estrogens, or other chemicals with estrogenic capacity, have been used to feminize tilapia. Both oral administration and immersion protocols were used with varying degrees of success (Table 8.5). Synthetic chemicals have been used for tilapia feminization at larger scales than natural steroids, with 17α-ethinylestradiol (EE) and diethylstilbestrol (DES) being the most common and most effective.

The relative effectiveness of steroids on feminization of tilapia depends on type of hormone, fish species, larval stage, dose and treatment timing and duration. For example,

TABLE 8.5 Production of female tilapia using natural and synthetic steroids (full names of the hormones are given in Table 8.3).

Species	Hormone	Route	Optimum dose (mg kg^{-1})	Fish age/size	Duration days	% females	Reference
Oreochromis niloticus	EE	Immersion	170–200 μg L^{-1}	Fry	18	100	Gilling et al. (1996)
	DES	Food	400	8.7 mm	28	80	Potts and Phelps (1995)
	EE	Food	100	7–12 mm	40	91	Mohamed et al. (2004)
O. mossambicus	DES	Food	100	10 d old	11	100	Varadaraj (1989)
	EE	Food	100	Yolk-sac fry	10	100	Rosenstein and Hulata (1994)
O. aureus	EE	Food	100	Yolk-sac fry	10	100	Rosenstein and Hulata (1994)
	EE + methallib	Food	100	Fry	42	95	Mair et al. (1987)
	EE	Food	100–200	Fry	40	93–98	Mélard (1995)
O. spilurus	EE	Food	100	9 mm	42	92	Ridha and Lone (1995)

Rosenstein and Hulata (1994) found that DES was more effective in feminizing blue tilapia (*O. aureus*) than EE, while the opposite was found in case of Nile tilapia (Gilling et al., 1996). Moreover, Rosenstein and Hulata (1992) failed to feminize *O. mossambicus* and *O. mossambicus* x *O. urolepis hornorum* hybrids by immersing eggs and fry in 17β-oestradiol (E2), progesterone, flutamide and progesterone + flutamide at different solutions and durations. However, these authors reported a 100% feminization when estrogens (DES and EE) were orally administered to these fishes. On the other hand, EE, DES, E2 successfully feminized Nile tilapia fry using immersion technique (Gilling et al., 1996). It appears from these results that more work is needed to verify whether oral administration or immersion technique is more effective and would produce higher all-female populations.

8.10.2 Hybridization

Hybridization of two different species has been extensively and successfully applied to produce monosex populations. There are several conditions affecting the success of hybridization of related fish taxa, including (1) external fertilization; (2) unequal abundance of two parental species; (3) weak behavioural isolating mechanisms; (4) competition for limited spawning habitat and (5) decreasing habitat complexity (Scribner et al., 2001). These factors are very likely to fit with most tilapias; therefore, tilapia have received a good deal of attention and have become the best-known example of hybrid production in aquaculture, since they are characterized with short life cycles and frequent spawning.

A substantial amount of information is now available on all-male and all-female tilapia hybrids (Tables 8.6 and 8.7). Most of the crosses carried out for the production of monosex tilapia have been between maternal mouthbrooders (Wohlfarth and Hulata, 1983; Beardmore et al., 2001). Most of crosses between pure mouthbrooding tilapias result in all-male or nearly all-male hybrids (Lovshin, 1982; McAndrew, 1993; Penman and McAndrew, 2000) (Table 8.6). All-male progenies have been produced from the following crosses: male *O. hornorum* × female *O. niloticus* (Lee, 1979), male *O. aureus* × female *O. niloticus* (Wohlfarth, 1994), male *O. mossambicus* × female *O. aureus* (Pierce, 1980), male *O. hornorum* × female *O. mossambicus* (Hickling, 1960) and male *O. mossambicus* × female *O. spilurus niger* (Pruginin, 1967). Other crosses resulted in 50%–98% males (Table 8.6). The failure to produce all-male progenies, in many cases, has been attributed to poor segregation of broodfish by sex and species, and also to the introduction of hybrids into broodstock ponds (Beardmore et al., 2001). Tilapia strains may also influence the results of tilapia hybridization, as reported by Marengoni et al. (1998). These authors found that, when Nile tilapia females were bred with

TABLE 8.6 Hybridization of different tilapia species to produce all-male populations.

Species hybridized			
Male	Female	% males	Reference
Oreochromis niloticus	*O. aureus*	75–95	Pruginin (1967)
	O. spilurus niger	93–98	Pruginin (1967)
	O. hornorum	75	Pruginin (1967)
O. aureus	*O. niloticus*	50–100	Lee (1979), Wohlfarth (1994)
	O. niloticus (Stirling strain)	100	Marengoni et al. (1998)
	O. niloticus (Uganda strain)	96–100	Pruginin et al. (1975)
	O. mossambicus	100	Beardmore et al. (2001)
	Tilapia vulcani	93–98	Pruginin et al. (1975)
O. mossambicus	*O. aureus*	70–75	Pierce (1980)
O. hornorum	*O. niloticus*	100	Lee (1979), Wohlfarth et al. (1990)
	O. mossambicus	100	Hickling (1960)
	O. aureus	90–100	Pruginin (1967), Lee (1979)
	O. spilurus	100	Pruginin (1967)
O. macrochir	*O. mossambicus*	100	Majumdar et al. (1983)
	O. spilurus	97.9	Majumdar et al. (1983)
	O. niloticus	100	Pruginin (1967)

TABLE 8.7 Hybridization of different tilapia species to produce all-female populations.

Species hybridized			
Male	Female	% females	Reference
Oreochromis mossambicus	*Sarotherodon melanotheron*	100	Peters (1963), Bauer (1968)
	Tilapia tholloni	100	Peters (1963), Bauer (1968)
O. niloticus	*S. melanotheron*	100	Peters (1963), Bauer (1968)
	T. tholloni	100	Peters (1963), Bauer (1968)
O. andersonii	*T. zillii*	100	Beardmore et al. (2001)

blue tilapia males, only the Stirling strain of Nile tilapia produced 100% males, while a Japan strain produced only 91% males.

8.11 Seed production

Global tilapia culture has witnessed a gradual, but continuous, switch from low input semi-intensive systems to more input-demanding, intensive systems during the last 2 decades. However, tilapia seed production industry did not pace with this imposed change; and still lags far behind. As mentioned earlier (Section 8.1; Introduction), the shortage of quality seed supply in many parts of the world, especially in Sub-Saharan Africa, together with poor seed production facilities and poor hatchery management are among the major obstacles limiting the expansion of intensive tilapia culture.

Information about tilapia hatching systems, broodstock management (described earlier), egg composition, hatchability, yolk-sac absorption, and larval rearing, water quality and other hatchery management measures is essential for sustainable and cost-effective quality seed supply. However, published data on most of these parameters are limited, inconsistent and sometimes controversial. Therefore, extensive efforts should be expended to face these challenges and better understand the optimum requirements for larval rearing of tilapia.

8.11.1 Hatching systems

8.11.1.1 Earthen ponds

Spawning in earthen ponds is the oldest method used for seed production of tilapia and still widely used in different regions of the world, especially in developing countries (Hepher and Pruginin, 1981; Macintosh and Little, 1995; Little and Hulata, 2000). Tilapia can spawn easily in ponds, regardless of pond size and depth, once the environmental requirements (temperature, salinity, etc.) and biological criteria (stocking density, sex ratio, etc.) are met. However, pond size, shape and depth affect harvest efficiency and seed production. Earthen ponds can be used for producing mixed-sex pure tilapia (Little et al., 1994), monosex hybrids (Hepher and Pruginin, 1981) and first feeding fry for sex-reversal (Verdegem and McGinty, 1987). Eggs and fry are usually harvested, either partially or completely, at varying intervals ranging from 6 to 60 days (Fig. 8.3). It has been reported, however, that shorter harvesting intervals lead to better results. Sorting of the seeds and removal of larger fry also reduces cannibalism and results in higher production of similar-sized fry (Little, 1989). Partial harvest is carried out by dip-netting, seining or trapping, without draining the ponds, while complete harvest requires checking of broodfish for seed incubation, along with draining of the pond and harvesting all seeds at once (Little and Hulata, 2000).

The main limitations of breeding ponds are the lack of sustainability, predation of small fry by other fish, cannibalism by older fry, asynchronous spawning and reduction of spawning frequency with overcrowding. Most of these limitations can be overcome through sound management such as increasing water fertility, decreasing sediment concentration, preventing the entry of wild predatory fishes and regular seed harvesting (Little, 1989; Macintosh and Little, 1995).

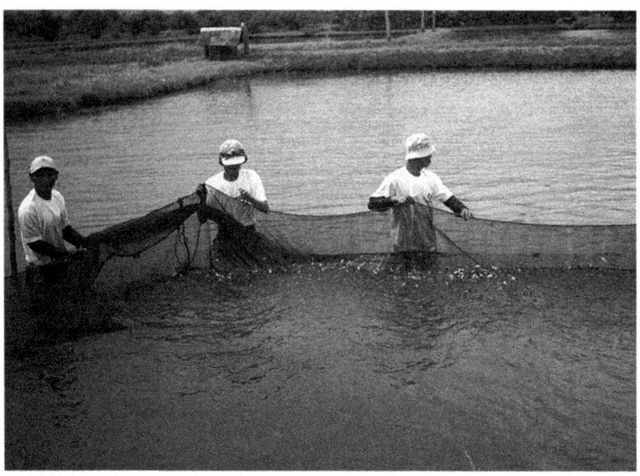

FIGURE 8.3 Harvesting tilapia fry from earthen ponds in the Philippines. *Photograph by A.-F. El-Sayed.*

8.11.1.2 Concrete tanks

Concrete tanks are currently among the most widely used spawning units for production of tilapia seeds (Fig. 8.2), especially for intensive culture in areas where fresh water is limited. Tanks have many advantages over earthen ponds, including high yield per unit area, easy harvest and better water management through exchange and/or filtration, while their main disadvantage is the higher cost. Spawning efficiency can be affected by tank size, dimensions, shape, colour, depth and construction material. Reproductive performance of Nile tilapia was found to be better in deep tanks (one to two m) than in shallow (0.5 m) tanks (El-Sayed et al., 1996). Courtship, spawning intensity and seed production of tilapia can also be related to artificial spawning shelters. Baroiller et al. (1997) found that the seed production of Nile tilapia was five times higher in raceways (12 m^2) containing artificial shelters (three breeze blocks) than in unsheltered raceways. The authors suggested that artificial shelters stimulated and synchronized reproductive activity of the fish. On the other hand, Duponchelle and Legendre (1997) reported that absolute fecundity of Nile tilapia females reared in tanks provided with artificial reefs was lower than in naked tanks. However, this result is questionable because the study was conducted for only 2 months, whereas a much longer period is required for concrete results.

8.11.1.3 Hapas

The use of hapas (Fig. 8.4) as a hatching system for tilapia has been tried in Asia (the Philippines, Thailand, Vietnam, etc.), the Americas (the United States, Brazil, Puerto Rico) and Africa (Malawi) (Little and Hulata, 2000), with varying degrees of success. Hapas have many attributes that make them an excellent hatchery system for tilapia, especially in developing countries. These include easy construction, easy management, easy seed harvest and low cost. Hapas can also be suspended in fertilized earthen ponds, deep water bodies and concrete tanks supplied with clear water. However, they need continuous maintenance and cleaning of fouling. Fouling leads to blocking the mesh netting of the hapas and deteriorating water quality inside them (Little and Hulata, 2000).

The spawning of tilapia in hapas suspended in ponds depends on broodstock density and sex ratio, broodstock

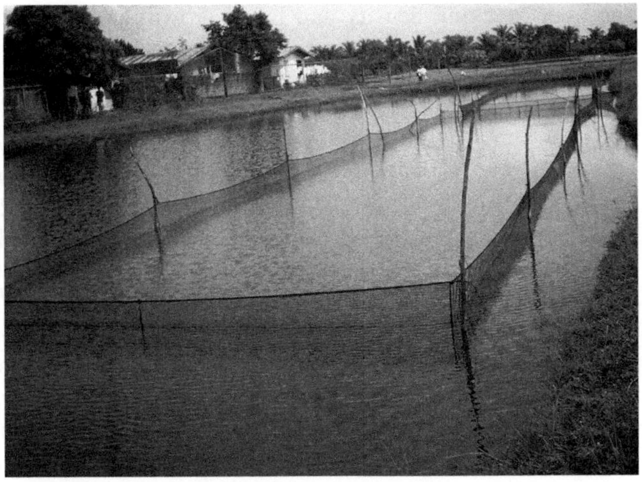

FIGURE 8.4 Breeding Nile tilapia in hapas fixed in earthen ponds in the Philippines. *Photograph by A.-F. El-Sayed.*

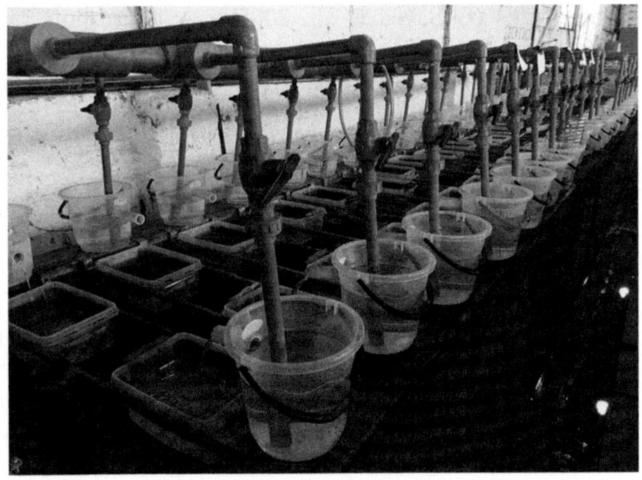

FIGURE 8.5 Tilapia hatchery in Congo. *Photo provided by Mohamed Marzouki.*

exchange, wind, water turbidity and varying water level. The use of double hapa system, where broodfish are stocked in an inner net having larger mesh size that allows free access of produced swim-up fry to the outer fine mesh hapa or directly to the surrounding water tanks/ponds, has been studied. This system was found effective in reducing the disturbance of brooding fish and fry and decreasing cannibalism, but the performance was not very encouraging (Guerrero and Garcia, 1983; Costa-Pierce and Hadikusumah, 1995). On the other hand, large amounts of Nile tilapia seeds are produced using hapas-in-pond systems by rural households in NW Bangladesh, leading to significant social and economic benefits (Barman and Little, 2011).

8.11.1.4 Artificial incubation

The removal of eggs and sac fry from the mouths of females and incubating them artificially is an effective method of tilapia seed production. Artificial incubation is preferable to natural incubation due to (1) elimination of cannibalism; (2) high production of even-sized fry; (3) increased spawning synchrony; (4) shortened interspawning intervals; (5) reduction of hatching time and (6) facilitation of research on tilapia genetics and reproduction.

The incubation units of tilapia eggs can range from simple, inexpensive and easy-to-make units, such as soft drink bottles and round-bottom containers such as carboys and plastic containers to commercial, more advanced conical upwelling jars (Fig. 8.5). The efficiency of an incubator depends on its type, size and shape, developmental stages of eggs, and water quality and flow. Rana (1986) found that round-bottom incubator caused higher survival than conical containers (85% compared to 60%), while the time to hatch was shorter in conical vessels than in round-bottom vessels (Macintosh and Little, 1995). Furthermore, Rana and Suliman (1993) found that hatching time and survival rates of tilapia fry were significantly better in downwelling round-bottom incubators than in upwelling conical chambers.

8.12 Egg hatching and yolk-sac absorption

The development time that the fertilized eggs of tilapia takes to hatch ranges from <3 to >6 days. Hatching time is affected by a number of factors, including water temperature (Rana, 1990b, 1990c; Hui et al., 2014), salinity (El-Sayed et al., 2005a; Hui et al., 2014), pH (Hui et al., 2014), water flow (Rab, 1989; El-Sayed et al., 2005b) and broodstock nutrition (Gunasekera et al., 1996a, 1996b; Siddiqui et al., 1997; El-Sayed et al., 2003; El-Sayed and Kawanna, 2008). The optimum temperature for best hatching and survival rates ranges from 25 to 32°C. The decrease in water temperature below 22°C in subtropical areas can lead to a delay or decrease in seed production, as has been reported in Nile tilapia in Vietnam (Green et al., 1997) and Egypt (El-Naggar et al., 2000). Improving water temperature through heating, increasing pond depth, shading, deep hapas, etc., improves reproduction efficiency and seed production. On the other hand, high ambient water temperature (33–35°C) was found to reduce spawning efficiency, egg quality and hatchability of Nile tilapia in central Thailand during hot seasons (Little et al., 1997).

Water flow was also found to affect spawning efficiency and larval growth of tilapia. The time taken to yolk sac-absorption of Nile tilapia eggs to reach swim-up fry was reduced with increasing water flow (El-Sayed et al., 2005b). A flow rate of about 8 L min^{-1} in a 20 L hatching unit was found optimal for yolk sac absorption of Nile tilapia eggs (El-Sayed et al., 2005b). A lower flow rate (3.6 L min^{-1}), at a stocking density of three females m^{-2} and a feeding level of 1% BW day^{-1}, was suggested by Tsadik and Bart (2007) for improving tilapia seed production.

A number of studies have considered the effects of water salinity on hatchability and larval rearing of tilapia. Hatching success of *O. niloticus* females was comparable at 5‰ to that in fresh water, while increasing salinity to 10 and 15‰ lowered hatching success, and no hatching occurred in full seawater (Watanabe and Kuo, 1985). Al-Ahmad et al. (1988) also found that egg hatching success and fry survival of *O. spilurus* was twice as high in groundwater (4‰) as in seawater (40‰). On the contrary, Uchida and King (1962) found that fry production of *O. mossambicus* was three times higher in brackish water (8.9–15.2‰) than in fresh water.

It has also been reported that broodstock nutrition significantly affects spawning efficiency, egg hatchability and larval growth. El-Sayed et al. (2003) found that the hatchability of Nile tilapia eggs hatched at different salinities (0–14‰) was linearly increased with increasing dietary protein levels from 25% to 40%. Eggs produced from broodstock fed 25% protein at 7 and 14‰ needed more time for hatching and yolk-sac absorption and resulted in poorer larval weight than those reared in fresh water. Furthermore, at high dietary protein levels (35%–40%), *O. niloticus* eggs took about 3–4 days to hatch, while at lower protein level (25%) hatching occurred after 4–6 days. Similar results have been reported on *O. niloticus* fed 20% and 35% protein at 26°C (Gunasekera et al., 1996a). In addition, as mentioned earlier, dietary lipid source and water salinity may have interactive effects on spawning, egg hatchability and larval performance and survival. El-Sayed et al. (2005a) found that Nile tilapia broodfish reared in brackish water (7 and 14‰) require a source of dietary n-3 HUFA (FO) for optimal egg hatchability and larval performance, while plant oil (SBO) met the requirements of broodfish reared in fresh water.

8.13 Larval rearing and growth

The growth of tilapia fry depends on many factors, including stocking density, food and feeding regimes, photoperiods, and water flow and replacement. The following sections briefly discuss these factors.

8.13.1 Stocking density

The effects of stocking density on larval performance are not well documented. Varying, and sometimes controversial, results have been reported concerning the relationship between stocking density and larval growth and survival. Dambo and Rana (1992) found that the growth rates of Nile tilapia fry were negatively correlated with stocking density ranging from 2 to 20 fry L^{-1}. They suggested that 5–10 fry L^{-1} be adopted as the optimum stocking density. Rana (1981) suggested also 8 fry L^{-1} as an optimal stocking density of *O. mossambicus*. El-Sayed (2002) found that the growth of Nile tilapia fry decreased with increasing stocking density from 3 to 20 fry L^{-1}, but no significant difference was found between 3 and 5 fry L^{-1}. Therefore, 5 fry L^{-1} was suggested as optimal for hatchery-reared Nile tilapia fry. This result is in agreement with that of Silva et al. (2000) who reported that the growth of tetra hybrid red tilapia decreased with increasing stocking density. On the contrary, much higher stocking densities have been reported by a number of authors. Gall and Bakar (1999) reported that body size of tilapia fry was not affected by stocking densities ranging from 10 to 200 fry L^{-1} when water flow was uniform. Luz et al. (2012) reported that up to 30 larvae L^{-1} can be successfully reared in a 2‰ water. Furthermore, Macintosh and De Silva (1984) found that the relationship between stocking density and survival of *O. mossambicus* and *O. niloticus* female × *O. aureus* male fry was not consistent. It is evident that more work is needed alongside this line.

The negative correlation between growth rates and stocking density of tilapia fry has been investigated by a number of authors. Macintosh and De Silva (1984) reported that increasing stocking density of *O. mossambicus* fry might have led to diminishing social dominance. This usually leads to 'social stress' and cause a 'chronic stress response', which, in turn, impairs fish growth, possibly due to the mobilization of dietary energy by the physiological alterations provoked by the stress response (Dambo and Rana, 1992; Kebus et al., 1992). Increasing stocking density may also cause deterioration in water quality, leading to stressful conditions (Barton and Iwama, 1991; Pankhurst and van der Kraak, 1997).

The high stocking density of tilapia fry may also cause excessive cannibalism, leading to high mortality. This phenomenon has been reported with Nile tilapia (Dambo and Rana, 1992; El-Sayed, 2002), *O. mossambicus* (Uchida and King, 1962; Macintosh and De Silva, 1984) and tilapia hybrids (Macintosh and De Silva, 1984). Abdel-Tawwab et al. (2006) reared Nile tilapia fry (1.2 g) at two densities (100 or 200 fish m^{-3}) with 50 fish m^{-3} of larger sizes (5–30 g). The cannibalistic rate increased as the size difference increased, where bigger fish were more cannibalistic than smaller fish. Cannibalism also increased with increasing larval density. These studies demonstrated that cannibalism can be a main cause of tilapia fry mortality. Continuous grading of the fry in nursing units to separate large fry and using broodstock of approximately similar ages and sizes to produce eggs and fry of similar sizes are a common practice to reduce cannibalism among tilapia fry.

8.13.2 Food and feeding regimes

The protein and energy requirements of tilapia fry have been discussed in Chapter 7. About 35%–45% crude protein is required for optimum larval performance, depending on protein and energy sources, fish species and culture systems. The effects of feeding levels on performance of tilapia fry are also well documented, although the results are controversial. El-Sayed (2002) found that Nile tilapia fry fed a larval test diet at 10%–35% BW d^{-1} attained their optimum performance at 35% level, while Santiago et al. (1987) found that the growth of Nile tilapia fry increased with increasing feeding levels up to 65%. However, no significant differences in growth rates and survival were found between 30% and 65% feeding level. These authors recommended a feeding rate of 30%–45% BW d^{-1} as optimal for Nile tilapia fry. The growth rates of red tilapia fingerlings (0.56 g) were increased, while feed conversion ratios were impaired with increasing feeding levels from 4% to 16% (Sirol et al., 2000).

The effects of food colour on growth and feed efficiency of tilapia fry is not well understood. Arumugam (1997) found that tilapia fry showed no preference to diet colour. In contrast, El-Sayed et al. (2013) found that feed colour significantly affected the growth and feed utilization efficiency of Nile tilapia fry (0.01 g). The fish were fed test diets with six different colours (dark blue, dark green, dark red, dark brown, yellow and light brown (control)). The best growth rates, feed efficiency, survival and body protein were achieved in larvae fed dark-coloured diets (dark blue, dark green, dark red and dark brown), while light-coloured diets (yellow and light brown) resulted in lower performance (Fig. 8.6). This result suggests that Nile tilapia larvae are visual feeders, and they prefer dark-coloured diets to light-coloured diets.

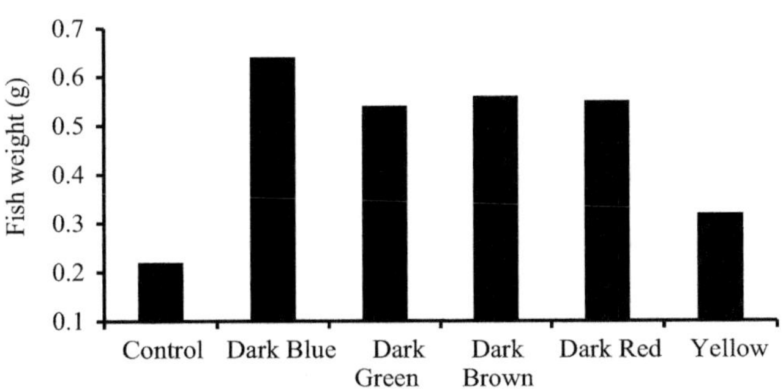

FIGURE 8.6 Effect of feed colour on growth rate of Nile tilapia fry.

8.13.3 Photoperiod

It has been suggested that freshwater fish species show more of a response to photoperiod than marine and diadromous species (Imsland et al., 1995). However, the response of marine species to photoperiods has been well investigated, while little attention has been paid to freshwater species. The available information indicates that the response of tilapia to photoperiod cycles depends on fish developmental stage and sex. El-Sayed and Kawanna (2004) found that larval stage of Nile tilapia was more sensitive to photoperiod than fingerling and juvenile stages. Fish fry subjected to long photoperiods (24 and 18 h) had significantly better performance than those exposed to intermediate or short photoperiods (12 or 6 h). Similar results have been reported on several marine fish larvae, where the growth rates were improved with increasing photoperiods (Tandler and Helps, 1985; Barlow et al., 1995; Hart et al., 1996).

One possible explanation of the decreased growth of tilapia fry during shorter photoperiods is that during these short light phases insufficient time was available for the establishment of a 'robust rhythmicity', as has been reported by Biswas and Takeuchi (2002) and Biswas et al. (2002). The effect of photoperiod on synchronizing an endogenous rhythm to the external environment may also require more energy in the shorter photoperiods, leading to a reduction of somatic fish growth (Biswas and Takeuchi, 2002; Biswas et al., 2002).

8.13.4 Water flow and replacement

Partial or total replacement of culture water may significantly affect the performance of tilapia fry. Absalom and Omenaihe (2000) reared Nile tilapia fry (1.14 g) using the following water replacement treatments: no water replacement, daily replacement, replacement every 3 days and every 6 days. They found that growth rates were not significantly affected by water replacement and suggested that less frequent water replacement may be better for larval growth and survival. The growth and survival of swim-up fry reared in 20 L fibre glass tanks in closed system, under different water flows (1, 2, 3, 4, and 8 L min^{-1}) were not affected by water flow of up to 4 L min^{-1} (El-Sayed et al., 2005b). Further increase in the water flow to 8 L min^{-1} caused extremely poor growth and high mortality (Fig. 8.7). However, the effects of water flow should be considered in relation to tank size. In other words, the water exchange rate has the major effect rather than water flow per se.

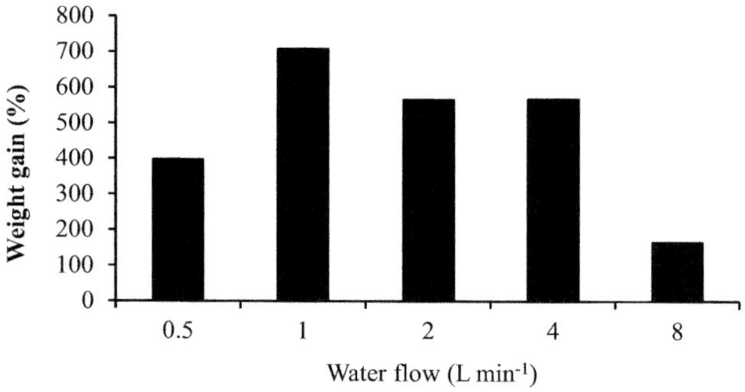

FIGURE 8.7 Effect of water flow on percent weight gain of Nile tilapia fry.

8.14 Closing remarks

1. Removal of eggs and fry from females' mouths accelerates vitellogenesis, shortens the intervals between successive spawnings. A 5-day cycle of seed removal from females' mouths is a common practice in commercial tilapia hatcheries in Thailand.
2. Exchange of tilapia male and female broodfish, after a period of conditioning, could be an effective tool of improving seed production, spawning synchrony and spawning frequency. A 5–15-day resting may be appropriate.
3. The ratio between dietary protein and energy (P:E ratio) in tilapia feeds is important for ensuring adequate use of energy and spare protein for anabolic processes and preventing the accumulation of excessive fat that would adversely affect the health of reproducing fish.
4. Partial or complete water change of spawning units, at frequent intervals, is suggested. This process may improve seed output and spawning synchrony of tilapia.
5. Immersing fish fry in hormone solutions for short periods of time could be a safe alternative for oral administration, but timing, duration and number of immersions should be carefully determined.
6. A 100% Nile tilapia males can be produced by suppressing aromatase activity, using AIs such as fadrozole.
7. Phytoestrogens (plant-derived substances with estrogenic activity) may affect reproductive development and sex differentiation in fish. SBM and other plant protein sources containing high levels of phytoestrogens should be avoided as protein sources for Nile tilapia larvae during sex reversal treatments.
8. The effects of stocking density of tilapia fry on larval performance are not well documented. The stocking density for optimum performance has been controversial; and more work is needed to verify this dispute.
9. Feed colour could be a key factor for feed acceptance in Nile tilapia. These fish appear to prefer dark-coloured feeds than light-coloured feeds during their larval stages, but no colour preference may exist during fingerling and adult stages.
10. Nile tilapia larvae may be more sensitive to photoperiod than fingerlings and juveniles, and they appear to perform better under long photoperiods (24 and 18 h).

References

Abdel-Tawwab, M., El-Marakby, H.I., Ahmad, M.H., 2006. Cannibalism in *Oreochromis niloticus* (Linnaeus): effect of stocking density, feed quality and submerged macrophytes. Indian Journal of Fisheries 53, 245–251.

Absalom, K.V., Omenaihe, O., 2000. Effects of water replacement rate on growth and survival of the Nile tilapia *Oreochromis niloticus* fry. Journal of Aquatic Sciences 15, 19–22.

Afonso, L.O.B., Leboute, E.M., 2003. Sex reversal in Nile tilapia: is it possible to produce all male stocks through immersion in androgens? World Aquaculture 34 (3), 16–19.

Afonso, L.O.B., Wassermann, G.J., De Oliveira, R.T., 2001. Sex reversal in Nile tilapia (*Oreochromis niloticus*) using a nonsteroidal aromatase inhibitor. Journal of Experimental Zoology 290, 177–181.

Akar, A.M., 2012. Effect of sex ratio on reproductive performance of broodstock Nile tilapia (*Oreochromis niloticus*) in suspended earthen pond hapas. Journal of the Arabian Aquaculture Society 7, 19–28.

Al-Ahmad, T.A., Ridha, M., Al-Ahmad, A.A., 1988. Reproductive performance of the tilapia *Oreochromis spilurus* in seawater and brackish ground-water. Aquaculture 73, 323–332.

Al-Feky, S.S.A., El-Sayed, A.-F.M., Ezzat, A.A., 2016. Dietary taurine improves reproductive performance of Nile tilapia (*Oreochromis niloticus*) broodstock. Aquaculture Nutrition 22, 392–399.

Andersen, L., Bjerregaard, P., Korsgaard, B., 2003. Vitellogenin induction and brain aromatase activity in adult male and female zebrafish exposed to endocrine disrupters. Fish Physiology and Biochemistry 28, 319–321.

Arumugam, P.T., 1997. Suitability of a continuous-flow chamber for investigating fish larvae/fry growth responses. Aquaculture 151, 365–370.

Barlow, C.G., Pearce, M.G., Rodgers, L.J., Clayton, P., 1995. Effects of photoperiod on growth, survival and feeding periodicity of larval and juvenile barramundi *Lates calcarifer* (Bloch). Aquaculture 138, 159–168.

Barman, B.K., Little, D.C., 2011. Use of hapas to produce Nile tilapia (*Oreochromis niloticus* L.) seed in household foodfish ponds: a participatory trial with small-scale farming households in Northwest Bangladesh. Aquaculture 317, 214–222.

Baroiller, J.F., Desprez, D., Carteret, Y., Tacon, P., Borel, F., Hoaraeu, M.C., et al., 1997. Influence of environmental and social factors on the reproductive efficiency in three tilapia species, *Oreochromis niloticus, O. aureus*, and the red tilapia (Red Florida Strain). In: Fitzsimmons, K. (Ed.), Tilapia Aquaculture. Proceedings from the Fourth International Symposium on Tilapia in Aquaculture. Northeast Regional Agriculture Engineering Service, Ithaca, NY, USA, pp. 238–252.

Bart, A., 2002. The application of ultrasound to produce all-male tilapia using immersion protocol. In: McElwee, K., Lewis, K., Nidiffer, M., Buitrago, P. (Eds.), Nineteenth Annual Technical Report. Pond Dynamics/Aquaculture CRSP. Oregon State University, Corvallis, OR, USA, pp. 53–57.

Barton, B.A., Iwama, G.K., 1991. Physiological changes in fish from stress in aquaculture with emphasis on the response and effects of corticosteroids. Annual Review of Fish Diseases 10, 3–26.

Bauer, J., 1968. Vergleichende Untersuchungen zum Kontaktverhalten verschiedener Arten der Gattung *Tilapia* (Cichlidae, Pisces) und ihrer Bastarde. Zeitschrift für Tierpsychologie 25, 22–70.

Beardmore, J.A., Mair, G.C., Lewis, R.I., 2001. Monosex male production in finfish as exemplified by tilapias: applications, problems and prospects. Aquaculture 197, 283–301.

Behrends, L.L., Smitherman, R.O., 1983. Use of warm water effluents to induce winter spawning of tilapia in a temperate climate. In: Fishelson, L., Yaron, Z. (Eds.), Proceedings of the International Symposium on Tilapia in Aquaculture. Tel-Aviv University, Israel, pp. 446–454.

Bennetau-Pelissero, C., Breton, B., Bennetau, B., Corraze, G., LeMenn, E., Davail-Cuisset, B., et al., 2001. Effect of Genistein-enriched diets on the endocrine process of gametogenesis and on reproduction efficiency of the rainbow trout *Onchohynchus mykiss*. General and Comparative Endocrinology 121, 173–187.

Bevis, R., 1994. The Effect of Artificial Nests on Reproductive Performance in Nile tilapia (*Oreochromis niloticus*, L.) Spawned in Net Hapas (M.Sc. thesis). Asian Institute of Technology, Bangkok, Thailand.

Bhujel, R.C., 1999. Management of Nile tilapia (*Oreochromis niloticus*) Broodfish for Commercial Seed Production in Thailand (Ph.D. thesis). Asian Institute of Technology, Bangkok, Thailand.

Bhujel, R.C., 2000. A review of strategies for the management of Nile tilapia broodfish in seed production systems, especially hapa-based systems. Aquaculture 181, 37–59.

Bhujel, R.C., Yakupitiyage, A., Turner, W.A., Little, D.C., 2001. Selection of a commercial feed for Nile tilapia (*Oreochromis niloticus*) broodfish breeding in a hapa-in-pond system. Aquaculture 194, 303–314.

Bhujel, R.C., Little, D.C., Hossain, A., 2007. Reproductive performance and the growth of pre-stunted and normal Nile tilapia (*Oreochromis niloticus*) broodfish at varying feeding rates. Aquaculture 273, 71–79.

Biswas, A.K., Takeuchi, T., 2002. Effect of different photoperiod cycles on metabolic rate and energy loss of both fed and unfed adult tilapia *Oreochromis niloticus*: Part II. Fisheries Science 68, 543–553.

Biswas, A.K., Endo, M., Takeuchi, T., 2002. Effect of different photoperiod cycles on metabolic rate and energy loss of both fed and unfed young tilapia *Oreochromis niloticus*: Part I. Fisheries Science 68, 465–477.

Biswas, A.K., Morita, T., Yoshizaki, G., Maita, M., Takeuchi, T., 2005. Control of reproduction in Nile tilapia *Oreochromis niloticus* (L.) by photoperiod manipulation. Aquaculture 243, 229–239.

Boeuf, G., Le Bail, P., 1999. Does light have an influence on fish growth? Aquaculture 177, 129–152.

Bombardelli, R.A., dos Reis Goes, E.S., de Negreiros Sousa, S.M., Syperreck, M.A., Goes, M.D., de Oliveira Pedreira, A.C., et al., 2017. Growth and reproduction of female Nile tilapia fed diets containing different levels of protein and energy. Aquaculture 479, 817–823.

Bromage, N., Porter, M., Randall, C., 2001. The environmental regulation of maturation in farmed finfish with special reference to the role of photoperiod and melatonin. Aquaculture 197, 63–98.

Broussard, M.C., Reyes, R., Raguindin, F., 1983. Evaluation of hatchery management schemes for large-scale production of *Oreochromis niloticus* fingerlings in Central Luzon, Philippines. In: Fishelson, L., Yaron, Z. (Eds.), Proceedings of the International Symposium on Tilapia in Aquaculture. Tel-Aviv University, Israel, pp. 414–424.

Bunthawin, S., Sornsilpa, T., Tuantranont, A., Jaruwongrungsee, K., Ritchie, R.J., 2015. Monosex-male sex reversal of Nile tilapia eggs using pulse-electric field inductions. Journal of Computational and Theoretical Nanoscience 12, 724–728.

Cagauan, A.G., Baleta, F.N., Abucay, J.S., 2004. Sex reversal of Nile tilapia *Oreochromis niloticus* L. by egg immersion technique: the effect of hormone concentration and immersion time. In: Bolivar, R., Mair, G., Fitzsimmons, K. (Eds.), Proceedings of the Sixth International Symposium on Tilapia in Aq1uaculture, Manila, Philippines, pp. 127–136.

Campos-Mendoza, A., McAndrew, B.J., Coward, K., Bromage, N., 2004. Reproductive response of Nile tilapia (*Oreochromis niloticus*) to photoperiodic manipulation; effects on spawning periodicity, fecundity and egg size. Aquaculture 231, 299–314.

Cao, T.B., 1998. Development of Pond Culture of Thai Nile tilapia (*Oreochromis niloticus* L.) and Its Marketability in Hanoi, Vietnam (Ph.D. thesis). Asian Institute of Technology, Bangkok, Thailand.

Carvalho, P.L.P.F., Koch, J.F.A., Cintra, F.T., Fernandes Júnior, A.C., Sartori, M.M.P., Barros, M.M., et al., 2018. Available phosphorus as a reproductive performance enhancer for female Nile tilapia. Aquaculture 486, 202–209.

Chervinski, J., 1982. Environmental physiology of tilapias. In: Pullin, R.V.S., Lowe-McConnell, R.H. (Eds.), The Biology and Culture of Tilapias. ICLARM Conference Proceedings No. 7. ICLARM, Manila, Philippines, pp. 119–128.

Chervinski, J., Yashouv, A., 1971. Preliminary experiments on the growth of *Tilapia aurea* in seawater ponds. Bamidgeh 23, 125–129.

Chervinski, J., Zorn, M., 1974. Note on the growth of *Tilapia aurea* and *Tilapia zillii* in seawater ponds. Aquaculture 4, 249–255.

Cissé, A., 1988. Effects of varying protein levels on spawning frequency and growth of *Sarotherodon melanotheron*. In: Pullin, R.S.V., Bhukaswan, T., Tonguthai, K., Maclean, J.L. (Eds.), Proceedings of the Second International Symposium on Tilapia in Aquaculture. ICLARM Proceedings No. 15. Department of Fisheries, Bangkok, Thailand, and ICLARM, Manila, Philippines, pp. 329–333.

Cornish, D.A., Smit, G.L., Campbell, I.M., 1997. Seasonal fluctuations in gonadotropin levels in the plasma and gonads of male and female tilapia, *Oreochromis mossambicus*. Water South Africa 23, 263–270.

Corre, V.L., 1981. Culture of Nile Tilapia in Brackishwater Ponds Using Supplemental Feeds Containing Various Levels of Protein (M.Sc. thesis). University of the Philippines, Holio City, Philippines.

Costa-Pierce, B.A., Hadikusumah, H., 1995. Production management of double-net tilapia *Oreochromis* spp. Hatcheries in a eutrophic tropical reservoir. Journal of the World Aquaculture Society 26, 453–459.

Coward, K., Bromage, N.R., 1998. Histological classification of ovarian growth and the dynamics of ovarian recrudescence in *Tilapia zillii* (Gervais), a substrate-spawning cichlid. Journal of Fish Biology 53, 285–302.

Coward, K., Bromage, N.R., 1999. Spawning periodicity, fecundity and egg size in laboratory-held stocks of a substrate-spawning tilapiine, *Tilapia zillii* (Gervais). Aquaculture 171, 251–267.

Coward, K., Bromage, N.R., 2000. Reproductive physiology of female tilapia broodstock. Reviews in Fish Biology and Fisheries 10, 1–25.

Dambo, W.B., Rana, K.J., 1992. Effects of stocking density on growth and survival of Nile tilapia *Oreochromis niloticus* (L.) fry in the hatchery. Aquaculture and Fisheries Management 23, 71–80.

Dan, N.C., Little, D., 2000. Overwintering performance of Nile tilapia Oreochromis niloticus (L.) broodfish and seed at ambient temperaturesin northern Vietnam. Aquaculture Research 31, 485–493.

De Graaf, G.J., Galemoni, F., Huisman, E.A., 1999. Reproductive biology of pond-reared Nile tilapia, *Oreochromis niloticus* L. Aquaculture Research 30, 25–33.

de Oliveira, M.M., Ribeiro, T., Orlando, T.M., de Oliveira, D.G., Drumond, M.M., de Freitas, R.T., et al., 2014. Effects of crude protein levels on female Nile tilapia (*Oreochromis niloticus*) reproductive performance parameters. Animal Reproduction Science 150, 62–69.

De Silva, S.S., Radampola, K., 1990. Effect of dietary protein level on the reproductive performance of *Oreochromis niloticus*. In: Hirano, R., Hanyu, I. (Eds.), Proceedings of the Second Asian Fisheries Forum. Asian Fisheries Society, Manila, Philippines, pp. 559–563.

Desprez, D., Géraz, E., Hoareau, M.C., Mélard, C., Bosc, P., Baroiller, J.F., 2003. Production of a high percentage of male offspring with a natural androgen, 11β-hydroxyandrostenedione (11βOHA4), in Florida red tilapia. Aquaculture 216, 55–65.

Duponchelle, F., Legendre, M., 1997. Influence of space structure on reproductive traits of *Oreochromis niloticus* females. In: Fitzsimmons, K. (Ed.), Proceedings from the Fourth International Symposium on Tilapia in Aquaculture. Northeast Regional Agriculture Engineering Service, Ithaca, New York, USA, pp. 305–314.

Duponchelle, F., Legendre, M., 2000. *Oreochromis niloticus* (Cichlidae) in Lake Ayame, Côte d'Ivoire: life history traits of a strongly diminished population. Cybium 24, 161–172.

Duponchelle, F., Panfili, J., 1998. Variations in size and age at maturity of female Nile tilapia, *Oreochromis niloticus*, populations from man-made lakes of Côte d'Ivoire. Environmental Biology of Fishes 52, 453–465.

Duponchelle, F., Pouyaud, L., Legendre, M., 1997. Variation in reproductive characteristics of *Oreochromis niloticus* populations: genetic or environmental effects? In: Fitzsimmons, K. (Ed.), Proceedings from the Fourth International Symposium on Tilapia in Aquaculture. Northeast Regional Agricultural Engineering Services, Ithaca, NY, USA, pp. 253–261.

El-Gamal, A.E., El-Greisy, Z.A., El-Ebiary, E.H., 2007. Synergistic effects of vitamins C and E and selenium on the reproductive performance of Nile tilapia, *Oreochromis niloticus*. Journal of Applied Sciences Research 3, 564–573.

El-Naggar, G.O., El Nady, M.A., Kamar, M.G., Al-Kobabay, A.I., 2000. Effect of photoperiod, dietary protein and temperature on reproduction in Nile Tilapia (*Oreochromis niloticus*). In: Fitzsimmons, K., Filho, J.C. (Eds.), Tilapia Culture in the 21st Century. Proceedings from the Fifth International Symposium on Tilapia Aquaculture. American Tilapia Association and ICLARM, Rio de Janeiro, Brazil, pp. 352–358.

El-Sayed, A.-F.M., 2002. Effects of stocking density and feeding levels on growth and feed efficiency of Nile tilapia, *Oreochromis niloticus* (L.) fry. Aquaculture Research 33, 621–626.

El-Sayed, A.-F.M., Garling Jr., D.L., 1988. Carbohydrate-to-lipid ratio in diets for *Tilapia zillii* fingerlings. Aquaculture 73, 157–163.

El-Sayed, A.-F.M., Kawanna, M., 2004. Effects of photoperiod on the performance of farmed Nile tilapia *Oreochromis niloticus*: I. Growth, feed utilization efficiency and survival of fry and fingerlings. Aquaculture 231, 393–402.

El-Sayed, A.-F.M., Kawanna, M., 2007. Effects of photoperiod on growth and spawning efficiency of Nile tilapia (*Oreochromis niloticus* L.) broodstock in a recycling system. Aquaculture Research 38, 1242–1247.

El-Sayed, A.-F.M., Kawanna, M., 2008. Effects of dietary protein and energy levels on spawning performance of Nile tilapia (*Oreochromis niloticus*) broodstock in a recycling system. Aquaculture 280, 179–184.

El-Sayed, A.-F.M., El-Ghobashy, A., Al-Amoudi, M.M., 1996. Effects of pond depth and water temperature on the growth, mortality and body composition of Nile tilapia, *Oreochromis niloticus* (L.). Aquaculture Research 27, 681–687.

El-Sayed, A.-F.M., Mansour, C.R., Ezzat, A.A., 2003. Effects of dietary protein levels on spawning performance of Nile tilapia (*Oreochromis niloticus*) broodstock reared at different water salinities. Aquaculture 220, 619–632.

El-Sayed, A.-F.M., Mansour, C.R., Ezzat, A.A., 2005a. Effects of dietary lipid source on spawning performance of Nile tilapia (*Oreochromis niloticus*) broodstock reared at different water salinities. Aquaculture 248, 187–196.

El-Sayed, A.-F.M., Kawanna, M., Mudar, M., 2005b. Effects of water flow rates on growth and survival of Nile tilapia fry. World Aquaculture 36 (1), 5–6.

El-Sayed, A.-F.M., Abdel-Aziz, E.H., Abdel-Ghani, H.M., 2012. Effects of phytoestrogens on sex reversal of Nile tilapia (*Oreochromis niloticus*) larvae fed diets treated with 17α-Methyltestosterone. Aquaculture 360–361, 58–63.

El-Sayed, A.F.M., El-Ghobashy, A.E., El-Mezayen, M.M., 2013. Effect of feed colour on growth and feed utilization of Nile tilapia (*Oreochromis niloticus* L.) larvae and fingerlings. Aquaculture Nutrition 19, 870–876.

Ernst, D.H., Watanabe, W.O., Ellingson, L.J., 1991. Commercial-scale production of Florida red tilapia seed in low-and brackish-salinity tanks. Journal of the World Aquaculture Society 22, 36–44.

FAO (Food and Agriculture Organization of the United Nations), 2019. FAO Fisheries and Aquaculture Statistics. http://www.fao.org/fishery/statistics/en.

Faunce, C.H., 2000. Reproduction of black tilapia, *Sarotherodon melanotheron*, within an impounded mangrove ecosystem in east-central Florida. Environmental Biology of Fishes 57, 353–361.

Fineman-Kalio, A.S., 1988. Preliminary observations on the effect of salinity on the reproduction and growth of freshwater Nile tilapia, *Oreochromis niloticus* (L.), cultured in brackishwater ponds. Aquaculture and Fisheries Management 19, 313–320.

Fryer, G., Iles, T.D., 1972. The Cichlid Fishes of the Great Lakes of Africa: Their Biology and Evolution. T.F.H. Publishing, Neptune City, New Jersy. Also published by Oliver and Boyd, Edinburgh.

Gale, W.L., Fitzpatrick, M.S., Lucero, M., Contreras-Sánchez, W.M., Schreck, C.B., 1999. Masculinization of Nile tilapia (*Oreochromis niloticus*) by immersion in androgens. Aquaculture 178, 349–357.

Gall, G.A.E., Bakar, Y., 1999. Stocking density and tank size in the design of breed improvement programs for body size of tilapia. Aquaculture 173, 197–205.

Galman, O.R., Moreau, J., Avtalion, R., 1988. Breeding characteristics and growth performance of Philippines red tilapia. In: Pullin, R.S.V., Bhukaswan, T., Tonguthai, K., Maclean, J.L. (Eds.), Proceedings of the Second International Symposium on Tilapia in Aquaculture. ICLARM Conference Proceedings No. 15. Department of Fisheries, Bangkok, Thailand, and ICLARM, Manila, Philippines, pp. 169–175.

Galvez, J.I., Morrison, J.R., Phelps, R.P., 1996. Efficacy of trenbolone acetate in sex inversion of the blue tilapia *Oreochromis aureus*. Journal of the World Aquaculture Society 27, 483–486.

Gauthaman, K., Adaikan, P.G., Prasad, R.N.V., 2002. Aphrodisiac properties of *Tribulus terrestris* extract (Protodioscin) in normal and castrated rats. Life Sciences 71, 1385–1396.

Getinet, G.T., 2008. Effects of maternal age on fecundity, spawning interval, and egg quality of Nile tilapia, *Oreochromis niloticus* (L.). Journal of the World Aquaculture Society 39, 671–677.

Gilling, C.J., Skibinski, D.O.F., Beardmore, J.A., 1996. Sex reversal of tilapia fry by immersion in water containing estrogens. In: Pullin, R.S.V., Lazard, J., Legendre, M., Amon Kottias, J.B., Pauly, D. (Eds.), Proceedings of the Third International Symposium on Tilapia in Aquaculture. ICLARM Conference Proceedings No. 41. ICLARM, Penang, Malaysia, pp. 314–319.

Goncalves-de-Freitas, E., Nishida, S.M., 1998. Sneaking behaviour of the nile tilapia. Boletim Tecnico do CEPTA 11, 71–79.

Green, C.C., Kelly, A.M., 2009. Effects of the estrogen mimic genistein as a dietary component on sex differentiation and ethoxyresorufin-O-deethylase (EROD) activity in channel catfish *Ictalurus punctatus*. Fish Physiology and Biochemistry 35, 377–384.

Green, B.W., Verrica, K.L., Fitzpatrick, M.S., 1997. Fry and fingerling production. In: Egna, H.S., Boyd, C.E. (Eds.), Dynamics of Pond Aquaculture. CRC Press, Boca Raton, USA, pp. 215–243.

Guerrero III., R.D., 1975. Use of androgens for the production of all-male tilapia *Tilapia aurea* (Steindachner). Transactions of the American Fisheries Society 104, 342–348.

Guerrero III., R.D., 1982. Control of tilapia reproduction. In: Pullin, R.S.V., Lowe-McConnell, R.H. (Eds.), The Biology and Culture of Tilapias. ICLARM Conference Proceedings No. 7. ICLARM, Manila, Philippines, pp. 309–316.

Guerrero III., R.D., Garcia, A.M., 1983. Studies on the fry production of *Sarotherodon niloticus* in a lake-based hatchery. In: Fishelson, L., Yaron, Z. (Eds.), Proceedings of the International Symposium on Tilapia in Aquaculture. Tel-Aviv University, Israel, pp. 388–393.

Guerrero III, R.D., Guerrero, L.A., 1988. Feasibility of commercial production of sex-reversed Nile tilapia fingerlings in the Philippines. In: Pullin, R.S.V., Bhukaswan, T., Tonguthai, K., Maclean, J.L. (Eds.), Proceedings of the Second International Symposium on Tilapia in Aquaculture. ICLARM Conference Proceedings No. 15. Department of Fisheries, Bangkok, Thailand, and ICLARM, Manila, Philippines, pp. 183–186.

Gunasekera, R.M., Lam, T.J., 1997. Influence of dietary protein level on ovarian recrudescence in Nile tilapia, *Oreochromis niloticus* (L.). Aquaculture 149, 57–69.

Gunasekera, R.M., Shim, K.F., Lam, T.J., 1995. Effect of dietary protein level on puberty, oocyte growth and egg chemical composition in the tilapia, *Oreochromis niloticus* (L.). Aquaculture 134, 169–183.

Gunasekera, R.M., Shim, K.F., Lam, T.J., 1996a. Effect of dietary protein level on spawning performance and amino acid composition of eggs of Nile tilapia, *Oreochromis niloticus* (L.). Aquaculture 146, 121–134.

Gunasekera, R.M., Shim, K.F., Lam, T.J., 1996b. Influence of protein content of broodstock diets on larval quality and performance in Nile tilapia, *Oreochromis niloticus* (L.). Aquaculture 146, 245–259.

Gunasekera, R.M., Shim, K.F., Lam, T.J., 1997. Influence of dietary protein content on the distribution of amino acids in oocytes, serum and muscle of Nile tilapia, *Oreochromis niloticus* (L.). Aquaculture 152, 205–221.

Gwahaba, J.J., 1973. Effects of overfishing on *Tilapia nilotica* populations of Lake George, Uganda, over the past 20 years. East African Wildlife Journal 11, 317–328.

Hajizadeh, A., Shinn, A., 2016. An experimental analysis of the effects of dietary lipid sources and feeding ration on the reproductive performance, egg and larval quality of Nile tilapia, *Oreochromis niloticus* (L.). Iranian Journal of Fisheries Sciences 15, 1187–1201.

Hart, P.R., Hutchinson, W.G., Purser, G.J., 1996. Effects of photoperiod, temperature and salinity on hatchery-reared larvae of the greenback flounder (*Rhombosolea tapirina* Gunther, 1862). Aquaculture 144, 303–311.

Hepher, B., Pruginin, Y., 1981. Commercial Fish Farming with Special Reference to Fish Culture in Israel. Wiley-Interscience, New York, p. 261.

Hickling, C.E., 1960. The Malacca *Tilapia* hybrids. Journal of Genetics 57, 1–10.

Hickling, C.E., 1963. The cultivation of tilapia. Scientific America 208, 143–152.

Hines, G.A., Watts, S.A., 1995. Non-steroidal chemical sex manipulation of tilapia. Journal of the World Aquaculture Society 26, 98–102.

Hughes, D.G., Behrends, L.L., 1983. Mass Production of *Tilapia nilotica* seed in suspended net enclosures. In: Fishelson, L., Yaron, Z. (Eds.), Proceedings of the International Symposium on Tilapia in Aquaculture. Tel-Aviv University, Israel, pp. 394–401.

Hui, W., Xiaowen, Z., Haizhen, W., Jun, Q., Pao, X., Ruiwei, L., 2014. Joint effect of temperature, salinity and pH on the percentage fertilization and hatching of Nile tilapia (*Oreochromis niloticus*). Aquaculture Research 45, 259–269.

Imsland, A., Folkvord, A.F., Steffansson, S.O., 1995. Growth, oxygen consumption and activity of juvenile turbot (*Scophthalmus maximus*) reared under different temperatures and photoperiods. Netherlands Journal of Sea Research 34, 149–159.

Kanazawa, A., Teshima, S., Imai, K., 1980. Biosynthesis of fatty acids in *Tilapia zillii* and the puffer Fish. Memoirs of Faculty of Fisheries Kagoshima University 29, 313–318.

Kebus, M.J., Collins, M.T., Brownfield, M.S., Amundson, C.H., Kayes, T.B., Malison, J.A., 1992. Effects of rearing density on stress response and growth of rainbow trout. Journal of Aquatic Animal Health 4, 1–6.

Kuwamura, T., 1987. Male mating territory and sneaking in a maternal mouthbrooder, *Pseudosimochromis curvifrons* (Pisces; Cichlidae). Journal of Ethology 5, 203–206.

Kwon, J.Y., Haghpanah, V., Kogson-Hurtado, L.M., McAndrew, B.J., Penman, D.J., 2000. Masculinization of genetic female Nile tilapia (*Oreochromis niloticus*) by dietary administration of an aromatase inhibitor during sexual differentiation. Journal of Experimental Zoology 287, 46–53.

Kwon, J.Y., McAndrew, B.J., Penman, D.J., 2002. Treatment with an aromatase inhibitor suppresses high-temperature feminization of genetic male (YY) Nile tilapia. Journal of Fish Biology 60, 625–636.

Lee, J.C., 1979. Reproduction and Hybridization of Three Cichlid Fishes, *Tilapia aurea*, *T. hornorum* and *T. nilotica* in Aquaria and in Plastic Pools (Ph.D. thesis). Auburn University, Auburn, AL, USA.

Lester, L.J., Abell, T.A., Palada, M.S., Keus, H.J., 1988. Genetic variation in size and sexual maturation of *Oreochromis niloticus* under hapa and cage culture conditions. In: Pullin, R.S.V., Bhukaswan, T., Tonguthai, K., Maclean, J.L. (Eds.), Proceedings of the Second International Symposium on Tilapia in Aquaculture. ICLARM Conference Proceedings No. 15. Department of Fisheries, Bangkok, Thailand, and ICLARM, Manila, Philippines, pp. 223–230.

Liao, I.C., Chang, S.L., 1983. Studies on the feasibility of red tilapia culture in saline water. In: Fishelson, L., Yaron, Z. (Eds.), Proceedings of the International Symposium on Tilapia in Aquaculture. Tel-Aviv University, Israel, pp. 524–533.

Likongwe, J.S., Stecko, T.D., Stauffer, J.R., Carline, R.F., 1996. Combined effects of water temperature and salinity on growth and feed utilisation of juvenile Nile tilapia *Oreochromis niloticus* (Linneaus). Aquaculture 146, 37–46.

Little, D.C., 1989. An Evaluation of Strategies for Production of Nile Tilapia (*Oreochromis niloticus* L.) Fry Suitable for Hormonal Treatment (Ph.D. thesis). Institute of Aquaculture, University of Stirling, Stirling, UK.

Little, D.C., 1992. The Development of Fry Production and Nursing Strategies for the Nile tilapia *Oreochromis niloticus*. Final Report. Asian Institute of Technology, Bangkok, Thailand, 24 pp.

Little, D.C., Hulata, G., 2000. Strategies for tilapia seed production. In: Beveridge, M.C.M., McAndrew, B.J. (Eds.), Tilapias: Biology and Exploitation. Kluwer Academic Publishers, Dordrecht/Boston/London, pp. 267–326.

Little, D.C., Macintosh, D.J., Edwards, P., 1993. Improving spawning synchrony in the Nile tilapia, *Oreochromis niloticus* (L). Aquaculture and Fisheries Management 24, 399–405.

Little, D.C., Sikawa, D., Juntana, J., 1994. Commercial production and marketing of Nile tilapia (*Oreochromis niloticus*) fry in Chonburi and Chachoengsao provinces, Thailand. NAGA: ICLARM Quarterly 17, 2–3.

Little, D.C., Bhujel, R.C., Turner, W.A., 1997. Commercialization of a hatchery process to produce MT-treated Nile tilapia in Thailand. In: Alston, D.E., Green, B.W., Clifford, H.C. (Eds.), Proceedings of the IV Symposium on Aquaculture in Central America: Focusing on Shrimp and Tilapia. National Honduran Aquaculturists and the Latin American Chapter of the World Aquaculture Society, Boca Raton, Florida, pp. 108–118.

Little, D.C., Coward, K., Bhujel, R.C., Pham, T.A., Bromage, N.R., 2000. Effect of broodfish exchange strategy on the spawning performance and sex steroid hormone levels of *Oreochromis niloticus* broodfish in hapas. Aquaculture 186, 77–88.

Lone, K.P., Ridha, M.T., 1993. Sex reversal and growth of *Oreochromis spilurus* (Guenther) in brackish and seawater by feeding 17α–methyltestosterone. Aquaculture and Fisheries Management 24, 593–602.

Lovshin, L.L., 1982. Tilapia hybridization. In: Pullin, R.S.V., Lowe-McConnell, R.H. (Eds.), The Biology and Culture of Tilapias. ICLARM Conference Proceedings No. 7. ICLARM, Manila, Philippines, pp. 279–308.

Lovshin, L.L., Ibrahim, H.H., 1988. Effects of broodstock exchange on *Oreochromis niloticus* egg and fry production in net enclosures. In: Pullin, R.S.V., Bhukaswan, T., Tonguthai, K., Maclean, J.L. (Eds.), Proceedings of the Second International Symposium on Tilapia in Aquaculture. ICLARM Conference Proceedings No. 15. Department of Fisheries, Bangkok, Thailand, and ICLARM, Manila, Philippines, pp. 231–236.

Lowe-McConnell, R.H., 1955. The fecundity of Tilapia species. East African Agricultural Journal 21, 45–52.

Lowe-Mcconnell, R.H., 1958. Observations on the biology of *Tilapia nilotica* L. in East African waters. Revue de Zoologie et de Botanique Africaines 57, 129–170.

Lowe-McConnell, R.H., 1959. Breeding behaviour patterns and ecological differences between tilapia species and their significance for evolution within the genus *Tilapia* (Pisces: Cichlidae). Proceedings of the Zoological Society of London 132, 1–30.

Lowe-Mcconnell, R.H., 1982. Tilapias in fish communities. In: Pullin, R.S.V., Lowe-McConnell, R.H. (Eds.), The Biology and Culture of Tilapias. ICLARM Conference Proceedings No. 7. ICLARM, Manila, Philippines, pp. 83–113.

Luz, R.K., de Souza e Silva, W., Filho, R.M., Santos, A.E.H., Rodrigues, L.A., Takata, R., et al., 2012. Stocking density in the larviculture of Nile tilapia in saline water. Revista Brasileira de Zootecnia 41, 2385–2389.

Macintosh, D.J., De Silva, S.S., 1984. The influence of stocking density and food ration on fry survival and growth in *Oreochromis mossambicus* and *O. niloticus* x *O. aureus* male hybrids reared in a closed circulated system. Aquaculture 41, 345–358.

Macintosh, D.J., Little, D.C., 1995. Nile tilapia (*Oreochromis niloticus*). In: Bromage, N.R., Roberts, R.J. (Eds.), Broodstock Management and Egg and Larval Quality. Blackwell Science, Oxford, UK, pp. 277–320.

Mair, G.C., Penman, D.J., Scott, A.G., Skibinski, D.O.F., Beardmore, J.A., 1987. Hormonal sex-reversal and the mechanisms of sex determination in *Oreochromis*. In: Tiews, K. (Ed.), Proceedings of the World Symposium on Selection, Hybridization and Genetic Engineering in Aquaculture, Vol. II. Heeneman, Berlin, pp. 301–312.

Mair, G.C., Estabillo, C.C., Sevilleja, R.C., Recometa, R.D., 1993. Small-scale fry production systems for Nile tilapia, *Oreochromis niloticus* (L.). Aquaculture and Fisheries Management 24, 229–235.

Majumdar, K.C., McAndrew, B.J., Fishelson, L., Yaron, Z., 1983. Sex ratios from interspecific crosses within the tilapias. In: Fishelson, L., Yaron, Z. (Eds.), Proceedings of the International Symposium on Tilapia in Aquaculture. Tel Aviv University, Tel Aviv, Israel, pp. 261–269.

Mansour, C.R., 2001. Nutritional Requirements of Nile Tilapia Broodstock Reared at Different Water Salinities (Ph.D. thesis). Alexandria University, Alexandria, Egypt.

Marengoni, N.G., Onoue, Y., Oyama, T., 1998. All-male tilapia hybrids of two strains of *Oreochromis niloticus*. Journal of the World Aquaculture Society 29, 108–113.

McAndrew, B.J., 1993. Sex control in tilapiines. In: Muir, J.J.F., Roberts, R.J. (Eds.), Recent Advances in Aquaculture. IV. Blackwell, London, UK, pp. 87–98.

Mélard, C., Ducarme, C., 1993. The tilapia intensive rearing technology in Europe. In: Kestemont, P., Billard, R. (Eds.), Proceedings of the Workshop on Aquaculture of Freshwater Species (Except Salmonids). Special Publication No. 20. European Aquaculture Society, Ostend, Belgium, pp. 24–28.

Mélard, C., Desprez, D., Philippart, J.C., 1995. Le comntrôle du sexe chez les tilapias: bilan etperspectives de recherche á la station de Tihange. Cahiers d'ethologie appliquée 13, 421–434.

Miranova, N.V., 1977. Energy expenditure on egg production in young *T. mossambica* and the influence of maintenance conditions on their reproductive intensity. Journal of Ichthyology 17, 627–633.

Mires, D., 1982. Study of the problems of the mass production of hybrid tilapia fry. In: Pullin, R.S.V., Lowe-McConnell, R.H. (Eds.), The Biology and Culture of Tilapias. ICLARM Conference Proceedings No. 7. ICLARM, Manila, Philippines, pp. 83–113.

Mohamed, G.A., Farag, M.E., Elghobashy, H.A., Ali, M.A., 2004. Feminization of sexually undifferentiated progeny of *Oreochromis niloticus* and *O. aureus*. Journal of Egyptian Academic Society for Environmental Development – C. Molecular Biology 5, 31–44.

Mohan, C.V., 2007. Seed quality in freshwater fish production. In: Bondad-Reantaso, M.G. (Ed.), Assessment of Freshwater Fish Seed Resources for Sustainable Aquaculture. FAO Fisheries Technical Paper. No. 501. Rome, Italy, pp. 499–517.

Msiska, O.V., Costa-Pierce, B.A., 1997. Factors affecting spawning success of *Oreochromis Karongae*. Aquaculture Research 28, 87–99.

Myers, J.M., Hershberger, W.K., 1991. Early growth and survival of heat-shocked and tetraploid-derived triploid rainbow trout (*Oncorhynchus mykiss*). Aquaculture 96, 97–107.

Nascimento, T.S.R., de Stéfani, M.V., Malheiros, E.B., Koberstein, T.C.D., 2014. High levels of dietary vitamin E improve the reproductive performance of female *Oreochromis niloticus*. Acta Scientiarum. Biological Sciences 36, 19–26.

Ng, W.-K., Wang, Y., 2011. Inclusion of crude palm oil in the broodstock diets of female Nile tilapia, *Oreochromis niloticus*, resulted in enhanced reproductive performance compared to broodfish fed diets with added fish oil or linseed oil. Aquaculture 314, 122–131.

Noakes, D.L.G., Balon, E.K., 1982. Life histories of tilapias: an evolutionary perspective. In: Pullin, R.S.V., Lowe-McConnell, R.H. (Eds.), The Biology and Culture of Tilapias. ICLARM Conference Proceedings No.7. ICLARM, Manila, Philippines, pp. 61–82.

Ojuok, J.E., Njiru, M., Ntiba, M.J., Mavuti, K.M., 2007. The effect of overfishing on the life-history strategies of nile tilapia, *Oreochromis niloticus* (L.) in the Nyanza Gulf of Lake Victoria, Kenya. Aquatic Ecosystem Health and Management 10, 443–448.

Okorie, O., 1973. Lunar Periodicity and the Breeding of *Tilapia nilotica* in the Northern Part of Lake Victoria. East African Freshwater Fish Research Organization, Annual Report, Appendix E, pp. 50–58.

Oliva-Teles, A., 2012. Nutrition and health of aquaculture fish. Journal of Fish Diseases 35, 83–108.

Omitoyin, B.O., Ajani, E.K., Sadiq, H.O., 2013. Preliminary investigation of *Tribulus terrestris* (Linn., 1753) extracts as natural sex reversal agent in *Oreochromis niloticus* (Linn., 1758) larvae. International Journal of Aquaculture 3, 133–137.

Pankhurst, N.W., van der Kraak, G., 1997. Effects of stress on reproduction and growth of fish. In: Iwama, J.K., Pickering, A.D. (Eds.), Fish Stress and Health in Aquaculture. Cambridge University Press, Cambridge, UK, pp. 73–93.

Payne, A.I., Collinson, R.I., 1983. A comparison of the biological characteristics of *Sarotherodon niloticus* (L.) with those of *S. aureus* (Steindachner) and other tilapia of the delta and lower Nile. Aquaculture 30, 335–351.

Penman, D.J., McAndrew, B.J., 2000. Genetics for the management and improvement of cultured tilapia. In: Beveridge, M.C.M., McAndrew, B.J. (Eds.), Tilapias: Biology and Exploitation. Kluwer Academic Publishers, Dordrecht/Boston/London, pp. 227–266.

Peters, H.M., 1963. Untersuchungen zum problem des angeborenen verhaltens. Naturwissenschaften 50, 677–686.

Peters, H.M., 1983. Fecundity, Egg Weight and Oocyte Development in tilapia (Cichlidae, Teleostei). In: ICLARM Translations 2. ICLARM, Manila, Philippines, 28 pp.

Philippart, J.-C.L., Ruwet, J.-C.L., 1982. Ecology and distribution of tilapias. In: Pullin, R.S.V., Lowe-McConnell, R.H. (Eds.), The Biology and Culture of Tilapias. ICLARM Conference Proceedings No. 7. ICLARM, Manila, Philippines, pp. 15–59.

Pierce, B.A., 1980. Production of hybrid tilapia in indoor aquaria. Progressive Fish-Culturist 42, 233–234.

Popma, T.J., Lovshin, L.L., 1996. Worldwide Prospects for Commercial Production of tilapia. In: Research and Development Series, No. 41. Department of Fisheries and Allied Aquaculture, Auburn University, Alabama, USA, 23 pp.

Potts, A.C., Phelps, R.P., 1995. Use of diethylstilbestrol and ethynylestradiol to feminize Nile tilapia, *Oreochromis niloticus*. Journal of Applied Ichthyology 11, 111–117.

Pruginin, Y., 1967. Report to the Government of Uganda on the Experimental Fish Culture Project in Uganda, 1965-1966. FAO/UNDP (Technical Assistance). Reports on Fisheries. TA Reports 2446. FAO, Rome, Italy, 19 pp.

Pruginin, Y., Rothbard, S., Wohlfarth, G., Halevy, A., Moav, R., Hulata, G., 1975. All-male broods of *Tilapia nilotica* and *T. aurea* hybrids. Aquaculture 6, 11–21.

Purchase, C.F., Boyce, D.L., Brown, J.A., 2000. Growth and survival of juvenile flounder *Pleuronectes ferrugineus* (Storer) under different photoperiods. Aquaculture Research 31, 547–552.

Purdom, C.E., 1995. Genetics and Fish Breeding. Chapman & Hall, London, UK, 291 pp.

Rab, M.A., 1989. Intensive nursing of Nile tilapia *(Oreochromis niloticus)* fry, (M.Sc. thesis). Asian Institute of Technology, Bangkok, Thailand.

Rana, K.J., 1981. Effects of Rearing Conditions, Age and Size on Performance of Normal Hormone-Treated Sarotherodon Mossambicus Fry, with Observations on Fry Abnormalities (M.Sc. thesis). University of Stirling, UK.

Rana, K., 1986. Tilapia Culture: Hatchery Methods for *Oreochromis mossambicus* and *O. niloticus* with Special Reference to All-Male Fry Production. Institute of Aquaculture, University of Stirling, Stirling, UK, 154 pp.

Rana, K., 1990a. Reproductive biology and the hatchery rearing of tilapia eggs and fry. In: Muir, J.F., Roberts, R.J. (Eds.), Recent Advances in Aquaculture, vol. 3. Croom Helm Ltd, London and Canberra, pp. 343–406.

Rana, K.J., 1990b. Influence of incubation temperature on *Oreochromis niloticus* (L.) eggs and fry. 1. Gross embryology, temperature tolerance and rates of embryonic development. Aquaculture 87, 165–181.

Rana, K.J., 1990c. Influence of incubation temperature on *Oreochromis niloticus* (L.) eggs and fry. 2. Survival, growth and feeding of fry developing solely on their yolk reserves. Aquaculture 87, 183–195.

Rana, K.J., Macintosh, D.J., 1988. A comparison of the quality of hatchery-reared *Oreochromis niloticus* and *O. mossambicus* fry. In:

Pullin, R.S.V., Bhukaswan, T., Tonguthai, K., Maclean, J.L. (Eds.), Proceedings of the Second International Symposium on Tilapia in Aquaculture. ICLARM Conference Proceedings No. 15. Department of Fisheries, Thailand, and ICLARM, Manila, Philippines, pp. 497–502.

Rana, K.J., Suliman, E.M., 1993. Artificial incubation of tilapia eggs and fry under semi-intensive and intensive aquaculture systems. In: Proceedings of the First International Symposium on Aquaculture Technology and Investment Opportunities. Ministry of Agriculture and Water, Riyadh, Saudi Arabia, pp. 208–218.

Ridha, M.T., Cruz, E.M., 1989. Effect of age on the fecundity of tilapia *Oreochromis spilurus*. Asian Fisheries Science 2, 239–247.

Ridha, M.T., Cruz, E.M., 1999. Effect of different broodstock densities on the reproductive performance of Nile tilapia, *Oreochromis niloticus* (L.), in a recycling system. Aquaculture Research 30, 203–210.

Ridha, M.T., Cruz, E.M., 2000. Effect of light intensity and photoperiod on Nile tilapia *Oreochromis niloticus*. Aquaculture Research 31, 609–617.

Ridha, M.T., Lone, K.P., 1990. Effect of oral administration of different levels of 17 α-methyltestosterone on the sex reversal, growth and food conversion efficiency of the tilapia *Oreochromis spilurus* (Guenther) in brackish water. Aquaculture and Fisheries Management 21, 391–397.

Ridha, M.T., Lone, K.P., 1995. Preliminary studies on feminization and growth of *Oreochromis spilurus* (Gaunter) by oral administration of 17 β-ethynyloestradiol in sea water. Aquaculture Research 26, 479–482.

Ridha, M.T., Cruz, E.M., Al-Ameeri, A., Al-Ahmad, A., 1998. Effect of controlling temperature and light duration on seed production in tilapia *Oreochromis spilurus* (Gunther). Aquaculture Research 29, 101–108.

Rosenstein, S., Hulata, G., 1992. Lack of sex inversion in tilapia immersed in estrogen solutions during embryonic development. Aquaculture '92- Book of Abstracts. World Aquaculture Society, Baton Rouge, LA, USA, p. 197.

Rosenstein, S., Hulata, G., 1994. Sex reversal in the genus *Oreochromis*: optimization of feminization protocol. Aquaculture and Fisheries Management 25, 329–339.

Rothbard, S.M., 1979. Observation on the reproductive behaviour of *Tilapia zillii* and several *Sarotherodon* spp. under aquarium conditions. Bamidgeh 31, 35–43.

Rothbard, S.M., Pruginin, Y., 1975. Induced spawning and artificial incubation of tilapia. Aquaculture 5, 315–321.

Rothbard, S., Solnik, E., Shabbath, S., Amado, R., Grabie, I., 1983. The technology of mass production of hormonally sex-inversed all male tilapia. In: Fishilson, L., Yaron, Z. (Eds.), International Symposium on Tilapia in Aquaculture. Tel-Aviv University, Israel, pp. 425–434.

Santiago, C.B., Laron, M.A., 2002. Growth and fry production of Nile tilapia, *Oreochromis niloticus* (L.), on different feeding schedules. Aquaculture Research 33, 129–136.

Santiago, C.B., Reyes, O.S., 1993. Effects of dietary lipid source on reproductive performance and tissue lipid levels of Nile tilapia *Oreochromis niloticus* (L.) broodstock. Journal of Applied Ichthyology 9, 33–40.

Santiago, C.B., Aldaba, M.B., Laron, M.A., 1983. Effect of varying dietary crude protein levels on spawning frequency and growth of *Sarotherodon niloticus* breeders. Fisheries Research Journal of Philippines 8, 9–18.

Santiago, C.B., Aldaba, M.B., Abuan, E.F., Laron, M.A., 1985. The effects of artificial diets on fry production and growth of *Oreochromis niloticus* breeders. Aquaculture 47, 193–203.

Santiago, C.B., Aldaba, M.B., Reyes, O.S., 1987. Influence of feeding rate and diet form on growth and survival of Nile tilapia (*Oreochromis niloticus*) fry. Aquaculture 64, 277–282.

Sarmento, N.L.A.F., Martins, E.F.F., Costa, D.C., Mattioli, C.C., da Costa Julio, G.S., Figueiredo, L.G., et al., 2018. Reproductive efficiency and egg and larvae quality of Nile tilapia fed different levels of vitamin C. Aquaculture 482, 96–102.

Schimittou, H.R., 1993. High-density Fish Culture in Low-Volume Cages. M.I.T.A. Publication Number 518. AQ41, 1993/7, 75 pp.

Schwank, E., 1987. Lunar periodicity in the spawning of *Tilapia mariae* in the Ethiop river, Nigeria. Journal of Fish Biology 30, 533–537.

Scribner, K.T., Page, K.P., Batron, M.L., 2001. Hybridization in freshwater fishes: a review of case studies and cytonuclear methods of biological inference. Reviews in Fish Biology and Fisheries 10, 293–323.

Siddiqui, A.Q., Harbi, A.H., 1997. Effects of sex ratio, stocking density and age of hybrid tilapia on seed production in concrete tanks in Saudi Arabia. Aquaculture International 5, 207–216.

Siddiqui, A.Q., Al-Harbi, A.H., Al-Hafedh, Y.S., 1997. Effects of food supply on size at first maturity, fecundity and growth of hybrid tilapia, *Oreochromis niloticus* (L.) x *Oreochromis aureus* (Steindachner), in outdoor concrete tanks in Saudi Arabia. Aquaculture Research 28, 341–349.

Siddiqui, A.Q., Al Hafedh, Y.S., Ali, S.A., 1998. Effect of dietary protein level on the reproductive performance of Nile tilapia, *Oreochromis niloticus* (L.). Aquaculture Research 29, 349–358.

Silva, P.C., Souza, V.L., Padua, D.M., Dalacorte, P.C., Goncalves, D.C., 2000. Effects of stocking density on growth and fillet composition of tetra hybrid red tilapia, Israeli strain. In: Fitzsimmons, K., Filho, J.C. (Eds.), Tilapia Aquaculture in the 21st Century. Proceedings from the Fifth International Symposium on Tilapia Aquaculture. Rio de Janeiro, Brazil, pp. 341–345.

Silva-Garcia, A.J., 1996. Growth of juvenile giltheadseabraem (*Sparus auratus L.*) reared under differentphotoperiod regimes. Israeli Journal of Aquaculture/Bamidgeh 48, 84–93.

Siraj, S.S., Smitherman, R.O., Castillo-Galluser, S., Dunham, R.A., 1983. Reproductive traits of three classes of *Tilapia nilotica* and maternal effects on their progeny. In: Fishelson, L., Yaron, Z. (Eds.), Proceedings of International Symposium on Tilapia in Aquaculture. Tel Aviv University Press, Israel, pp. 210–218.

Sirol, R.N., Andrade, D.R., Salaro, A.L., 2000. Growth and body composition of red tilapia fingerlings (*Oreochromis niloticus x O. aureus*) submitted to different feeding levels. In: Fitzsimmons, K., Filho, J.C. (Eds.), Tilapia Aquaculture in the 21st Century. Proceedings from Fifth International Symposium on Tilapia Aquaculture. Rio de Janeiro, Brazil, pp. 382–389.

Smith, E.S., Phelps, R.P., 1997. Reproductive efficiency, fry growth, and response to sex reversal of Nile and red tilapia. In: Fourteenth Annual Technical Report. Pond Dynamics/Aquaculture CRSP, Oregon State University, Corvallis, OR, pp. 112–119.

Smith, S.J., Watanabe, W.O., Chang, J.R., Ernst, D.H., Wicklund, R.I., Olla, B.L., 1991. Hatchery production of Florida red tilapia seed in brackishwater tanks: the influence of broodstock age. Aquaculture and Fisheries Management 22, 141–147.

Soliman, A.K., Jauncey, K., Roberts, R.J., 1986. The effects of dietary ascorbic acid supplementation on hatchability, survival rate and fry performance in *Oreochromis mossambicus*. Aquaculture 59, 197–208.

Sun, L.-N., Jiang, X.-L., Xie, O.-P., Yuan, J., Huang, B.-F., Tao, W.-J., et al., 2014. Transdifferentiation of differentiated ovary into functional testis by long-term treatment of aromatase inhibitor in Nile tilapia. Endocrinology 155, 1476–1488.

Suresh, A.V., Lin, C.K., 1992. Tilapia culture in saline waters: a review. Aquaculture 106, 201–226.

Tacon, P., Ndiaye, P., Cauty, C., Le Menn, F., Jalabert, F., 1996. Relationships between the expression of maternal behavior and ovarian development in the mouthbrooding cichlid fish *Oreochromis niloticus*. Aquaculture 146, 261–275.

Tandler, A., Helps, S., 1985. The effects of photoperiod and water exchange rate on growth and survival of gilthead seabream (*Sparus auratus*, Linnaeus; Sparidae) from hatching to metamorphosis in mass rearing systems. Aquaculture 48, 81–82.

Torrans, L., Meriwether, F., Lowell, F., Wyatt, B., Gwinup, P.D., 1988. Sex-reversal of *Oreochromis aureus* by immersion in Mibolerone, a synthetic steroid. Journal of the World Aquaculture Society 19, 97–102.

Trant, J.M., Gavasso, S., Ackers, J., Chung, B.C., Place, A.R., 2001. Developmental expression of cytochrome P450 aromatase genes (CYP19a and CYP19b) in zebrafish fry (*Danio rerio*). Journal of Experimental Zoology 290, 475–483.

Trewavas, E., 1983. Tilapiine Fishes of the Genera Sarotherodon, Oreochromis and Danakilia. British Museum (Natural History), London, UK, 340 pp.

Trippel, E.A., Neil, S.R.E., 2002. Effect of photoperiod and light intensity on growth and activity of juvenile haddock (*Melanogrammus aeglefinus*). Aquaculture 217, 633–645.

Tsadik, G.G., Bart, A.N., 2007. Effects of feeding, stocking density and water-flow rate on fecundity, spawning frequency and egg quality of Nile tilapia, *Oreochromis niloticus* (L.). Aquaculture 272, 380–388.

Tsai, C.-L., Wang, L.-H., Chang, C.-F., Kao, C.-C., 2000. Effects of gonadal steroids on brain serotogenic and aromatase activity during the critical period of sexual differentiation in tilapia, *Oreochromis* mossambicus. Journal of Neuroendocrinology 49, 894–898.

Turner, G.F., Robinson, R.L., 2000. Reproductive biology, mating systems and parental care. In: Beveridge, M.C.M., McAndrew, B.J. (Eds.), Tilapias: Biology and Exploitation. Kluwer Academic Publishers, Dordrecht/Boston/London, pp. 33–58.

Uchida, R.N., King, J.E., 1962. Tank culture of tilapia. US Fish and Wildlife Service Fisheries Bulletin 199, 21–47.

Ungsethaphan, T., 1995. An On-Farm Trial to Investigate Feeding Strategies for Nile Tilapia (*Oreochromis niloticus*) Broodfish (M.Sc. thesis). Asian Institute of Technology, Bangkok, Thailand.

Varadaraj, K., Pandian, T.J., 1987. Masculinization of *Oreochromis mossambicus* by administration of 17α-methyl-5-androsten-3β-17β-diol through rearing water. Current Science 56, 412–413.

Varadaraj, K., 1989. Feminization of *Oreochromis mossambicus* by the administration of diethylstilbestrol. Aquaculture 80, 337–341.

Vera-Cruz, E.M.V., Mair, G.C., 1994. Conditions for effective androgen sex-reversal in *Oreochromis niloticus* (L.). Aquaculture 122, 237–248.

Verdegem, M.C., McGinty, A.S., 1987. Effects of frequency of egg and fry removal on spawning of *Tilapia nilotica* in hapas. Progressive Fish-Culturist 49, 129–131.

Wardoyo, S.E., 1991. Effects of Different Salinity Levels and Acclimation Regimes on Survival, Growth, and Reproduction of Three Strains of Tilapia Nilotica and a Red Tilapia Nilotica Hybrid (Ph.D. thesis). Auburn University, Auburn, AL, USA.

Wassermann, G.J., Afonso, L.O.B., 2003. Sex reversal in Nile tilapia (*Oreochromis niloticus* Linnaeus) by androgen immersion. Aquaculture Research 34, 65–71.

Watanabe, T., 1985. Importance of the study of broodstock nutrition for further development of aquaculture. In: Cowey, C.B., Mackie, A.M., Bell, J.G. (Eds.), Nutrition and Feeding in Fish. Academic Press, London, pp. 395–414.

Watanabe, W.O., Kuo, C.-M., 1985. Observations on the reproductive performance of Nile tilapia (*Oreochromis niloticus*) in laboratory aquaria at various salinities. Aquaculture 49, 315–323.

Watanabe, W.O., Kuo, C.-M., Huang, M.-C., 1985. The ontogeny of salinity tolerance in the tilapias *Oreochromis aureus, O. niloticus* and *O. mossambicus x O. niloticus* hybrids, spawned and reared in freshwater. Aquaculture 47, 353–367.

Watanabe, W.O., Ellingson, L.J., Wicklund, R.I., Olla, B.L., 1988. The effects of salinity on growth, food consumption and conversion in juvenile, monosex male Florida red tilapia. In: Pullin, R.S.V., Bhukaswan, T., Tonguthai, K., Maclean, J.L. (Eds.), Proceedings of the Second International Symposium on Tilapia in Aquaculture. ICLARM Conference Proceedings No. 15. Department of Fisheries, Thailand, and ICLARM, Manila, Philippines, pp. 515–523.

Watanabe, W.O., Ernst, D.H., Chasar, M.P., Wicklund, R.I., Olla, B.L., 1993. The effects of temperature and salinity on growth and feed utilization of juvenile, sex-reversed male Florida red tilapia cultured in a recirculating system. Aquaculture 112, 309–320.

Wee, K.L., Tuan, N.A., 1988. Effects of dietary protein level on growth and reproduction of Nile tilapia (*Oreochromis niloticus*). In: Pullin, R.S.V., hukaswan, T., Tonguthai, K., Maclean, J.L. (Eds.), Proceedings of the Second International Symposium on Tilapia in Aquaculture. ICLARM Conference Proceedings No. 15. Department of Fisheries, Bangkok, Thailand and ICLARM, Manila, Philippines, pp. 401–410.

Wohlfarth, G.W., 1994. The unexploited potential of tilapia hybrids in aquaculture. Aquaculture and Fisheries Management 25, 781–788.

Wohlfarth, G.W., Hulata, G., 1983. Applied Genetics of Tilapia, second ed. In: ICLARM Studies and Reviews 6. ICLARM, Manila, Philippines. 26 pp.

Wohlfarth, G.W., Hulata, G., Halevy, A., 1990. Growth, survival and sex ratio of some tilapia species and their interspecific hybrids. European Aquaculture Society Special Publication 11. European Aquaculture Society, Bredene, Belgium, pp. 87–101.

Wootton, R.J., 1979. Energy costs of egg production and environmental determinants of fecundity of teleost fishes. In: Miller, P.J. (Ed.), Fish Phynology: Anabolic Adaptiveness in Teleosts. (Symposium of the Zoological Society of London), No. 44. Academic Press, London, pp. 133–159.

Chapter 9

Stress and diseases

Chapter outline

9.1 Introduction

Tilapia, like other aquatic animals, can be subjected to various infectious and noninfectious diseases. Tilapia diseases have attracted the attention in recent years, for the following reasons:

1. The wide expansion of tilapia culture which may increase the risk of diseases.
2. The extensive introduction of tilapia into many countries that would increase the chances of disease occurrence.
3. Increasing public awareness about the role of fish culture in the spread of human diseases.
4. Increasing public concern about environmental protection.
5. Increasing global exportation and importation of tilapia, with high quality standard.

It is no surprise, therefore, that fish health and disease control are now reviewed in integration with environmental protection, pollution control, human health, aquaculture technologies, sanitation of culture facilities, diagnosis and treatment of diseases of cultured species, formulation and implementation of regulatory measures to control the spread of diseases and development of disease-resistant aquatic strains (Pillay, 1990). This chapter addresses the major fish stressors and common diseases that infect wild and cultured tilapia, with emphasis on disease agents, symptoms and methods of treatments.

9.2 Stress

Stress is generally defined as the disturbance of internal equilibrium (homoeostasis) of fish. It is the first step toward disease occurrence, since it reduces fish resistance and

Tilapia Culture. https://doi.org/10.1016/B978-0-12-816541-6.00009-X
Copyright © 2020 Elsevier Inc. All rights reserved.

makes it more susceptible to diseases (Everitt and Leung, 1999). Therefore, the extent of stress and ability of fish to resist and maintain homoeostasis are most important for survival and growth. Stress can be caused by different factors, including the following:

- Nutritional differences (e.g. vitamin imbalances).
- Environmental quality and culture conditions.
- Well-being of cultured animal.
- Physical, chemical and biological interference (crowding, handling, transportation, pollution, organic enrichment, etc.).

Tilapia are well adapted to prevailing environmental conditions and can tolerate a wide range of environmental factors such as water temperature, salinity, dissolved oxygen, ammonia, etc. (see Chapter 4). However, stressful conditions adversely affect tilapia and make them more susceptible to different diseases, presumably due to immunosuppression. Foo and Lam (1993) found that handling stress caused a significant increase in serum cortisol levels of Mozambique tilapia (*Oreochromis mossambicus*), and the cortisol level depended on the severity of the stressor, duration of exposure and fish health status. The removal of the stressor resulted in a rapid return to the normal cortisol level. Barcellos et al. (1999a) studied the effects of acute stress on Nile tilapia (*Oreochromis niloticus*) previously exposed to chronic stress (handling stress). They found that fish exposed to chronic stress for 59 days had lower growth rates than nonstressed fish. Plasma cortisol in fish previously exposed to chronic stress (169 ng mL^{-1}) was significantly lower than that obtained from those exposed only to acute stress (9267 ng mL^{-1}). The authors concluded that Nile tilapia can adapt to chronic stress, and this adaptation reduces, but does not eliminate, their response to additional acute stress.

Inappropriate handling of farmed tilapia may induce stressful conditions, leading to poor performance and physiological functions, disease or mortality. For example, Akinrotimi et al. (2007) found that oxygen deficiency during transportation induces stress in blackchin tilapia (*Sarotherodon melanotheron*). Adult fish transported without oxygenation for 50 km suffered from a significant reduction in haemoglobin, packed cell volume (PCV), red blood cells (RBCs) and thrombocytes, compared to those transported in oxygenated water. In the mean time, total white blood cells (WBCs), neutrophils, lymphocytes and monocytes increased.

Upton and Riley (2013) investigated the effect of acute handling stress on food intake and neuroendocrine regulators of food intake in Mozambique tilapia. These regulators include the expression of neuropeptide Y (NPY), corticotropin-releasing hormone (CRH) and ghrelin (a gut hormone, produced by ghrelinergic cells, activates its receptor, growth hormone secretagogue receptors (GHSRs), leading to stimulatory effects on food intake and growth hormone release). The authors found that food intake was significantly reduced in fish exposed to a 30-min crowding and handling stress. Handling stress also led to an elevation in the ghrelin transcript in the telencephalon/preoptic area and elevation of its functional receptor (GHSR1a-LR) in the hypothalamic/optic tectum. This result suggests a rapid control of the ghrelin regulatory system in response to acute stress and indicates that ghrelin signalling is changed during acute stress.

An essential cause of chronic stress in tilapia is social interactions and hierarchies. A negative correlation between growth rates and stocking density of fish fry has been reported in tilapia fry (Macintosh and De Silva, 1984; Dambo and Rana, 1992; El-Sayed, 2002). Increasing fish density leads to what is known as 'social stress' causing 'chronic stress response'. This leads to impaired fish growth; presumably due to the mobilization of dietary energy by the physiological alterations provoked by the stress response (Kebus et al., 1992). As a result, resting plasma cortisol concentrations of Nile tilapia fingerlings were reported to have increased with increasing the stocking density indicating a chronic stress response, attributable to social stress (Barcellos et al., 1999b).

High stocking densities without water exchange may negatively affect fish performance, haematological and serum biochemical indices, as has been reported in genetically improved farmed tilapia (GIFT) (Kpundeh et al., 2013). Growth and survival rates and feed efficiency were significantly decreased in response to these stressors. Haematological indices, including RBCs, WBCs, haemoglobin content, haematocrit and platelet decreased as stocking density increased. The activity of liver enzymes, aspartate aminotransferase (AST) and alanine aminotransferase (ALT), was also significantly increased. In the mean time, high stocking densities with zero water exchange resulted in a decrease in serum protein, triglycerides, cholesterol and thyroxine.

Tilapia may also be exposed to secondary stress after medical (chemical) treatments. The response of Nile tilapia to secondary stress after treatment with a mixture of formalin, malachite green and methylene blue (FMC) has been investigated (Yavuzcan and Pulatsü, 1999). Treating the fish with FMC increased plasma glucose and haematocrit and reduced plasma phosphorus and calcium, while magnesium was not affected. These changes in blood chemistry were attributed to secondary stress response to FMC treatment. This indicates that therapeutic agents (such as FMC) are an 'under-recognized' stress source.

Reducing stress is, therefore, an important means of disease control and improvement of immunity in cultured fish. Endo et al. (2002) studied the stress and immune response of Nile tilapia under self-feeding and scheduled-feeding regimes. They found that self-fed fish had lower levels of plasma cortisol, higher phagocytic activity of their macrophages, higher antibody production and higher number of lymphocytes than scheduled-fed fish. The authors concluded that self-feeding regime is less stressful than scheduled feeding. Thus, it is evident that the best way of preventing, or at least reducing, tilapia diseases is the adoption of best management practices. These practices include improving and controlling culture environment, adopting proper handling and transportation techniques, reasonable stocking densities, using proper amounts of high-quality feed with the adoption of the right feeding regimes, using legal drugs judiciously and using the most effective vaccines (Plumb, 1999).

9.3 Major fish diseases

Some tilapia diseases such as bacterial and parasitic diseases have received considerable attention in recent years. Many articles describing the symptoms, diagnosis, treatment and prevention of these diseases appeared in specialized journals. On the other hand, much less work has been done on other disease groups, particularly fungal, viral and noninfectious diseases. For this reason, the reader may realize that this chapter covers parasitic and bacterial diseases in much more detail than other disease groups. The following sections address the major diseases that infect both wild and farmed tilapia.

9.4 Parasitic diseases

9.4.1 Protozoan diseases

Several external and internal protozoan parasites are known to live on (or inside) tilapia, causing illness, mortality and economic loss (Table 9.1). The severity of protozoan diseases depends on the number of parasites infesting the fish, culture systems and fish species, sex, size and health status. Protozoan parasites have been reported to cause serious mortality in wild and farmed tilapia, both in hatcheries and rearing facilities. The most important parasitic protozoan diseases of tilapia are summarized below.

9.4.1.1 *Ichthyophthirius multifiliis*

Ichthyophthirius multifiliis (Ich) is a ciliated protozoan with a round or ovoid body, small mouth and longitudinal rows of cilia on the body surface, converging at the anterior end (Pillay, 1990). It has a large, horseshoe-shaped macronucleus, a small micronucleus and many contractile vacuoles. The infective stage of this parasite is known as a theront or tomite. This disease is known as white spot because an infected fish is characterized by the appearance of white spots where the parasites live in the epidermis of the skin and gills (Ewing and Kocan, 1992). The optimum temperature for the growth of the parasite is 20–25°C at a high stocking density.

Infection of tilapia with *I. multifiliis* has been widely reported in the Americas (Lightner et al., 1988; Crosby, 2001; Straus and Griffin, 2001) and Asia (Lua et al., 1999; Te et al., 1999). Larval fish stages appear more susceptible than fingerling and adult stages. Subasinghe and Sommerville (1992) found that the effect of *I. multifiliis* on larval *O. mossambicus* was more severe than on fingerlings. Similar results have been reported with Nile tilapia, where the incidence of infection decreased with increasing fish size (Lua et al., 1999). The parasites were found in large numbers in the nares, pharynx, gills and skin of tilapia fry, causing severe mortality (Roberts and Sommerville, 1982). Similarly, El-Dien and Abdel-Gaber (2009) found that *I. multifiliis* infection induces apoptosis in different species of wild tilapia, with highest rate of infection being recorded in Nile tilapia, followed by blue tilapia, Galilee tilapia and *Tilapia zillii*. Apoptotic cells were aggregated on the apical and basal parts of the ciliated and nonciliated endothelial lining in the gill epithelium. The macrophage number of infected Nile tilapia was higher than noninfected fish. Ich-infected Galilee tilapia exhibited a marked decrease in splenic cells number.

The infection of tilapia with *I. multifiliis* does not only directly affect fish health and performance, but it can also increase fish susceptibility to other pathogens, as reported by Xu et al. (2014). These authors found that *I. multifiliis* parasitism of hybrid tilapia (*Oreochromis* spp.) enhanced *Flavobacterium columnare* invasion and resulted in higher fish mortality than nonparasitized fish. The bacterial loads of *F. columnare* were also much higher in parasitized tilapia than those of nonparasitized fish.

The confrontation of Ich, and other parasites, has received considerable attention in recent years. Potassium permanganate ($KMnO_4$) is widely used to control this disease throughout the world. Straus and Griffin (2001) determined the acute toxicity of $KMnO_4$ to *I. multifiliis* and the concentration required for preventing its infestation to juvenile blue tilapia (*Oreochromis aureus*) and channel catfish. They found that the lowest effective doses were 0.5 mg L^{-1} and 1.0 mg L^{-1} for tilapia and catfish. The protective immunity of tilapia against *I. multifiliis* has also been investigated. When *O. mossambicus* (120–200 g) were subjected to a trickle, sublethal infection of *I. multifiliis* tomites, they were free of the parasite 18 days after the initial infection, and remained free for 9 months in an infectious environment (Subasinghe and Sommerville, 1986). The survival of *O. mossambicus* fry obtained from adult females immunized against *I. multifiliis* and challenged with controlled infection was also better than the survival of these of challenged nonimmuned females (Subasinghe and Sommerville, 1989). Similarly, Sin et al. (1994) found that *O. aureus* fry obtained from broodstock

TABLE 9.1 A list of the common disease agents, symptoms and treatment protocols of tilapia.

Agent	Species (location)	Disease symptoms	Treatment protocols	References
Parasites				
Ichthyophthirius multifiliis	*O. m, O. a, T. z, O. m* x *O. h* (USA)	Low growth, white spots on fins and epidermis		Lightner et al. (1988)
	O. m fry (UK)	High mortality		Subasinghe and Sommerville (1986)
	O. a (USA)		0.5 mg L^{-1} $KMnO_4$, single dose	Straus and Griffin (2001)
Trichodina	*O. n* (Cameroon)	Loss of escape reaction, scraping against tank walls, rapid opercular movement, jumping out of water	**1** Formalin bath, 250 ppm for 35–49 min. **2** $KMnO_4$, 5 ppm for 10–15 min.	Nguenga (1988)
	O. m, O. a, T. z, O. m x *O. h* (USA)	Gill hyperplasia, eroded fins, epidermal ulcers, high mortality		Lightner et al. (1988)
Paratrichodina africana	*O. n* (Brazil)	Lesions in the gills, epithelial hyperplasia, desquamation and mononuclear and eosinophilic infiltrate		Valladão et al. (2013)
Epistylis sp.	*O. n* males (Brazil)	Inflammation, higher lymphocyte number, lower neutrophil numbers, erosions on the head and lateral line		Valladão et al. (2014)
	O. n (Vietnam)	Massive mortality in nursery stage		Lua et al. (1999)
Myxobolus ovariae	*O. n, S. g* (Nigeria)	Inflammatory reaction, reabsorption of ovary tissue, replacing gonads tissues with the spores, gonadal atrophy and low GSI	Culling infected fish, water filtration to eliminate the spores	Okaeme et al. (1989)
Myxobolus sp.	*Oreochromis* sp. (Mexico)	White nodules in the gills, dark skin, exophthalmia, loss of appetite, increased abdominal volume, congestion and thickening of intestines		de Ocampo and Camberos (1998)
Cryptobia branchialis (*Costia*)	*O. m* (USA)	Thick mucus on gill surface, swelling of gill filaments, reduction of respiratory lamellae and hypertrophy of respiratory epithelium		Kuperman et al. (2002)
Dactylogyrus sp.	*O. n* (Cameroon)	Rapid opercular movements, opercula held opened, thickened edges of gills and destruction of branchial epithelium	**1** A single dose of formalin (250 ppm for 35–40 min). **2** Two repeated doses of $KMnO_4$, 5 ppm for 10–15 min.	Nguenga (1988)

Alitropus typus	*O. n* (Thailand)	50%–100% mortality		Chinabut (2002)
Renocila thresherorum	*T. z* (Egypt)	Eroded gill filaments, degenerative lesions including destruction, detachment, hyperplasia and fusion of the primary and secondary gill lamellae		Ali and Aboyadak. (2018)
Lamproglena sp.	*O. n* (Ethiopia, Kenya and Uganda)	Gill damage, epithelial sloughing off and thick mucus secretion		Florio et al. (2009), Akoll et al. (2012a)
Acanthogyrus sp.	*O. n* (Philippines)	Decreased haematocrit volume and RBC, increased WBC, proliferation of lymphocytes and eosinophilic granulocytes, lesions and exfoliation of the mucosal layer		Pallet et al. (2016)
Bacteria				
Aeromonas hydrophila	*O. n* (China)	Erosion of skin and dorsal fin, body surface filled with blood, high mortality		Wang and Xu (1985)
	O. n (China)	Slow movement, caudal fin rot, swimming near water surface, poor appetite, mortality		Liu et al. (1993)
	O. n (Philippines)	Skin lesion, ulceration, fin rot, body discolouration, mouth sore, eye opacity, exophthalmia, dislodged eyeball, sluggishness		Yambot (1998)
Aeromonas jandaei and *Aeromonas veronii*	*O. n* (Thailand)	Mass mortality, dark body, abnormal swimming behaviour, loss of appetite, haemorrhage and liver blood congestion		Dong et al. (2017a)
Aeromonas sobria	*O. n* (China)	Fin rot, mass mortality, skin darkening, ascites with abdominal swelling, lack of feeding, hemorrhagic blots on the liver		Li and Cai (2011)
Pseudomonas sp.	*O. n* (Japan)	Fine white nodules in the spleen, abscesses in the swim bladder, exophthalmia, dark body, nodular lesions and focal necrosis in the liver, spleen, kidney and gills, inflamed swim bladder, abscess in the eyes, spleen and swim bladder		Miyashita (1984), Miyazaki et al. (1984)
Vibrio sp.	*O. s* (Kuwait)	Lethargy, dark body colour, dermal necrosis, high mortality		Saeed (1993)

Continued

TABLE 9.1 A list of the common disease agents, symptoms and treatment protocols of tilapia.—cont'd

Agent	Species (location)	Disease symptoms	Treatment protocols	References
Vibrio vulnificus	Hybrid (Taiwan)	Dark colouration, lethargy, skin haemorrhage and ulceration, liver splenomegaly and haemorrhagic lesions and septicaemia		Chen et al. (2006)
Streptococcus sp.	*O. n* (USA)	Hyperaemic gills, diffused epithelial tissue proliferation, lesions, dermal haemorrhage		Bowser et al. (1998)
	O. m (Taiwan)	Haemorrhage, exophthalmia, corneal opacity, dark colouration, abscess of trunk muscles	Erythromycin, doxycycline	Tung et al. (1987)
	O. n x *O. a* (Saudi Arabia)	Erratic swimming, melanosis, exophthalmia, haemorrhage around the jaws and base of pectoral and pelvic fins, ascetic fluid in the abdominal cavity		Al-Harbi (1994)
Streptococcus iniae	*O. n* (USA)	Darkened skin pigments, bottom swimming, rising and falling, side swimming, losing appetite		Evans et al. (2000)
	O. n (USA)	Dark skin pigmentation, abdominal distension, haemorrhage, erythema, eye lesion, lethargy, reduction or cessation of feeding, circular swimming, side swimming	Oxytetracycline (75–100 mg kg^{-1} feed	Darwish and Griffin (2002)
	O. n x *O. a* (USA)	Loss of orientation, exophthalmia, corneal opacity, petechia around the mouth and anus, fluid accumulation in the peritoneal cavity	- Tetracycline, Oxytetracycline - Sulfadimethoxine-ormitoprim (5:1)	Perera et al. (1994)
Streptococcus dysgalactiae	*O. n* (Brazil)	High mortality, anorexia, lethargy, tachypnoea and skin darkness		Netto et al. (2011)
Staphylococcus epidermis	*O. a* (Taiwan)	Lesions of spleen and kidney, apoptosis in lymphocytes and macrophages, brain, liver, gonads, mesentery, stomach, intestines and skeletal muscles		Huang et al. (2000)
Mycobacterium marinum	*O. n* x *O. m* x *O. a* (USA)	Small visceral granulomas, high epithelial macrophages and peripheral lymphocytes		Wolf and Smith (1999)

Mycobacterium fortuitum and *Mycobacterium marinum*	*O. n* (Mexico)	Body deformity, haemorrhage, exophthalmia, ulcers in head, mouth and skin, multiple granulomas with thick capsules on spleen, liver and stomach		Lara-Flores et al. (2014)
Flexobacter columnaris	*O. n* (USA), *Tilapia* sp. (Korea)	Respiratory disorder, fin erosion, body discolouration, lesion in muscles and skin, heavy mucus secretion	Oxytetracycline, tetracycline, chloramphenicol, amikacine erythromycine, kanamycin	Roberts and Sommerville (1982), Chun and Sohn (1985)
Edwardsiella tarda	*Oreochromis* spp. (Colombia)	Mortality, granulomatous inflammation, haemorrhage, necrotic meningitis, encephalitis, vasculitis with fibrinoid necrosis of the blood vessels walls, lesions in the brain, liver, kidney, spleen and pancreas		Iregui et al. (2012)
Edwardsiella ictaluri	*O. n.* (Chile)	Multifocal nodulation of the spleen, head kidney, hepatomegaly and inflammatory infiltrates in the spleen, head kidney and liver		Soto et al. (2012b)
Yersinia ruckeri	*O. n* (Egypt)	Mortality, haemorrhages on mouth, fin and skin, haemorrhagic gastroenteritis and congestion of the internal organs		Eissa et al. (2008)
Fungi				
Saprolegnia parasitica	*O. n* (Egypt)	Cotton-like growths on the skin and fins, listlessness, erratic swimming and rising near water surfaces or resting on the bottom	Potassium permanganate and hydrogen peroxide	Zahran et al. (2017), Sherif and Abdel–Hakim (2016)
Branchiomyces	*O. n* x *O. m*, *O. n* x *O. a* (Israel)	Damage of gill tissue, high mortality		Paperna and Smirnova (1997)
Branchiomyces demigrans	*O. n* (Egypt)	Massive mortality, gill tissue damage, rapid movement of gill operculum, hyphae and spores embedded in gill tissues	Clotrimazole and clove oil	El-Bouhy et al. (2014)

O. a, Oreochromis aureus; O. m, Oreochromis mossambicus; O. n, Oreochromis niloticus; O. s, Oreochromis spilurus; T. z, Tilapia zillii; S. g; Sarotherodon galilaeus.

previously vaccinated with ineffective live tomites of *I. multifiliis* exhibited 95% survival with mouthbrooding and 78.4% survival without mouthbrooding, compared to only 0% and 37.3% survival in nonvaccinated fish without and with mouthbrooding. The authors suggested that protective immunity against *I. multifiliis* in tilapia fry is derived from both the mother via eggs and acquired indirectly from mouth cavity during mouthbrooding.

Alongside the same line, Xu et al. (2008) evaluated the protective immunity of Nile tilapia against *I. multifiliis* post immunization with live theronts and sonicated trophonts by bath immersion and intraperitoneal (IP) injection. Serum anti-Ich antibody was significantly higher in tilapia immunized with live theronts by immersion or IP injection or with sonicated trophonts administered by IP injection than in tilapia immunized with sonicated trophonts by immersion. Host protection was acquired in fish immunized with live theronts by immersion or IP injection. Tilapia immunized with sonicated trophonts by IP injection were partially protected, achieving a survival rate of 57%–77%.

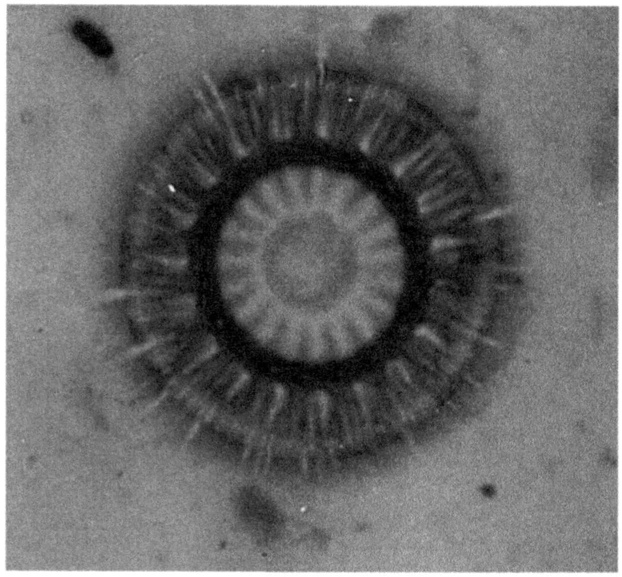

FIGURE 9.1 Trichodina; an internal parasite isolated from Nile tilapia. *Photo provided by M.Kh. Soliman.*

9.4.2 Other ciliates

Several other unicellular parasitic ciliates including *Trichodina*, *Tricodinella*, *Epistylis*, *Ichthyobodo*, *Apiosoma*, *Vorticella* and *Ambiphrya* are common among wild and cultured tilapia, especially when the fishes are farmed at high stocking densities (Lightner et al., 1988; Bondad-Reantaso and Arthur, 1989; Valladão et al., 2013, 2016; Abdel-Baki et al., 2014). *Trichodina* is the most documented ciliate in Nile tilapia in the Philippines (Natividad et al., 1986; Bondad-Reantaso and Arthur, 1989) and Vietnam (Lua et al., 1999), Mozambique tilapia, blue tilapia, tilapia hybrids and *T. zillii* in the United States (Lightner et al., 1988), Egypt (El-Tantawy and Kazaubski, 1986) and both Nile tilapia and Mozambique tilapia in Nigeria (Okaeme and Okojie, 1989; Bello-Olusoji et al., 2000).

Trichodina is a saucer-shaped parasite (Fig. 9.1) that attacks fish skin and gills. The typical signs of the disease include skin and gill damage, respiratory distress, loss of appetite and loss of scales. Skin and gill damage caused by this parasite may lead to the entry of other pathogens such as bacteria and fungus (Lightner et al., 1988; Plumb, 1997). Six species of trichodinids (*Trichodina centrostrigata*, *Trichodina migala*, *Trichodina heterodentata*, *Trichodina compacta*, *Tripartiella orthodens* and *Paratrichodina africana*) have recently been identified as parasites of Nile tilapia in Brazil (Valladão et al., 2016). Alterations were greater in number and more severe in the larvae than in the juveniles. The outer surfaces of the infected larvae (integument, eye and fins) were highly affected, whereas the juveniles were rarely affected. The use of formaldehyde ($0.5-1$ mL L^{-1}) and sodium chloride (0.5%–1%) for 15 min was highly effective in treating this parasite. This finding suggests that Nile tilapia larviculture is highly susceptible to trichodinids infection. Therefore, special attention should be given to the prevention and control of this type of parasites in the hatcheries. Preventive measures, including indoor production strategies during early life stages in the hatchery are highly recommended. The ciliated protozoan *P. africana* also caused lesions in the gills of farmed Nile tilapia in Brazil (Valladão et al., 2013), and the lesions were proportional to parasite intensity. Infected fish had proliferative disturbances, including epithelial hyperplasia, desquamation, and mononuclear and eosinophilic infiltrates that culminated in necrosis.

Trichodinids were also recorded in commercial tilapia farms and hatcheries in Uganda and were the most prevalent parasite (Akoll et al., 2012a). The infection of Nile tilapia juveniles reared in cages in Brazil by *Epistylis* sp. was also reported by Valladão et al. (2014). Heavily infected fish (>400 zooids per fish) showed higher lymphocyte and lower neutrophil numbers than the less infected group (<400). Heavily infected fish also exhibited inflammatory response, presumably due to the contact of *Epistylis* with fish skin. The presence of protozoan ciliates, *Ambiphrya* and *Vorticella* spp., in cultured Nile tilapia in a number of farms in the central region of Saudi Arabia was reported by Abdel-Baki et al. (2014).

The infection of the above-mentioned parasites is generally affected by tilapia species, size and sex, and season. Ramadan (1991) studied the infection of Lake Manzala (Egypt) fishes by different parasites. The prevalence of infection was higher in larger fish than smaller fish and in *T. zillii* than in Nile tilapia. Parasitism also increased with decreasing water temperature (i.e. the infection was higher in winter than in summer).

Most of ciliate parasites can be treated with table salt (NaCl), $KMnO_4$ (5 ppm for 10−15 min) (Nguenga, 1988) and formalin (30−50 mg L^{-1}) (Plumb, 1997; Natividad et al., 1986; Shoemaker et al., 2000). Treatment dose is affected by water quality (temperature, salinity, dissolved oxygen, ammonia concentration, etc.).

9.4.3 Flagellated protozoa

A number of parasitic flagellated protozoans have been reported to infect tilapia in fish farms as well as in the wild. *Ichthyobodo necator* (previously known as *Costia necatrix*) is probably the most important flagellated parasite infecting tilapia (Plumb, 1997; Shoemaker et al., 2000). Crosby (2001) reported that *Ichthyobodo* represented a major problem for tilapia farmers in Virginia, USA. Heavy infection of *O. mossambicus* with *Ichthyobodo* in marine fish hatcheries in Hawaii has also been reported (Brock et al., 1993). The general signs of the disease include flashing and scraping, listlessness and resting on the bottom, loose of appetite, presence of blue-grey sheen with thick mucus patches. *Ichthyobodo* sp. was also recorded in farmed Nile tilapia in Uganda (Akoll et al., 2012a).

Cryptobia branchialis is another unicellular flagellate that has been reported to cause severe damage for tilapia in fresh water and brackish water (Natividad et al., 1986; Kuperman et al., 2002). This parasite is pear-shaped or elongated, anteriorly rounded and tapered posteriorly. Kuperman et al. (2002) reported an infestation of young *O. mossambicus* in Salton Sea (a highly saline lake in California, USA) by *C. branchialis*. Disease symptoms included deposition of thick mucus on gill surface, swelling of gill filaments, reduction of respiratory lamellae and hypertrophy of respiratory epithelium. These changes lead to depression in oxygen consumption. Tilapia fry were more susceptible to this parasite than adult fish.

The infection of tilapia by other flagellate protozoans has been recorded recently. Kuperman and Matey (1999) reported massive infestation of young *O. mossambicus* in Salton Sea by *Amyloodinium ocellatum* (Dinoflagellida). Outbreaks of the infestation and the subsequent mortality was recorded when water temperature and salinity were 40°C and 46‰, respectively. Paull and Matthews (2001) suggested that *Spironucleus vortens* is a flagellate that possibly caused a hole-in-the-head disease in cichlid fishes in the UK. The parasite was isolated from the kidney, liver, spleen and head lesions, as well as from the intestines.

Trypanosoma mukasai has also been isolated and described from the peripheral blood of *O. mossambicus* in West Bengal, India (Sinha, 1986). Jesus et al. (2018) recorded a first outbreak of *Trypanosoma* in Nile tilapia in South America, causing mass mortality. Heavily infested fish showed skin darkening, tegument haemorrhage, decrease in the haematocrit, mast cell infiltrates in the gill and intestine and multifocal aggregates of melanomacrophages in the liver, pancreas, spleen and kidney. Similar prevalence of trypanosome infection in Nile tilapia and North African catfish from fish farms and reservoir of Jebel Aulia Dam in Sudan was also reported by Hamid and Babiker (2011).

9.4.4 Sporozoan diseases

Myxosporidian sporozoans are a class of protozoans that may cause serious diseases in fish culture. They commonly occur as cysts replete with spores in the tissues of most wild tilapias (Okaeme and Okojie, 1989; Gbankoto et al., 2001). Their pathological effects become higher in intensive earthen ponds, where the conditions facilitate the parasite's life cycle, since released spores require a period of initiation in pond mud prior to infectious stage (Roberts and Sommerville, 1982).

Myxobolus sp. is the most important myxosporidian affecting tilapia in fish farms. Okaeme et al. (1989) reported that *Myxobolus ovariae* was highly prevalent among the tilapias *O. niloticus* and *Sarotherodon galilaeus* in Nigeria, and ovaries were the most affected organs. Histological changes of infected fish revealed an inflammatory reaction, mechanical pressure, reabsorption of ovary tissues, gradual replacement of gonadal tissues by the spores, gonadal atrophy and a reduced gonadosomatic index. The same authors (Okaeme et al., 1989) recommended that infected fish should be culled and culture water should be sedimented and filtered to eliminate the spores. It was also found that *Myxobolus exiguus* infect the fry of different Nile tilapia strains (Thailand, GIFT and Vietnam strains) in North Vietnam (Lua et al., 1999). *Myxobolus* sp. also infested tilapia (*Oreochromis* sp.) in Mexico (de Ocampo and Camberos, 1998). Disease symptoms included loss of appetite, increase in abdominal size, congestion and thickening of the medial and posterior intestines. Gbankoto et al. (2001) reported an occurrence of six myxosporidian parasites in the gills of *S. melanotheron* and *T. zillii* from Lake Nokoué (Benin, West Africa). The two most common myxosporidians were *Myxobolus* sp. and *Myxobolus zillii*, which were located in the branchial filaments of *S. melanotheron* and *T. zillii*, respectively. Two other myxosporidians; *Myxobolus sarotherodoni* and *Myxobolus beninensis* were also recorded, but at lower levels, in the branchial arch cartilage of *S. melanotheron.* On the other hand, *Myxobolus dossoui* and *Myxobolus microcapsularis* were found in the branchial arch cartilage of *T. zillii* (Gbankoto et al., 2001). Control of the disease includes killing the spores through culling infected fish, water filtration and partial drainage of the water, followed by addition of chlorine (at about 10 ppm) and air drying of contaminated mud. Similarly, *Myxobolus* sp. infected the gills of farmed Nile tilapia in Uganda (Akoll et al., 2012a).

Five new myxosporean species infecting Nile tilapia in a Nile tributary in Nile Delta region, Egypt, were described by Abdel-Ghaffar et al. (2008). They were *Zschokkella nilei*, *Ortholinea africanus*, *Triangula egyptica*, *Myxobolus fomenai* and *Myxobolus branchiophilus*. Abdel-Baki et al. (2015a) also reported a new record of two myxosporidians, *Myxobolus brachysporus* and *Myxobolus israelensis*, in wild tilapia collected from the Nile River, Egypt. About 52% of sampled fish were infected with *M. brachysporus* and 25% with *M. israelensis*. Very high numbers of free spores were found in the kidney and spleen of infected fish. The authors speculated that since these parasites infected wild fish, it is very likely they will invade farmed tilapia, and necessary protective measurements should be taken. The same authors (Abdel-Baki et al., 2015b) described the infection in kidney of Nile tilapia collected from the River Nile, Egypt, by two *Myxobolus* spp., *Myxobolus. tilapiae* and *Myxobolus agolus*. The infection appeared as free spores in Bowman capsules and renal glomeruli. In some cases, the infection was shown as fibrous plasmodia-like structure containing degenerated developmental stages and spores in the interstitium. El-Gayar and Aly (2013) also found that 22% of farmed tilapia in Sharkia province, Egypt, were infected with *Myxobolus* sp.

Control of the disease includes killing the spores through culling of infected fish, water filtration, partial drainage of the water followed by addition of chlorine (at about 10 ppm) and air drying of contaminated mud. However, it appears, at least up until now, that there is no known effective treatment for myxosporidian diseases in tilapia. Avoiding the infective spores through water sedimentation and filtration, partial discharge, eventual pond drying and proper stocking densities have been the main controlling and protective measures. These methods have been tried with other farmed fish species, with varying degrees of success.

9.4.5 Metazoan parasites

9.4.5.1 Monogenetic trematodes

Monogenetic trematodes including *Gyrodactylus*, *Dactylogyrus* (Fig. 9.2) (known as *Cichlidogyrus* in Cichlid fishes (le Roux and Avenant-Oldewage, 2010) and *Cleidodiscus* have been reported to parasitize on tilapia, especially on gills and skin, both in farmed and wild fish (Ramadan, 1991; Plumb, 1997; Omoregie et al., 1995; Shoemaker et al., 2000). Roberts and Sommerville (1982) reviewed the occurrence of monogenetic and digenetic trematodes in cultured tilapia. Three species of monogenetic trematodes (*Cichlidogyrus sclerosus*, *Cichlidogyrus tilapiae* and *Gyrodactylus niloticus*) have been recorded in cultured tilapia in Vietnam (Te et al., 1999). Several cichlids, including *Sarotherodon*, *Haplochromis*, *Oreochromis*, *Tilapia* and *Tristramella* have been reported to host *Gyrodactylus cichlidarum* under natural (Shinn et al., 2010) and aquaculture conditions (Garcia-Vasquez et al. 2007). A new species of monogenetic trematodes (*Gyrodactylus malalai* sp. nov.) has been isolated and described from the fin surface of Nile tilapia and *T. zillii* in Lake Turkana (Kenya) and Blue Nile (Sudan) (Prikrylova et al., 2012).

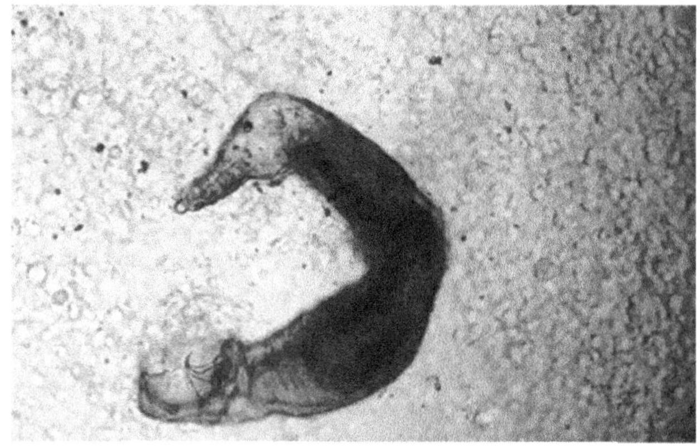

FIGURE 9.2 Dactylogyrus isolated from Nile tilapia reared in a RAS system, South Africa. *Photo provided by G. Taylor.*

Risk assessment of parasitic helminths on cage- or pond-cultured Nile tilapia in Uganda revealed that monogeneans (*C. tilapiae* and *C. sclerosus*) are high-risk parasites, particularly in pond-raised fish (Akoll et al., 2012b). *Gyrodactylus* infection of pond-reared tilapia was also recorded in Uganda, causing corneal damage (Fryer and Iles, 1972) and Kenya (C. Sommerville and R.D. Haller, unpublished results). Infection is usually associated with poor handling and high stocking density. Nguenga (1988) reported an infection of Nile tilapia with *Dactylogyrus* (*Cichlidogyrus*) sp. in Cameroon. Infested fish showed rapid opercular movements and the opercula held opened, thickened edges of the gills and destruction of branchial epithelium. *Cichlidogyrus* and *Gyrodactylus* have also been reported to infect tilapia in a number of fish farms in the eastern region of Saudi Arabia (FRRC, 2001). Infected fish suffered from difficulties in respiration, due to the damage of gills, haemorrhage, fin rot and increased mucus secretion.

The infection of tilapia by monogenetic trematodes is affected by fish species, sex and size and environmental conditions. Thus, monogenetic trematodes are considered as a bioindicator of the quality of culture conditions. Bad water quality, poor farm management and chemical pollution generally enhance the impact of these parasites. Sanchez-Ramirez et al. (2007) found that *C. sclerosus* and its host (Nile tilapia) exhibited significant numerical and physiological responses after exposure to sediments polluted with polycyclic aromatic hydrocarbons (PAHs), polychlorinated biphenyls and heavy metals. After 15 days of exposure, high sediment pollutant concentrations reduced the abundance of *C. sclerosus,* but suppressed the immune response in hosts, leading to increasing histological damage in hosts and allowing *C. sclerosus* infection. Consequently, hypertrophy and hyperplasia in secondary gill lamellae and the spleen melanomacrophage centres (MMCs) were significantly higher at extremely high sediment pollution compared with the controls. Spleen lymphocyte and monocyte counts were also significantly lower at extremely high sediment pollutant concentrations.

Madanire-Moyo et al. (2012) evaluated the diversity of metazoan parasites of the Mozambique tilapia as indicators of pollution in the Limpopo and Olifants River systems in South Africa. The fish were collected from unpolluted, moderately polluted and polluted lakes. The infection indices, including prevalence, mean abundance and mean intensity, and species richness and diversity indicated that the structure of parasite communities were related to the pollution levels of the water. The unpolluted site had the highest species richness and overall parasite abundance. The monogenean parasite *Cichlidogyrus halli* was found in or on Mozambique tilapia in all the sampled sites. On the other hand, the distribution of *C. sclerosus*, *Cichlidogyrus dossoui*, *C. tilapiae*, *Scutogyrus longicornis* and three *Enterogyrus* spp. was limited to the unpolluted and moderately polluted lakes.

Ramadan (1991) found also that *T. zillii* in Lake Manzala, Egypt, were more infected with *Dactylogyrus* than *O. niloticus*, and larger fish were also more infected than smaller fish. Furthermore, females were more susceptible to the disease than males, and the infection rate was higher in winter than in summer. The major factors associated with prevalence and abundance of the monogenean parasites *C. sclerosus*, *C. dossoui* and *Scutogyrus* sp. infecting the gills of farmed tilapia in Mexico were also investigated by Aguirre-Fey et al. (2015). *C. sclerosus* presented the highest abundance, and parasite burdens were highly negatively correlated with water temperature. The authors suggested that despite water high temperatures generally promoting faster egg hatching and propagation of monogenean parasites, increased temperature also impacts parasite longevity and enhances host immunity. Parasite numbers were not affected by host size and coefficient of body condition. However, significant negative correlation was found between parasite abundance and haematocrit values in juvenile fish, suggesting that infection is likely detrimental to hosts.

Dactylogyrus was successfully treated with a single dose of formalin (250 ppm for 35–40 min) or two repeated applications of potassium permanganate at a dose of 5 ppm in static water with a 2-day interval (Nguenga, 1988). Table salt (sodium chloride) is also commonly used in tanks for preventive measures at a rate of 25 g L^{-1} of water (Nguenga, 1988). A number of other chemicals have been reported to effectively control these parasites in other fish species. The list includes $KMnO_4$ bath, acriflavine, sodium hydroxide, methylene blue, formalin, magnesium sulphate, sodium perborate and many others (see Hoffman and Meyer, 1974 for details). The doses and methods of application depend on fish species and size and duration of treatment.

9.4.5.2 Digenetic trematodes

Digenetic parasitic trematodes can be very problematic to tilapia culture and can cause heavy loss among fingerling and juvenile fish (Roberts and Sommerville, 1982). The life cycle of these parasites involves three hosts: a snail, a fish and a fish-eating vertebrate. Therefore, they may not cause any problems in closed systems, since one or more of the hosts may not be available. In open systems, they can infest the fish when the circariae migrate to the target organ to develop into metacercariae (Shoemaker et al., 2000).

A number of digenetic trematodes have been associated with disease infection in cultured and wild tilapias. *Clinostomum* sp., which is generally known as 'yellow grub' or 'white grub', is one of the most important digenetic trematodes that infect tilapia. The metacercariae may encyst in different body sites (e.g. dermis, muscles, gills) or remain free in the body cavity. They cause bulging and distortion of fish body profile, spoiling their appearance and make them more susceptible to handling (Roberts and Sommerville, 1982). *Clinostomum* sp. has been recovered from wild tilapia (*Oreochromis leucostictus*) in Lake Naivasha, Kenya (Aloo et al., 1995) and *O. niloticus*, *S. galilaeus* and *T. zillii* in Kompienga's Lake (Burkina Faso) (Coulibaly and Salembere, 1998). The prevalence of the parasite was highest in *O. niloticus* (56.2%) followed by *S. galilaeus* (45.79%) and *T. zillii* (18.21%). Omoregie et al. (1995) recorded *C. tilapiae* in Nile tilapia from a fish farm and petroleum-polluted water in Nigeria. *Clinostomum* spp. was also isolated from the muscles of farmed Nile tilapia and North African catfish in Kenya (Mavuti et al., 2017).

It was reported that the metacercariae cysts of *C. tilapiae* on the skin of Nile tilapia are double walled (Adeyemo and Agbede, 2008; Ochieng et al., 2012). The metacercariae is suspected to produce the cyst as a form of protective mechanism and to prevent displacement. The cyst may also be produced by fish epithelia as a defensive mechanism to prevent further damage of tissue by the parasite (Ochieng et al., 2012). This may also lead to irritation on the sites of attachment, excess mucus secretions and inflammatory. Four digeneans (*Clinostomum cutaneum*, *Tylodelphys* sp., *Diplostomum* sp. and *Bolbophorus* sp.) were also recorded in farmed Nile tilapia in Uganda (Akoll et al., 2012b).

Another digenetic trematode, *Diplostomum* (eye fluke) was recorded in the same fish farm in Nigeria (Omoregie et al., 1995). Okaeme and Okojie (1989) found also that feral tilapia *O. niloticus* and *S. galilaeus* in Nigeria were infected with *Diplostomum tregenna*. In Mexico, *Diplostomum (Austrodiplostomum) compactum* was recorded in different tilapias, including *O. mossambicus*, *O. niloticus*, and *Oreochromis urolepis hornorum* (Pineda-López et al., 1985). *Diplostomum* spp. was also found in the eyes of farmed Nile tilapia in Kenya (Mavuti et al., 2017). This parasite can cause complete blindness and loss of reflex and pigmentation control when the number of metacercariae infecting the eye is high (Roberts and Sommerville, 1982).

The prevalence of *Diplostomum* infection is related to host species and size, stocking density and water quality. For example, Violante-González et al. (2009) found that the infection level of *D. compactum* in Nile tilapia was higher in cultured than in wild fish. The authors attributed this to higher fish densities in the culture systems and higher abundance of the snail *Biomphalaria cf. havanensis* (Pteiffer), which is the first intermediate host of this parasite in freshwater and brackish water systems. The infection level also decreased in cultured tilapia as total host length increased. The authors referred this to behavioural differences between fingerlings and adults in fish ponds. During early life stages, smaller fingerlings take refuge among the aquatic vegetation along the pond dikes, where they are in constant proximity to the snail *B. cf. havanensis*.

The black spot disease which is caused by *Neascus* metacercariae has also been reported in Nile tilapia and *S. galilaeus* in Lake Kainji, Nigeria (Okaeme and Okojie, 1989), in wild and farmed Nile tilapia in Kenya and Uganda, and in wild tilapia in Ethiopia (Florio et al., 2009). *Neascus* metacercariae stimulate the accumulation of the host capsule in the skin, resulting in obvious black spots that can be easily observed (Roberts and Sommerville, 1982). The real effect of this parasite is that it makes the fish unmarketable if the infection is heavy. *Haplorchis* sp. is another digenetic trematode that is found in a wide range of freshwater fishes including tilapia, in many countries, such as Egypt, Kenya, Israel, the Philippines, China and Japan (Roberts and Sommerville, 1982). Mass penetration of fish skin by large numbers of cercariae and the migration of metacercariae to accumulate at fin bases may lead to the loss of skin function and cause fish mortality (Roberts and Sommerville, 1982).

As far as I know, no specific drugs have been suggested for controlling digenetic trematodes in tilapia. However, di-*N*-butyl tin oxide has been effective in salmonids. Sand–gravel filtration of culture water has also been effective (Hoffman and Meyer, 1974). Above all, snail control remains the best method of controlling digenetic trematodes.

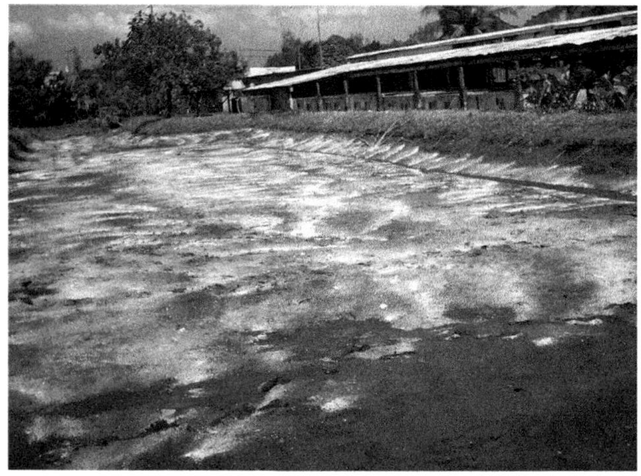

FIGURE 9.3 Drying and liming earthen ponds in the Philippines to eliminate trematodes and other parasites that might have been present in the pond water and mud. *Photograph by A.-F. El-Sayed.*

In this regard, fish ponds should be dried and limed prior to stocking to eliminate any trematodes that might have been present in pond water and/or mud. This practice is widely applied in the Philippines (Fig. 9.3). In addition, removal or eradication of snails from the pond and preventing bird access to the farm would reduce the infection of these parasites. Farm management may also play a significant role in the prevalence of trematodes. Li et al. (2013) assessed the risks for fishborne zoonotic trematodes (FZTs) in tilapia production systems in Guangdong province, China. FZT identified included intestinal flukes (*Haplorchis* spp., *Procerovum varium* and *Metagonimus* spp.) and metacercariae (*Clonorchis sinenesis*). The occurrence of FZT in wild fish was higher than in farmed fish, suggesting that the current tilapia culture management systems are generally effective in preventing transmission of these parasites into tilapia production systems. Similar evidences of FZT were reported in Thailand, where the prevalence of metacercariae of FZT in wild-caught Nile tilapia (53.3%) was much higher than in cage-cultured (2.5%) and pond-cultured fish (10%) (Wiriya et al., 2013). *Stellantchasmus falcatus*, *Haplorchis pumilio* and *P. varium* were most common zoonotic species. The high prevalence of FZT in wild-caught tilapia suggests that the potential for FZT transfer from wild reservoirs is high and the need for vigilance and good management practices by the tilapia farmers is necessary.

9.4.5.3 Parasitic nematodes, cestodes and acanthocephalans

Several nematode species have been reported in wild and cultured tilapia, but little information is available on their parasitic significance (Fryer and Iles, 1972; Scott, 1977). The nematode *Contacaecum* sp. have been reported to cause pathological effects and growth retardation in

Sarotherodon grahami and Nile tilapia in Kenya (Scott, 1977; Mavuti et al., 2017). They have also been recorded in *O. leucostictus* in Lake Naivasha in Kenya (Aloo et al., 1995), where males were more parasitized than females. This parasite can also be a problem to the consumer, since it occurs as large encysted worm throughout fish muscles. Another nematode (*Paracamallanus* spp.) was isolated from the intestines of farmed Nile tilapia in Kenya (Mavuti et al., 2017). Cestodes, nematodes and acanthocephalans were also prevalent in wild and caged Nile tilapia in Kenya, Uganda and Ethiopia (Florio et al., 2009). The prevalence was higher in wild tilapia than in caged fish. This was mainly due to the difference in feeding habits; since wild fish feed on natural zooplankton which may contain larval stages of these parasites. On the other hand, caged tilapia feed on pelleted diets with a reduced intake of plankton and, in turn, a reduced risk of parasitic infection.

Limited information is also available on the parasitic effects of cestodes and acanthocephalans on tilapia, despite the fact that they have been reported in wild and farmed tilapia (Fryer and Iles, 1972; Ramadan, 1991; Aloo et al., 1995; Omoregie et al., 1995). Omoregie et al. (1995) isolated two cestodes, *Eubothrium tragenna* and *Polyonchobothrium* sp. from farmed Nile tilapia and oil-polluted water. The infection was concentrated in the intestines, stomach, liver, brain, while the muscles and gonads were significantly infected in adult and sub-adult fish. The acanthocephalan *Polycanthorhynchus kenyensis* was also recorded in *O. leucostictus* in Lake Naivasha, Kenya (Aloo et al., 1995) and *T. zillii* and *S. galilaeus* in Lake Manzala in Egypt (Ramadan, 1991). *Acanthosentis tilapiae* also infested the intestines of commonly farmed tilapia: *O. niloticus*, *O. aureus* and wild *T. zillii* in Egypt (El-Mansy et al., 2011). The parasite proboscis was deeply embedded with its hooks in intestinal epithelia, causing severe rupture of tissue at the attachment sites.

Acanthocephalans may also act as bioindicators of aquatic chemical pollution. This assumption has recently been tested by Paller et al. (2016). The authors investigated the potential use of acanthocephalan *Acanthogyrus* sp., recovering from Nile tilapia, as a bioindicator of Lead (Pb) pollution in Sampaloc Lake, Laguna, the Philippines. Significantly higher levels of Pb were detected in the parasites relative to the fish host tissues. The prevalence rate of *Acanthogyrus* sp. was extremely high (74%). This rate was much higher than the values reported by de la Cruz et al. (2013) in cultured Nile tilapia in the same Sampaloc Lake (29%). This difference could be attributed to the differences in their feeding habits and host mobility. Heavy infestation of *Acanthogyrus* sp. was also observed by Paller et al. (2016) in the posterior region of the small intestine in Nile tilapia in the Philippines. Infected fish showed significant haematological changes. Haematocrit volume and RBC count decreased, while WBC increased, with increasing the intensity of infection. Proliferation of lymphocytes and eosinophilic granulocytes was also observed around the infected area, indicating an immune response by the host. The invasion of the parasite in the intestinal submucosal layer caused lesions and exfoliation of the mucosal layer.

9.4.6 Parasitic crustaceans

Parasitic crustaceans, including the copepods *Ergasilus*, *Lernaea*, *Caligus* and *Lamperoglena*, the branchiurans *Argulus* and *Dolops* and the isopod *Alitropus typus*, are very common among wild and farmed tilapia. Most of these parasites can cause serious damage in cultured tilapias, and in turn lead to severe loss to tilapia farmers. They can also infect wild tilapia, as has been reported by Doueellou and Erlwanger (1994) who recorded an infection of the tilapias *Sarotherodon macrocephalus* and *Tilapia rendalli* in Lake Kariba (Zimbabwe) by *Lamperoglena monodi* and *Dolops ranarum.*

Parasitic copepods are among the most serious pathogen in fish culture. *Lernaea* sp. are sedentary parasites, that have been found to cause varying losses of farmed tilapia in Nigeria, Israel, Malawi, Brazil, and Indonesia (Roberts and Sommerville, 1982; Tavares-Dias et al., 2001). Fryer and Iles (1972) reported that *Lernaea tilapiae* are restricted to tilapia in Lake Malawi. The heads of *Lernaea* are deeply embedded in fish skin and muscles, causing severe inflammatory lesions, interference with feeding and mouthbrooding, reduction in fish growth and rendering the fish unmarketable. An infestation by *Ergasilus* sp. has been reported in polyculture of carps, mullets and tilapia in Israel (Sarig, 1971). However, the infection of tilapia was lower than the other two groups. Lin et al. (1996) described the developmental stages of *Caligus epidemicus* that infect cultured tilapia in Taiwan.

The fish lice (*Argulus* sp.) are a mobile branchiuran that has been found on tilapias, especially in stagnant water (Sarig, 1971; Tavares-Dias et al., 2001). Experimental infection of Mozambique tilapia by hatched *Argulus americanus* larvae has been successful (Shimura and Asai, 1984). In addition to the damage that *Argulus* sp. can cause to the fish, the open wounds they cause are responsible for facilitating secondary infection by bacteria or fungi (Roberts and Sommerville, 1982).

Parasitic *Lamproglena* sp. are lernaeid copepods which can attach on fish gills and interfere with respiration of their host fishes. Their egg sacs are elongated, and eggs are arranged in a string rather than in a clump as in *Lernaea*. *Lamproglena* sp. was recorded in wild and farmed Nile tilapia in Kenya and Ethiopia (Florio et al., 2009) and Uganda (Akoll et al., 2012a). In the infected gills, the attachment area exhibited epithelial sloughing off and thick mucus secretion, suggesting that this parasite can cause gill damage and hamper oxygen intake at heavy infestation.

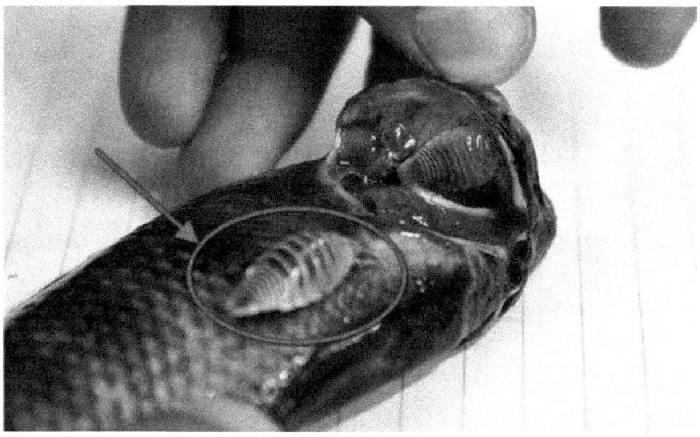

FIGURE 9.4 Isopods on the skin and gills of *Tilapia zillii* in Lae Qaroun, Egypt. *Photo provided by A. Younis.*

Alitropus typus are a parasitic isopod that can cause extensive damage to tilapia culture. They feed by sucking the blood of their host. A severe infestation of Nile tilapia cage culture by *A. typus* in central Thailand has recently been recorded (Chinabut, 2002). This parasite caused 50%−100% mortality within 2−7 days after initial infestation, leading to economic loss estimated between US$ 234−468 $cage^{-1}$.

Two cymothoid isopods (*Nerocila orbegnyi* and *Renocila thresherorum*) were found on the skin and gills of *T. zillii* in Lake Qarun, Egypt (Fig. 9.4), with a high rate of infestation (51%) (Abdelkhalek et al., 2017; Mahmoud et al., 2017). The gills of infected fish showed sever congestion, oedema and deformity of the gill arch (Abdelkhalek et al., 2017). Various degrees of degenerative lesions were observed in the gills of infested fish, including destruction, detachment, hyperplasia and fusion of the primary and secondary gill lamellae (Ali and Aboyadak, 2018).

Hoffman and Meyer (1974) listed a number of chemicals that are widely used for controlling crustacean parasites (copepods) in many fish species. Sodium chloride, potassium permanganate, lindane, ammonium chloride, DDT, Dipterex and benzene hexachloride were among the most effective drugs in controlling *Argulus* and *Lernaea*. Of course, the dose, method of application and treatment duration depend on fish species and size and drug concentration. However, the farmer should consult the authority in-charge before using any of these drugs because some of them may have been banned due to their carcinogenic effects and severe environmental impacts.

9.5 Bacterial diseases

Bacteria are found naturally in the intestine of tilapia and may become infective when environmental and culture conditions become favourable. Al-Harbi and Naim Uddin (2004) isolated and identified 17 bacterial genera from the intestine of hybrid tilapia (*O. niloticus* x *O. aureus*) reared in earthen ponds in Saudi Arabia. Despite the fact that many of these bacteria are pathogenic to tilapia, none of the sampled fish exhibited any bacterial disease symptoms or was dead. Nonetheless, increased attention has been paid to bacterial diseases of tilapias in recent years. Several studies have investigated the effects of bacterial infection of wild and farmed tilapia in different parts of the world. Both Gram-negative and Gram-positive bacteria have been associated with disease of tilapia. The significance of bacterial infection depends mainly on water quality, organic load and culture intensification. The following groups of bacteria have been reported to infect wild and farmed cichlids.

9.5.1 Motile *Aeromonas* septicaemia

The Gram-negative motile bacteria, *Aeromonas* (Fig. 9.5), are probably the most common bacteria that infect wild and cultured tilapia. They cause ‘fin rot’ or ‘skin rot’ diseases and may lead to heavy mortality in cultured tilapia (Roberts and Sommerville, 1982). Infected fish usually have dark colour, lose appetite, develop ulcers or hyperaemia at the bases of pectoral and pelvic fins (Scott, 1977), ascitis and exophthalmia (Soliman, Alexandria, 2005; personal communication). Internal symptoms include pale liver and presence of many focal haemorrhagic necrosis in the liver, heart, skeletal muscles and over the visceral and peritoneal surfaces. Massive losses of tilapia due to *Aeromonas* infection have been reported worldwide. Considerable attention has therefore been paid to this disease, for the sake of reducing its potential in tilapia farms.

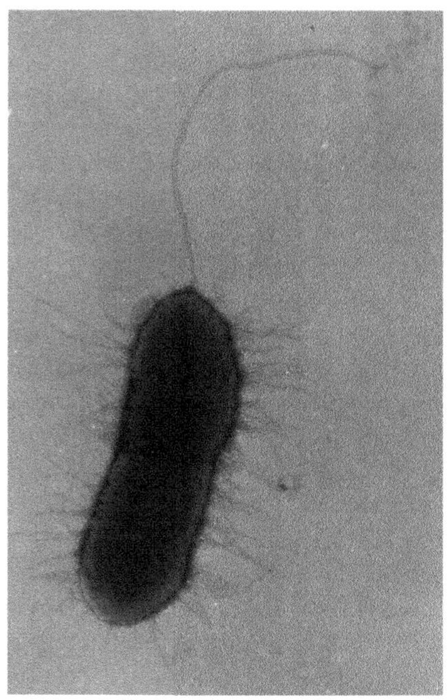

FIGURE 9.5 *Aeromonas hydrophila* isolated from Nile tilapia. *Photo provided by M.Kh. Soliman.*

Outbreaks of caudal fin rot caused by *Aeromonas hydrophila* have caused 80%−100% mortality in farmed Nile tilapia in South China (Liu et al., 1993). Infected fish showed slow movements, rotted caudal fin, swimming near the surface and poor appetite. Similar infection of Nile tilapia by *A. hydrophila* (biotype 1) was reported in wintering ponds in some districts of China (Wang and Xu, 1985). The major symptoms included the presence of circular or elliptic erosion of skin, 'rotten skin' and dorsal fin. In early infection stages, the body surface was haemorrhagic. Another outbreak of caudal fin rot induced by *Aeromonas sobria* occurred in farmed juvenile Nile tilapia in China, causing mass mortality (Li and Cai, 2011). In addition to fin rot signs, skin darkening, ascites with abdominal swelling or distention, lack of feeding and haemorrhage on the liver were observed in infected fish. *A. hydrophila* have also been isolated from Nile tilapia during fish disease outbreaks in various aquaculture farms and projects in the Philippines between 1994 and 1996 (Yambot, 1998). The occurrence of the disease was observed in low-volume and high-density aquaculture of Nile tilapia during the rainy season and cold months when water temperature was low. Infected fish suffered from skin lesion, ulceration, fin rot, body discolouration, mouth sore, eye opacity, exophthalmia, dislodged eyeball and sluggishness. High mortality was also observed in cage culture of Nile tilapia during the rainy season and cold months. The bacteria were isolated from the liver, kidney, spleen, gall bladder and opaque eyes of infected fish.

Garcia et al. (1999) isolated *A. hydrophila*, *Aeromonas schubertii* and *A. sobria* from cultured *O. mossambicus* and hybrid tilapia (*O. mossambicus* x *O. niloticus*) in Venezuela. The bacteria were isolated from the kidney, liver and dermal lesions of infected fishes. *Aeromonas salmonicida* also caused mass mortality of wild common carp and *O. mossambicus* in Kalyani reservoir in India (Reddy et al., 1994). The infection of blue tilapia with *A. hydrophila* was also recorded in Mexico (Constantino Casas et al., 1997). Stress and lack of proper culture conditions were the major contributors to the development of the disease.

Apart from *A. hydrophila* and *A. sobria*, several other *Aeromonas* species associated with disease in tilapia have been reported, including *Aeromonas dhakensis* (*A. hydrophila* subsp. *dhakensis*) (Soto-Rodriguez et al., 2013), *Aeromonas veronii* (synonyms are *Aeromonas ichthiosmia*, *Aeromonas culicicola* and *Aeromonas allosaccharophila*) (Dong et al., 2015, 2017a; Eissa et al., 2015) and *Aeromonas jandaei* (Dong et al., 2017a). Experimental infection of *A. jandaei* and *A. veronii* at high doses killed 100% of Nile tilapia within 24 h (Dong et al., 2017a). Diseased fish exhibited dark bodies, abnormal swimming behaviour, loss of appetite and severe haemorrhage and blood congestion mainly in the liver. A disease outbreak caused by *A. veronii*, leading to mass mortality of farmed Nile tilapia in Sharkia Province, Egypt, was reported by Eissa et al. (2015). Infected fish suffered from skin haemorrhages, ulcers with muscular necrosis, septicaemic lesions, including congestion in the gas bladder, kidney, liver, spleen, gall bladder, heart, brain and intestines.

Experimental infection of Mozambique tilapia held in seawater by *A. hydrophila* via intramuscular injection has been tested (Azad et al., 2001). Experimentally infected fish developed ulceration leading to open wounds, dermal necrosis and liquefying muscular degeneration, with infiltration of cellular and serum factors to the site of injection. The major histpathological manifestations were focal necrosis, loss of submucosa and sloughing of the intestinal microvillii. Similar experimental infection of tilapia by *Aeromonas* was reported by Liu et al. (1990) in Taiwan. As previously mentioned, experimental infection of Nile tilapia with *A. jandaei* and *A. veronii* was also evaluated by Dong et al. (2017a). Blue tilapia, *O. aureus*, infected with *A. hydrophila* exhibited a significant damage in the gills, liver and intestine (AlYahya et al., 2018). A moderate aggregation of haemocytes with cell necrosis occurred in the gills; while a massive aggregation of haemocytes and pyknotic nuclei appeared in the hepatopancreas of the infected fish.

A number of studies have been conducted on the resistance of carps to *Aeromonas*, based on nonspecific immunity functions, including the intra-species and inter-species variations (Cai and Sun, 1994, 1995). Studies on the potential heterosis for disease resistance of tilapia are almost lacking, despite the fact that the resistance of tilapia to bacterial infection may vary from one tilapia species to the other. Cai et al. (2004) studied the resistance of Nile tilapia, blue tilapia and their hybrids (male blue tilapia x female Nile tilapia) to *A. sobria*. Based on LD_{50}, functions of nonspecific immunity, the authors found that the hybrids have the highest resistance to the disease, while blue tilapia were the lowest resistant.

Several methods of treatment of and protection from *Aeromonas* disease have been tested, with varying effectiveness. Jirawong (2000) studied the toxicity of copper sulphate ($CuSO_4$) to *A. hydrophila.* He found that a concentration of 0.5−1.0 ppm $CuSO_4$ killed 90%−99% of the bacteria within 2−8 h, while 100% was killed within 2 h at 2 ppm. The immune response of tilapia (*Oreochromis* sp.) immunized with formalin-killed *A. hydrophila*, by intramuscular injection (IM) and direct immersion (DI), was significantly increased when the fish were fed with diets containing ascogen (5 g kg^{-1} feed) (Ramadan et al., 1994). The survival of challenged fish after IM and DI vaccination was 89.80% and 40.82%, respectively, in ascogen-fed groups compared to 75.51% and 10.20% in the vaccinated, non ascogen-treated groups, respectively.

Protective vaccination against *Aeromonas* in other tilapias has also been successful. Ruangpan et al. (1986) found that Nile tilapia vaccinated with formalin-killed bacterial vaccines showed a 53%–61% protection within 1 week after vaccination, while 100% of the fish were protected within 2 weeks. Nonspecific immune systems of tilapia have been shown to be stimulated by different polysaccharides. Similar results were obtained by Aly et al. (2015), where formalin-killed *A. hydrophila* bacteria significantly improved the immune response of Nile tilapia fingerlings (1.5 g). Vaccinated fish showed higher antibody titre and nitro blue tetrazolium activity than the control group. The protection level of vaccinated tilapia after challenge infection with *A. hydrophila* was also higher than unvaccinated fish.

Wang and Wang (1997) examined the efficacy of 11 polysaccharides in the protection of blue tilapia and grass carp against bacterial infection of *A. hydrophila* and *Edwardsiella tarda*. They found that four glycans, namely, Bar (glycan extracted from barely), Krestin, scleroglucan and Zymosan significantly increased the survival rates of tilapia (80%, 60%, 70% and 60%, respectively) and grass carp (60%, 70%, 90% and 60%, respectively). Vaccination of Nile tilapia with lipopolysaccharide (LPS) prepared from *A. hydrophila* was also investigated (Fernandez et al., 2014). The fish were immersed in the vaccine for different exposure durations (30–120 s) and then challenged intraperitoneally with 0.1 mL of virulent *A. hydrophila* suspension. Fish survival increased linearly with vaccination duration, where exposure for 120 s showed the highest survival rate. This result suggests that LPS vaccination can be used for the protection of Nile tilapia against *A. hydrophila*.

Nonspecific immune response of Nile tilapia clones was also investigated (Sarder et al., 2001). Serum lysozyme activity, phagocytosis and natural resistance to *A. hydrophila* infection by bacterial challenge were compared between fully inbred clones (ICs) of Nile tilapia (produced by gynogenesis and sex reversal) and crosses between these lines (outbred clones). The results showed a positive correlation between the level of infection and the nonspecific immune parameters measured. Cumulative mortality showed also that the cross between resistant IC and IC susceptible to *A. hydrophila* resulted in a progeny with intermediate levels of resistance to that of their parents.

9.5.2 Streptococcosis

Streptococcosis is a disease caused by Gram-positive, nonmotile bacteria *Streptococcus* sp. This disease is a major cause of damage to global aquaculture industry, with an economic loss exceeding US$ 250 million annually (Klesius et al., 2008). Streptococcosis caused a loss of US$ 40 million in tilapia industry in China alone in 2011 (Chen et al., 2012). These bacteria are opportunistic pathogens that are widely spread in aquaculture environments because of their dependence on stress to assert pathogenicity (Bunch and Bejerano, 1997). They have been isolated from pond water, bottom mud, organic manure used for pond fertilization and contaminated fish (Bunch and Bejerano, 1997). *Streptococcus* gain access to fish body by ingestion, injured skin and experimental injection (Evans et al., 2000; McNulty et al., 2003). It is no surprise, therefore, that streptococcosis is one of the most widely studied pathogens in aquaculture, and in tilapia culture in particular.

One other major concern about *Streptococcus* is that it can be transmitted from fish to humans. *Streptococcus iniae* has been reported to infect people who have handled fresh, whole fish (mostly tilapia) from fish farms in Toronto, Canada (Getchell, 1998). The patients, who were of Asian origin, cleaned and ate the fish, and some of them had injured their hands during fish cleaning, when the bacteria may have entered their bodies through the wounds. This particular accident indicates that tilapia infected with *Streptococcus* should be carefully handled and treated.

The infection of tilapia by *Streptococcus* sp. has been widely reported, but *S. iniae* and *Streptococcus agalactiae* are among the most serious pathogens affecting tilapia culture industry (Evans et al., 2006a; Zamri-Saad et al., 2010; Wang et al., 2013; Li et al., 2014; Oda et al., 2016). Stressful culture conditions including low or high water temperature, high salinity and alkalinity ($pH > 8$), low dissolved oxygen, high nitrite and ammonia concentration and high stocking density increase the susceptibility of tilapia to streptococcal infection (Chang and Plumb, 1996a, 1996b; Bunch and Bejerano, 1997; Perera et al., 1994, 1997; Shoemaker et al., 2000; Evans et al., 2006b; Zhou et al., 2008; Mian et al., 2009; Kayansamruaj et al., 2014).

Several natural outbreaks of streptococcal infection in different tilapia species and hybrids have been reported in different geographical regions of the world, including Malaysia (Abuseliana et al., 2011; Musa et al., 2009), Thailand (Jantrakajorn et al., 2014), Saudi Arabia (Al-Harbi, 1994), Colombia (Hernández et al., 2009), Brazil (Filho et al., 2009; Figueiredo et al., 2012), USA (Berridge et al., 1998; Perera et al., 1997), Indonesia (Yuasa et al., 2008) and Egypt (Aly, 2013). Stressful culture conditions, bad water quality and poor farm management were a major cause of these outbreaks. Symptoms of infected fish included heavy mortality, haemorrhage, hyperaemic gills, diffused epithelial tissue proliferation, lesions, exophthalmia, dark colouration, abscess, erratic swimming, losing appetite, abdominal distension, and lethargy (see Table 9.1).

Tung et al. (1987) reported epizootics of streptococcal infections in cage-cultured Mozambique tilapia in Taiwan, which resulted in heavy moralities, reaching 50%–60%

within 1 month. The major pathological signs of the disease included haemorrhage and exophthalmia with corneal opacity, dark body colouration, with nodular or abscess formation on the trunk and/or peduncle muscles (Figs. 9.6 and 9.7). Similar disease symptoms and mass mortality were found in the same species infected with *S. iniae* in brackishwater ponds in India (Mukhi et al., 2001). When healthy fish were injected with the pathogen (10^{5-8} cell ml^{-1}), 10% mortality was observed within 7 days of infection. Incidences of infection caused by *Streptococcus* sp. and *Enterococcus* sp. have also been associated with endemic mortality of tilapia hybrids in commercial freshwater farms in Colombia (Pulido et al., 1999). In addition, Berridge et al. (1998) reported periodical outbreaks of Streptococcosis caused by *S. iniae* and *Streptococcus difficile* in hybrid tilapia (*O. aureus* x *O. niloticus*) in Texas, USA. The authors observed that the rapid and marked mortality of market fish were associated with transferring fish from production units to market tanks. McNulty et al. (2003) studied the haematological changes in Nile tilapia infected with *S. iniae* by nare inoculation. Infected fish had increased pigmentation, eye opacity, erratic swimming and lethargy. The authors suggested that two stressors may have resulted from the infection: the loss of the oxygen carrying capacity and increase in iron levels. The identification and characterization of *S. iniae* in two, isolated populations of farmed blue tilapia (*O. aureus*) in Mexico has recently been reported by Ortega et al. (2018). The authors referred the new appearance of this pathogen to intensified aquaculture activities in the country. Affected fish showed various external signs, including exophthalmia and cachexia, whereas internal symptoms were granulomatous septicaemia and interstitial nephritis.

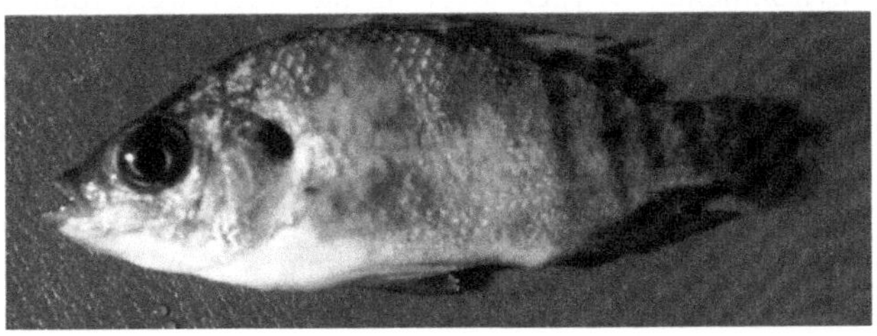

FIGURE 9.6 Severe haemorrhage and fin erosion in Nile tilapia caused streptococcal infection. *Photo provided by M.Kh. Soliman.*

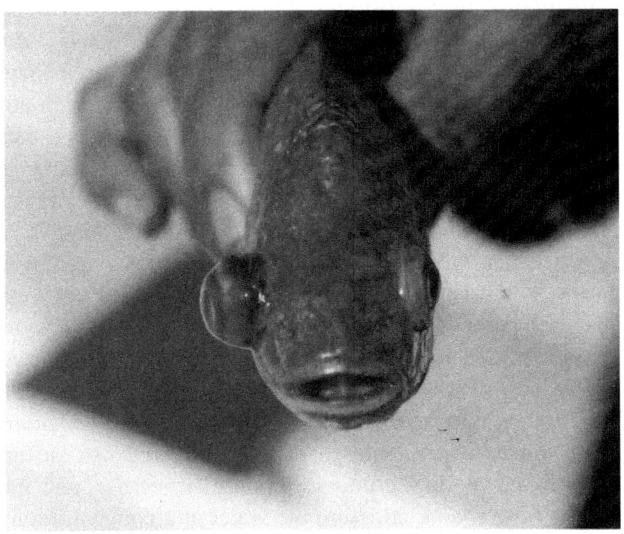

FIGURE 9.7 Exophthalmia (Popeye) in Nile tilapia caused by streptococcal infection. *Photo provided by M.Kh. Soliman.*

Apart from *S. iniae* and *S. agalactiae*, other streptococcus species, such as *Streptococcus dysgalactiae*, *Streptococcus milleri*, *Streptococcus ictaluri*, *Streptococcus faecelis*, *Streptococcus sanguis*, *Streptococcus pyogenes*, *Streptococcus pluranimalium* and *Streptococcus parauberis*, are known to induce infection in tilapia. It has been suggested that *S. dysgalactiae* is restricted to farmed marine fish in Japan (Nomoto et al., 2004). However, disease infections and outbreaks caused by this pathogen in Nile tilapia farms in several states in Brazil have been reported (Mian et al., 2009; Netto et al., 2011). The main symptoms of this disease include anorexia, lethargy, tachypnoea and skin darkness. Intramuscular and intraperitoneal injection caused rapid progress of the disease, leading to mass mortality (100% and 83%, respectively). *S. sanguis*, *S. milleri* III and *S. pyogenes* have also been isolated from wild and farmed tilapia in Egypt (Abou El-Gheit, 2005). Infected fish showed septicaemic clinical signs, exophthalmia with occasional corneal opacity. *S. pluranimalium*, *S. dysgalactiae*, and *S. anginosus* also infected wild and cultured Nile tilapia in different areas in Egypt (Osman et al., 2017).

Several drugs have been tested for treatment of *Streptococcus*. Antibiotic treatment is generally ineffective, and the need for a proper vaccine becomes a must (Klesius et al., 2000). However, Darwish and Griffin (2002) found that Oxytetracycline was effective in controlling *S. iniae* in blue tilapia (*O. aureus*). Oxytetracycline was incorporated into the feed at 0, 25, 50, 75 and 100 mg kg^{-1} body weight. The 75- and 100-mg dose significantly increased the survival of the infected fish from 7% in the infected non-medicated to 85% and 98%, respectively. Abou El-Gheit (2005) found that streptococcal isolates from Nile tilapia were highly sensitive to ciprofloxacin and oxytetracycline; but resistant to penicillin. Fish treated with ciprofloxacin and oxytetracycline showed a significant decrease in mortality; while mortality stopped completely after 4–5 days of treatment.

Aerococcus viridans, which belongs to the Family Streptococcaceae, has been recognized as a new etiological agent in aquaculture. However, little information is available on *A. viridans* as a new potential pathogen in wild and farmed tilapia. Only Ke et al. (2012) identified and characterized *A. viridans* isolated from diseased Nile tilapia in

Southeast China. Infected fish suffered from heavy mortality (30%−40%), congestive gill and abdomen, swelling gall bladder and a severe diffusion in the liver.

Passive immunization in Nile tilapia by vaccination with anti-*S. iniae* whole sera has been successful in treating this pathogen (Klesius et al., 2000, 2001; Shelby et al., 2002a). Immunized fish developed significant antibacterial responses and sharp reduction in abnormal behaviour and morphology. Furthermore, Shelby et al. (2002b) found that intraperitoneally injected Nile tilapia with anti-*Streptococcus* whole sera developed secondary antibody response and immunity to *S. iniae* with 100% survival after challenge with *S. iniae*.

Many research studies were also carried out to develop effective *S. agalactiae* vaccines for tilapia. Among the various vaccines developed, whole-cell inactivated *S. agalactiae* vaccines showed high protection efficiency (see Liu et al. (2016), for review). Inactivated *S. agalactiae* vaccines provided significant protection and survival to tilapia when challenged with homologous strains after immunization by intraperitoneal injection (Pretto-Giordano et al., 2010; Chen et al., 2012). DNA vaccines could also protect tilapia against *S. agalactiae* (Zhu et al., 2017). Oral vaccination of Nile tilapia by recombinant DNA vaccine SL7207-pVAX1-sip significantly enhanced innate immune responses, including total serum protein, superoxide dismutase activity, lysozyme activity, complement C3 concentration in serum, serum antibacterial activity, and interleukin 1b and tumour necrosis factor-a. In addition, vaccinated fish had higher survival rates than the control group. However, the vaccine efficacy is affected by immunization duration and number, fish species and size and challenge dose. With regards to vaccination method, injecting the vaccine into tilapia provided the most effective immunoprotection.

The efficacy of *S. agalactiae* vaccine in preventing streptococcosis in tilapia broodstock (species not provided) has been evaluated (Sukenda et al., 2018). The fish were vaccinated, through intraperitoneal injection, 2 and 3 weeks before spawning, using a whole-cell vaccine, an extracellular product (ECP) vaccine, and a combination of both (1:1). Produced larvae were challenged against *S. agalactiae* for 30 min, at ages 7, 14, 21, and 28 days post hatching. The broodstock treated with the combined vaccine, 3 weeks before spawning, showed better antibody levels, lysozyme activity, and haematology profiles, than the other treatments. The larvae produced from broodstock subjected to the combined vaccine, and challenged with the pathogenic *S. agalactiae* at ages 7, 14, 21, and 28 days, had relative percent survival values of 95.24%, 83.33%, 72.22% and 56.02%, respectively. These results conclude that the administration of a combination of ECP and whole-cell vaccines to tilapia broodstock in the 3 weeks before spawning can increase specific and nonspecific immunity in the broodstock and protect the larvae from *S. agalactiae* infection.

9.5.3 Vibriosis

Vibriosis, a bacterial disease caused by the Gram-negative bacteria *Vibrio*, can affect freshwater and saltwater fishes. This bacterium could constitute a serious health hazard for cultured tilapia. Several incidences of *Vibrio* infections were reported in tilapia, with varying levels of damage. The susceptibility of tilapia to vibriosis depends on tilapia species, bacteria species and strains, environmental conditions, water quality (oxygen, salinity, temperature, etc.) and culture systems. For example, Chen et al. (2006) found that the infection of hybrid tilapia (*Oreochromis* sp.) by *Vibrio vulnificus* in Taiwan was only found in fish in ponds with a salinity <10 ppt, whereas tilapia raised at higher salinities were not affected. External signs of infection included dark colouration, lethargy and skin haemorrhage and ulceration, while splenomegaly and severe haemorrhagic lesions in the liver were the most prominent internal signs. On the other hand, Plumb (1999) pointed out that *V. vulnificus* is common in saltwater, while *Vibrio cholerae* is found in fresh water, and *Vibrio parahaemolyticus* could be found in both environments. Oxygen levels in the water were found to modulate immune response in tilapia. When Nile tilapia were acclimatized to chronic moderate hypoxia (55% DO) or normoxia (85% DO), and immunized with inactivated *Vibrio anguillarum*, normoxic fish showed better immune response than hypoxic fish (Gallage et al., 2016). The absolute blood lymphocyte counts and serum bactericidal activities against *V. anguillarum* were significantly higher in normoxic fish.

Sakata and Hattori (1988) isolated and characterized three strains of *V. vulnificus* from infected, pond-cultured Nile tilapia in Kagoshima, Japan. Different *Vibrio* species, including *V. vulnificus*, *Vibrio harveyi* and *Vibrio mimicus*, have also been isolated from diseased red tilapia, blue tilapia and their hybrids in brackish water floating cages in the Philippines (Aban et al., 1999). Infected fishes showed body lesions and high mortality. This secondary infection was attributed to the great fluctuation of water salinity (18−35‰) at cage sites. In Saudi Arabia, it was reported that the outbreak of vibriosis among tilapia in fish farms in the eastern region was mainly due to stress and external parasite infection (FRRC, 2001). Disease symptoms included exophthalmia, scale loss, haemorrhage and increased mucus secretion. In a similar case, Saeed (1993) reported an outbreak of *Vibrio* sp. in *Oreochromis spilurus* reared in seawater tanks in Kuwait. Infected fish suffered from lethargy, dark colouration, dermal necrosis and mortality. Terramycin, added to the water at a concentration of 45 mg L^{-1} for 7 days, successfully controlled the disease and improved fish survival.

The susceptibility of Nile tilapia to a *V. vulnificus* strain with a high degree of virulence for eels has been investigated (Fouz et al., 2002). Infected fish developed a septicaemia similar to eel vibriosis. This result suggested that when tilapia are co-cultured with eels, they should be vaccinated against *V. vulnificus* (biotype 2) to prevent the occurrence of the disease and improve fish survival under adverse environmental conditions. In another study, the nonspecific immunity of red and black strains of Nile tilapia was compared following challenge with the bacterium *Vibrio parahaemolyticus* (Balfry et al., 1997). The results revealed a significant effect of tilapia strain on immune response (e.g. serum lysozyme and phagocytic activities). Phagocytic activity increased while lymphocyte numbers decreased following the bacterial challenge.

Similar to *Streptococcus*, *Vibrio* can be transmitted from fish to human. A fatal case of *V. vulnificus* was reported in a Canadian patient (58-year-old man) with chronic hepatitis B and chronic renal failure (Vinh et al., 2006). Diagnosis was made by isolation of the pathogen by blood culture. The patient's family recounted that he had handled and ingested tilapia in the hours preceding his hospitalization. This particular case stresses the need to educate patients with liver disease (and certain other chronic diseases) about the precautions that should be taken when handling or consuming seafood.

9.5.4 Pseudomonas

Pseudomonas are Gram-negative bacteria that have been reported to infect cichlid fishes in different geographical regions. *Pseudomonas fluorescens* were found to cause chronic mortality in farmed Nile tilapia in Japan (Miyashita, 1984). Infected fish were characterized by fine white nodules in the spleen and abscesses in the swim bladder. The infection occurred mainly in winter and spring, with peak mortality at low water temperatures (15–20°C). Miyazaki et al. (1984) also found that pond-farmed Nile tilapia infected with *Pseudomonas* in Japan suffered from exophthalmia, dark body colouration, nodular lesions, focal necrosis in the liver, spleen, kidney and gills, inflamed swim bladder, abscesses in the eyes, spleen and swim bladder and granuloma formation. *Pseudomonas* spp. have also been recorded in red tilapia, blue tilapia and their hybrids in brackish water aquaculture in the Philippines, causing dermal lesions and increased mortality in infected fish (Aban et al., 1999).

Soto-Rodriguez et al. (2013) isolated *Pseudomonas mosselii* from diseased, cage-cultured Nile tilapia in Mexico. Sick fish exhibited lethargy, erratic swimming, skin discolouration, scale loss, lateral blindness, red or opaque eyes and/or exophthalmia. The pathogenicity of *P. mosselii* to Mozambique tilapia (*O. mossambicus*) IP injected with washed bacterial cells or ECPs (3.1×10^6 CFU g^{-1}) was evaluated. Infected fish suffered from mass mortality (up to 100%), erratic swimming and skin darkening. It was concluded that this strain's ECPs were lethal to tilapia because they contain potential virulence factors, such as gelatinase and cytotoxic and haemolytic compounds. Four *Pseudomonas* species, namely *Pseudomonas fluorescens biovar I, II, III*, *Pseudomonas anguilliseptica*, *Pseudomonas putida* and *Pseudomonas aeruginosa* were isolated form wild Nile tilapia collected from Lake Qaroun and El Rayan Depression in Egypt (Eissa et al., 2010). Challenge tests revealed that *P. anguilliseptica* was the most pathogenic, inducing 97% mortality.

Antibiotics have been commonly used for treatment of *Pseudomonas* septicaemia in aquaculture. Zaki et al. (2011) found that both florfenicol and enrofloxacin can be used in combating *P. fluorescens* infection; however, enrofloxacin was more effective than florfenicol. Avatryl and Amikicin were also suggested for treating Nile tilapia infected with *Pseudomonas* (Eissa et al., 2010). However, there is an increasing public awareness regarding the use of antimicrobials for disease control due to their human health and environmental problems. As result, the search for alternative, unconventional and more environmentally friendly disease treatments and control strategies is increasing. In this regard, several herbs or their extracts have been investigated as alternatives to antimicrobial drugs in aquaculture. The aqueous extracts of six plants, *Andrographis paniculata*, *Cassia alata*, *Centella asiatica*, *Garcinia mangostana*, *Punica granatum* and *Psidium guajava*, were investigated as antimicrobial agents against *P. anguilliseptica* in Nile tilapia in Thailand (Phumkhachorn and Rattanachaikunsopon, 2015). Among the tested plant extracts, the *C. alata* extract had the strongest inhibitory effect. When Nile tilapia, infected with *P. anguilliseptica*, were exposed to a bath of the *C. alata* at 100 ppm, fish mortality was eliminated completely.

9.5.5 Staphylococcosis

Staphylococcus epidermidis is another bacterium that has been reported to infect tilapia. Huang et al. (1999) described the epizootiology and pathogenicity of *S. epidermidis* in cultured tilapia (*Oreochromis* spp.) in Taiwan. Diseased fish showed splenomegaly with diffusion of several white nodules and lesions in the spleen and anterior kidney. When blue tilapia (*O. aureus*) were challenged with viable *S. epidermidis* and its supernatant, apoptosis was predominantly detected in the lymphocytes and macrophages in the spleen and kidney, and occasionally in the brain, liver, gonads, mesentery, stomach, intestine and skeletal muscles (Huang et al., 2000). This particular study indicated that the pathogenicity of *S. epidermidis* for tilapia is due to the toxicity of the bacterial product, which induces the apoptosis.

Another methicillin-resistant species; *Staphylococcus aureus*, was isolated from diseased, cage-cultured Nile tilapia in Malaysia (Atyah et al., 2010), especially from fish eye (Najiah et al., 2012). Tetracycline, nitrofurantoin and erythromycin were found to be effective against *S. aureus*. This pathogen was reported to increase the susceptibility of tilapia to infection by *S. agalactiae* (Amal et al., 2008). *Staphylococcus* spp. were also isolated from tilapia pond water in Trinidad (Newaj-Fyzul et al., 2008), while three species; *S. epidermidis*, *Staphylococcus galinarum and Staphylococcus xylosus* were recovered from tilapia farm waters during dry and rainy seasons in Brazil (Resende et al., 2015).

9.5.6 Mycobacteriosis

Mycobacteriosis or 'fish tuberculosis' is a chronic bacterial disease caused by *Mycobacterium* spp. The disease can infect a wide range of freshwater and marine fish. The infection of wild and cultured tilapia by *Mycobacterium* is well documented. Three pathogenic agents, *Mycobacterium marinum*, *Mycobacterium fortuitum* and *Mycobacterium chelonae*, have been reported to cause the disease (Chen et al., 1998). *M. fortuitum* has been reported in the tilapias *Sarotherodon andersonii* and *Tilapia sparrmanii* from the Okavangu swamp in Botswana (Roberts and Matthiessen, 1979). The infection of farmed Nile tilapia in intensive culture in Kenya with *M. fortuitum* (Roberts and Sommerville, 1982) and the infection of tilapia hybrids (*O. niloticus* × *O. mossambicus* × *O. aureus*) with *M. marinum* (Wolf and Smith, 1999) was also reported. Affected fish showed focal granulomata in the liver, spleen, kidney and viscera; a high proportion of epithelial macrophages and more peripheral lymphocytes.

An outbreak of farmed Nile tilapia, caused by *M. fortuitum* and *M. marinum* was reported in Campeche, Mexico (Lara-Flores et al., 2014). Clinical signs of infected fish included body deformity, necrotic and haemorrhagic areas in the fins and gills, exophthalmia and ulcers in head, mouth and skin. Histological examination of spleen, liver and stomach revealed multiples granulomas with thick capsules, walled off by epithelial cells and robust acid-fast rods on the necrotic centre. Ranzani-Paiva et al. (2004) investigated the effects of *M. marinum* on blood parameters of Nile tilapia. The fish were inoculated intraperitoneally with 10^8 c.f.u. of *M. marinum*, and blood parameters, including haematocrit (Hct), haemoglobin concentration (Hgb), total erythrocytes count (RBC), haematological indexes (mean corpuscular volume (MCV), mean corpuscular haemoglobin (MCH) and mean corpuscular haemoglobin concentration (MCHC), thrombocyte count (Tr), leucocyte count (WBC) and leucocyte differential count, were estimated. The result revealed that *M. marinum* injection did not affect Hct, Hgb, MCH and MCHC. On the other hand, the values for RBC and Hct decreased, and the MCV and MCH increased, in inoculated fish. Bacterial injection also increased neutrophilia, lymphocytosis, neutropenia and monocytosis.

The effects of ECPs of *Mycobacterium* spp. on the nonspecific immune response of Nile tilapia have been examined by Chen et al. (1998). The fish were immunized by injecting their swim bladders with ECP, Freund's complete adjuvant (FCA) and Freund's incomplete adjuvant. The results revealed that ECPs from *Mycobacterium* spp. and the adjuvants used in the study provided good stimulation of nonspecific immune response in Nile tilapia.

9.5.7 Edwardsiellosis

Edwardsiellosis is a bacterial disease caused by *E. tarda*, which are short-rod, Gram-negative bacteria belonging to family Enterobacteriaceae. *E. tarda* have been isolated from reptiles, fishes, amphibians, freshwater and integrated aquaculture (Muratori et al., 2000). The pathogenicity of *E. tarda* to fish increases under stressful conditions, especially at high water temperature (>30°C) and high organic contents (even at low water temperature).

The infection of tilapia by *E. tarda* has been reported by a number of authors. Miyashita (1984) recorded chronic mortalities in Nile tilapia in some farms in Japan due to the infection of *E. tarda* and *Pseudomonas*. Muratori et al. (2000) also isolated *E. tarda* from skin, gills, fins, intestines and muscles of Nile tilapia reared in integrated fish farm fertilized with pig manure. External surfaces (skin, gills and fins) were more affected than other organs. Pathological signs of the disease include haemorrhage, corneal opacity (Fig. 9.8) and chronic mortality. *E. tarda* caused heavy mortalities in commercially farmed red tilapia (*Oreochromis* spp.) in Colombia (Iregui et al., 2012). Infected fish showed granulomatous inflammation, necrotic meningitis, encephalitis and vasculitis with fibrinoid necrosis of the blood vessels walls, and lesions in the brain, liver, kidney,

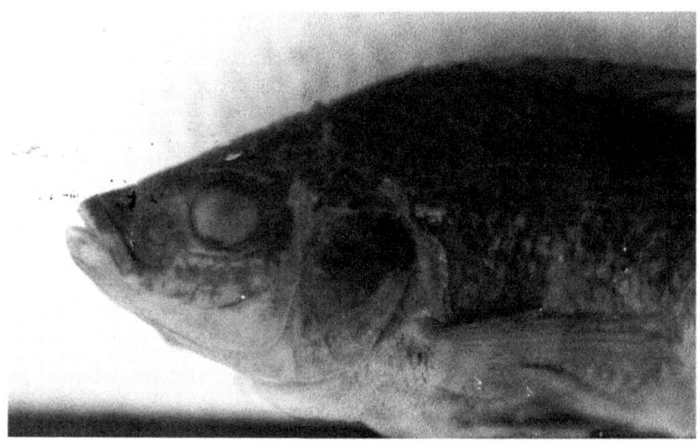

FIGURE 9.8 Corneal opacity of Nile tilapia caused by *Edwardsiella* infection. *Photo provided by M.Kh. Soliman.*

spleen and pancreas. Severe gastritis and necrotic and hemorrhagic enteritis were also found with abundant mucus production.

Another bacterial species, *Edwardsiella ictaluri*, was reported as a causative agent of mass mortality in pond-farmed Nile tilapia in Chile (Soto et al., 2012a). The pathogen was isolated from the spleens, livers, and head kidneys of diseased fish. Diseased fish showed multifocal nodulation of the spleen, head kidney and hepatomegaly and a reduced fat reserve in the liver and peritoneal cavity. Internal clinical signs included inflammatory infiltrates in the spleen, head kidney and liver. Healthy Nile tilapia challenged with *E. ictaluri* through intraperitoneal injection (at 10^6 CFU $fish^{-1}$) showed 100% mortality. Fish injected with 10^3 CFU $fish^{-1}$ exhibited bloody ascites, splenomegaly, and renomegaly, multifocal white nodules in anterior kidney and spleen with increased numbers and sizes of melanomacrophage centers (MMCs) and moderate to severe inflammatory infiltrate.

The resistance of tilapia to *E. tarda* infection has also been investigated, with contradictory results. When Nile tilapia were intraperitoneally injected with a protein-bound polysaccharide preparation (PS–K), at a dose of 0.1 mg g^{-1} body weight, maximal resistance was developed in the fish 1 week after the injection (Park and Jeong, 1996). PS-K-injected fish showed increased phagocytic activity of the pronephros cells. These results suggested that PS-K activated the nonspecific immune system of injected tilapia. Similarly, Wang and Wang (1997) evaluated the effectiveness of 11 polysaccharides in the protection of blue tilapia against *E. tarda*. They found that four glycans (Bar, Krestin, Scleroglucan and Zymosan) improved fish resistance and survival rates. In conflict with the above results, Lio-Po and Wakabayashi (1986) found that Nile tilapia immunized with formalin-killed *E. tarda* through intraperitoneal injection were not effectively protected from infection by *E. tarda*.

Mozambique tilapia immunized with *E. tarda* ghosts (ETG) and formalin-killed *E. tarda* (FKC) vaccines showed significantly higher serum agglutination titres than control group. Serum agglutination titres of ETG-immunized fish did not differ from that of fish immunized with FKC (Kwon et al., 2006). However, fish immunized with ETG showed significantly higher bactericidal activity and protection than fish immunized with FKC.

9.5.8 Columnaris disease

Columnaris disease or 'gill rot' is caused by the aquatic myxobacterium *Flexobacter columnaris*, which can affect cold water and warm water fish worldwide. *F. columnaris* is the most common myxobacterial disease in tilapia culture and is usually associated with stressful culture conditions, especially high or low water temperature and high ammonia concentration (Roberts and Sommerville, 1982; Amin et al., 1988). *F. columnaris* has been isolated from Nile tilapia (Amin et al., 1988) and *Tilapia* spp. (Chun and Sohn, 1985). The disease symptoms included respiratory disorder, body discolouration, heavy mucus secretion, fin and gill erosion and lesions in the skin and muscles. Sebastião et al. (2011) found also that Nile tilapia naturally infected with *F. columnare* showed a reduction in erythrocytic variables (total erythrocyte count, haemoglobin content, haematocrit percentage, MCH, MCHC and MCV), while a significant increase occurred in the numbers of defence blood cells, lymphocytes and neutrophils. Growth rates of infected fish were also significantly lower in diseased fish than in noninfected fish.

Improving the quality of culture water is the best way of protecting the fish from columnaris disease. Meanwhile, *F. columnaris* are susceptible to antibiotics such as oxytetracycline, chloramphenicol and erythromycine (Amin et al., 1988) and kanamycin, tetracycline and amikacine, but resistant to sulfa drugs (Chun and Sohn, 1985). Vaccination by intraperitoneal (IP) injection or immersion immunization with formalin-killed or whole cell preparations may induce antibody responses. Nile tilapia immunized with formalin-killed sonicated cells in FCA injected intraperitoneally showed a significant systemic humoral response within 2 weeks and antibody levels increased by three folds following secondary immunization (Grabowski et al., 2004). Antibody titre remained significantly high after 10 weeks post immunization, and antibodies were also found in cutaneous mucus of these fish after 6 and 8 weeks post vaccination.

9.5.9 Other bacterial diseases

Incidences of bacterial infection by other species of bacteria have been reported in tilapia. Paperna et al. (1996) found that overwintered tilapia hybrids (*O. aureus* x *O. niloticus*) had focal white lesions in the liver, filled with amoeboid organisms inside and outside the host cells. The lesions were granulomata comprising degenerating epithelial cells surrounding an expanding necrotic core. The susceptibility of Mozambique tilapia to the toxins (types A–E) produced by *Clostridium botulinum* (an anaerobic spore-forming Gram-positive bacillus) was also investigated by Lalitha and Gopakumar (2001). All five toxins were found to be toxic to the fish. The authors emphasized that proper hygiene should be maintained in fish farms to minimize bacterial contamination. *C. botulinum* (Type C) was also detected in Mozambique tilapia (Nol et al., 2004).

Francisella noatunensis subsp. *orientalis* (syn. *Francisella asiatica*), a member of the genus *Francisella*, is a causative agent of piscine francisellosis in warm water fish. Francisellosis has been diagnosed in several farmed aquaculture species, including tilapia. Francisellosis syndrome in tilapia can be acute with high mortality or moderate to chronic syndrome with nonspecific clinical signs (Soto et al., 2011). Fish injected intracoelomically with low numbers (<10 CFUs) can cause colonization and lesions in the anterior kidney and spleen, while injection of slightly higher numbers (23 CFUs) leads to mortality (Soto et al., 2009). Little information is available on the effects of environmental conditions on the pathogenicity of *F. noatunensis*. Only Soto et al. (2012b) assessed the effect of temperature and salinity on the infectivity of this bacterium in Nile tilapia. Fish were challenged with *F. noatunensis* at 25 and 30°C in fresh water and seawater. At 25°C the fish developed francisellosis and had higher mortality and splenic bacterial concentrations than the control group. Increasing the water temperature from 25 to 30°C alleviated the development of clinical signs and stopped mortality in *Francisella*-challenged fish. On the other hand, salinity had no effect on the pathogenicity of *F. noatunensis*.

Shewanella has been reported to cause mortalities in a wide variety of freshwater and marine fish species, including tilapia (Lu and Levin, 2010). *Shewanella putrefaciens* were isolated from farmed Nile tilapia and red tilapia hybrid (*O. niloticus* × *O. mossambicus*) in Thailand (Suebsing et al., 2015). The highest prevalence was recorded in fish gonads (55%) and fertilized eggs (55%), indicating that *S. putrefaciens* could be transferred from broodstock to fry. The highest colonization by *S. putrefaciens* in infected fish was observed in the spleen.

A disease outbreak caused by *Yersinia ruckeri* was recorded in Nile tilapia farmed in earthen ponds in Sharkiya Governorate, Egypt, in 2007, with a prevalence of 67% (Eissa et al., 2008). It was suggested that the mortality was due to the sharp fluctuation in water temperature, fish predation caused by migratory birds and fish crowding due high stocking density. Clinical symptoms of infected fish included mortality; haemorrhages on mouth, fin and skin; haemorrhagic gastroenteritis and congestion of the internal organs.

9.6 Fungal diseases

Fungal diseases are considered 'secondary diseases' because they are generally opportunistic, taking advantage of necrotic tissues associated with injuries, bacterial or parasitic lesions, dead and decaying eggs and poor culture conditions (Pillay, 1990). Several fungal species have been isolated from wild and farmed tilapia and organic fertilizers used for pond fertilization. El-Sharouny and Badran (1995) recovered 17 fungal species from Nile tilapia and *S. galilaeus* in Egypt. Similarly, Okaeme and Olufemi (1997) isolated 18 fungal species in tilapia culture ponds in Nigeria, 8 of them having originated from the organic manure used for pond fertilization. Although many of these fungi are infectious to tilapia, the following fungal diseases are the most important and also the most documented.

9.6.1 Saprolegniasis

Saprolegniasis is a disease caused by *Saprolegnia* and *Achlya* spp. and appears as white cotton-like patches on the necrotic tissues of infected fish, mainly skin, gills, fins, eyes and mouth. The clinical signs of saprolegniasis include haemorrhagic ulceration; erosion of skin, fins, gills and muscles; systemic mycosis of the liver, spleen, eyes and kidney and massive mortality (Okaeme and Olufemi, 1997). Low water temperature is a main reason for the spread of this disease. Lightner et al. (1988) reported 100% mortality of *O. mossambicus*, *O. aureus* and tilapia hybrids (*O. mossambicus* × *O urolepis hornorum*) caused by *Saprolegnia* due to low water temperature (<15°C). The tilapia hybrids were the most susceptible to the fungal infection, followed by *O. mossambicus*, while *O. aureus* was the most resistant because of its higher cold tolerance. Severe infection caused by *Saprolegnia* was also reported in Nile tilapia eggs and crowded fish in Kenya (Arrumm, 1987) and *T. zillii* in freshwater ponds in Nigeria (Ogbonna and Alabi, 1991). Similarly, El-Sharouny and Badran (1995) found that Nile tilapia and *S. galilaeus* infected with *Saprolegnia ferax* and *Saprolegnia parasitica* suffered from high mortality, but *S. galilaeus* was more susceptible to fungal infection than Nile tilapia.

Two different pathogenic strains of *S. parasitica* (named ManS22 and ManS33), associated with high mortalities in Nile tilapia, have recently been identified and characterized in Egypt, with ManS22 being a newly described strain (Zahran et al., 2017). Both strains were tested for pathogenicity, and they were highly pathogenic. When healthy tilapia were exposed to zoospores of both strains, cumulative mortalities reached 88.9% (for ManS22) and 95.6% (for ManS33) over 9 days. Diseased fish showed signs of water mould infection, including cotton-like growths on the skin and fins, listlessness, erratic swimming and rising near water surfaces or resting on the bottom.

A mass mortality caused by *S. parasitica* was also reported in Egyptian fish farms in Kafr El-Sheikh Governorate during overwintering (Noor El-Deen et al., 2018). Affected fish suffered from cotton wool-like masses on the head and gills, ulceration on the body surface and congestions in internal organs. The fungus was successfully treated with humic acid at a dose of 125 ppm for 10–12 min, for 3 successive days. Potassium permanganate ($KMnO_4$) and hydrogen peroxide (H_2O_2) were also effective in treating *S. parasitica* infection in the same region (Sherif and Abdel–Hakim, 2016). $KMnO_4$ also plays a protective role against oxidative stress in Nile tilapia infected with *S. ferax* (Zahran and Risha, 2013). Measured stress indicators, including Nitric Oxide (NO), glutathione (GSH) and superoxide dismutase (SOD), and biochemical parameters, including total protein, albumin, globulin, aspartate aminotranseferase (AST), and alanine aminoranferase (ALT) were all reduced in $KMnO_4$-treated fish compared with non-treated group. In addition, Freund's complete adjuvant (FCA) can modulate the oxidative stress response in infected fish and, therefore, enhance fish immune response against *S. ferax* infection.

9.6.2 Branchiomyces

Infection by *Branchiomyces* spp. is generally known as 'bad-management disease' since it flourishes in poor-quality water with high levels of organic matter. As expected, water re-use systems (closed systems) are more susceptible to its infection than other culture systems. The fungus invades the gill via branchial vessels or the epithelium and can cause massive destruction of respiratory surfaces. *Branchiomyces*-like fungus sp. have been isolated from red tilapia (*O. niloticus* x *O. mossambicus*) and green tilapia (*O. niloticus* x *O. aureus*) in intensive farming in Israel (Paperna and Smirnova, 1997). Severe infection resulted in the loss of 85% of the fish.

El-Bouhy et al. (2014) isolated *Branchiomyces demigrans* from farmed Nile tilapia in Behaira, Egypt. The infected fish suffered from massive mortality, gill tissue damage, rapid movement of gill operculum. Nonseptated hyphae and spores were embedded between the gill tissues of infected fish. Both clotrimazole and clove oil were effective in treating *B. demigrans*; but clotrimazole was more effective than clove oil. Using a mix of both drugs led to higher lysozyme and phagocytic activities. Another species, *B. demigrans*, causing similar pathogenic symptoms, was isolated from farmed Nile tilapia and common carps in different aquaculture regions in Egypt (Khalil et al., 2015). Water quality at the sites of infection, including ammonia, nitrite and organic matter, was poor, suggesting that environmental stress could be a major cause of this fungal infection.

9.6.3 Aspergillus

Aspergillus flavus produces aflatoxins that are toxic to fish. Poor storage of fish feeds leads to the growth of this mould. Farmed tilapia fed with feed contaminated with aflatoxins B_1 and B_2 showed severe haemorrhage in the branchial muscles below the dorsal commissure of the operculum, intestinal haemorrhage, haemopoiesis and massive accumulation of haemosiderin in splenic and renal melanomacrophage centres (Roberts and Sommerville, 1982). The genotoxic potential of the spores isolated from *Aspergillus niger*, *Aspergillus ochraceus* and *Helminthosporium oryzae* in intraperitoneally injected tilapia (*O. mossambicus*) was found to be positive for the frequency of chromosome aberration in gill epithelia and primary spermatocyte metaphase (Manna and Sadhukhan, 1991).

Different chemicals such as malachite green, potassium permanganate, quick lime, copper sulphate, formalin, mercurochrome and sodium chloride have been effective in treating fungal disease. However, improving water quality, culture conditions and developing management practices are the key factors in preventing fungal diseases.

9.7 Viral diseases

Despite the damage that viral diseases may cause to infected fishes, information available in the literature on their effects on cichlid fishes in general, and tilapia in particular, is very limited. Only a few studies have considered the viral diseases of cichlid fishes. The limitation of viral infection in tilapia may be attributed to the fact that tilapia are reared in warm water environments, which are not favourable for viral multiplication (Soliman, Alexandria, 2005; personal communication).

Iridovirus (*Bohle iridovirus*, BIV), which causes lymphocystic diseases, was first reported and described in wild tilapia from East African lakes in the early 1970s (Paperna, 1974). This virus has been suggested to have caused 100% mortality of *O. mossambicus* fry over a period of 60 days (Ariel and Owens, 1997). Infected fish showed rapid corkscrew-like swimming patterns ('spinning'), a symptom that renders them more susceptible to cannibalism. An outbreak of viral diseases, including an *Iridovirus*-like agent, has also been reported in cultured Nile tilapia in Canada (McGrogan et al., 1998). Infected fish were characterized by a dark colour, lethargy, slow swimming or resting on the bottom, exophthalmia, marked pallor of the gills and visceral organs, particularly the liver, erythema of the submandibular skin, severe abdominal ascites and haemorrhages in the liver. In addition to these symptoms, Smith et al. (1998) found that Nile tilapia fingerlings infected with this virus exhibited necrosis and inflammation of several organs, including the choroid of the eye, heart, intestines, kidney, liver and spleen. The most severe change was necrosis of the haematopoietic tissue of the spleen, kidney and heart. Similarly, iridoviral disease caused gill pallor, degeneration of tissue cells, the presence of intranuclear inclusion bodies and progressive weakness of the chromide cichlid *Etroplus maculatus*, leading to the death of the fish (Armstrong and Ferguson, 1989).

Rhabdovirus is a viral agent of cichlid fishes that has been isolated and described from the cichlids *Cichlasoma cyanoguttatum*, *Cichlasoma nigrofaciatum* and *T. zillii* (Lautenslager, 1986). This agent causes fatal diseases of these hosts. Skliris and Richards (1999) studied the susceptibility of Mozambique tilapia to another viral agent, nodavirus, isolated from naturally infected European sea bass, *Dicentrarchus labrax*. The authors suggested that nodavirus might be transmitted to seawater-reared tilapia. Another virus, birnavirus, was described and isolated from Mozambique tilapia in Taiwan in the early 1980s (Hedrick et al., 1983). The virus was widespread and may have led to secondary effects on the fish, such as increasing their susceptibility to other infectious agents. In addition, Avtalion and Shlapobersky (1994) reported that the larvae of blue tilapia, Nile tilapia and Galilee tilapia were highly susceptible to 'unidentified' whirling viral disease. Disease symptoms included whirling, followed by darkening of the skin and anorexia.

Betanodaviruses, which belong to Family Nodaviridae, are known to cause viral nervous necrosis disease in many marine and freshwater fish species, including tilapia (Bigarré et al., 2009; Keawcharoen et al., 2015). The disease has been considered as one of the most serious viral diseases, especially in hatchery-reared larvae and juveniles. An outbreak of betanodavirus infection in tilapia larvae was recorded in a western European fish farm (Bigarré et al., 2009). Infected fish suffered from erratic swimming and histological lesions, while experimentally infected fish showed lethargy, anorexia and darkness in colour. However, some fish showing these signs recovered completely after a few days of infection. Betanodavirus was also isolated from farmed Nile tilapia larvae in central Thailand (Keawcharoen et al., 2015). The larvae exhibited mass mortality (90%—100%), together with signs of neurological disorders, including loss of balance and corkscrew-like swimming behaviour prior to death. Extensive vacuolar degeneration and neuronal necrosis were also observed in infected fish.

Megalocytivirus is another infectious spleen and kidney necrosis virus (ISKNV), which can induce fatal systemic diseases in different fish species. Subramaniam et al. (2016) reported Megalocytivirus infection in Nile tilapia cultured in the Midwest United States. Diseased fish displayed lethargy, gill pallor and ascites causing distension of the coelomic cavity. Internal signs included abundance of intravascular megalocytes, especially in the gills, kidney, spleen, liver and intestinal submucosa. These results suggest that ISKNV can be a real threat to tilapia aquaculture. Tilapia larvae encephalitis virus (TLEV) is a newly discovered herpes-like virus, belonging to Family Herpesviridae. An outbreak of acute TLEV, causing high mortality rate in laboratory-reared tilapia larvae, was reported by Shlapobersky et al. (2010).

There are no reported effective treatments for viral diseases of tilapia except the removal and destruction of infected fish. The best protective treatment is the quarantine of larval fish and the avoidance of introducing fish with viral disease histories into culture facilities (Shoemaker et al., 2000).

9.7.1 Tilapia lake virus

Starting in the summer of 2009, disease outbreaks with massive losses of tilapia were recorded in fish farms all over Israel, due to unknown reason (Eyngor et al., 2014). A histological analysis of infected fish revealed the presence of augmented melanomacrophage centers (MMCs). Other pathological signs included gross lesions, opacity of the lens (cataract), ruptured lenses with phacoclastic induced uveitis or endophthalmitis accompanied by the formation of a cyclitic membrane, swelling of the eyeball (buphthalmia), loss of globe integrity with occasional perforated cornea and loss of ocular functioning. Other lesions included skin erosions, haemorrhages in the leptomeninges, congestion of the spleen and kidney, foci of gliosis, encephalitis and mild perivascular cuffing by lymphocytes in the brain (Eyngor et al., 2014; Fathi et al., 2017). These symptoms are certainly due to a pathological source. In order to elucidate the cause of these symptoms, attempts were first made in Israel to culture and identify a probable infectious agent that might trigger this disease (Eyngor et al., 2014). Infection of this virus was also restricted to fertilized eggs, yolk-sac larvae, fingerlings and juvenile stages (Dong et al., 2017b).

In 2014, the virus was identified and named as tilapia lake virus (TiLV) or syncytial hepatitis of tilapia (SHT). However, the taxonomic affiliation of TiLV has not been confirmed (Eyngor et al., 2014; OIE, 2017). Nonetheless, the genetic composition of this emerging novel virus was similar to that of orthomyxoviruses; therefore, it is grouped with the viruses of the Family Orthomyxoviridae. In addition, syncytial hepatitis, a novel viral disease of tilapia (SHT), has been suggested as a cause of the mortality in tilapia. The ultrastructural morphology of SHT is associated with TiLV (Del-Pozo et al., 2017). Therefore, the disease associated with TiLV infection is currently known as 'tilapia lake virus disease' (TiLVD) (OIE, 2017) and SHT (Ferguson et al., 2014; Del-Pozo et al., 2017).

Since its first appearance in Israel in 2009, TiLV has been a cause of several outbreaks with massive loss of farmed tilapia in many counties worldwide. These include Colombia, Ecuador, Israel (Ferguson et al., 2014; Bacharach et al., 2016), Egypt (Fathi et al., 2017; Nicholson et al., 2017), Thailand (Dong et al., 2017b, 2017c), India (Behera et al., 2018), Malaysia (Amal et al., 2018) and the Philippines (OIE, 2017). TiLV outbreaks in Thailand during 2015 and 2016 resulted in 20%—90% mortalities of farmed Nile tilapia and red tilapia hybrid (Dong et al., 2017b, 2017c). In Egypt, mortality of farmed Nile tilapia during the summer months in recent years, presumably due to TiLV, resulted in an economic loss of around USD 100 million in 2015 (Fathi et al., 2017). However, the lack of accurate investigations and reporting of global TiLV disease incidents suggests that the geographic distribution of TiLV is wider than what is currently reported. For example, Ghana and Zambia declared that mortality of tilapia in 2016 has not been caused by TiLV, despite that the available information indicating that the presence of the virus in these two countries has not been investigated (OIE, 2017).

Published research studies indicated that mortalities caused by TiLV in wild and cultured tilapia have been reported in wild Galilee tilapia (*S. galilaeus*), farmed Nile tilapia (*O. niloticus*) and commercial hybrid tilapia (*O. niloticus* X *O. aureus*) (Eyngor et al., 2014; Ferguson et al., 2014; Bacharach et al., 2016; Fathi et al., 2017). Current evidences also indicate that only tilapias are susceptible to TiLV, and it is not known whether it is transmittable to other fishes. In Egypt, for example, the vast majority of tilapia farmers grow tilapia with mullets (*Mugil cephalus* and *Liza ramada*) in a polyculture system. Yet, only 8% of tilapia farms practicing tilapia monoculture were affected, whereas 73% farms practicing tilapia/mullet polyculture were not affected (Fathi et al., 2017). Mullets were also resistant to TiLV, but their role in the disease transmission remains unknown. It should also be mentioned that certain genetic strains of tilapia may be more resistant to TiLV than others. Ferguson et al. (2014) found that the level of infection in genetically male Nile tilapia was significantly lower than another Nile tilapia strain 'Chitralada strain'.

It has been suggested that TiLV is horizontally transmitted through the movement of live fish. For example, as Egypt shares a border with Israel (in which TiLV has been confirmed) and is on a bird migration route passing through Israel, the disease could have been easily transmitted to Egypt (Fathi et al., 2017).

Global attention and awareness have been given to TiLVD during the past few years because of the huge risk it may pose to tilapia industry worldwide. A technical disease card for TiLV has been released recently by the OIE (OIE, 2017). A Network of Aquaculture Centres in Asia–Pacific (NACA) disease alert (NACA, 2017), a CGIAR Research Program on Fish Agri-food Systems (CGIAR, 2017; Jansen and Mohan, 2017) Factsheet, an FAO Global Information and Early Warning System (GIEWs) Special Alert 388 (FAO, 2017) have also been released (Jansen and Mohan, 2017). In addition, several website warnings have been issued. These publications and warnings clearly demonstrate the increasing concern about TiLV, the urgent need for further knowledge on its implications and the importance of international collaboration.

It is, therefore, imperative that tilapia producing countries should be fully aware of TiLV and take the necessary risk management measures (e.g. enhanced diagnostic testing of imported stocks and unexplained tilapia mortalities and reporting to biosecurity authorities, active surveillance, public information campaigns and contingency plans) to reduce the further spread and potential socio-economic impacts of this emerging disease (FAO, 2017). Since transportation of live or processed tilapias between countries is increasing, it may pose a threat by TiLV. Reliable diagnostic tools for TiLV are currently available, and it should be used to rule out TiLV as the causative agent of unexplained mortalities.

The following measures have been suggested by FAO (2017) in countries with confirmed cases of TiLV:

- Initiate an active surveillance programme to determine the geographical extent of the infection and undertake mitigation measure to restrict the spread of infection; identify risk factors that may assist in appropriate interventions.
- Initiate public information campaigns to advise aquaculturists of the threat posed by TiLV, its clinical signs, potential economic and social impacts, and the need to report unexplained large-scale mortalities to biosecurity authorities.
- Conduct appropriate diagnostic testings, where unexplained mortalities of tilapias occur, particularly if clinical signs similar to those reported for TiLV are observed.

On the other hand, countries with unknown status of TiLV should do the following:

- Initiate an active surveillance programme to determine if TiLV is present as well as to identify the susceptible species and country distribution.
- Initiate public information campaigns to advise aquaculturists of the threat posed by TiLV, its clinical signs and the need to report unexplained large-scale mortalities to biosecurity authorities.

9.8 Noninfectious diseases and disorders

Tilapia, like other farmed aquatic animals, may be subjected to unfavourable conditions, leading to health problems and noninfectious diseases. Unfortunately, the information which is available on noninfectious disorders of tilapia is very limited. Only nutritional disorders, gas bubble diseases and the disorders caused by pollutants are reasonably documented. The following sections briefly discuss these disorders.

9.8.1 Gas bubble disease

Excessive aeration in intensive aquaculture systems may result in supersaturating culture water with dissolved gases. When these gases are absorbed by the fish during respiration, they cause a change in partial pressure, leading to gas accumulation (gas bubbles) at different sites of the fish body. In tilapia fry, gas bubbles are concentrated in the yolk sac, while in older fish they are found in the gills and under the skin (Roberts and Sommerville, 1982).

Outbreaks of gas bubble disease have been reported in farmed saltwater juvenile tilapia, *O. spilurus* (52.5 g), in Saudi Arabia (Saeed and Al-Thobaiti, 1997). About 50% of fish populations were affected, resulting in 30% mortality. Another outbreak occurred in adult Nile tilapia (270 g) in brackish water, affecting about 40% of the fish population, with 40% mortality. Affected Nile tilapia were heavily infected with monogenetic trematodes. In all cases, the total gas was higher than 111% saturation, nitrogen was supersaturated and oxygen undersaturated. The disease symptoms were overcome by reducing the gas pressure through splashing the water and using water with lower gas pressure.

9.8.2 Nutritional diseases

The deficiency of certain nutrients in the diets of farmed fish may lead to disease symptoms and health problems. The effects of dietary vitamin deficiency on farmed tilapia are well documented (see Chapter 7 for more details). Blue tilapia fed pantothenic acid-deficient diets exhibited poor growth, haemorrhage, sluggishness, anaemia, hyperplasia in epithelial cells of gill lamellae and high mortality (Soliman and Wilson, 1992a). Anorexia, low growth, fin erosion, loss of body colour, cataract and mortality were also observed in fish fed with riboflavin-deficient diets (Soliman and Wilson, 1992b). Similar deficiency symptoms have been reported in tilapia hybrids fed test diets deficient in niacin, pyridoxine and thiamine (Lim and Leamaster, 1991; Shiau and Suen, 1992; Shiau and Hsieh, 1997). Fish fed diets devoid of thiamin suffered from high mortality, neurological disorders, anorexia, poor growth rates and low RBC count and haematocrit (Ht) (Lim et al., 2011). In the meantime, Lim and Klesius (2001) reported low growth and reduced RBC and total cell counts in Nile tilapia fed diets deficient in folic acid.

Guimarães et al. (2014) found that Nile tilapia fed diets deficient in vitamin A exhibited significantly low growth performance, haemorrhages, operculum deformity, fin erosion, darker body colouration, lethargy and low haematological parameters (except WBC count) compared to fish fed vitamin A-supplemented diets. The resistance of erythrocytes to haemolysis in hypotonic solutions was lowest in fish fed vitamin A-unsupplemented diet and increased with increasing vitamin A supplementation. When vitamin A was supplemented at 3910 IU kg^{-1}, these deficiency signs disappeared. In addition, low vitamin E contents in the diets resulted in poor growth and FCR, skin haemorrhage, muscle dystrophy, impaired erythropoiesis and abnormal skin colouration (Roem et al., 1990). Fish fed vitamin E-deficient diet had significantly lower growth, feed efficiency and survival rate than those fed vitamin E-supplemented diets (Wu et al., 2017). Vitamin E deficiency also reduced texture cohesiveness and chewiness.

On the other hand, the addition of certain feed elements to tilapia feeds may play a significant protective role in the fish, especially when they are cultured at a high stocking density and under deteriorated water quality. Schlechtriem et al. (2004) studied the effects of dietary L-carnitine on tilapia hybrids (*O. niloticus* × *O. aureus*) reared under intensive pond-culture conditions. The fish were fed diets containing either 150 or 450 ppm of L-carnitine. Histological examinations revealed that fish fed 150 ppm carnitine showed the lowest permeability to fluorescein in gills, gut and skin epithelia, the highest activity in the system of active transport for organic anions and the highest levels of the multixenobiotic resistance transporter (MXRtr) for lipophilic/amphiphilic xenobiotics, compared to the control and the 450-ppm treated fish. The MXRtr activity in the liver bile canaliculi and renal proximal tubules of this group of fish was much higher than that of the other groups except those from the indoor tank. The intralysosomal accumulation of neutral red in their head–kidney macrophages was also significantly higher. The authors suggested that even a low level of L-carnitine enrichment can provide considerable protective effects in fish reared under intensive pond-culture conditions.

9.8.3 Disorders caused by pollutants

Aquatic environments receive a wide variety of agricultural run-offs, including pesticides, herbicides, fungicides, fertilizer residues and heavy metals. Considerable amounts of various industrial wastes, human wastes, molluscicides and oil compounds are also discharged into aquatic environments. These organic and inorganic compounds are very likely to cause environmental impacts such as bio-accumulation, eutrophication, environmental degradation and imbalance of aquatic biodiversity. Farmed and wild fish, including tilapia, are therefore expected to be adversely affected by these pollutants. Such impacts depend on fish species and size, type and concentration of pollutant, duration of exposure and environmental conditions. However, little attention has been paid to the impacts of environmental pollution on farmed tilapia. Despite the fact that hundreds of chemical compounds are likely to be hazardous to these fish, even at low concentrations, only a few compounds have been considered.

Phenolic compounds are among the most serious organic pollutants in the aquatic environments. These chemicals are highly toxic to aquatic animals and can cause severe ecological and economic losses. For example, Hart et al. (1998) found that Nile tilapia subjected to the carcinogenic PAH 7,12-dimethylbenzanthracene suffered from reduced spleen, pronephros and total WBC counts. The fish also exhibited reduced swimming activity and feeding activity and increased skin pigmentation and mortality. In another study, Mehrim (2001) evaluated the maximum tolerable level of phenol for fingerling Nile tilapia, and the effects of chronic exposure on growth performance and feed utilization efficiency. He found that 30 ppm was the maximum tolerable level, and beyond that level fish exhibited a respiratory manifestation and hyperirritability, followed by lethargy, lesions, increased mucus secretion, skin darkness, fin erosion, gill and liver congestion and distension of the gall bladder. Fish exposed to the maximum tolerable level (30 ppm) had significantly reduced growth, survival and feed utilization efficiency. The addition of Biogen as a feed supplement to the diets has significantly overcome the symptoms mentioned.

The effects of different concentrations of another phenolic compound, 4-nonylphenol (NP), on the structure and functions of Nile tilapia gonads were investigated in a series of studies (El-Sayed Ali et al., 2014a; 2014b; 2017). The results indicated that NP at a concentration of $60-100\ \mu g\ L^{-1}$ resulted in impaired female gonadal development and differentiation, due to the significant effect of NP on 11-ketotestosterone, 17β-oestradiol and vitellogenin synthesis (El-Sayed Ali et al., 2014a). In case of males, NP-exposed fish had oestrogenic potency and induced marked alteration in the male sexual development, including inhibition in testicular growth and deformation in the sperms (El-Sayed Ali et al., 2014b). In addition, when Nile tilapia fingerlings were exposed to NP, vitellogenin was observed in the plasma of all fish (El-Sayed Ali et al., 2017). A dose-dependent tendency in the gonadosomatic index in NP-exposed groups was also found. As in adult fish, NP impaired gonadal growth and induced intersex state in the fish. Along the same line, acute exposure of Nile tilapia to high dose of NP ($500\ \mu g\ L^{-1}$) showed anorexia, sluggish movement, erythema of the skin, loss of scales and severe skin haemorrhagic ulcers, leading to exposing the viscera (Ismail and Mahboub, 2016). A significant increase was observed in serum total proteins and globulins levels; ALT and AST activities; triglycerides, cholesterol and creatinine levels and RBCs count and PCV values. On the other hand, serum testosterone and 17β-oestradiol levels were significantly decreased.

Bayluscide is another phenolic compound that is widely used as a molluscicide. It is one of the chloronitrophenol derivatives (niclosamide ethanolamine salt) (5,2-dichloro-4 nitro salicylic-anilide). This compound is frequently used for eradication of the intermediate host snails of Schistosomiasis (Bilharzia) and fascioliasis in Egypt. It is very toxic to snails, but it can be toxic to fishes as well. Acute toxicity of Nile tilapia intoxicated with Bayluscide included erratic and nervous swimming, continuous opening of mouth and gill cover, haemorrhage under the scales and at the base of the fins and degenerative and necrotic changes in the liver, kidney, spleen, heart and gills (Nafady et al., 1986; Marzouk and Bakeer, 1991; Khalil, 1998). Khalil (1998) found that $0.3\ mg\ L^{-1}$ was lethal to Nile tilapia, while $0.1\ mg\ L^{-1}$ was sublethal. Fish exposed to $0.15\ mg\ L^{-1}$ (50% of LC_{50}) suffered from nervous and respiratory manifestation; corneal opacity; decrease in red and WBC counts, haemoglobin concentration and phagocytic activity and high accumulation of Bayluscide in the gills, liver and muscles.

Several other organophosphorus compounds, including Diazinon, Endosulfan, Dichlobenil, and many others, are widely used as insecticides, molluscicides, herbicides and therapeutic agents for many diseases. As expected, these compounds can pose a wide range of impacts on cultured and wild tilapias. Since it would be difficult to go through all these impacts in details in the text, they are summarized in Table 9.2.

Rajavarthini and Michael (1996) found that exposure to Nuvalron caused dose-dependent suppression of antibody response in Mozambique tilapia. *T. rendalli* exposed to Endosulfan suffered from hepatic lesion, encephalitis, meningitis, oedema and inflammatory infiltrate of eosinophilic granular cells in the brain (Makhiessen and Roberts, 1982). When Nile tilapia were exposed to Diazinon, they exhibited lethargic behaviour, loss of coordination, dark red gills, pale liver, distended gall bladder with dilated bile ducts, dilated arterioles and lamellar capillaries (El-Khateib and Afifi (1993). Similarly, Nile tilapia exposed to a high dose of Metrifonate showed respiratory manifestation, loss of pigmentation, dark body colouration, protrusion of anal opening and haemorrhage (El-Gohary, 2004). Chronic symptoms included darkness of body colour, haemorrhage, decrease in phagocytic activity, necrotic and degenerative changes in the kidney, liver, spleen, heart and brain.

The above results clearly indicate that water pollution can have harmful impacts on tilapia. The use of the different chemicals and drugs for controlling pests, insects, snails, herbs, etc. should be carefully regulated and managed. In addition, culture water should be analyzed prior to, and continuously monitored during, culture practices to investigate whether it contains any traces of pollutants and whether the levels of these pollutants are hazardous to farmed tilapia. In the late 1990s, a sudden, tragic, mass mortality occurred in Nile tilapia, cage-cultured in a waterway close to El-Salam Canal in Lake Manzala, Egypt, within the 'Cages-for-Graduates Project', which was funded by the Social Development Fund (El-Sayed, Mansoura, 1999; personal observation). This massive mortality was attributed to increased levels of pesticides in the canal from land run-offs. In fact, the owners of these cages faced a serious problem because they had to pay back the loans they had taken from the Social Development Fund. Only governmental interference saved them from prison. This particular example stresses the

TABLE 9.2 A list of the common pollutants and their impacts on wild and farmed tilapia.

Compound name	Fish species	Levels tested/LC_{50}	Impact	References
Nuvalron	*Oreochromis mossambicus*		Suppression of antibody response	Rajavarthini and Michael (1996)
Endosulfan (OCs)	*O. mossambicus*	3.6 $\mu g\,L^{-1}$	Oxidative tissue damage, increase in anti-oxidative enzymes activity. Acute toxicity, reduced neurotransmission and depleted RBCs, WBCs and haemoglobin and caused stress and immune suppression.	Kumar et al. (2011)
Endosulfan	*Oreochromis niloticus*	4.0 and 7.0 $\mu g\,L^{-1}$	Acute exposure (4.0 and 7.0 $\mu g\,L^{-1}$) decreased phagocytic index and the percentage of active cells in peripheral blood.	Girón-Pérez et al. (2008)
Diazinon	*O. niloticus*	3.85 $mg\,L^{-1}$	Alteration of immunological response and induction of oxidative stress. Low concentrations (0.39 and 0.78 $mg\,L^{-1}$) have no effects. Higher levels (1.96 $mg\,L^{-1}$) increased respiratory burst and IgM concentration.	Girón-Pérez et al. (2009)
Diazinon (organophosphorus pesticides)	*O. niloticus*	0.97, 1.95, 3.95 ppm	Oxidative damage in liver and gill proteins, decrease in total proteins.	Toledo-Ibarra et al. (2016)
Chlorpyrifos	*O. niloticus*	Tested at 15 and 75 $\mu g\,L^{-1}$	Decreased RBCs, serum bactericidal and lysozyme activity. Increased blood packed cell volume (PCV), mean corpuscular volume (MCV), total leukocytes, lymphocytes and neutrophil counts, antioxidant enzyme activity in liver and gills and whole blood respiratory burst.	Zahran et al. (2018)
Glyphosate herbicide ($C_3H_8NO_5P$)	*O. niloticus*	Exposure for 3 months to sublethal concentrations (5 and 15 ppm)	Gill filaments proliferation, lamellar cell hyperplasia, lamellar fusion, epithelial lifting and aneurysm, vacuolation of liver hepatocytes, kidney lesions and accumulation of hyaline droplets in the tubular epithelial cells.	Jiraungkoorskul et al. (2003)
Nonylphenol	*O. niloticus*	500 $\mu g\,L^{-1}$	Increasing: serum total proteins and globulins levels, alanine aminotransferase and aspartate aminotransferase activities, triglycerides, cholesterol, creatinine levels and RBC count and PCV. Serum testosterone and 17β-oestradiol levels decreased.	Ismail and Mahboub (2016)
Folidol 600 organophosphate pesticide	*O. niloticus*	LC_{50} (96h) 2.7 $mg\,L^{-1}$	Increase of haematological parameters, inhibition of cholinesterases activity (AChE, BChE and PChE) in plasma of fish exposed to the higher concentrations, increase in ammonia excretion.	Barbieri and Ferreira (2011)
1-Nitropyrene (polycyclic aromatic hydrocarbons or nitroarenes)	*O. niloticus*	250, 2500 or 25,000 $pg\,L^{-1}$	Oxidative stress, micronucleus and other nuclear abnormalities, induction of genotoxicity.	Bacolod et al. (2017)
Pendimethalin-based herbicide (Stomp)	*O. niloticus*	4.92 $mg\,L^{-1}$	Acute exposure induced leucocytosis, hyperglobulinaemia, hyperglycaemia and increased lipid peroxidation. Low levels reduced glutathione and antioxidant enzymes (superoxide dismutase, catalase, and glutathione reductase in both liver and gill tissues).	El-Sayed et al. (2015)

necessity of regular monitoring of culture water, especially in areas where the water may receive pollutants from various sources.

9.9 Closing remarks

1. Stressful conditions adversely affect tilapia and make them more susceptible to different diseases. Essential causes of chronic stress in tilapia are inappropriate handling and social interactions and hierarchies. Reducing stress is an important tool for disease control and improvement of immunity in cultured tilapia.
2. Tilapia have been reported to be subjected to parasitic, viral, fungal and bacterial diseases, in addition to a number of noninfectious diseases.
3. Protozoan parasitic ciliates and flagellates have been reported to widely infect wild and farmed tilapia. Most of ciliate parasites can be treated with table salt and formalin (30–50 mg L^{-1}).
4. Monogenetic trematodes can parasitize on wild and farmed tilapia. Bad water quality, poor farm management and chemical pollution generally enhance the impact of these parasites. *Gyrodactylus* infecting tilapia was successfully treated with a single dose of formalin (250 ppm for 35–40 min) or two repeated applications of potassium permanganate at a dose of 5 ppm in static water with a 2-day interval.
5. Digenetic parasitic trematodes can be very problematic to tilapia culture. Removal or eradication of snails from the pond and preventing bird access to the farm would reduce the infection of these parasites. Farm management also plays a significant role in the prevalence of these trematodes.
6. Little information is available on the parasitic effects of cestodes and acanthocephalans on tilapia, despite that they have been reported in wild and farmed tilapia. Acanthocephalans may act as bioindicators of aquatic chemical pollution.
7. Parasitic crustaceans including the copepods *Eragasillus*, *Lernaea*, *Caligus* and *Lamperoglena*, the branchiuran *Argulus* and *Dolops* and the isopod *A. typus* are among the most serious pathogens in tilapia culture.
8. The significance of bacterial infection of tilapia depends on water quality, organic load and culture intensification. Most of infectious bacteria can cause massive losses of farmed tilapia. Several methods of treatment including copper sulphate ($CuSO_4$), vaccination against the bacteria with formalin-killed bacterial vaccines, antibiotics and passive immunization by vaccination with anti-bacterial whole sera, have been used with varying levels of effectiveness.
9. Despite the damage that viral diseases may cause to infected tilapia, very limited information is available on their effects. There are no effective treatments for these diseases except the removal and destruction of infected fish. The quarantine of larval fish and the avoidance of introducing fish with viral disease histories into culture facilities are the most effective protective treatment.
10. TiLV has been a cause of several outbreaks with massive loss of farmed tilapia in many counties all over the world. The disease associated with TiLV infection is currently known as 'tilapia lake virus disease (TiLVD) and 'syncytial hepatitis of tilapia (SHT)'. Global attention and awareness have been given to TiLVD during the past few years because of the huge risk it may pose to tilapia industry worldwide. Tilapia producing countries must take the necessary risk management measures in order to reduce the spread of TiLV.
11. The organic and inorganic compounds discharged into aquatic environments are very likely to cause adverse environmental impacts on farmed and wild tilapia. Controlling the use of these compounds, together with regular monitoring of culture water, is necessary for controlling such impacts.

References

Aban, S.M., Ba-ad, E.G.V., Parreno, S.C., Garcia, A.C., 1999. Bacterial diseases and salinity tolerance of red tilapia *Oreochromis aureus* and their hybrids (*Red tilapia* x *Oreochromis aureus*). In: Paper Presented at the Fourth Symposium on Diseases in Asian Aquaculture: Aquatic Animal Health for Sustainability. Cebu City, Philippines.

Abdel-Baki, A.A., Gewik, M.M., Al-Quraishy, S., 2014. First records of *Ambiphrya* and *Vorticella* spp. (Protozoa, Ciliophora) in cultured Nile tilapia (*Oreochromis niloticus*) in the Central region of Saudi Arabia. Saudi Journal of Biological Sciences 21, 520–523.

Abdel-Baki, A.A., Zayed, E., Sakran, T., Al-Quraishy, S., 2015a. A new record of *Myxobolus brachysporus* and *M. israelensis* in the tilapia (*Oreochromis niloticus*) collected from the Nile River, Egypt. Saudi Journal of Biological Sciences 22, 539–542.

Abdel-Baki, A.A., Abdel-Haleem, H.M., Sakran, T., Zayed, E., Ibrahim, K.E., Al-Quraishy, S., 2015b. Two *Myxobolus* spp. infecting the kidney of Nile tilapia (*Oreochromis niloticus*) in the River Nile at Beni-Suef governorate, Egypt, and the associated renal changes. Parasitological Research 114, 1107–11012.

Abdel-Ghaffar, F., El-Toukhy, A., Al-Quraishy, S., Al-Rasheid, K., Abdel-Baki, A.S., Hegazy, A., et al., 2008. Five new *myxosporean* species (Myxozoa: Myxosporea) infecting the Nile tilapia *Oreochromis niloticus* in Bahr shebin, Nile tributary, Nile Delta, Egypt. Parasitological Research 103, 1197–1205.

Abdelkhalek, N., El-Adl, M., Salama, M., Al-Araby, M., 2017. Mass mortalities associated with isopoda infestation as a result of uncontrolled biosecurity measures in Lake Qarun, Egypt. Book of Abstracts, World Aquaculture 2017, Cape Town, RSA.

Abou El-Gheit, E.N., 2005. *Streptococcus* infections among farmed and wild tilapia fish in Egypt. Egyptian Journal of Experimental Biology (Zoology) 1, 1–7.

Abuseliana, A.F., Daud, H.M., Aziz, S.A., Bejo, S.K., Alsaid, M., 2011. Pathogenicity of *Streptococcus agalactiae* isolated from a fish farm in Selangor to juvenile red tilapia (*Oreochromis* sp.). Journal of Animal and Veterinary Advances 10, 914–919.

Adeyemo, A.O., Agbede, S.A., 2008. Histopathology of Tilapia tissues harbouring *Clinostomum tilapiae* parasites. African Journal of Biomedical Research 11, 115–118.

Aguirre-Fey, D., Benítez-Villa, G.E., De León, G.P., Rubio-Godoy, M., 2015. Population dynamics of *Cichlidogyrus* spp. and *Scutogyrus* sp. (Monogenea) infecting farmed tilapia in Veracruz, México. Aquaculture 443, 11–15.

Akinrotimi, O.A., Ansa, E.J., Owhonda, K.N., Onunkwo, D.N., Edun, O.M., Anyanwu, P.E., et al., 2007. Effects of transportation stress on haematological parameters of blackchin tilapia *Sarotherodon melanotheron*. Journal of Animal and Veterinary Advances 6, 841–845.

Akoll, P., Konecny, R., Mwanja, W.W., Nattabi, J.K., Agoe, C., Schiemer, F., 2012a. Parasite fauna of farmed Nile tilapia (*Oreochromis niloticus*) and African catfish (*Clarias gariepinus*) in Uganda. Parsitological Research 110, 315–323.

Akoll, P., Konecny, R., Mwanja, W.W., Schiemer, F., 2012b. Risk assessment of parasitic helminths on cultured Nile tilapia (*Oreochromis niloticus*, L.). Aquaculture 356–357, 123–127.

Al-Harbi, A.H., 1994. First isolation of *Streptococcus* sp. from hybrid tilapia (*Oreochromis niloticus* x *O. aureus*) in Saudi Arabia. Aquaculture 128, 195–201.

Al-Harbi, A.H., Naim Uddin, M., 2004. Seasonal variations in the intestinal bacterial flora of hybrid tilapia (*Oreochromis niloticus* x *Oreochromis aureus*) cultured in earthen ponds in Saudi Arabia. Aquaculture 229, 37–44.

Ali, N.G., Aboyadak, I.M., 2018. Histopathological alterations and condition factor deterioration accompanied by isopod infestation in *Tilapia zilli, Mugil capito* and *Solea aegyptiaca* from Lake Qaroun. Egyptian Journal of Aquatic Research 44, 57–63.

Aloo, P., Okelo, R.O., Ntiba, M.J., 1995. Helminth parasites of *Oreochromis leucostictus* (Trewavas) in Lake Naivasha, Kenya. Pan African Fisheries Congress on Sustainable Development of Fisheries in Africa, FSA, Nairobi, Kenya, 31 July–4 August, Abstract No. 172.

Aly, S.M., 2013. A Review of Fish Diseases in the Egyptian Aquaculture Sector. Working Report. WorldFish, 25 pp.

Aly, S.M., Albutti, A.S., Rahmani, A.H., Abdel Atti, N.M., 2015. The response of New-season Nile tilapia to *Aeromonas hydrophila* vaccine. International Journal of Clinical and Experimental Medicine 8, 4508–4514.

AlYahya, S.A., Ameen, F., Al-Niaeem, K.S., Al-Sa'adi, B.A., Hadi, S., Mostafa, A.A., 2018. Histopathological studies of experimental *Aeromonas hydrophila* infection in blue tilapia, *Oreochromis aureus*. Saudi Journal of Biological Sciences 25, 182–185.

Amal, A.M.N., Zamri-Saad, M., Siti-Zahrah, A., Nur-Nazifah, M., Nurazlan, W., Shahidan, H., 2008. Bacterial isolation pattern from tilapia infected with *Streptococcus agalactiae. Proceedings of the 1st International Congress of Aquatic Animal Health Management and Diseases. Tehran, Iran Veterinary Organization.* https://www.civilica.com/Paper -ICAAHMD01-ICAAHMD01_211.html.

Amal, M.N.A., Koh, C.B., Nurliyana, M., Suhaiba, M., Nor-Amalina, Z., Santha, S., et al., 2018. A case of natural co-infection of Tilapia Lake Virus and *Aeromonas veronii* in a Malaysian red hybrid tilapia (*Oreochromis niloticus* × *O. mossambicus*) farm experiencing high mortality. Aquaculture 485, 12–16.

Amin, N.E., Abdallah, I.S., Faisal, M., Easa, E.M., Alaway, T., Alyan, S.A., 1988. *Columnaris* infection among cultured Nile tilapia *Oreochromis niloticus*. Antonie van Leeuwenhoek 54, 509–520.

Ariel, E., Owens, L., 1997. Epizootic mortalities in tilapia *Oreochromis mossambicus*. Diseases of Aquatic Organisms 29, 1–6.

Armstrong, R.D., Ferguson, H.W., 1989. Systematic viral disease of the chromide cichlid *Etroplus maculatus*. Diseases of Aquatic Organisms 7, 155–157.

Arrumm, A., 1987. Effects of parasite Contracaecum on tilapia (*Oreochromis niloticus*). Annual Report: Kenya Marine Fisheries Research Institute 1986/1987, 21 pp.

Atyah, M.A., Zamri-Saad, M., Siti-Zahrah, A., 2010. First report of methicillin-resistant *Staphylococcus aureus* from cage-cultured tilapia (*Oreochromis niloticus*). Veterenary Microbiology 144, 502–504.

Avtalion, R.R., Shlapobersky, M., 1994. A whirling viral disease of tilapia larvae. Israeli Journal of Aquaculture Bamidgeh 46, 102–104.

Azad, I.S., Rajendran, K.V., Rajan, J.J.S., Vijayan, K.K., Santiago, T.C., 2001. Virulence and histopathology of *Aeromonas hydrophila* (Sah 93) in experimentally infected tilapia, *Oreochromis mossambicus* (L.). Journal of Aquaculture in the Tropics 16, 265–275.

Bacharach, E., Mishra, N., Briese, T., Zody, M.C., Tsofack, J.E.K., Zamostiano, R., et al., 2016. Characterization of a novel orthomyxo-like virus causing mass die-offs of tilapia. mBio 7 e00431–16.

Bacolod, E.T., Uno, S., Villamor, S.S., Koyama, J., 2017. Oxidative stress and genotoxicity biomarker responses in tilapia (*Oreochromis niloticus*) exposed to environmental concentration of 1-nitropyrene. Marine Pollution Bulletin 124, 786–791.

Balfry, S.K., Shariff, M., Iwama, G.K., 1997. Strain differences in non-specific immunity of tilapia (*Oreochromis niloticus*) following challenge with *Vibrio parahaemolyticus*. Diseases of Aquatic Organisms 30, 77–80.

Barbieri, E., Ferreira, L.A.A., 2011. Effects of the organophosphate pesticide Folidol 600® on the freshwater fish, Nile tilapia (*Oreochromis niloticus*). Pesticide Biochemistry and Physiology 99, 209–214.

Barcellos, L.J.G., Nicolaiewsky, S., de Souza, S.M.G., Lulhier, F., 1999a. Plasmatic levels of cortisol in the response to acute stress in Nile tilapia, *Oreochromis niloticus* (L.), previously exposed to chronic stress. Aquaculture Research 30, 437–444.

Barcellos, L.J.G., Nicolaiewsky, S., de Souza, S.M.G., Lulhier, F., 1999b. The effects of stocking density and social interaction on acute stress response in Nile tilapia (*Oreochromis niloticus*) fingerlings. Aquaculture Research 30, 887–892.

Behera, B.K., Pradhan, P.K., Swaminathan, T.R., Sood, N., Paria, P., Das, A., et al., 2018. Emergence of tilapia lake virus associated with mortalities of farmed Nile tilapia *Oreochromis niloticus* (Linnaeus 1758) in India. Aquaculture 484, 168–174.

Bello-Olusoji, O.A., Aderiye, B.K., Borede, A.A., Oyekanmi, F.B., 2000. Ectoparasitic studies of pond cultured and wild tilapia in major cocoa producing area of Nigeria. In: Fitzsimmons, K., Filho, J.C. (Eds.), Tilapia Culture in the 21st Century. Proceedings from the Fifth International Symposium on Tilapia Aquaculture. American Tilapia Association and ICLARM, Rio de Janeiro, Brazil, pp. 496–498.

Berridge, B.R., Gonzalez, M., Frelier, P.F., 1998. Outbreak of *S. difficile* in hybrid tilapia (*Oreochromis aura X O. nilotica*) persistently infected with *S. iniae*. In: Book of Abstracts – Aquaculture '98. World Aquaculture Society, Baton Rouge, Louisiana, USA, pp. 186–187.

Bigarré, L., Cabon, J., Baud, M., Heimann, M., Body, A., Lieffrig, F., Castric, J., 2009. Outbreak of betanodavirus infection in tilapia, *Oreochromis niloticus* (L.), in fresh water. Journal of Fish Diseases 32, 667–673.

Bondad-Reantaso, M.G., Arthur, J.R., 1989. Trichodinids (Protozoa: Ciliophora: Peritrichida) of Nile tilapia (*Oreochromis niloticus*) in the Philippines. Asian Fisheries Science 3, 27–44.

Bowser, P.R., Wooster, G.A., Getchell, R.G., Timmons, M.B., 1998. *Streptococcus iniae* infection of tilapia *Oreochromis niloticus* in a recirculation production facility. Journal of the World Aquaculture Society 29, 335–339.

Brock, J.A., LeaMaster, B.R., Lee, C.-S., 1993. An overview of pathogens and diseases in marine finfish hatcheries in Hawaii with comments on strategies for health management and disease prevention. In: Lee, C.-S., Su, M.S., Liao, I.C. (Eds.), Proceedings of Finfish Hatchery in Asia '91. Tungkang Marine Laboratory, TFRI, Keelung, Taiwan, pp. 221–238.

Bunch, E.C., Bejerano, I., 1997. The effect of environmental factors on the susceptibility of hybrid tilapia, *Oreochromis niloticus* x *Oreochromis aureus*, to *streptococcosis*. Israeli Journal of Aquaculture Bamidgeh 49, 67–76.

Cai, W.-Q., Sun, P.F., 1994. Within species variation of resistance of common carp in the case of outbreak fish disease. Journal of Fisheries of China 18, 290–301.

Cai, W.-Q., Sun, P.F., 1995. Among species variation of resistance of grass carp, bighead carp and silver carp to the case of outbreak fish disease. Journal of Fishery Sciences of China 2, 71–75.

Cai, W.-Q., Li, S.-f., Ma, J-y., 2004. Disease resistance of Nile tilapia (*Oreochromis niloticus*), blue tilapia (*Oreochromis aureus*) and their hybrid (female Nile tilapia x male blue tilapia) to *Aeromonas sobria*. Aquaculture 229, 79–87.

CGIAR Research Program on Fish Agri-food Systems, 2017. Tilapia Lake Virus (TiLV): What to Know and Do? Factsheet: FISH-2017-03. https://fish.cgiar.org/publications/tilapia-lake-virus-tilv-what-know-and-do.

Chang, P.H., Plumb, J.A., 1996a. Effects of salinity on *Streptococcus* infection of Nile tilapia, *Oreochromis niloticus*. Journal of Applied Aquaculture 6, 39–46.

Chang, P.H., Plumb, J.A., 1996b. Histopathology of experimental *Streptococcus* sp. infection in tilapia, *Oreochromis niloticus* (L.) and Channel catfish *Ictalurus punctatus* (Rafinesque). Journal of Fish Diseases 19, 235–241.

Chen, S.-C., Yoshida, T., Adams, A., Thompson, K.D., Richards, R.H., 1998. Non-specific immune response of Nile tilapia, *Oreochromis nilotica*, to the extracellular products of *Mycobacterium* spp. and to various adjuvants. Journal of Fish Diseases 21, 39–46.

Chen, C.-Y., Chao, C.-B., Bowser, P.R., 2006. Infection of tilapia *Oreochromis* sp. by *Vibrio vulnificus* in freshwater and low-salinity environments. Journal of the World Aquaculture Society 37, 82–88.

Chen, M., Li, L.-P., Wang, R., Liang, W.-W., Huang, Y., Li, J., et al., 2012. PCR detection and PFGE genotype analyses of streptococcal clinical isolates from tilapia in China. Veterinary Microbiology 159, 526–530.

Chinabut, S., 2002. A case study of isopod infestation in tilapia cage culture in Thailand. In: Arthur, J.R., Phillips, M.J., Subasinghe, R.P., Reantaso, M.B., MacRae, I.H. (Eds.), Primary Aquatic Animal Health Care in Rural, Small-Scale, Aquaculture Development. FAO Fisheries Technical Paper No. 406. FAO, Rome, pp. 201–202.

Chun, S.-K., Sohn, S.-G., 1985. Characteristics of *Flexibacter columnaris* isolated from tilapia (*Tilapia* sp.). Bulletin of the Korean FIsheries Society 18, 369–373.

Constantino Casas, F., Armijo Ortiz, A., Osorio Sarabia, D., Chavez Soriano, L.A., 1997. Clinical and pathological descriptions of an infection due to *Aeromonas hydrophila* and *Ichthyophthirius multifiliis* in rainbow trout (*Oncorhynchus mykiss*, Walbaum) and tilapia (*Oreochromis aureus*, L). Veterinaria México 28, 59–62.

Coulibaly, N.D., Salembere, S., 1998. La biocenose terrestre des zones humids et ses incidences sur l'infestion des Poissons Cichlides du lac de Kompienga *Clinostomum* sp (Trematode: Clinostomatidae). In: Coetzee, L., Kulongowski, C. (Eds.), African Fisheries Diversity and Utilization. Paradi Association and the Fisheries Society of Africa. FISA/Paradi, Grahamstown, South Africa, p. 352.

Crosby, D., 2001. Fish Health Issues and Problems in Virginia's Aquaculture industry. In: Book of Abstracts – Aquaculture 2001. World Aquaculture Society, Baton Rouge, Louisiana, USA, p. 145.

Dambo, W.B., Rana, K.J., 1992. Effects of stocking density on growth and survival of Nile tilapia *Oreochromis niloticus* (L.) fry in the hatchery. Aquaculture and Fisheries Management 23, 71–80.

Darwish, A.M., Griffin, B.R., 2002. Study shows Oxytetracycline controls *Streptococcus* in tilapia. Global Aquaculture Advocate 5 (6), 34–35.

de la Cruz, C.P.P., Bandal Jr., M.Z., Avila, A.R.B., Paller, V.G.V., 2013. Distribution pattern of *Acanthogyrus* sp. (Acanthocephala: Quadrigyridae) in nile tilapia (*Oreochromis niloticus* L.) from Sampaloc Lake, Philippines. Journal of Nature Studies 12, 11–17.

de Ocampo, A.A., Camberos, L.O., 1998. Histopatologica de la respuesta de la tilapia (*Oreochromis* sp) a una infeccion mixta por myxosporidios. Estudio en un caso natural. Veterinaria México 29, 213–216.

Del-Pozo, J., Mishra, N., Kabuusu, R., Cheetham, S., Eldar, A., Bacharach, E., et al., 2017. Syncytial hepatitis of tilapia (*Oreochromis niloticus* L.) is associated with orthomyxovirus-like virions in hepatocytes. Veterinary Pathology 54, 164–170.

Dong, H.T., Nguyen, V.V., Le, H.D., Sangsuriya, P., Jitrakorn, S., Saksmerprome, V., et al., 2015. Naturally concurrent infections of bacterial and viral pathogens in disease outbreaks in cultured Nile tilapia (*Oreochromis niloticus*) farms. Aquaculture 448, 427–435.

Dong, H.T., Techatanakitarnan, C., Jindakittikul, P., Thaiprayoon, A., Taengphu, S., Charoensapsri, W., et al., 2017a. *Aeromonas jandaei* and *Aeromonas veronii* caused disease and mortality in Nile tilapia, *Oreochromis niloticus* (L.). Journal of Fish Diseases 40, 1395–1403.

Dong, H.T., Siriroob, S., Meemetta, W., Santimanawong, W., Gangnonngiw, W., Pirarat, N., et al., 2017b. Emergence of tilapia lake virus in Thailand and an alternative semi-nested RT-PCR for detection. Aquaculture 476, 111–118.

Dong, H.T., Ataguba, G.A., Khunrae, P., Rattanarojpong, T., Senapin, S., 2017c. Evidence of TiLV infection in tilapia hatcheries from 2012 to 2017 reveals probable global spread of the disease. Aquaculture 479, 579–583.

Doueellou, L., Erlwanger, K.H., 1994. Crustacean parasites of fishes in Lake Kariba, Zimbabwe, preliminary results. Hydrobiologia 287, 233–242.

Eissa, A.E., Moustafa, M., Abdelaziz, M., Ezzeldeen, N.A., 2008. *Yersinia ruckeri* infection in cultured Nile tilapia, *Oreochromis niloticus*, at a semi-intensive fish farm in lower Egypt. African Journal of Aquatic Science 33, 283–286.

Eissa, N.M.E., Abou El-Ghiet, E.N., Shaheen, A.A., Abbass, A., 2010. Characterization of *Pseudomonas* species isolated from tilapia "*Oreochromis niloticus*" in Qaroun and Wadi-El-Rayan lakes, Egypt. Global Veterinaria 5, 116–121.

Eissa, I.A.M., El-lamei, M., Sherif, M., Desuky, E., Zaki, M., Bakry, M., 2015. *Aeromonas veronii biovar sobria* a causative agent of mass mortalities in cultured Nile tilapia in El-Sharkia governorate, Egypt. Life Science Journal 12, 90–97.

El-Bouhy, Z.M., Shaheen, A.A., Hassanin, M.E., Mahboub, H.H., 2014. Branchiomyosis in Nile tilapia (*Oreochromis niloticus)* in Behiera governorate with trials for treatment. Zagazig Veterenary Journal 42, 29–42.

El-Dien, A.H., Abdel-Gaber, R.A., 2009. *Ichthyophthirius multifiliis* infection induces apoptosis in different species of tilapia. Journal of the Egyptian Society of Parasitology 39, 665–678.

El-Gayar, K., Aly, S.M., 2013. Studies on some protozoan parasites and encysted metacercarial infection of freshwater fishes in Egypt. Egyptian Veterinary Medical Society of Parasitology Journal (EVMSPJ) 9, 31–43.

El-Gohary, M.S.A., 2004. Effects Of Some Organophosphorus Compounds on Some Cultured Freshwater Fishes. PhD Thesis. Alexandria University, Alexandria, Egypt.

El-Khateib, T., Afifi, S.H., 1993. Inspection of (*Tilapia nilotica*) Nile fish exposed to organophosphorus compound (Diazinon). Assut Veterinary Medical Journal 29, 119–124.

El-Mansy, A., Hamada, S., Hasan, S., El-Sarnagawy, D., 2011. Histopathology of farmed freshwater fish infested with different helminthes. Egyptian Journal of Aquatic Biology and Fisheries 15, 1110–1131.

El-Sayed, A.-F.M., 2002. Effects of stocking density and feeding levels on growth and feed efficiency of Nile tilapia, *Oreochromis niloticus* (L.) fry. Aquaculture Research 33, 621–626.

El-Sayed Ali, T., Abdel-Aziz, S.H., El-Sayed, A.-F.M., Zeid, S., 2014a. Structural and functional effects of early exposure to 4-nonylphenol on gonadal development of Nile tilapia (*Oreochromis niloticus*): a-histological alterations in ovaries. Fish Physiology and Biochemistry 40, 1495–1507.

El-Sayed Ali, T., Abdel-Aziz, S.H., El-Sayed, A.-F.M., Zeid, S., 2014b. Structural and functional effects of early exposure to 4-nonylphenol on gonadal development of Nile tilapia (*Oreochromis niloticus*): b-histological alterations in testes. Fish Physiology and Biochemistry 40, 1509–1519.

El-Sayed Ali, T., Abdel-Aziz, S.H., El-Sayed, A.-F.M., Zeid, S., 2017. Effects of nonylphenol on plasma steroids, vitellogenin synthesis and sex reversal in Nile tilapia (*Oreochromis niloticus*) fingerlings. Indian Journal of Geo Marine Sciences 46, 521–528.

El-Sayed, Y.S., Samak, D.H., Abou-Ghanema, I.Y., Soliman, M.K., 2015. Physiological and oxidative stress biomarkers in the freshwater monosex Nile tilapia, *Oreochromis niloticus* L., exposed to Pendimethalin-based herbicide. Environmental Toxicology 30, 430–438.

El-Sharouny, H.M., Badran, R.A.M., 1995. Experimental transmission and pathogenicity of some zoosporic fungi to tilapia fish. Mycopathologia 132, 95–103.

El-Tantawy, S.A.M., Kazaubski, S.L., 1986. The trichodinid ciliates from fish, *Tilapia nilotica* from the Nile Delta (Egypt). Acta Protozoologica 25, 439–444.

Endo, M., Kumahara, C., Yoshida, T., Tabata, M., 2002. Reduced stress and increased immune responses in Nile tilapia kept under self-feeding conditions. Fisheries Science 68, 253–257.

Evans, J.J., Shoemaker, C.A., Klesius, P.H., 2000. Experimental *Streptococcus iniae* infection of hybrid striped bass (*Morone chrysops* x *Morone saxatilis*) and tilapia (*Oreochromis niloticus*) by nares inoculation. Aquaculture 189, 197–210.

Evans, J.J., Klesius, P.H., Shoemaker, C.A., 2006a. An overview of *Streptococcus* in warmwater fish. Aquaculture Health International 7, 10–14.

Evans, J.J., Pasnik, D.J., Brill, G.C., Klesius, P.H., 2006b. Un-ionized ammonia exposure in Nile tilapia: toxicity, stress response, and susceptibility to *Streptococcus agalactiae*. North American Journal of Aquaculture 68, 23–33.

Everitt, S., Leung, C.-F.A., 1999. Fish disease in Hong Kong. Paper Presented at the Fourth Symposium on Diseases in Asian Aquaculture: Aquatic Animal Health for Sustainability. 22–26 November, Cebu City, Philippines.

Ewing, M.S., Kocan, K.M., 1992. Invasion and development strategies of *Ichthyophthirius multifiliis*, a parasitic ciliate of fish. Parasitology Today 8, 204–208.

Eyngor, M., Zamostiano, R., Kembou Tsofack, J.E., Berkowitz, A., Bercovier, H., Tinman, S., et al., 2014. Identification of a novel RNA virus lethal to tilapia. Journal of Clinical Microbiology 52, 4137–4146.

FAO (Food and Agriculture Organization of the United Nations), 2017. Outbreaks of Tilapia Lake Virus (TiLV) Threaten the Livelihoods and Food Security of Millions of People Dependent on Tilapia Farming. FAO/Global Information and Early Warning System (GIEWS). Special Alert No. 338. http://www.fao.org/3/a-i7326e.pdf.

Fathi, M., Dickson, C., Dickson, M., Leschen, W., Baily, J., Muir, F., et al., 2017. Identification of Tilapia Lake virus in Egypt in Nile tilapia affected by 'summer mortality' syndrome. Aquaculture 473, 430–432.

Ferguson, H.W., Kabuusu, R., Beltran, S., Reyes, E., Lince, J.A., Del Pozo, J., 2014. Syncytial hepatitis of farmed tilapia, *Oreochromis niloticus* (L.): a case report. Journal of Fish Diseases 37, 583–589.

Fernandez, J.B., Yambot, A.V., Almeria, O., 2014. Vaccination of Nile tilapia (*Oreochromis niloticus*) using lipopolysaccharide (lps) prepared from *Aeromonas hydrophila*. International Journal of Fauna and Biological Studies 1, 01–03.

Figueiredo, H.C.P., Nobrega Netto, L., Leal, C.A.G., Pereira, U.P., Mian, G.F., 2012. *Streptococcus iniae* outbreaks in Brazilian Nile tilapia (*Oreochromis niloticus* L.) farms. Brazilian Journal of Microbiology 43, 576–580.

Filho, C.I., Muller, E.E., Pretto-Giordano, L.G., Bracarense, A.F.R.L., 2009. Histological findings of experimental *Streptococcus agalactiae* infection in Nile tilapias (*Oreochromis niloticus*). Brazilian Journal of Veterinary Parasitology 2, 12–15.

Florio, D., Gustinelli, A., Caffara, M., Turci, F., Quaglio, F., Konecny, R., et al., 2009. Veterinary and public health aspects in tilapia (*Oreochromis niloticus niloticus*) aquaculture in Kenya, Uganda and Ethiopia. Ittiopatologia 6, 51–93.

Foo, J.T.W., Lam, T.J., 1993. Serum cortisolresponse to handling stress and the effect ofcortisol implantation on testosterone level in thetilapia, *Oreochromis mossambicus*. Aquaculture 115, 145–158.

Fouz, B., Alcaide, E., Barrera, R., Amaro, C., 2002. Susceptibility of Nile tilapia (*Oreochromis niloticus*) to vibriosis due to *Vibrio vulnificus* biotype 2 (Serovar E). Aquaculture 212, 21–30.

FRRC (Fisheries Resources Research Centre at Qatif), 2001. The most common diseases in fish farms and some marine fishes in the eastern region, Saudi Arabia. Ministry of Agriculture and Waters, Extension News Bulletin No. 225/226, Qatif, 15 pp, (in Arabic).

Fryer, G., Iles, T.D., 1972. The Cichlid Fishes of the Great Lakes of Africa: Their Biology and Evolution. T.F.H. Publishing, Neptue City, New Jersy. Also published by Oliver and Boyd, Edinburgh.

Gallage, S., Katagiri, T., Endo, M., Futami, K., Endo, M., Maita, M., 2016. Influence of moderate hypoxia on vaccine efficacy against *Vibrio anguillarum* in *Oreochromis niloticus* (Nile tilapia). Fish & Shellfish Immunology 51, 271–281.

Garcia, C.L., Clavijo, A.M., Santander, J., 1999. Incidence of *aeromonas* spp. in some cultured fish species in the states of Aragua, Carabobo, Monagas and Cojedes in Venezuela. In: Cabrera, T., Jory, D., Silva, M. (Eds.), Aquaculture 99. Congreso sur American de Acuicultura, World Aquaculture Society/Latin American Chapter, Puerto la Cruz, Venezuela, pp. 218–222.

Garcia-Vasquez, A., Hansen, H., Shinn, A.P., 2007. A revised description of *Gyrodactylus cichlidarum* Paperna, 1968 (Gyrodactylidae) from the Nile tilapia, *Oreochromis niloticus niloticus* (Cichlidae), and its synonymy with *G. niloticus* Cone, Arthur et Bondad- Reantaso, 1995. Folia Parasitologica 54, 129–140.

Gbankoto, A., Pampoulie, C., Marques, A., Sakiti, G.N., 2001. Occurrence of myxosporean parasites in the gills of two tilapia species from Lake Nokoué (Bénin, West Africa): effect of host size and sex, and seasonal patterns of infection. Diseases of Aquatic Organisms 44, 217–222.

Getchell, R., 1998. *S. iniae* causes tilapia infection. Fish Farming News 6, 16.

Girón-Pérez, M.I., Montes-López, M., García-Ramírez, L.A., Romero-Bañuelos, C.A., Robledo-Marenco, M.L., 2008. Effect of sub-lethal concentrations of endosulfan on phagocytic and hematological parameters in Nile tilapia (*Oreochromis niloticus*). Bulletin of Environmental Contamination and Toxicology 80, 266–269.

Girón-Pérez, M.I., Velázquez-Fernández, J., Díaz-Resendiz, K., Díaz-Salas, F., Canto-Montero, C., Medina-Díaz, I., et al., 2009. Immunologic parameters evaluations in Nile tilapia (*Oreochromis niloticus*) exposed to sublethal concentrations of diazinon. Fish & Shellfish Immunology 27, 383–385.

Grabowski, L.D., LaPatra, S.E., Cain, K.D., 2004. Systemic and mucosal antibody response in tilapia, *Oreochromis niloticus* (L.), following immunization with *Flavobacterium columnare*. Journal of Fish Diseases 27, 573–581.

Guimarães, I.G., Lim, C., Yildirim-Aksoy, M., Li, M.H., Klesius, P.H., 2014. Effects of dietary levels of vitamin A on growth, hematology, immune response and resistance of Nile tilapia (*Oreochromis niloticus*) to *Streptococcus iniae*. Animal Feed Science and Technology 188, 126–136.

Hamid, S.H.A., Babiker, E.M., 2011. Prevalence of trypanosome infection in *Oreochromis niloticus* and *Clarias lazera* from fish farms and reservoir of Jebel Aulia Dam in Sudan. World's Veterinary Journal 1, 14–16.

Hart, L.J., Smith, S.A., Smith, B.J., Robertson, J., Besteman, E.G., Holladay, S.D., 1998. Subaccute immunotoxic effects of the polycyclic aromatic hydrocarbon (PAH), 7,12-dimethylbenzanthracene (DMBA) on spleen and pronephros leukocytic cell counts and phagocytic cell activity in tilapia *Oreochromis niloticus*. Aquatic Toxicology 41, 17–29.

Hedrick, R.P., Fryer, J.L., Chen, S.N., Kou, G.H., 1983. Characteristics of four birnaviruses isolated from fish in Taiwan. Fish Pathology 18, 91–97.

Hernández, E., Figueroa, J., Iregui, C., 2009. Streptococcosis on a red tilapia, *Oreochromis* sp., farm: a case study. Journal of Fish Diseases 32, 247–252.

Hoffman, G.L., Meyer, F.P., 1974. Parasites of Freshwater Fishes, 224 pp. T.F.H. Publications, Inc. Ltd, Neptune City, New Jersy, USA. https://enaca.org/?id=870&title=urgent-update-on-possible-worldwide-spread-of-tilapia-lake-virus-tilv.

Huang, S.-L., Chen, W.C., Shei, M.C., Liao, I.C., Chen, S.N., 1999. Studies on epizootiology and pathogenicity of *Staphylococcus epidermidis* in tilapia (*Oreochromis* spp.) cultured in Taiwan. Zoological Studies 38, 178–188.

Huang, S.-L., Liao, I.-C., Chen, S.-N., 2000. Induction of apoptosis in tilapia, *Oreochromis aureus* Steindachner, and in TO-2 cells by *Staphylococcus epidermidis*. Journal of Fish Diseases 23, 363–368.

Iregui, C.A., Guarin, M., Tibata, V.M., Ferguson, H.W., 2012. Novel brain lesions caused by *Edwardsiella tarda* in a red tilapia (*Oreochromis* spp.). Journal of Veterinary Diagnostic Investigation 24, 446–449.

Ismail, H.T., Mahboub, H.H., 2016. Effect of acute exposure to nonylphenol on biochemical, hormonal, and hematological parameters and muscle tissues residues of Nile tilapia; *Oreochromis niloticus*. Veterenary World 9, 616–625.

Jansen, M.D., Mohan, C.V., 2017. Tilapia lake virus (TiLV): literature review. Working Paper: FISH-2017-04. CGIAR Research Program on Fish Agri-Food Systems, Penang, Malaysia.

Jantrakajorn, S., Maisak, H., Wongtavatchai, J., 2014. Comprehensive investigation of Streptococcosis outbreaks in cultured Nile tilapia, *Oreochromis niloticus*, and red tilapia, *Oreochromis* sp., of Thailand. Journal of the World Aquaculture Society 45, 392–402.

Jesus, R.B., Gallani, S.U., Valladão, G.M.R., Pala, G., da Silva, T.F.A., da Costa, J.C., et al., 2018. Trypanosomiasis causing mortality outbreak in Nile tilapia intensive farming: identification and pathological evaluation. Aquaculture 491, 169–176.

Jiraungkoorskul, W., Upatham, E.S., Kruatrachue, M., Sahaphong, S., Vichasri-Grams, S., Pokethitiyook, P., 2003. Biochemical and histopathological effects of glyphosate herbicide on Nile tilapia (*Oreochromis niloticus*). Environmental Toxicology 18, 260–267.

Jirawong, P., 2000. Toxicity of Copper Sulfate to Fishes, Phytoplankton, and Bacteria, Aeromonas Hydrophila. MSc Thesis. Kasetsart University, Bangkok, Thailand.

Kayansamruaj, P., Pirarat, N., Hirono, I., Rodkhum, C., 2014. Increasing of temperature induces pathogenicity of *Streptococcus agalactiae* and the up-regulation of inflammatory related genes in infected Nile tilapia (*Oreochromis niloticus*). Veteranary Microbiology 172, 265–271.

Ke, X., Lu, M., Ye, X., Gao, F., Zhu, H., Huang, Z., 2012. Recovery and pathogenicity analysis of *Aerococcus viridans* isolated from tilapia (*Orecohromis niloticus*) cultured in southwest of China. Aquaculture 342–343, 18–23.

Keawcharoen, J., Techangamsuwan, S., Ponpornpisit, A., Lombardini, E.D., Patchimasiri, T., Pirarat, N., 2015. Genetic characterization of a betanodavirus isolated from a clinical disease outbreak in farm-raised tilapia *Oreochromis niloticus* (L.) in Thailand. Journal of Fish Diseases 38, 49–54.

Kebus, M.J., Collins, M.T., Brownfield, M.S., Amundson, C.H., Kayes, T.B., Malison, J.A., 1992. Effects of rearing density on stress response and growth of rainbow trout. Journal of Aquatic Animal Health 4, 1–6.

Khalil, R.H., 1998. Effect of Bayluscide® on Some Cultured Freshwater Fish (*Oreochromis niloticus*). PhD Thesis. Alexandria University, Egypt.

Khalil, R.H., Saad, T.T., Abo Selema, T.A.M., Abdel-Latif, H.M.R., 2015. *Branchiomyces Demigrans* infection in farm-reared common carp (*Cyprinus Carpio L.*) and Nile tilapia (*Oreochromis Niloticus*) at different localities in Egypt, with special emphasis to the role of environmental stress factors. International Journal of Innovative Studies in Aquatic Biology and Fisheries 1, 15–23.

Klesius, P.H., Shoemaker, C.A., Evans, J.J., 2000. Efficacy of single and combined *Streptococcus iniae* isolate vaccine administered by intraperitoneal and intramuscular routes in tilapia (*Oreochromis niloticus*). Aquaculture 188, 237–246.

Klesius, P.H., Shoemaker, C.A., Evans, J.J., 2001. Efficacy of *Streptococcus Iniae* Vaccine Administered in Nile tilapia *Oreochromis niloticus*. *Sixth Asian Fisheries Forum*. Book of Abstracts. Asian Fisheries Society, Quezon City, Philippines, p. 130.

Klesius, P.H., Shoemaker, C.A., Evans, J.J., 2008. Streptococcus: a worldwide fish health problem. In: Elghobashy, H., Fitzsimmons, K., Diab, A. (Eds.), The 8th International Symposium on Tilapia in Aquaculture. Cairo, Egypt. Central Laboratory for Aquaculture Research, Abbasa, pp. 83–107.

Kpundeh, M.D., Xu, P., Yang, Y., Qiang, J., He, J., 2013. Stocking densities and chronic zero culture water exchange stress effects on biological performances, hematological and serum biochemical indices of GIFT tilapia juveniles (*Oreochromis niloticus*). Journal of Aquaculture Research & Development 4, 189. https://doi.org/10.4172/2155- 9546.1000189.

Kumar, N., Antony Jesu Prabhu, P., Pal, A.K., Remya, S., Aklakur, M., Rana, R.S., et al., 2011. Anti-oxidative and immuno-hematological status of Tilapia (*Oreochromis mossambicus*) during acute toxicity test of endosulfan. Pesticide Biochemistry and Physiology 99, 45–52.

Kuperman, B.I., Matey, V.E., 1999. Massive infestation by *Amyloodinium ocellatum* (Dinoflagellida) of fish in a highly saline lake, Salton Sea, California, USA. Diseases of Aquatic Organisms 39, 65–73.

Kuperman, B.I., Matey, V.E., Barlow, S.B., 2002. Flagellate *Cryptobia branchialis* (Bodonida: Kinetoplastida), ectoparasite of tilapia from the Salton Sea. Hydrobiologia 473, 93–102.

Kwon, S.R., Nam, Y.K., Kim, S.K., Kim, K.H., 2006. Protection of tilapia (*Oreochromis mosambicus*) from edwardsiellosis by vaccination with *Edwardsiella tarda* ghosts. Fish & Shellfish Immunology 20, 621–626.

Lalitha, K.V., Gopakumar, K., 2001. Sensitivity of Tilapia (*Oreochromis mossambicus*) to *Clostridium botulinum* toxins. Aquaculture Research 32, 761–764.

Lara-Flores, M., Aguirre-Guzman, G., Balan-Zetina, S.B., Sonda-Santos, K.Y., Zapata, A.A., 2014. Identification of *Mycobacterium* agent isolated from tissues of Nile tilapia (*Oreochromis niloticus*). Turkish Journal of Fisheries and Aquatic Sciences 14, 575–580.

Lautenslager, G.T., 1986. Cichlid Infectious Agent Virus: A Characterization of a New Rhabdovirus of Cichlid Fish. PhD Thesis. Lehigh University, Bethlehem, Pennsylvania.

le Roux, L.E., Avenant-Oldewage, A., 2010. Checklist of the fish parasitic genus *Cichlidogyrus* (Monogenea), including its cosmopolitan distribution and host species. African Journal of Aquatic Science 35, 21–36.

Li, Y., Cai, S.H., 2011. Identification and pathogenicity of *Aeromonas sobria* on tail-rot disease in juvenile tilapia *Oreochromis niloticus*. Current Microbiology 62, 623–627.

Li, K., Clausen, J.H., Murrell, K.D., Liu, L., Dalsgaard, A., 2013. Risks for fishborne zoonotic trematodes in tilapia production systems in Guangdong province, China. Veterinary Parasitology 198, 223–229.

Li, Y.W., Liu, L., Huang, P.R., Fang, W., Luo, Z.P., Peng, H.L., et al., 2014. Chronic streptococcosis in Nile tilapia, *Oreochromis niloticus* (L.), caused by *Streptococcus agalactiae*. Journal of Fish Diseases 37, 757–763.

Lightner, D., Redman, R., Mohney, L., Dickenson, G., Fitzsimmons, K., 1988. Major diseases encountered in controlled environment culture of tilapias in fresh- and brackishwater over a three-year period in Arizona. In: Pullin, R.S.V., Bhukaswan, T., Tonguthai, K., Maclean, J.L. (Eds.), Proceedings of the Second International Symposium on Tilapia in Aquaculture. ICLARM Conference Proceeding No. 15. Department of Fisheries, Thailand, and ICLARM, Manila, Philippines, pp. 111–116.

Lim, C., Klesius, P.H., 2001. Influence of dietary levels of folic acid on growth response and resistance of Nile tilapia *Oreochromis niloticus* to *Streptococcus iniae*. In: Sixth Asian Fisheries Forum. Book of Abstracts. Asian Fisheries Society, Quezon City, Philippines, p. 150.

Lim, C., Leamaster, B., 1991. Thiamine requirements of red hybrid tilapia grown in seawater. Journal of the World Aquaculture Society 22, 36A.

Lim, C., Yildirim-Aksoy, M., Barros, M.M., Klesius, P., 2011. Thiamin requirement of nile tilapia, *Oreochromis niloticus*. Journal of the World Aquaculture Society 42, 824–833.

Lin, C.-L., Ho, J.-S., Chen, S.-N., 1996. Developmental stages of *Caligus epidemicus* Hewitt, a copepod parasite of tilapia culture in brackish water. Journal of Natural History 30, 661–684.

Lio-Po, G., Wakabayashi, H., 1986. Immuno-response in tilapia *Sarotherodon niloticus* with *Edwardsiella tarda* by hyperosmotic infiltration method. Veterinary Immunology and Immunopathology 12, 351–357.

Liu, C.I., Huang, J.L., Hung, H.H., Pen, C.F., 1990. The experimental infection of *Streptococcus* and/or *Aeromonas* to induce bacterial septicemia in cultured tilapia. Council of Agriculture Fisheries Series 24, 40–45.

Liu, X., Zhou, X., Mo, X., 1993. Characteristics on pathogen of caudal fin rot disease of tilapia (*Oreochromis niloticus*) in mariculture. Tropic Oceanography Redai Haiyang 12, 100–103.

Liu, G., Zhu, J., Chen, K., Gao, T., Yao, H., Liu, Y., et al., 2016. Development of *Streptococcus agalactiae* vaccines for tilapia. Diseases of Aquatic Organisms 122, 163–170.

Lu, S., Levin, R.E., 2010. *Shewanella* in a tilapia fish farm. Journal of FisheriesSciences.com 4, 159–170.

Lua, D.T., Te, B.Q., Thanh, N.V., 1999. A study on parasites in different stages of three strains of cultured Nile tilapia (*Oreochromis niloticus*): Thai strain, GIFT strain and Viet strain in North Vietnam. Paper Presented at the Fourth Symposium on Diseases in Asian Aquaculture: Aquatic Animal Health for Sustainability. November 22–26, Cebu City, Philippines.

Macintosh, D.J., De Silva, S.S., 1984. The influence of stocking density and food ration on fry survival and growth in *Oreochromis mossambicus* and *O. niloticus* x *O. aureus* male hybrids reared in a closed circulated system. Aquaculture 41, 345–358.

Madanire-Moyo, G.N., Luus-Powell, W.J., Olivier, P.A., 2012. Diversity of metazoan parasites of the Mozambique tilapia, *Oreochromis mossambicus* (Peters, 1852), as indicators of pollution in the Limpopo and Olifants River systems. Onderstepoort Journal of Veterinary Research 79 (1), E1–E9.

Mahmoud, N.E., Fahmy, M.M., Abuowarda, M., 2017. An investigation of cymothoid isopod invasion in Lake Qarun fishes with preliminary trial for biological control. International Journal of ChemTech Research 10, 409–416.

Makhiessen, P., Roberts, R.J., 1982. Histopathological change in the liver and brain of fish exposed to endosulfan insecticide during tsetse fly control operations in Botswana. Jornal of Fish Diseases 5, 153–159.

Manna, G.K., Sadhukhan, A., 1991. Genotoxic potential of the spores of three species of fungi experimented on cichlid fish, *Oreochromis mossambicus*. Kromosomo 2, 2129–2134.

Marzouk, M.S., Bakeer, A., 1991. Some investigations in Nile tilapia exposed to sublethal concentration of Bayluscide. Journal of Egyptian Veterinary Medicine Association 51, 97–107.

Mavuti, S.K., Waruiru, R.M., Mbuthia, P.G., Maina, J.G., Mbaria, J.M., Otieno, R.O., 2017. Prevalence of Ecto- and Endo-Parasitic Infections of Farmed tilapia and Catfish in Nyeri County, vol. 29. Livestock Research for Rural Development, Kenya (6). Article # 122. http://www.lrrd.org/lrrd29/6/stek29122.htm.

McGrogan, D.G., Ostland, V.E., Byrne, P.J., Ferguson, H.W., 1998. Systemic disease involving an iridovirus-like agent in cultured tilapia, *Oreochromis niloticus* L. – a case report. Journal of Fish Diseases 21, 149–152.

McNulty, S.T., Klesius, P.H., Shoemaker, C.A., 2003. Hematological changes in Nile tilapia (*Oreochromis niloticus*) infected with *Streptococcus iniae* by nare inoculation. Journal of the World Aquaculture Society 34, 418–422.

Mehrim, A.I.M., 2001. Effects of Some Chemical Pollutants on Growth Performance, Feed and Nutrient Utilization of Tilapia. MSc Thesis. Alexandria University, Egypt.

Mian, G.F., Godoy, D.T., Leal, C.A., Yuhara, T.Y., Costa, G.M., Figueiredo, H.C., 2009. Aspects of the natural history and virulence of *S. agalactiae* infection in Nile tilapia. Veterinary Microbiology 136, 180–183.

Miyashita, T., 1984. *Pseudomonas fluorescens* and *Edwardsiella tarda* isolated from diseased tilapia. Fish Pathology 19, 45–50.

Miyazaki, T., Kubota, S.S., Miyashita, T., 1984. A histopathological study of *Pseudomonas fluorescens* infection in tilapia. Fish Pathology 19, 161–166.

Mukhi, S.K., Chandrika, V., Madhavi, B., Nayak, B.B., 2001. Incidence of β-haemolyctic streptococcal infection associated with mass mortalities of cultured tilapia, *Oreochromis mossambicus* in brackishwater ponds in India. Journal of Aquaculture in the Tropics 16, 373–383.

Muratori, M.C.S., de Oliveira, A.L., Leite, R.C., Costa, A.P.R., da Silva, M.C.C., 2000. *Edwardsiella tarda* isolated in integrated fish farming. Aquaculture Research 31, 481–483.

Musa, N., Wei, L.S., Musa, N., Hamdan, R.H., Leong, L.K., Wee, W., et al., 2009. Streptococcosis in red hybrid tilapia (*Oreochromis niloticus*) commercial farms in Malaysia. Aquaculture Research 40, 630–632.

NACA (Network of Aquaculture Centres in Asia-Pacific), 2017. Urgent Update on Possible Wordlwide Spread of Tilapia Lake Virus.

Nafady, A., Shahata, A., Ibrahim, I.A., Shabaan, A.A., 1986. Clinical signs, post-mortem findings and histopathological changes in *Tilapia nilotica* fish intoxicated with Bayluscide. Assut Veterinary Medical Journal 17, 126–132.

Najiah, M., Aqilah, N.I., Lee, K.L., Khairulbariyyah, Z., Mithun, S., Jalal, K.C.A., et al., 2012. Massiva mortality associated with *Streptococcus agalactiae* infection in cage-cultured red hybrid tilapia *Oreochromis niloticus* in Como River, Kenyir Lake, Malaysia. Journal of Biological Sciences 12, 438–442.

Natividad, J.M., Bondad-Reantaso, M.G., Arthur, J.R., 1986. Parasites of Nile tilapia (*Oreochromis niloticus*) in the Philippines. In: Maclean, J.L., Dizon, L.B., Hosillos, L.V. (Eds.), Proceedings of the First Asian Fisheries Forum. Asian Fisheries Society, Manila, Philippines, pp. 255–259.

Netto, L.N., Leal, C.A., Figueiredo, H.C., 2011. *Streptococcus dysgalactiae* as an agent of septicaemia in Nile tilapia, *Oreochromis niloticus* (L.). Journal of Fish Diseases 34, 251–254.

Newaj-Fyzul, A., Mutani, A., Ramsubhag, A., Adesiyun, A., 2008. Prevalence of bacterial pathogens and their anti-microbial resistance in tilapia and their pond water in Trinidad. Zoonoses Public Health 55, 206–213.

Nguenga, D., 1988. A note on infestation of *Oreochromis niloticus* with *Trichodina* sp. and *Dactylogyrus* sp. In: Pullin, R.S.V., Bhukaswan, T., Tonguthai, K., Maclean, J.L. (Eds.), Proceedings of the Second International Symposium on Tilapia in Aquaculture. ICLARM Proceedings No. 15. Deaprtment of Fisheries, Thailand, and ICLARM, Manila, Philippines, pp. 117–119.

Nicholson, P., Fathi, M.A., Fischer, A., Mohan, C., Schieck, E., Mishra, N., et al., 2017. Detection of Tilapia Lake Virus in Egyptian fish farms experiencing high mortalities in 2015. Journal of Fish Diseases 40, 1925–1928.

Nol, P., Williamson, J.L., Rocke, T.E., Yuill, T.M., 2004. Detection of *Clostridium botulinum* type C cells in the gastrointestinal tracts of Mozambique tilapia (*Oreochromis mossambicus*) by Polymerase chain reaction. Journal of Wildlife Diseases 40, 749–753.

Nomoto, R., Munasinghe, L.I., Jin, D.-H., Shimahara, Y., Yasuda, H., Nakamura, A., et al., 2004. Lancefield group C *Streptococcus dysgalactiae* infection responsible for fish mortalities in Japan. Journal of Fish Diseases 27, 679–686.

Noor El-Deen, A.N., Osman, H.M., Zaki, M.S., Abo-State, H.A., 2018. Mass mortality in cultured Nile tilapia *Oreochromis niloticus* in Kafr El-Sheikh province, Egypt, due to Saprolegniosis with emphasis on treatment trials. Journal of Biological Sciences 18, 39–45.

Ochieng, V.O., Matolla, G.K., Khyria, S.K., 2012. A Study of *Clinostomum* affecting *Oreochromis niloticus* in small water bodies in Eldoret-Kenya. International Journal of Scientific Engineering and Research 3, 1–6.

Oda, S.S., Tohamy, H.G., Massoud, R.G., 2016. Pathological alterations in Nile tilapia experimentally infected with *Streptococcus iniae* and *Candida albicans*. Turkish Journal of Fisheries and Aquatic Sciences 16, 779–788.

Ogbonna, C.I.C., Alabi, R.O., 1991. Studies on species of fungi associated with mycotic infections of fish in a Nigerian freshwater fish pond. Hydrobiologia 220, 131–135.

OIE, 2017. Tilapia Lake Virus (TiLV)- A Novel Orthomyxo-like Virus. http://www.oie.int/fileadmin/Home/eng/Internationa_Standard_Setting/docs/pdf/A_TiLV_disease_card.pdf.

Okaeme, A.N., Okojie, P.U., 1989. Parasites and diseases of feral *Oreochromis niloticus*, *Sarotherodon galilaeus* and *Clarias* sp. of Lake

Kainja. Annual Report, National Institute of Freshwater Fisheries Research, New Bussa, Nigeria, pp. 41–44.

Okaeme, A.N., Olufemi, B.E., 1997. Fungi associated with tilapia (*Oreochromis niloticus*) culture ponds in Nigeria. Journal of Aquaculture in the Tropics 12, 267–274.

Okaeme, A.N., Obiekezie, A., Okojie, P.U., Agbontale, J.J., 1989. Histopathology of normal and infected organs of tilapia by *Myxobolus ovariae*. Annual Report, National Institute of Freshwater Fisheries Research, New Bussa, Nigeria, pp. 37–40.

Omoregie, E., Ufodike, E.B.C., Onwuliri, C.O.E., 1995. A comparative survey of helminth parasites of the Nile tilapia, *Oreochromis niloticus* from a fish farm and petroleum polluted freshwater. Journal of Aquatic Sciences 10, 7–14.

Ortega, C., Garcia, I., Irgang, R., Fajardo, R., Tapia-Cammas, D., Acosta, J., et al., 2018. First identification and characterization of *Streptococcus iniae* obtained from tilapia (*Oreochromis* aureus) farmed in Mexico. Journal of Fish Diseases 41, 773–782.

Osman, K.M., Al-Maary, K.S., Mubarak, A.S., Dawoud, T.M., Moussa, I.M.I., Ibrahim, M.D.S., et al., 2017. Characterization and susceptibility of streptococci and enterococci isolated from Nile tilapia (*Oreochromis niloticus*) showing septicaemia in aquaculture and wild sites in Egypt. BMC Veterinary Research 13, 357. https://doi.org/10.1186/s12917-017-1289-8.

Paller, V.G., Resurreccion, D.J., de la Cruz, C.P., Bandal Jr., M.Z., 2016. Acanthocephalan parasites (*Acanthogyrus* sp.) of Nile tilapia (*Oreochromis niloticus*) as biosink of lead (Pb) contamination in a Philippine freshwater lake. Bulletin of Environmental Contamination and Toxicology 96, 810–815.

Pallet, V.G.V., Sy, R.A.R., Bandal Jr., M.Z., 2016. Hematology and histopathology of nile tilapia (*Oreochromis niloticus* L.) infected with *Acanthogyrus* sp. (Acanthocephala: Quadrigyridae). Ecology Environment and Conservation 22, 493–500.

Paperna, I., 1974. Lymphocystis in fish from East african lakes. Journal of Wildlife Diseases 9, 331–335.

Paperna, I., Smirnova, M., 1997. *Branchiomyces*-like infection in a cultured tilapia (*Oreochromis* hybrid, Cichlidae). Diseases of Aquatic Organisms 31, 233–238.

Paperna, I., Kim, S.H., Hammerschlag, E., 1996. Liver lesions in cultured *Oreochromis* hybrids caused by amoeboid organisms similar to the aetiological agent of goldfish kidney granuloma. Diseases of Aquatic Organisms 25, 151–153.

Park, K.H., Jeong, H.D., 1996. Enhanced resistance against *Edwardsiella tarda* infection in tilapia (*Oreochromis niloticus*) by administration of protein-bound polysaccharide. Aquaculture 143, 135–143.

Paull, G.C., Matthews, R.A., 2001. *Spironucleus vortens*, a possible cause of hole-in thehead-disease in cichlids. Diseases of Aquatic Organisms 45, 197–202.

Perera, R.P., Johnson, S.K., Collins, M.D., Lewis, D.H., 1994. *Streptococcus iniae* associated with mortality of *Tilapia nilotica* x *T. aurea* hybrids. Journal of Aquatic Animal Health 6, 335–340.

Perera, R.P., Johnson, S.K., Lewis, D.H., 1997. Epizootiological aspects of *Streptococcus iniae* affecting tilapia in Texas. Aquaculture 152, 25–33.

Phumkhachorn, P., Rattanachaikunsopon, P., 2015. Use of *Cassia alata* aqueous extract as a bath treatment to control *Pseudomonas anguilliseptica* infection in tilapia (*Oreochromis niloticus*). Archives of Biological Sciences 67, 1165–1172.

Pillay, T.V.R., 1990. Aquaculture Principles and Practices. Blackwell Science Ltd, Fishing News books, Oxford, Edinburgh, London, 575 pp.

Pineda-López, R., Andrade-Salas, O., Páramo-Delgadillo, S., Trejo, P.L., Almeida-Artigas, J., Osorio-Sarabia, D., et al., 1985. Estudio del control sanitario de la piscifactoría Benito Juárez y en los Vasos de las Presas la Angostura y Malpaso. Dirección de Acuacultura, Secretaría de Pesca, México, 309 pp.

Plumb, J.A., 1997. Infectious diseases of tilapia. In: Costa-Pierce, B.A., Rakocy, J.E. (Eds.), Tilapia Aquaculture in the Americas, vol. 1. World Aquaculture Society, Baton Rouge, Louisiana, USA, pp. 212–228.

Plumb, J.A., 1999. Overview of warmwater fish diseases. Journal of Applied Aquaculture 9, 1–10.

Pretto-Giordano, L.G., Müller, E.E., Klesius, P., da Silva, V.G., 2010. Efficacy of an experimentally inactivated *Streptococcus agalactiae* vaccine in Nile tilapia (*Oreochromis niloticus*) reared in Brazil. Aquaculture Research 41, 1539–1544.

Prikrylova, I., Radim, B., Gelnar, M., 2012. *Gyrodactylus malalai* sp. nov. (Monogenea, Gyrodactylidae) from nile tilapia, *Oreochromis niloticus* (L.) and Redbelly tilapia, *Tilapia zillii* (Gervais) (Teleostei, Cichlidae) in the Lake Turkana, Kenya. Acta Parsitologica 57, 122–130.

Pulido, A.B., Iregui, C.C., Figueroa, J., 1999. Report of *Streptococcus* in tilapia cultivated in Colombia. In: Cabrera, T., Jory, D., Silva, M. (Eds.), Aquaculture 99. Congreso sur American de Acuicultura, Puerto la Cruz, Venezuela, pp. 229–239.

Rajavarthini, P.B., Michael, R.D., 1996. The effect of monocrotophos (Nuvacron) on the antibody response to bovine serum albumin in *Oreochromis mossambicus* (Peters). Journal of Aquaculture in the Tropics 11, 27–32.

Ramadan, H.H., 1991. Effect of host species, sex, length, diet and different seasons on the parasitic infection of *Tilapia* fish in Lake Manzala. Journal of King Abdulaziz University - Marine Sciences 2, 81–91.

Ramadan, A., Afifi, N.A., Mostafa, M.M., Samy, A.M., 1994. The effect of ascogen on the immune response of tilapia fish to *Aeromonas hydrophila* vaccine. Fish & Shellfish Immunology 4, 159–165.

Ranzani-Paiva, M.J.T., Ishikawa, C.M., das Eiras, A.C., da Silveira, V.R., 2004. Effects of an experimental challenge with *Mycobacterium marinum* on the blood parameters of Nile tilapia, *Oreochromis niloticus* (Linnaeus, 1757). Brazilian Archives of Biology and Technology 47, 945–953.

Reddy, T.V., Ravindranath, K., Sreeraman, P.K., Rao, M.V.S., 1994. *Aeromonas salmonicida* associated with mass mortality of *Cyprinus carpio* and *Oreochromis mossambicus* in a freshwater reservoir in Andhra Pradesh, India. Journal of Aquaculture in the Tropics 9, 259–268.

Resende, J.A., Silva, V.L., Cesar, D.E., Del'duca, A., Fontes, C.O., Diniz, C.G., 2015. Seasonal dynamics of microbial community in an aquaculture system for Nile tilapia (*Oreochromis niloticus*). Aquaculture Research 46, 1233–1240.

Roberts, R.J., Matthiessen, P., 1979. Pathological Findings in Fishes of the Okavangu Swamp, Botswana, Following Endosulphan Spraying. ODM Special Report. UK Ministry of Overseas Development, London, 9 pp.

Roberts, R.J., Sommerville, C., 1982. Diseases of tilapias. In: Pullin, R.S.V., Lowe-McConnell, R.H. (Eds.), The Biology and Culture of Tilapias, ICLARM Conference Proceedings No. 7. ICLARM, Manila, Philippines, pp. 247–262.

Roem, A.J., Kohler, C.C., Stickney, R.R., 1990. Vitamin E requirements of the blue tilapia *Oreochromis aureus* (Steindachner), in relation to dietary lipid levels. Aquaculture 87, 155–164.

Ruangpan, L., Kitao, T., Yoshida, T., 1986. Protective efficacy of *Aeromonas hydrophila* vaccines in Nile tilapia. Veterinary Immunology and Immunopathology 12, 346–350.

Saeed, M.O., 1993. Efforts to control outbreaks of diseases among cultured fish in Kuwait. In: Proceeding of the First International Aquaculture Symposium: Technologies and Investment Opportunities. Ministry of Agriculture and waters, Riyadh, Saudi Arabia, pp. 400–409.

Saeed, M.O., Al-Thobaiti, S.A., 1997. Gas bubble disease in farmed fish in Saudi Arabia. The Veterinary Record 140, 682–684.

Sakata, T., Hattori, M., 1988. Characteristics of *Vibrio vulnificus* isolated from diseased tilapia. Fish Pathology 23, 33–40.

Sanchez-Ramirez, C., Vidal-Martinez, V.M., Aguirre-Macedo, M.L., Rodriguez-Canul, R.P., Gold-Bouchot, G., Sures, B., 2007. *Cichlidogyrus sclerosus* (Monogenea: Ancyrocephalinae) and its host, the Nile tilapia (*Oreochromis niloticus*), as bioindicators of chemical pollution. Journal of Parsitology 93, 1097–1106.

Sarder, M.R.I., Thompson, K.D., Penman, D.J., McAndrew, J., 2001. Immune response of Nile tilapia (*Oreochromis niloticus* L) clones: 1. Non-specific responses. Developmental & Comparative Immunology 25, 37–46.

Sarig, S., 1971. Diseases of Warmwater Fishes. T.F.H. Publications, Neptune City, New Jersey.

Schlechtriem, C., Bresler, V., Fishelson, L., Rosenfeld, M., Becker, K., 2004. Protective effects of dietary l-carnitine on tilapia hybrids (*Oreochromis niloticus* x *Oreochromis aureus*) reared under intensive pond-culture conditions. Aquaculture Nutrition 10, 55–63.

Scott, P.W., 1977. Preliminary Studies on Disease in Intensively Farmed Tilapia in Kenya. MSc. Thesis. University of Stirling, Scotland.

Sebastião, F.A., Nomura, D., Sakabe, R., Pilarski, F., 2011. Hematology and productive performance of Nile tilapia (*Oreochromis niloticus*) naturally infected with *Flavobacterium columnare*. Brazilian Journal of Microbiology 42, 282–289.

Shelby, R.A., Shoemaker, C.A., Klesius, P.H., 2002a. Detection of humoral response to *Streptococcus iniae* infection of Nile tilapia, *Oreochromis niloticus,* by a monoclonal antibody-based ELISA. Journal of Applied Aquaculture 12, 23–31.

Shelby, R.A., Klesius, P.H., Shoemaker, C.A., Evans, J.J., 2002b. Passive immunization of tilapia, *Oreochromis niloticus* (L.), with anti-*Streptococcus iniae* whole sera. Journal of Fish Diseases 25, 1–6.

Sherif, A.H., Abdel–Hakim, S.A., 2016. Treatment trails of saprolegniosis in *Oreochromis niloticus*. Alexandria Journal of Veterinary Sciences 49, 99–104.

Shiau, S.-Y., Hsieh, H.L., 1997. Vitamin B6 requirements of tilapia, *Oreochromis niloticus* × *O. aureus* fed two dietary protein concentrations. Fisheries Science 63, 1002–1007.

Shiau, S.-Y., Suen, G.S., 1992. Estimation of the niacin requirements for tilapia fed diets containing glucose or dextrin. Journal of Nutrition 122, 2030–2036.

Shimura, S., Asai, M., 1984. *Argulus americanus* (Crustacea: Branchiura) parasite on the bowfin, *Amia calva*, imported from North America. Fish Pathology 18, 199–213.

Shinn, A.P., Harris, P.D., Cable, J., Bakke, T.A., Paladini, G., Bron, J.E. (Eds.), 2010. GyroDb. World Wide Web Electronic Publication. www.gyrodb.net.version(06/2010).

Shlapobersky, M., Sinyakov, M.S., Katzenellenbogen, M., Sarid, R., Don, J., Avtalion, R.R., 2010. Viral encephalitis of tilapia larvae: primary characterization of a novel herpes-like virus. Virology 399, 239–247.

Shoemaker, C.A., Evans, J.J., Klesius, P.H., 2000. Density and dose: factors affecting mortality to *Streptococcus iniae*-infected tilapia (*Oreochromis niloticus*). Aquaculture 188, 229–235.

Sin, Y.M., Ling, K.H., Lam, T.J., 1994. Passive transfer of protective immunity against *Ichthyophthirius* from vaccinated mother to fry in tilapia, *Oreochromis aureus*. Aquaculture 120, 229–237.

Sinha, C.K., 1986. Occurrence of *Trypanosoma mukasai* Hoare, 1932 in *Tilapia mossambica* (Peters) from India. Acta Protozoologica 25, 449–452.

Skliris, G.P., Richards, R.H., 1999. *Nodavirus* isolated from experimentally infected tilapia, *Oreochromis mossambicus* (Peters). Journal of Fish Diseases 22, 315–318.

Smith, C.E., Ramsey, D., Speer, C.A., 1998. Histopathology associated with an irido-like virus infection of tilapia, *Tilapia nilotica*. In: Aquaculture'98 – Book of Abstracts. World Aquaculture Society, Baton Rouge, Louisiana, p. 504.

Soliman, A.K., Wilson, R.P., 1992a. Water-soluble vitamin requirements of tilapia. 1. Pantothenic acid requirement of blue tilapia, *Oreochromis aureus*. Aquaculture 104, 121–126.

Soliman, A.K., Wilson, R.P., 1992b. Water-soluble vitamin requirements of tilapia. 2. Riboflavin requirement of blue tilapia, *Oreochromis aureus*. Aquaculture 104, 309–314.

Soto, E., Hawke, J.P., Fernandez, D., Morales, J.A., 2009. *Francisella* sp., an emerging pathogen of tilapia, *Oreochromis niloticus* (L.), in Costa Rica. Journal of Fish Diseases 32, 713–722.

Soto, E., Baumgartner, W., Wiles, J., Hawke, J.P., 2011. *Francisella asiatica* as the causative agent of piscine francisellosis in cultured tilapia (*Oreochromis* sp.) in the United States. Journal of Veterinary Diagnostic Investigation 23, 821–825.

Soto, E., Griffin, M., Arauz, M., Riofrio, A., Martinez, A., Cabrejos, M.E., 2012a. *Edwardsiella ictalurias* as the causative agent of mortality in cultured Nile tilapia. Journal of Aquatic Animal Health 24, 81–90.

Soto, E., Abrams, S.B., Revan, F., 2012b. Effects of temperature and salt concentration on *Francisella noatunensis* subsp. *orientalis* infections in Nile tilapia *Oreochromis niloticus*. Diseases of Aquatic Organisms 101, 217–223.

Soto-Rodriguez, S.A., Cabanillas-Ramos, J., Alcaraz, U., Gomez-Gil, B., Romalde, J.L., 2013. Identification and virulence of *Aeromonas dhakensis, Pseudomonas mosselii* and *Microbacterium paraoxydans* isolated from Nile tilapia, *Oreochromis niloticus*, cultivated in Mexico. Journal of Applied Microbiology 115, 654–662.

Straus, D.L., Griffin, B.R., 2001. Prevention of an initial infestation of *Ichthyophthirius multifiliis* in channel catfish and blue tilapia by potassium permanganate treatment. North American Journal of Aquaculture 63, 11–16.

Subasinghe, R.P., Sommerville, C., 1986. Acquired immunity of *Oreochromis mossambicus* to the ciliate ectoparasite *Ichthyophthirius multifiliis* (Fouquet). In: Maclean, J.L., Dizon, L.B., Hosillos, L.V. (Eds.), Proceedings of the First Asian Fisheries Forum. Asian Fisheries Society, Manila, Philippines, pp. 279–283.

Subasinghe, R.P., Sommerville, C., 1989. An experimental study into possible protection of fry from *Ichthyophthirius multifiliis* (Fouquet) infections during mouthbrooding of *Oreochromis mossambicus* (Peters). Journal of Fish Diseases 12, 143–149.

Subasinghe, R.P., Sommerville, C., 1992. Susceptibility of *Oreochromis mossambicus* (Peters) fry to the ciliate ectoparasite *Ichthyophthirius multifiliis* (Fouquet). In: Shariff, M., Subasinghe, R.P., Arthur, J.R. (Eds.), Proceedings of the First Symposium on Diseases in Asian Aquaculture. Asian Fisheries Society, Manila, Philippines, pp. 355–360.

Subramaniam, K., Gotesman, M., Smith, C.E., Steckler, N.K., Kelley, K.L., Groff, J.M., et al., 2016. Megalocytivirus infection in cultured Nile tilapia *Oreochromis niloticus*. Diseases of Aquatic Organisms 119, 253–258.

Suebsing, R., Kampeera, J., Sirithammajak, S., Pradeep, P.J., Jitrakorn, S., Arunrut, N., et al., 2015. *Shewanella putrefaciens* in cultured tilapia detected by a new calcein-loop-mediated isothermal amplification (Ca-LAMP) method. Diseases of Aquatic Organisms 117, 133–143.

Sukenda, S., Rahman, R., Nisaa, K., Hidayatullah, D., Vinasyiam, A., 2018. The efficacy of *Streptococcus agalactiae* vaccine preparations, administered to tilapia broodstock, in preventing streptococcosis in their offspring, via transfer of maternal immunity. Aquaculture International 26, 785–798.

Tavares-Dias, M., Moraes, F.R., Martins, M.L., Kronka, S.N., 2001. Parasitic fauna of cultivated fishes in feefishing farm of Franca, Sao Paulo. II. Metazoans. Revista Brasiliera de Zoologia 18, 81–95.

Te, B.Q., Lua, D.T., Viet, N.V., Thanh, N.V., 1999. Parasitic fauna of cultured tilapia (*Oreochromis* spp) in Vietnam. Paper Presented at the Fourth Symposium on Diseases in Asian Aquaculture: Aquatic Animal Health for Sustainability. Cebu City, Philippines, 22–26 November 1999.

Toledo-Ibarra, G.A., Díaz Resendiz, K.J.G., Ventura-Ramón, G.H., González-Jaime, F., Vega-López, A., Becerril-Villanueva, E., et al., 2016. Oxidative damage in gills and liver in Nile tilapia (*Oreochromis niloticus*) exposed to diazinon. Comparative Biochemistry and Physiology – Part A 200, 3–8.

Tung, M.-C., Chen, S.-C., Tsai, S.-S., 1987. General septicemia of streptococcal infection in cage-culture tilapia, *Tilapia mossambica*, in Southern Taiwan. In: COA Fisheries Series, 10, pp. 187–197.

Upton, K.R., Riley, L.G., 2013. Acute stress inhibits food intake and alters ghrelin signaling in the brain of tilapia (*Oreochromis mossambicus*). Domestic Animal Endocrinology 44, 157–164.

Valladão, G.M.R., Pádua, S.B., Gallani, S.U., Menezes-Filho, R.N., Dias-Neto, J., Martins, M.L., et al., 2013. *Paratrichodina africana* (Ciliophora): a pathogenic gill parasite in farmed Nile tilapia. Veterinary Parasitology 197, 705–710.

Valladão, G.M.R., Levy-Pereira, N., Viadanna, P.H.O., Gallani, S.U., Farias, T.H.V., Pilarski, F., 2014. Haematology and histopathology of Nile tilapia parasitised by *Epistylis* sp., an emerging pathogen in South America. Bulletin of the European Association of Fish Pathologists 35, 14–20.

Valladão, G.M.R., Alves, L.O., Pilarski, F., 2016. Trichodiniasis in Nile tilapia hatcheries: diagnosis, parasite:host-stage relationship and treatment. Aquaculture 451, 444–450.

Vinh, D.C., Mubareka, S., Fatoye, B., Plourde, P., Orr, P., 2006. *Vibrio vulnificus* septicemia after handling tilapia species fish: a Canadian case report and review. The Canadian Journal of Infectious Diseases & Medical Microbiology 17, 129–132.

Violante-González, J., García-Varela, M., Rojas-Herrera, A., Guerrero, S.G., 2009. Diplostomiasis in cultured and wild tilapia *Oreochromis niloticus* in Guerrero state, Mexico. Parsitological Research 105, 803–807.

Wang, W.-S., Wang, D.-H., 1997. Enhancement of the resistance of tilapia and grass carp to experimental *Aeromonas hydrophila* and *Edwardsiella tarda* infections by several polysaccharides. Comparative Immunology, Microbiology and Infectious Diseases 20, 261–270.

Wang, Z.-G., Xu, B.-H., 1985. Studies on the pathogenic bacteria of the "rotten-skin" diseases of the Nile tilapia (*Tilapia nilotica*). Journal of Fisheries of China/Shuichan Xuebao 9, 217–221.

Wang, K., Chen, D., Huang, L., Lian, H., Wang, J., Xiao, D., et al., 2013. Isolation and characterization of *Streptococcus agalactiae* from Nile tilapia *Oreochromis niloticus* in China. African Journal of Microbiology Research 7, 317–323.

Wiriya, B., Clausen, J.H., Inpankaew, T., Thaenkham, U., Jittapalapong, S., Satapornvanit, K., et al., 2013. Fish-borne trematodes in cultured Nile tilapia (*Oreochromis niloticus*) and wild-caught fish from Thailand. Veterinary Parasitology 198, 230–234.

Wolf, J.C., Smith, S.A., 1999. Comparative severity of experimentally induced mycobacteriosis in striped bass *Morone saxatilis* and hybrid tilapia *Oreochromis* spp. Diseases of Aquatic Organisms 38, 191–200.

Wu, F., Jiang, M., Wen, H., Liu, W., Tian, J., Yang, C., et al., 2017. Dietary vitamin E effects on growth, fillet textural parameters, and antioxidant capacity of genetically improved farmed tilapia (GIFT), *Oreochromis niloticus*. Aquaculture International 25, 991–1003.

Xu, D.-H., Klesius, P.H., Shoemaker, C.A., 2008. Protective immunity of Nile tilapia against *Ichthyophthirius multifiliis* post-immunization with live theronts and sonicated trophonts. Fish & Shellfish Immunology 25, 124–127.

Xu, D.-H., Shoemaker, C.A., Lafrentz, B.R., 2014. Enhanced susceptibility of hybrid tilapia to *Flavobacterium columnare* after parasitism by *Ichthyophthirius multifiliis*. Aquaculture 430, 44–49.

Yambot, A.V., 1998. Isolation of *Aeromonas hydrophila* from *Oreochromis niloticus* during fish disease outbreaks in the Philippines. Asian Fisheries Science 10, 347–354.

Yavuzcan, Y.H., Pulatsü, S., 1999. Evaluation of the secondary stress response in healthy Nile tilapia (*Oreochromis niloticus* L.) after treatment with a mixture of formalin, malachite green and methylene blue. Aquaculture Research 30, 379–383.

Yuasa, K., Kamaishi, T., Hatai, K., Bahnnan, M., Borisutpeth, P., 2008. Two cases of streptococcal infections of cultured tilapia in Asia. In: Bondad-Reantaso, M.G., Mohan, C.V., Crumlish, M., Subasinghe, R.P. (Eds.), Diseases in Asian Aquaculture VI. Asian Fisheries Society, Manila, Philippines, pp. 259–268.

Zahran, E., Risha, E., 2013. Protective role of adjuvant and potassium permanganate on oxidative stress response of Nile tilapia (*Oreochromis niloticus*) challenged with *Saprolegnia ferax*. SpringerPlus 2 (1), 94. https://doi.org/10.1186/2193-1801-2-94.

Zahran, E., Hafez, E.E., Mohd Altaf Hossain, F., Elhadidy, M., Shaheen, A.A., 2017. Saprolegniosis in Nile tilapia: identification, molecular characterization, and phylogenetic analysis of two novel pathogenic Saprolegnia Strains. Journal of Aquatic Animal Health 29, 43–49.

Zahran, E., Risha, E., Awadin, W., Palić, D., 2018. Acute exposure to chlorpyrifos induces reversible changes in health parameters of Nile tilapia (*Oreochromis niloticus*). Aquatic Toxicology 197, 47–59.

Zaki, M.M., Eissa, A.E., Saeid, S., 2011. Assessment of the immune status in Nile tilapia (*Oreochromis niloticus*) experimentally challenged with toxogenic/septicemic bacteria during treatment trial with Florfenicol and Enrofloxacin. World Journal of Fish and Marine Sciences 3, 21–36.

Zamri-Saad, M., Amal, M.N., Siti-Zahrah, A., 2010. Pathological changes in red tilapias (*Oreochromis* spp.) naturally infected by *Streptococcus agalactiae*. Journal of Comparative Pathology 143, 227–229.

Zhou, K., Cui, T.T., Li, P.L., Liang, N.J., Liu, S.C., Ma, C.W., et al., 2008. Modelling and predicting the effect of temperature, water activity and pH on growth of *Streptococcus iniae* in tilapia. Journal of Applied Microbiology 105, 1956–1965.

Zhu, L., Yang, Q., Huang, L., Wang, K., Wang, X., Chen, D., et al., 2017. Effectivity of oral recombinant DNA vaccine against *Streptococcus agalactiae* in Nile tilapia. Developmental & Comparative Immunology 77, 77–87.

Chapter 10

Harvesting, processing, economics and value chain

Chapter outline

10.1 Introduction

As indicated in Chapter 1 of this book, the production of farmed tilapia has been rapidly expanding in the past few years. Most of this production is used directly for local markets, mainly as a cheap, good-quality animal protein source in rural areas. Because tilapia was considered to be a low-value product, little attention has been paid to their harvesting and handling, for many years. Tilapia have also not been identified as a trade item according to the International Standard Statistical Classification (ISSC). As a result, information on tilapia exports and imports has been very limited. However, the international trade in tilapia and tilapia products started to gain increased global attention. Thus, it is essential to shed some lights on the factors that may affect tilapia production, costs, trade and overall economics, with emphasis on harvesting, handling, processing and economics, in order to adopt the best cost-effective production strategies.

10.2 Harvesting

Tilapia culture is dominated by small-scale rural farms, especially in developing countries, and most of the production is consumed in local areas. There is no specific harvesting method for farmed tilapia. The information available on tilapia harvesting methods is also very limited. Moreover, polyculture with other aquatic species makes it more difficult to adopt specific harvesting techniques for tilapia. For these reasons, small-scale farmers in different regions may adopt different, but simple harvesting techniques.

Harvesting methods depend on pond size, culture systems and levels of technology applied. For example, small-scale tilapia farmers in many parts of Africa and Asia cannot easily get harvesting nets and other equipment required for complete harvesting of their ponds. To overcome this problem, many farmers adopt partial harvesting techniques, using locally available gears (Fig. 10.1) (Brummett, 2002). Large-scale tilapia produces adopt more advanced harvesting tools such as winches because they generally prefer batch harvesting (Fig. 10.2). Sometimes they anesthetize the fish before harvesting to reduce stress and to comply with the animal welfare regulations (Fig. 10.3). Partial harvesting is usually designed to remove large fish and provide smaller fish with more space for growth (Hepher and Pruginin, 1981). Yet, many questions regarding this system remain unanswered: (1) Is this system preferable to batch harvesting methods? (2) At what size and harvesting intervals should the fish be harvested? (3) How much fish (as a percent of total density) should be harvested each time? (4) Should harvested fish be replaced

Tilapia Culture. https://doi.org/10.1016/B978-0-12-816541-6.00010-6
Copyright © 2020 Elsevier Inc. All rights reserved.

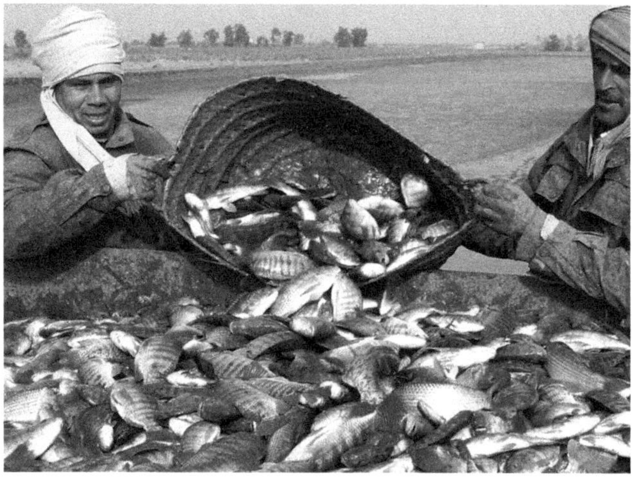

FIGURE 10.1 Manual harvesting of Nile tilapia from earthen ponds in Egypt. *Photo provided by A. Hamdeen.*

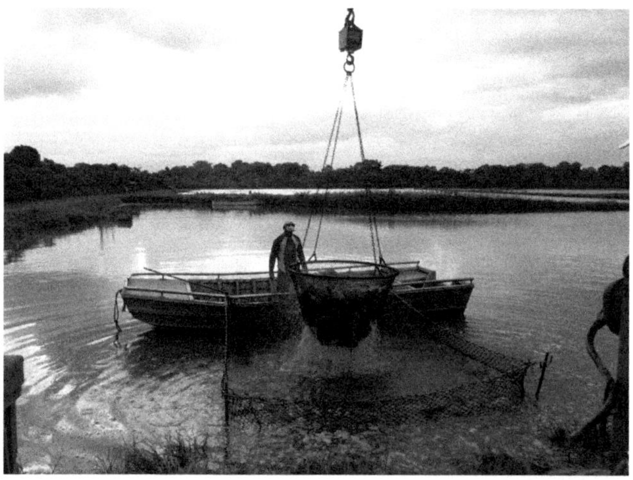

FIGURE 10.2 Mechanical harvesting of pond-raised tilapia in Ecuador. *Photograph by A.-F.M. El-Sayed.*

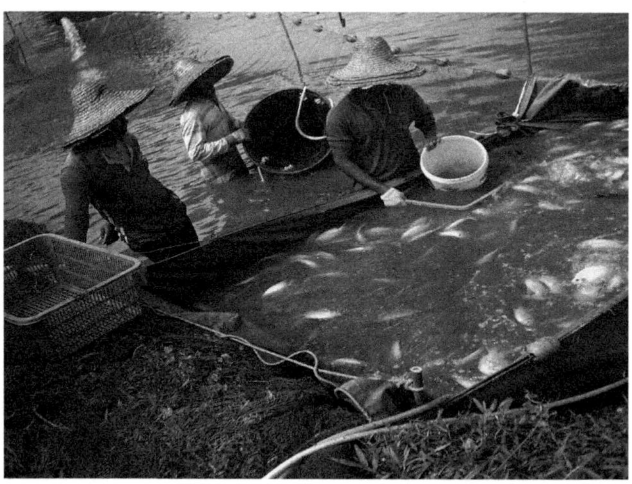

FIGURE 10.3 Harvesting red tilapia in Malaysia. Fish are anesthetized to reduce stress. *Photograph by A.-F.M. El-Sayed.*

with new fish? (5) What is the best fish size that will replace the harvested portion? and (6) What are the best harvesting methods for this system?. To the extent that these questions are not answered, the system may not lead to the outputs that the farmers hope to get and may also fail to increase overall yield (Knud-Hansen and Lin, 1996). Therefore, finding answers to these questions is necessary in order to evaluate and improve partial harvesting methods.

The limited information available may suggest the use of partial harvest as a more cost-effective harvesting method than using single harvest techniques. Nitithamyong et al. (1990) compared partial harvest and batch harvest of Nile tilapia reared in monoculture systems or in integration with pigs. Marketable-size fish were harvested monthly (multiple harvest) from one monoculture system and from the integrated system, while another monoculture system was harvested only once at the end of the study. Total fish production from monoculture and integrated systems using the multiple harvesting techniques was higher than from the monoculture system with a single harvest. However, despite higher yields, the integrated system with multiple harvest provided a significantly lower return than the monoculture system, probably because of the higher labour cost. This result indicated that the supposed benefits to be gained from employing the partial harvesting may be misleading, and therefore, it should be evaluated biologically and economically.

Saiti et al. (2007) found that when mixed-sex tilapia (*Oreochromis shiranus*) were subjected to different harvesting scenarios; the lowest yield was obtained when no partial harvesting was carried out and the fish were harvested only once after 365 days. On the other hand, maximum yield was obtained when partial harvesting was applied every 90 days starting with a first harvest of fish weighing 60 g. However, maximum profits were achieved when the fish were partially harvested at 120-day intervals, with the first harvest at day 90 and removing all fish weighing 60 g or more.

McGinty and Alston (1993) reported that the annual yield of all-male tilapia reared in polyculture with juvenile freshwater prawn (*Macrobrachium rosenbergii*) and partially harvested monthly was similar to that from a batch harvest system. The authors suggested that partial harvesting offers good potential for small farmers who need to supply markets on a regular basis. This system also facilitates meeting the demands for fish fry since all the fish for stocking are not required at the same time. Again, evaluating tilapia harvesting methods must consider technical, biological, economic and socioeconomic factors.

In many rural areas, fish harvesting methods are one of the major bottlenecks to the development of rural aquaculture. In Malawi, for example, most fish farmers have been completely dependent on the government by borrowing harvesting nets from Fisheries Departments

(Kaunda and Costa-Pierce, 1993). In this context, cheap and locally available harvesting tools are an important prerequisite to the success of rural aquaculture. Brummett (2002) tackled this issue and evaluated the effectiveness of various local fishing gears as partial harvesting methods in small tilapia (*O. shiranus*) ponds in Malawi. The fish (13.7 g) were stocked in 200-m^2 ponds ($20 \times 10 \times 0.6$ m $= 120$ m^3) at a density of 2.5 fish m^{-3} and fed local feed sources (maize, bran and vegetable leaves). After 122 days, the ponds were assigned to (1) weekly seining with a reed fence; (2) weekly fishing for 4 h with hook and line by a single fisherman; (3) weekly fishing for 9 h with two basket traps and (4) no fishing (control). The partial harvesting methods continued for 20 weeks. The author found that hook and line fishing and fishing with a reed fence partially harvested significantly greater weights of fish than trapping. Partial removal of tilapia juveniles had the highest impact on increased yield. The partial removal of tilapia juveniles (not fry or adults) is probably the main limiting factor in increasing productivity of fish ponds.

10.3 Handling

Tilapia is generally marketed in rural areas and local markets in developing countries, either fresh or iced, with little handling and processing. However, the global tilapia market is growing sharply, not only in producing regions (mainly South East Asia, the Far East and Africa) but also in many nonproducing regions, such as the United States, Europe and Australia. More attention should therefore be paid to tilapia handling and processing in order to maintain quality and meet the quality standards required by external markets. Poor handling and holding conditions, inadequate processing and the use of inappropriate processing methods can seriously affect the quality of tilapia and increase post-harvest losses. For example, Enujiugha and Nwanna (1998) reported that more than 20% of Nile tilapia and African catfish yields were lost in Nigeria as a result of inadequate handling and processing.

Live tilapia have become an important product in the market in many parts of the world where consumers prefer to buy live rather than iced or frozen fish (Singh and Daud, 2001). It is becoming common to find live tilapia in display tanks and aquaria in seafood restaurants and supermarkets in countries like Singapore, Thailand and Malaysia (Singh and Daud, 2001). However, live food systems require effective support systems, including live holding containers, specially equipped trucks, live holding centres and other infrastructure components. Consumers prefer to pay higher prices in order to get live fish. In Malaysia, for example, the price of live red tilapia is 37%–40% higher than that of chilled tilapia (Singh and Daud, 2001). The price of live tilapia in Egypt, particularly in large cities such as Cairo and Alexandria, is 50%–75% higher than that of iced fish of similar sizes (El-Sayed, Alexandria, 2004; personal observation).

Singh and Daud (2001) described the different steps and processes involved in the handling and marketing of tilapia in Malaysia, including transport, distribution, display and holding facilities. A modern technology has been developed by the Malaysian Agricultural Research and Development Institute (MARDI) for the transport of live fish such as tilapia in a minimum quantity of water (Wan Johari et al., 1999). The system involves transferring the fish into tanks at a temperature of 21°C for about 10 h to reduce stress. The water in the tanks is gradually cooled to 11°C, with the addition of ice, to reduce fish activity. The fish are then packed in plastic bags with water and oxygen at a fish:water ratio of 1:1. The bags are tied and placed in polystyrene boxes, which are sealed and transferred to refrigerated trucks maintained at 15°C and transported to their final destination. On arrival, the fish are stocked in holding facilities and left to regain their normal physiological functions as the temperature gradually rises. By using this technique, live tilapia can be transported for a journey of 12 h without any mortality on arrival (Singh and Daud, 2001).

Different handling, slaughtering and pre-processing techniques have been proposed, in order to reduce stress and improve the quality and shelf life of the fish and their products. Factors such as pre-slaughter conditions and slaughter weight may have significant impacts on the physical properties and quality of harvested fish. For example, Goes et al. (2015) evaluated the effect of pre-slaughter stress (both stocking density and transportation times) on serum cortisol levels, pH, colourimetry, water-holding capacity (WHC) and gene expression of ryanodine (RyR1 and RyR3) in the Nile tilapia. Ryanodine is a chemical compound that allows the liberation of calcium from the endoplasmic reticulum (ER) lumen through ER-ryanodine receptor. The authors found that transportation time alone (not stocking density) reduced cortisol levels up to 180 min of transportation, followed by increased WHC and mRNA expression of RyR1 and RyR3. These results clearly demonstrate that pre-slaughter stress can lead to increased WHC in tilapia fillets.

Even the weight of slaughtered fish may affect meat quality of tilapia; and therefore, modifying the slaughter weight can achieve targeted meat quality. Kayan et al. (2015) assessed the effects of different slaughter weights (600, 800 and 1200 g per fish) of Nile tilapia on the meat quality. The results showed that protein content of the 600-g fish was the highest, while fat content of the 1200-g fish was significantly higher than that of the 600-g fish. Drip loss percentage of the fillet of 600 g was the highest, whereas boiling loss percentage was the highest in the 1200-g fish. Shear force values of raw and cooked fillets were highest with the 1200-g fish. The total collagen content, flavour, juiciness, tenderness and acceptability of the fillet of the 1200-g fish was highest. This study clearly concludes that fat content, fillet firmness and flavour improvement increased with increasing the slaughter weight of Nile tilapia.

10.3.1 Stunning and killing

A 'Protocol on the Protection and Welfare of Animals' in the EU was a result of the Amsterdam Treaty (EFSA–AHAW/04-027, 2004). This treaty requires that full consideration should be paid to welfare requirements of animals in formulation and implementation of EU regulations. Accordingly, all animals, including fish, should be protected from stress, pain or suffering during transport, restraint, stunning, slaughtering or killing. This simply means that higher standards of welfare for fish at slaughter should be adopted in tilapia harvesting and handling. This includes improvements in the methods used in transportation and killing of the fish. Crowding during transportation is one of the major causes of poor welfare during harvest due to the physiological disorders caused by oxygen deficiency.

A number of studies revealed that fish have pain sensory pathways, indicating that they have the capacity to experience pain, suffering and fear (Sneddon, 2003; Chandroo et al., 2004). However, most of farmed fish are killed without prior stunning, mainly by cold shock, by asphyxiating them in air or in ice slurry. Ice slurry is a convenient method because it cools and preserves the fish, while killing them with no additional cost. But this method is considered nonhumane. Species which are tolerant of low oxygen levels, such as tilapia, may suffer and therefore require a more follow-up killing method (e.g. immediate bleeding to avoid recovery) (Lines and Spence, 2014). In this case, it is necessary to sever all of the gill arches on at least one side of the head, immediately after stunning.

Stunning is generally applied to animals to induce unconsciousness and insensibility to pain stimuli for sufficient duration to assure that slaughtered animal does not recover during killing or bleeding. Stunning should be induced immediately to optimize animal welfare and also to minimize any possible negative effect of these handling techniques on meat quality. Different stunning methods of farmed fish have been applied worldwide, including elctrostunning, carbon dioxide (CO_2), carbon monoxide (CO) and thermal shock. The effects of these methods on the welfare, stress, and meat quality and colour were tested by a number of authors.

de Oliveira Filho et al. (2015a) evaluated the effects of two stunning methods (iced water and CO_2 narcosis) on the quality of tilapia meat which was refrigerated in ice (4°C) for up to 26 days. Tilapia stunned by CO_2 narcosis showed less stress compared to iced water, indicated by the higher muscle adenosine triphosphate (ATP) and better meat colour (higher lightness and lower redness values). These results demonstrated that stunning of tilapia by CO_2 narcosis can be an alternative to the traditional iced water method. In support, the same authors (de Oliveira Filho et al., 2015b) further evaluated the effect of electrical stunning, CO_2 narcosis and iced water on stress indicators in Nile tilapia, including muscle ATP, enzymatic antioxidants (catalase, lactate dehydrogenase and glutathione reductase) and plasma cortisol. CO_2 narcosis caused less stress than other tested methods, suggesting that the stunning with CO_2 is in accordance with good practices of animal welfare. A similar comparison was carried out on the effects of CO_2 narcosis and thermal shock on the physicochemical properties of Nile tilapia fillets stored frozen (−18°C) for up to 6 months (de Oliveira Filho et al., 2017). The properties of frozen tilapia fillets stunned by CO_2 narcosis were more desirable than those stunned by thermal shock. Tilapia fillets subjected to CO_2 narcosis had higher lightness and whiteness, lower redness and higher hardness values than tilapia subjected to thermal shock. It is evident, therefore, that CO_2 narcosis can be a potential tilapia stunning alternative for thermal shock.

Electrostunning of farmed animals has also been recognized as a humane slaughter practice, as it ensures unconsciousness of the slaughtered animal. Electric current of sufficient strength can cause complete suppression of nerve function, resulting in immediate unconsciousness and insensibility to stress and pain. This technique has been tried in different farmed fish species, including tilapia. Lambooij et al. (2008) found that Nile tilapia can be humanely electrostunned. However, the direction of the fish towards the electric field is important for effective stunning. When the fish was electrostunned side-to-side, 1.0 A_{rms} dm^{-2} (50 Hz AC) top-to-bottom in freshwater was needed for stunning. The electric current can be reduced to 0.4 A_{rms} dm^{-2} (at 50 Hz AC) if a head-to-tail current was applied. When a square wave pulsed alternating current (density of 0.6 A_{rms} dm^{-2}, 133 Hz and 43% duty cycle) was applied side-to-side, instead of a top-to-bottom current (50 Hz sinusoidal), the overall current density can be reduced from 1 to 0.6 A_{rms} dm^{-2}. The authors recommend that electrostunning of Nile tilapia followed by killing in ice water, rather than by bleeding by gill cutting, should be adopted to achieve the maximum protection of welfare of the fish at slaughter. Venturini et al. (2018) also found that higher-frequency (1200 Hz) electronarcosis improved Nile tilapia welfare during slaughtering.

10.3.2 Nitric oxide euthanasia

As mentioned above, animal welfare legislation in many countries requires that the fish should be euthanatized before bleeding. CO_2, CO and isoeugenol have been traditionally used as anaesthetics for euthanatizing farmed fish (Mantilla et al., 2008; Bjørlykke et al., 2011; Guan et al., 2017). However, some authors claim that CO_2 euthanizing is not an optimal slaughter technique, since the fish remains under considerable stress because they do not lose their consciousness immediately (Van de Vis et al., 2003). Therefore, some countries decided to stop the use of CO_2 for euthanasia of farmed fish and replace it with nitric oxide (NO). NO has recently been emerged as an alternative method for euthanatizing farmed fish prior to slaughter.

Several studies investigated the effect of NO euthanasia on the quality of tilapia fillets such as pH values, rigor index, drip loss, muscle colour and animal welfare. Wang et al. (2017) evaluated the effect of euthanasia using direct saturated NO on the muscle colour and animal welfare of Nile tilapia. NO euthanasia led to an improved muscle red colour, a shorter euthanasia time and less stress, and in turn, improved the welfare of the fish. The same authors (Wang et al., 2018a) found that NO postmortem treatment significantly prolonged the shelf life of Nile tilapia fillets and improved their muscle colours and colour stability during the storage. Furthermore, Wang et al. (2018b) investigated the effect of NO euthanasia on the quality of Nile tilapia fillets and estimated the safety of NO euthanasia and NO postmortem treatment for the application of NO technology in industrial processing of tilapia. They found that fillets obtained from fish euthanized by NO showed a later decrease of muscle pH, a later onset of rigor mortis postmortem and less drip loss during the refrigerated storage than the control, untreated fish. NO treatment also caused less total volatile basic nitrogen (TVBN) than control, leading to prolonged shelf life of tilapia fillets. These studies clearly demonstrate that both NO euthanasia and NO postmortem treatment improved the quality of tilapia fillets and reduced their safety threats. NO has also been reported to inhibit microbial growth (Skibsted, 2011).

10.4 Processing

Fish processing is becoming increasingly important due to the increasing demand for processed fish in global markets. Traditionally, processed freshwater fishes, supplied in various simple forms, have increased consumer choice. Normally, small processors sell their products directly to consumers. In many provinces of Thailand, for example, processed fish, mostly in dried and salted form, are sold along highways to serve domestic travellers. On the other hand, large fish processors usually sell their products to the wholesale fish markets in Bangkok and to retailers as well. Sometimes, processed fish, such as fish balls and minced fish, are resold in supermarkets.

Marketing of processed tilapia is also gaining high popularity in some South East Asian countries. Indonesia and Thailand, for instance, export filleted tilapia to the US market (Guerrero and Guerrero, 2001). Other products of processed tilapia, such as dried, smoked and canned tilapia; fish balls; sausages; surimi; fish flour; fish burgers; fish fingers; fish noodles; sashimi and various breaded, battered and marinated products are now well accepted by Asian consumers (Irianto and Irianto, 1997). These products are more convenient for working households, where family members come home late from work and may not have time to clean and cook fish. This simply means that tilapia can be an ideal raw material for producing value-added products. This approach is likely to create more jobs, generate more income and improve the standard of living, especially in rural areas. As a result, the export of prepared or preserved tilapia products amounted to 113,957 t in 2016, representing 23% of total tilapia exports (FAO, 2018).

Typically, the processing of tilapia includes one or more of the following techniques: (1) cooling (icing, refrigeration, freezing, etc.); (2) filleting; (3) radiation and (4) industrial processing (drying, smoking, canning, fish balls and sausages, etc.). A number of precautions must be taken into consideration during processing in order to ensure a good-quality product. These include the following:

1. Assurance of the total removal of off-flavour in the flesh either during the culture of the fish or during processing.
2. Proper purging and bleeding.
3. Careful heading to avoid damage to the fish and subsequent contamination by internal organs such as the gall bladder.
4. Fillets must not contain excess fats.

10.4.1 Cooling

Icing, chilling and refrigeration are the most common methods used for the storage of tilapia. However, cool storage is usually done improperly and without considering scientific, quality and hygienic standards. This generally leads to reducing the quality and shelf life of the fish and increasing health risks. It is therefore essential that proper temperature and processing methods are adopted for the storage of tilapia.

The effect of storage temperature on the quality and shelf life of tilapia (*Tilapia* spp.) in Sri Lanka has been evaluated by Rajaratnam and Balasundaram (2001). Gutted and gut retaining fish and shrimp (*Penaeus monodon*) were stored at 0, 4 and 28°C (room temperature). The authors found that freezing significantly reduced the microbial populations, while the initial bacterial population increased by 300% after 72 h of storage at room temperature. Spoilage rate was also more rapid in gut-retaining than gutted fish and headed shrimp. It was concluded that shelf life and quality acceptance could be extended up to 25 days when the products are stored at 0 and 4°C. It was also suggested that tilapia and shrimp should be gutted and headed before refrigeration. Similarly, Irianto and Irianto (1997) reported that icing is an effective method for extending shelf life of tilapia and improving their quality.

A number of studies evaluated the effects of chilled storage on the physicochemical properties of tilapia, including sensory changes, pH, microbial counts, proximate composition and shelf life. Rodrigues et al. (2008) found that the values for the volatile nitrogen bases (VNB) and trimethylamine of Nile tilapia stored in ice for 28 days were within the permissible limits (30 mg $100\ g^{-1}$ and 4 mg $100\ g^{-1}$, respectively) for 22 days of storage. The microbial counts were also within the legal range for up to 18 days. The authors concluded that tilapia could be stored in ice for up to 18 days. In another, long-term study, Emire and Gebremariam (2010) evaluated the effects of storage duration on the proximate composition, pH, VNB and microbiology of Nile tilapia fillets frozen for up to 90 days. Protein, moisture and ash contents decreased, while lipid content increased, with storage. Both VNB and pH increased, and the total bacterial count decreased after 90 days of frozen storage. However, despite the decrease in fillet quality, it was still valid for human consumption.

10.4.2 Filleting

Among commercial aquaculture species, tilapia is the most difficult to process and has a relatively low fillet yield (33%) compared to salmon (>50%), catfish (>38%), striped bass (>40%), sea bream, sea bass and others (Snir, 2001). The main product of tilapia processing is the fillet (Fig. 10.4). Filleting yield depends on machinery efficiency, operator experience, fish shape and filleting method. Souza and Macedo-Viegas (2000) evaluated the effects of four different filleting methods on the processing yield of Nile tilapia in Brazil. The filleting methods were (1) skinning and filleting the whole fish; (2) filleting the whole fish and then removing the skin; (3) skinning and filleting headless fish and (4) filleting headless fish and then removing the skin. The best fillets and total eatable yield (36.59% and 42.15%, respectively) were obtained with skinning the whole fish before filleting, followed by filleting and skinning headless fish. Skinning and filleting the whole fish also produced thicker and longer fillets compared to other methods. The type of head cut used during processing may also affect the dressout and yield of tilapia, as reported by Souza et al. (2000). These authors found that contour and oblique head cuts produced better dressout and yield than straight head cuts.

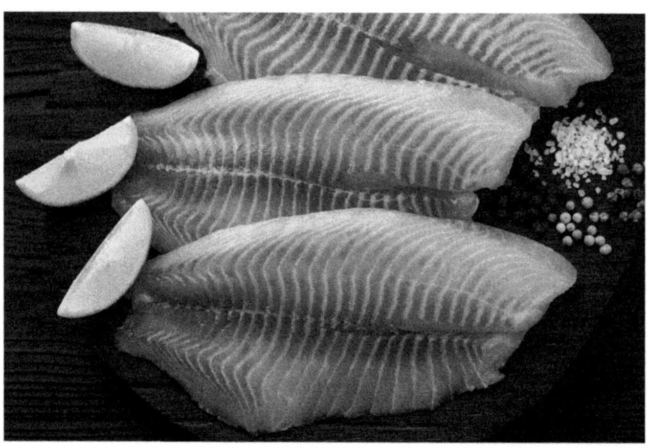

FIGURE 10.4 Tilapia fillet. *Source: Shutterstock.*

The retail market of tilapia fillets has been rapidly developing during the past decades. The consumers' demand for fresh products has also been increasing progressively. Therefore, the need for prolonged shelf life of fresh fillets has become imperative. The quality, freshness and shelf life of tilapia fillets have been evaluated under different storage and processing conditions. The shelf life of air and modified atmosphere-packaged fresh Nile tilapia fillets stored under chilled and superchilled conditions was assessed (Cyprian et al., 2013). Harvested fish were filleted, de-skinned, and packaged in air and 50% CO_2/50% N_2 prior to chilling and superchilling storage at 1°C and −1°C. Sensory analysis of cooked samples, total viable counts and pseudomonad counts indicated that air packaging in a high-barrier film bag at −1°C storage maintained the best fillet quality and longest shelf life. The use of ozonated water as a disinfectant for removing microorganisms in Nile tilapia was also investigated (de Mendonça Silva and Gonçalves, 2017). Whole fish and fish fillets were immersed in cold water (11°C), with 0.0, 0.5, 1.0 and 1.5 ppm ozone for 0, 5, 10, and 15 min. The most efficient ozone concentration for microbiological contamination reduction of the whole fish and fillet was 1.5 ppm for 15 min. These results prove that the use of ozone technology during fish processing is an effective way of reducing the microbial load and maintaining the quality of the fish.

10.4.3 Drying

Drying is a technology commonly used in processing and preservation of agricultural and aquatic products. Heat drying, osmotic dehydration and chemical extraction of moisture are the major drying methods (Duan et al., 2011), with heat drying with hot air being the most popular (Fig. 10.5). However, prolonged hot-air drying and high drying temperature may lead to deterioration of product quality, flavour, colour and rehydration rate, in addition to increased energy consumption in processing.

A number of studies have considered the use of different drying techniques in drying tilapia, including solar tunnel dryer (Kituu et al., 2010), hot air-microwave heating (Duan et al., 2011; Zhi-qiang et al., 2012), heat pump drying (Li et al., 2017), sun drying and microwave drying (Chaijan et al., 2017) and osmotic dehydration (Liu et al.,

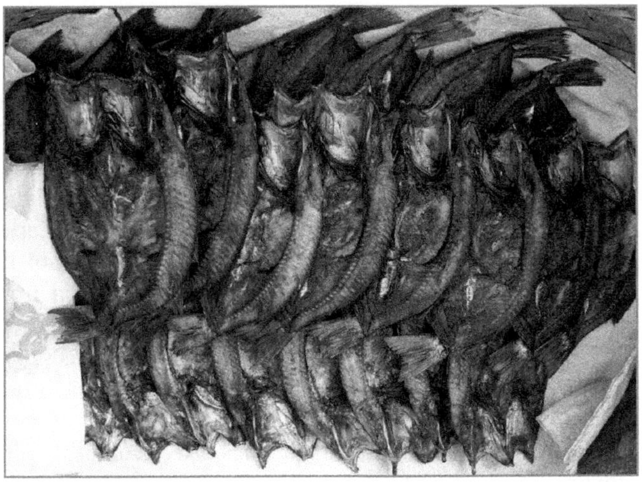

FIGURE 10.5 Heat-dried tilapia (*Oreochromis shiranus*) in Malawi. *Photograph by A.-F. M. El-Sayed.*

2018). Duan et al. (2011) evaluated the effect of hot air-microwave heating on the dryness and quality of fresh tilapia fillets. The fillets were dried in hot air at two air temperatures (40 and 50°C) and then exposed to three microwave powers (200, 400 and 600 W). At the same exposure time, the increase in microwave power resulted in a decrease in final moisture content, whereas the dehydration rate increased with increasing hot air temperature. The shrinkage and rehydration ratios increased, but the recovery ratio decreased, as the microwave power and air temperature increased. The authors concluded that lower hot air temperature and microwave power are better for maintaining the quality of tilapia fillets.

Sun drying is a popular method for drying tilapia, particularly in tropical and subtropical regions. However, this method can lead to significant deterioration of fish quality and may pose health risks. Chaijan et al. (2017) investigated the effect of sun drying and microwave drying at different effective powers on the physicochemical changes of semidried Nile tilapia. The analysis included lipid deterioration, protein oxidation and discolouration of fish muscle. The results indicated that these quality parameters were influenced by drying methods. The pH of microwaved tilapia increased with increasing microwave power and was higher than that of the sun-dried fish. Sun drying led to higher lipid oxidation and lipolysis levels than microwave drying. Muscle protein carbonyl content was also higher in microwaved tilapia than in sun-dried fish; and this component increased with increasing microwave power. In addition, sun drying resulted in a brown discolouration associated with high metmyoglobin formation, whereas microwave drying caused a green discolouration.

Liu et al. (2018) developed a novel drying method based on vacuum-microwave dehydration to investigate the effects of microwave gap ratios (MGRs), microwave times, power densities and degrees of vacuum after osmotic pretreatment on tilapia fillets. They found that the fillet moisture decreased with increasing drying time, power density and vacuum degree. The rehydration ratio, shrinkage ratio and total colour change increased with elevated microwave time and power density. The overall fillet quality was improved at higher degrees of vacuum. The authors concluded that osmotically pre-treated tilapia fillets can retain their original quality properties at MGR = 2; microwave time = 10 min; power density = 20 W g^{-1} and vacuum degree = 0.08 MPa.

10.4.4 Rigor mortis

It is important to throw some light on rigor mortis phenomenon in order to assure that the quality of the product is retained during production, processing and storage. Rigor mortis is the rigidity or stiffness of the fish body that occurs after death. The onset of rigor mortis may vary from about 10 min to several hours after death. This natural phenomenon may therefore influence the appearance and structure of fish muscles and render it unsuitable for filleting. Jarding et al. (2000) examined the occurrence of rigor mortis in farmed Nile tilapia at a commercial processor in Zimbabwe. Live fish were killed by cranial fracture or bleeding for 10 min after severance of the gills and/or the ventral aorta, and rigor mortis was then measured. The fish were left at an ambient temperature (20 ± 3°C) or iced at 2−5°C. The occurrence of rigor mortis took place within 1−1.5 h and was faster for fish stored on ice than those stored at ambient temperature, while the effects of killing methods were not different. It has also been reported that stressed fish go into rigor mortis more rapidly than unstressed fish and also generate more tension in their muscles postmortem (Nakayama et al., 1992). Similarly, Viegas et al. (2013) evaluated the physicochemical changes in Nile tilapia refrigerated for up to 92 h and in their frozen fillets. Tilapia were slaughtered by iced water shock (1:1) in a temperature of about 2°C for 30 min and refrigerated at 4°C in ice-containing polystyrene boxes. The fish were then filleted, and the fillets were weighed, frozen and the drip loss and protein were determined after 23 days. All fish were in full rigor mortis after 4 h of storage. The muscle pH decreased for up to 45 h of the storage period. The fillets obtained from tilapia stored for over 72 h lost more weight and protein. The authors concluded that tilapia filleting or processing should be done before 72 h of cold storage, since deterioration of the fish starts to occur after this period. The rapid rigor mortis may render filleting tilapia difficult or even impossible, due to the stiffness of the muscles and their inability to appear in a relaxed stage after entering stiffening phase (Jarding et al., 2000).

It is clear that filleting tilapia during rigor mortis is not a good idea and it is not recommended since it has an adverse effect on fillet quality. Tilapia stay in rigor mortis for at least 1 week, leading to decreased shelf life. Therefore, they must be processed before rigor mortis because waiting for filleting after the end of rigor mortis may lead to fish spoilage. It is also necessary to freeze the fish prior to rigor mortis because they usually develop gaping when they are frozen. It appears from this discussion that the low fillet yield of tilapia (35%—43%) and the problem of rigor mortis make the fillet market difficult to enter and develop.

10.4.5 Radiation

Radiation can be an effective tool for maintaining high fish quality and enhancing the shelf life of processed fish. Radiation is generally combined with cooling. Cozzo-Siqueira et al. (2003) evaluated the effects of combining ionizing radiation and refrigeration with minimal processing on the shelf life of processed Nile tilapia in Brazil. The physical, chemical, nutritional and microbiological characteristics of the fish were studied in eviscerated samples and in commercial cuts. The fish were irradiated with 0, 1.0, 2.2 and 5 kGy and stored at temperatures ranging from 0.5 to 2°C for 20 and 30 days. During storage, the level of moisture in the nonirradiated samples decreased and the levels of protein and lipid increased, while the irradiated samples remained stable. Muscle amino acids and fatty acids remained stable in the irradiated samples but decreased in the nonirradiated samples. The levels of total volatile base (TVBN) and nonprotein nitrogen increased in the nonirradiated samples but tended to remain stable in the irradiated fish samples. The microbiological content in the irradiated samples was below the levels established by Brazilian seafood legislation, whereas the nonirradiated samples had a higher microbiological content. In addition, lipid oxidation tended to increase with increasing irradiation dose.

Monteiro et al. (2018) investigated the separate or combined effects of high hydrostatic pressure (HHP) and ultraviolet radiation (UV-C) on the physical, chemical and bacterial characteristic of Nile tilapia fillets stored at 4°C for 2 weeks. UV-C was applied at a dose of 0.103 J cm^{-2}, and HHP at a pressure of 220 MPa for 10 min at 25°C. Fillet samples were analyzed for total aerobic mesophilic count, total aerobic psychrotrophic count, Enterobacteriaceae count, pH, lipid oxidation, TVBN, ammonia (NH_3) and biogenic amines. Both UV-C and HHP, separate or combined, reduced bacterial growth and delayed the increase in pH, TVBN, NH_3 and biogenic amines during refrigerated storage. The shelf life of refrigerated tilapia fillets were extended at least 2.5 times. Lipid oxidation was not affected by UV-C radiation; however, it was decreased by HHP and UV-C + HHP. These results demonstrate that HHP alone or combined with UV-C show high potential benefits for tilapia fillets preservation.

10.5 Economics

Typically, tilapia marketing is controlled by the following factors: (1) production systems; (2) operating costs; (3) competition among producers; (4) degree of processing; (5) production scale and (6) consumer demand. For example, production costs in the United States and Canada are higher than those in Central America, Latin America, the Caribbean and other tropical regions due to the high cost of labour, energy and operating costs. Importing tilapia from these regions would be more profitable than farming them in North America (Watanabe et al., 2002). This gives tropical producers a competitive advantage over US and Canadian producers.

However, this disadvantage can be overcome by optimizing resource utilization, such as using fertilization for the production of tilapia fingerlings, and improving production management (Hargreaves and Behrends, 1997; Watanabe et al., 2002).

Since the production system is probably the most important factor affecting tilapia marketing and economics, it is discussed further in the following section. The cost-effectiveness of some farming systems is also described under various culture conditions, in order to help tilapia farmers and farm operators and managers adopt the most economically sound farming system.

10.5.1 System economics

Tilapia are cultured mostly in semi-intensive systems, where operating costs are low and culture inputs are minimal. Intensive tilapia culture with high investment and maximum inputs is also practiced in many countries, but at smaller scales. The expected outputs of culture practices are therefore a function of the culture systems adopted and the inputs to these systems. A number of studies have been carried out to evaluate and analyze the economic returns of different farming systems in different geographical locations. Such analyses would certainly help fish farmers and farm managers adopt the most sustainable and economically feasible systems.

Samonte et al. (1991) compared the economic feasibility of the polyculture of tiger shrimp (*P. monodon*) with Nile tilapia in brackish-water ponds in the Philippines. A stocking combination of 6000 shrimp and 4000 tilapia ha^{-1} produced the highest total yields and net income compared to monoculture of tilapia or shrimp. Two crops per year provided a 70% return on investment and 1.2 years payback. Sensitivity analysis revealed that shrimp/tilapia polyculture was profitable up to a 20% decrease in the selling price of both species.

The feasibility of small-scale hapa culture of Nile tilapia as an additional income source for rice farmers in northeast Thailand has also been evaluated (Middendorp and Verreth, 1992) using different production scenarios. Rice farmers stocked tilapia at an initial weight of 50 g to reach marketable size after 85 days. Investment costs were about 5% of total operating costs. Fingerling costs (about 25% of total costs) could be reduced significantly when fingerlings were collected from backyard ponds or from the hapas. Feed costs, which represented about 70% of total costs, could also be reduced by optimizing the feeding regime and using home-mixing of fish feed and extending the rearing period to 100 days. A density of 14 fish (50 g) m^{-3} was suggested to reach a market size of 216 g in 100 days. If smaller sizes (<50 g) are stocked, two rearing cycles (about 200 days) will be needed to reach market size. In this way, rice farmers may increase their household income by about 20%.

The economics and profitability of artisanal and commercial tilapia culture in Malawi is another example of the importance of system analysis (Stewart, 1993). Considering the local support services including fry and fingerling supply and local market development, it was found that polyculture of Nile tilapia and African catfish (*Clarias gariepinus*) in earthen ponds was more cost-effective than other culture systems.

The economic and engineering evaluation of tilapia production in a small recirculating culture system using computer simulation model has been described in the United States (Losordo and Westerman, 1994). Sensitivity analysis indicated that, among all operational variables tested, reducing feed cost and improving FCR were the most effective variables in reducing the production costs. Increasing productive capacity or decreasing the investment cost also increased system profitability. Head et al. (1996) found that feed, processing and distribution and sex-reversed fry represented the highest variable costs in commercial scale, seawater pond production of Florida red tilapia in Puerto Rico, while salaries and depreciation accounted for the highest fixed costs. At a stocking density of 2 fish m^{-2}, the proposed production was not economical, while increasing the density to 3.5 and 4 fish m^{-2} increased the profitability of the operation. Using locally prepared feed together with the integration of hatchery and grow-out operations are also suggested for reducing operational costs and increasing return.

Similarly, Head and Watanabe (1995) evaluated the economics of a commercial scale, recirculating, brackish-water hatchery for Florida red tilapia (*Oreochromis urolepus hornerum* x *Oreochromis mossambicus*) in the Bahamas, using previously collected production data. Salaries and benefits were the largest fixed costs. Airfreight shipping to Miami, Florida, represented the largest variable cost when air charters were used. The study indicated that the system is economically feasible if fry can be sold year-round, while seasonal market demand may limit the economic return. The authors reported also that more economic success can be achieved if more economical building construction, modifications in rearing tank design, and vertical integration of hatchery and grow-out operations, with external sales of excess fry and broodstock are adopted. When the economic and technical feasibility of tilapia cage culture in Ghana were investigated, using least cost easily available local inputs (Oduro-Boateng, 1998), the sensitivity analysis indicated that the internal rate of return was 58%, meaning that the investment in tilapia cage culture in Ghana is highly profitable, especially in rural areas, where the system can be easily adopted by rural farmers.

In Egypt, which is a major tilapia producer (third in the world after China and Indonesia), tilapia is practiced mainly in semi-intensive systems in earthen ponds. Intensive farming of tilapia in ponds, tanks and cages and recirculating aquaculture systems is also practiced at various scales. The cost and cost—benefit ratio of tilapia farms vary considerably and are dependent on the culture system, the availability and costs of inputs and the geographical region. However, all farming systems appear cost-effective with varying degrees of profitability. In semi-intensive systems, the benefit—cost ratio (BCR) ranged from 1.3 to 1.5. Intensive culture in ponds and cages exhibit much better BCR (Table 10.1). This is mainly due to the better access that intensive tilapia farmers have to funds, technology and production inputs, and thus they can operate systems with much higher operational and capital investment (El-Sayed, 2017). In contrast, the limited access of small-scale semi-intensive farmers to funding and production inputs leads to low total costs, revenue and BCR; however, this practice is still very profitable to these farmers.

These results clearly indicate that system analysis is necessary for successful rural aquaculture practices. This is simply because each geographical location has it own unique characteristics. In other words, the culture inputs that may be limiting in one place may not be so in another. Accordingly, system analysis would provide the farmer with different culture scenarios, so that he can choose the most cost-effective scenario.

10.5.2 Risk analysis

It is evident from the above examples that economic analyses applied to tilapia culture enterprises are specific to the culture system. This means that each system has its own risk and therefore enterprises that generate higher returns must accept higher risks. Thus, economic analyses that indicate higher economic return must also report the higher risk, so that the producer can be aware of such risks. Nevertheless, most economic studies concerning tilapia culture are directed to technical and economic practices and incentives (as mentioned in the previous sections), with

TABLE 10.1 Economic performance of tilapia farming in Egypt.

Costs and returns (US$)	SI (earthen ponds)[1]	Intensive systems		
		Cages[2]	Concrete tanks[2]	Recirculating aquaculture systems[3]
Farm size	8.3 ha	600 m^3	4.2 ha	140 m^3
Total variable costs (TVC):	14,664	14,756	19,336	7,704
Seeds	606	262	545	4,333
Feeds	12,000	13,630	16,364	2,327
Fertilizers	991	0.0	0.0	0.0
Labour	629	364	727	522
Energy and fuel	255	0.0	700	522
Miscellaneous costs	183	500	1,000	0.0
Total fixed costs (TFC):	543	300	2,680	486
Depreciation:	366	300	1,000	486
Construction depreciation	123	NA*	NA	NA
Equipment depreciation	243	NA	NA	NA
Land use cost (rental)	177	0.0	1,680	NA
Total costs (TC) = TVC + TFC	15,384	15,056	22,016	8,190
Total gross revenue (GR)	21,221	29,000	32,000	11,230
Net return (NR) = GR − TC	5,837	13,944	9,984	3,040
Benefit–cost ratio (BCR) = GR/TC	1.38	1.93	1.45	1.37

SI, semi-intensive system; *NA*, not available.
[1]*Naziri (2011);*
[2]*El-Sayed (2013);*
[3]*Radwan and Leschen (2011).*
Adapted from El-Sayed (2017).

little attention to economic risk. It is essential that economic analyses of aquaculture projects consider not only economic benefits but also the 'down-side' risk and risk potential.

In an earlier study, El-Sayed (1990) evaluated feeding Nile tilapia with cottonseed meal (CSM) containing different protein levels compared with a fish meal (FM)-based diet. Fish fed hulled CSM (25% crude protein (cp)) resulted in the lowest fish performance. However, cost–benefit analyses indicated that this diet was economically the best, followed by the dehulled CSM (40% cp), while the FM-based diet had the lowest economic return. Similarly, Hatch and Falck (2001) evaluated alternative production systems of tilapia in Honduras, in terms of profitability and risks. They developed "user friendly tools" to assess the economic performance of these systems, and at what level of risk to tilapia producers. Economic indicators of profitability and risk were determined using baseline production data such as nutrient inputs, stocking rates, etc., in addition to the prices of nutrient inputs and sale prices of fish. The authors concluded that this evaluation procedure will allow researchers to use their limited resources more efficiently through directing their research to production strategies that are likely to be profitable at an acceptable risk level.

A number of studies have analyzed the risk of tilapia culture in Kenya. Veverica et al. (2001) compared the performance and economic benefits of polyculture of Nile tilapia and African catfish in earthen ponds in Kenya, under different feeding and fertilization regimes, using low-cost, locally available resources. In addition to fertilization, the fishes received rice bran (RB), pig finisher pellets (PFPs) or a test diet (20% cp) for 180 days. The RB produced the lowest growth, while PFP resulted in the highest performance. Relative profitability analysis indicated that PFP was economically the best, followed by RB. However, RB had the lowest break-even price and the least investment cost. This result revealed that using low-cost ingredients such as RB in semi-intensive polyculture of tilapia could be highly profitable with minimal risks, especially in developing countries where resources are limited.

In another study, the polyculture of Nile tilapia and African catfish in earthen ponds in Kenya was reassessed under other feeding and fertilization regimes (Omondi et al., 2001). The fishes received the following combinations of RB and fertilizer in order to realize the least-cost combination: (1) urea and diammonium phosphate (DAP) to provide 16 kg of N and 4 kg of P ha^{-1} wk^{-1}, (2) urea and DAP to provide 8 and 4 kg of N and P ha^{-1} per wk, respectively, in addition to RB fed at 60 kg ha^{-1} per day, (3) RB fed at 120 kg ha^{-1} per day and (4) RB at 120 kg ha^{-1} per day plus urea and DAP at 8 kg of N and 4 kg P ha^{-1} per week. The economic analyses indicated that the net profits of polyculture were lower than that of monoculture of Nile tilapia and catfish, but were higher for treatment (1) followed by treatment (2) and significantly reduced in treatments (3) and (4) because of the high cost of feed and fingerlings. This study indicated that the inclusion of RB was less cost-effective than fertilizer alone. Similarly, Neira et al. (2009) evaluated the profitability and risks of tilapia culture industry in Kenya. Information collected from pond experiments, on-farm trials and farm surveys was used for a risk analysis for nine production scenarios, including (1) monoculture of all-male tilapia fed either RB, a pelleted experimental diet, or a pelleted pig finisher diet; (2) African catfish monoculture fed with each of the three mentioned diets and (3) tilapia—catfish polyculture fed with each of the three diets. Economic analysis indicated that the highest net profits were achieved in catfish and tilapia, respectively, in monoculture system, followed by polyculture practice, while the lowest net return was obtained with catfish fed RB.

The above results look contradictory to that of Veverica et al. (2001) who recommended the use of RB as a low-cost ingredient for tilapia polyculture systems. This controversy could be attributed to the differences in the cost of culture inputs (seeds, feed, fertilizer, transportation, labour, etc.) between the studies. Once again, this controversy means that economic analyses are system specific, and each system has its own risk.

In China, the economic efficiency of small-scale tilapia farms in Guangxi has been analyzed (Zongli et al., 2017) using Data Envelopment Analysis. The mean technical (under the constant returns-to-scale and Voluntary Retirement Scheme), allocative and economic efficiencies of small-scale tilapia farms were 0.89, 0.97, 0.71 and 0.68, respectively. Economic efficiency analysis indicated that when small-scale tilapia farms are inefficient, they will need to increase production by 32% in order to achieve performance comparable to the farms which adopt the best aquaculture practice. Allocative inefficiency was the main cause of the overall economic inefficiency. Positive relationships existed between economic inefficiency and age, culture mode and farming period, while family members, farmer's experience and technology support were negatively correlated with economic efficiency. Another comprehensive study was carried out to analyze the economic profitability of tilapia farming in the major tilapia producing provinces in China (Guangdong, Hainan, Guangxi, Fujian and Yunnan) (Yuan et al., 2017). Small (<1 ha), medium (1—10 ha) and large (>10 ha) tilapia farms were used to estimate the costs and benefits in monoculture, polyculture and integrated farming systems. The analysis revealed that large farms achieved the highest costs and the highest cost—benefit margin, followed by medium-size farms, while small farms have the lowest cost and lowest profit margin. The BCR of small, medium and large farms was 1.26, 1.33 and 1.37, respectively. However, sensitivity analysis indicated that the net profit of tilapia farming in these provinces is flexible to the change of price, feed, rent and fixed costs, of which price elasticity was the highest, followed by the feed, rent and fixed costs.

The above results clearly demonstrate that the practice that may produce the best yield may not necessarily be the most cost-effective. This emphasizes the need for economic and risk analyses for tilapia culture projects concomitant with biological and technical analyses, prior to the start of the project. Such analyses will help the farmer use the available resources in a sustainable manner and adopt the most efficient production strategy.

10.6 The value chain analysis of farmed tilapia

A value chain (VC) is defined as a chain of practices and services taking place to bring a product or service from its conception to final customers, and final disposal after use (Hellin and Meijer, 2006). In this concept, VCs must include all stakeholders; from suppliers through producers, processors to final end users, supported by technical, business and financial service providers. Value chain analysis (VCA) is a multidimensional analytical tool for understanding and assessing the performance of each component of the VC, including the analysis of product flows, information flows and management of the whole VC. VCA has been used to assess the performance in different systems, including the factors affecting competitiveness, the costs and earnings of each cycle of the VC, identifying and analyzing gaps and weaknesses in VC performance and suggesting appropriate upgrading, management and development strategies to improve VC performance (Macfadyen et al., 2012).

Aquaculture is currently one of the fastest growing and most important food production systems in the world. The analysis of aquaculture VC, with emphasis on the creation and synthesis of new knowledge and perspectives is necessary. VC in aquaculture has a number of benefits such as providing policymakers, fisheries and aqua farm managers with a systematic tool which enables them to understand and analyze the processes and added values in the industry. Value addition is an important concept in fisheries and aquaculture as it promotes better profit, more stable market conditions, job opportunities and product diversification (Russell and Haanoomanjae, 2012).

Despite the importance of tilapia culture as a key player in global aquaculture production, market and trade, only a handful of studies have analyzed their VCs in just a few countries. In Egypt, for example, the tilapia VC is simple and short, but rather efficient. It takes only 1 to 2 days from harvest to the final consumer, with low post-harvest loss (Macfadyen et al., 2012). The local distribution system is also quite efficient, mainly because most production sites are located near heavily populated areas (Rothuis et al., 2013). Tilapia VC in Egypt includes only three main categories before reaching the final end user, namely fish producers (input production, farming, harvesting, handling and transportation), fish traders (wholesalers) and retailers. The components of each ring of the whole VC of tilapia culture in Egypt are listed in Fig. 10.6.

Anane-Taabeah et al. (2016) assessed the VC of farmed tilapia in Ghana to identify the key actors, flow of products and information, costs and profit margins, and relationships among the various actors. They found that, except fish farmers, all major chain actors identified (input suppliers, traders and food services) have positive profit margins. Most of the margins generated along the chain go to input suppliers. The authors concluded that the efficiency and profitability of tilapia VC in Ghana can be improved through establishing well-defined payment transaction with customers, persistent relationships with customers and good information management system. Fish farmers should reduce their variable costs, price their fish using a cost plus or percentage markup in order to be more profitable.

In another study, also in Ghana, the VC of the tilapia aquaculture sector was analyzed (Asiedu et al., 2016). Particular areas of intervention and development opportunities to achieve food security and nutrition needs, safety, quality and trade benefits were identified. The analysis indicated that most tilapia supplies come from cage culture (85%) and all farmed tilapia products are locally consumed. The demand for tilapia in the domestic market is increasing, especially among middle and lower classes. The marketing channel involves farmers selling to wholesalers/retailers and also to consumers and restaurants in nearby villages or secondary towns. Only sun drying and small-size smokers are the processing technologies adopted. Processed farmed tilapia, especially smoked and salted fish, have the potential for export. In order to achieve this, a practical guide for aquaculture exporters should be developed and the capacity of public institutions should be strengthened to properly deal with the export requirements of aquaculture products.

Ndanga (2012) evaluated the VC for tilapia and catfish products and the opportunities for female participation in Kenya. The study found that input supply is a major constraint for all VC actors in aquaculture industry. Tilapia and catfish production is dominated by males, but with full engagement of women. Women participation is restricted to harvesting, post-harvest fish handling and marketing. The study identified the opportunities for female participation in different aspects of the tilapia and catfish VC. Women participation depends on the woman's characteristics and objectives. For example, female participants seeking flexibility and liquidity should join fish marketing, while those with good educational and technical backgrounds who seek financial strength should consider input supply and those looking for long-term stability should consider fish farming.

The major actors involved in the VC of farmed Nile tilapia in Tanzania (Coast, Dar es Salaam, Mwanza and Geita regions) were also identified, characterized and mapped (Ayubu, 2017), and the areas of upgrade and improvement in VC were defined. Marketing margins of the different subsectors along the VC from tilapia farmers to consumers were also analyzed, and key constraints affecting different actors were identified. The major constraints facing tilapia farmers in the country include shortage of water, unavailability and/or high cost of farming inputs (e.g. seeds, feeds and fertilizers, gas, electricity), limited knowledge on the knowhow of fish farming, marketing difficulties and low security. The study concluded that farmers need training on farm-made feed production using locally available ingredients. The study further suggested that actors at each level in the chain should be grouped in order to access loans, and farmers should be given financial capital assistance.

The VC of tilapia in southern region of Bangladesh has been evaluated by the WorldFish (2012). Results revealed that the demand for tilapia in local markets may not be met in the short run, meaning that the market will absorb all produced tilapia. In the long run, the market demand will possibly be saturated, leading to a decrease in sale prices. The region should look for tilapia export; this would provide a chance for processing plants to play a role in tilapia fillet market. However, extensive efforts are needed to enter the export market, including basic research on export competitiveness, establishment of support industries to utilize fillet by-products and market promotion. The main constraint of tilapia in local market is that the sale prices are much higher than the international market prices. Tilapia is produced in polyculture systems with other local fishes, mainly in homestead small ponds, where women engagement is high, especially in unpaid labour activities, such as feeding. These small farmers rely on their own sources,

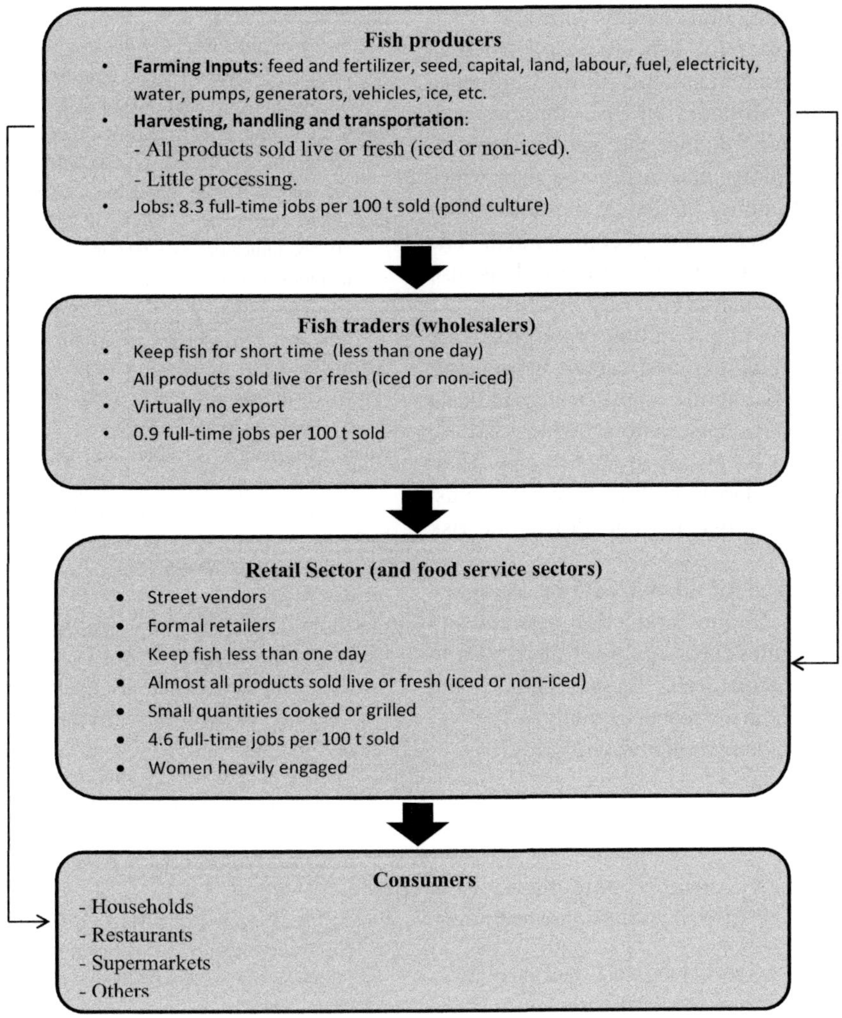

FIGURE 10.6 Value chain of tilapia culture in Egypt. *Modified from El-Sayed (2017).*

with limited access to finance, whereas large farmers, who have adequate properties, are accessible to bank loans.

10.7 Closing remarks

1. There is no specific harvesting system for farmed tilapia, but partial harvest may be the best cost-effective, but this technique should be evaluated biologically and economically. Cheap and locally available harvesting tools should also be adopted.
2. Different handling, slaughtering and pre-processing techniques are used in tilapia culture. Poor handling, inadequate processing and holding conditions, and inappropriate processing methods may deteriorate the quality of tilapia and increase post-harvest losses. Proper handling, transportation and displaying should, therefore, be used.
3. Fish should be protected from stress, pain or suffering during transport, restraint, stunning, slaughter or killing.
4. Stunning should be applied to the fish to induce unconsciousness and insensibility to pain stimuli for sufficient duration to assure that they do not recover during killing or bleeding. Stunning should be induced immediately to optimize animal welfare and also to minimize possible negative effects of these procedures on meat quality.
5. Cooling (icing, refrigeration, freezing, etc.), filleting, radiation and industrial processing (drying, smoking, canning, fish balls and sausages, etc.) are commonly used for processing tilapia.
6. Tilapia guts should be removed before refrigeration, because the spoilage rate is more rapid in gut-containing fish than in gutless fish.
7. Tilapia are difficult to process and have relatively low fillet yield. Skinning off the whole fish before filleting may produce the best fillet and total eatable yield. Contour and oblique head cuts may also produce better fillet yield than straight head cuts.

8. Rigor mortis takes place immediately within 1−1.5 h after death and is faster for fish stored on ice than those stored at ambient temperatures. It may influence the appearance and structure of fish muscles and render it unsuitable for filleting. Stressed fish go into rigor mortis more rapidly than unstressed fish. Rigor mortis reduces fillet quality of tilapia, therefore filleting during rigor mortis is not recommended. The fish must be processed before rigor mortis. It is also necessary to freeze the fish prior to rigor mortis.
9. Economic analyses of tilapia culture enterprises are specific to the culture system and cannot be generalized to all systems. Economic analyses that indicate higher economic return must report higher risk, so that the producer can be aware of such a risk. Economic analyses of tilapia culture projects must consider both economic benefits and down-side risk and risk potential.
10. Despite the importance of tilapia culture as a key player in global aquaculture production, market and trade, only a few studies have analyzed their VCs in a few countries (Bangladesh, Egypt, Ghana and Kenya). More studies are needed to analyze the VC of farmed tilapia in other producing countries.

References

Anane-Taabeah, G., Quagrainie, K., Amisah, S., 2016. Assessment of farmed tilapia value chain in Ghana. Aquaculture International 24, 903−919.

Asiedu, B., Failler, P., Beyens, Y., 2016. Enhancing aquaculture development: mapping the tilapia aquaculture value chain in Ghana. Reviews in Aquaculture 8, 394−402.

Ayubu, S., 2017. Value Chain Analysis of Farmed Nile Tilapia in Selected Areas, Tanzania (M.Sc. thesis). Sokoine University of Agriculture, Morogoro, Tanzania, p. 186.

Bjørlykke, G.A., Roth, B., Sørheim, O., Kvamme, B.O., Slinde, E., 2011. The effects of carbon monoxide on Atlantic salmon (*Salmo salar* L). Food Chemistry 127, 1706−1711.

Brummett, R.E., 2002. Comparison of African tilapia partial harvesting systems. Aquaculture 214, 103−114.

Chaijan, M., Panpipat, W., Nisoa, M., 2017. Chemical deterioration and discoloration of semi-dried tilapia processed by sun drying and microwave drying. Drying Technology 35, 642−649.

Chandroo, K.P., Duncan, I.J.H., Moccia, R.D., 2004. Can fish suffer?: perspectives on sentience, pain, fear and stress. Applied Animal Behaviour Science 86, 225−250.

Cozzo-Siqueira, A., Oetterer, M., Gallo, C.R., 2003. Effects of irradiation and refrigeration on the nutrients and shelf-life of tilapia (*Oreochromis niloticus*). Journal of Aquatic Food Product Technology 12, 85−102.

Cyprian, O., Lauzon, H.L., Jóhannsson, R., Sveinsdóttir, K., Arason, S., Martinsdóttir, E., 2013. Shelf life of air and modified atmosphere-packaged fresh tilapia (*Oreochromis niloticus*) fillets stored under chilled and superchilled conditions. Food Science & Nutrition 1, 130−140.

de Mendonça Silva, A.M., Gonçalves, A.A., 2017. Effect of aqueous ozone on microbial and physicochemical quality of Nile tilapia processing. Journal of Food Processing and Preservation 41 e13298. https://doi.org/10.1111/jfpp.13298.

de Oliveira Filho, P.R.C., Oliveira, C.A.F., Sobral, P.J.A., Balieiro, J.C.C., Natori, M.M., Viegas, E.M.M., 2015a. How stunning methods affect the quality of Nile tilapia meat. CyTA - Journal of Food 13, 56−62.

de Oliveira Filho, P.R.C., Giraro, P.J.M., de Melo, M.P., Viegas, E.M.M., 2015b. Indicators of stress in tilapia subjected to different stunning methods. Boletim do Instituto de Pesca Sao Paulo 41, 335−343.

de Oliveira Filho, P.R.C., do Amaral Sobral, P.J., de Carvalho Balieiro, J.C., Viegas, E.M.M., 2017. Comparison of stunning methods on the physicochemical properties of frozen Nile tilapia (*Oreochromis niloticus*) fillets. Journal of Aquatic Food Product Technology 26, 325−334.

Duan, Z.H., Jiang, L.N., Wang, J.I., Yu, X.Y., Wang, T., 2011. Drying and quality characteristics of tilapia fish fillets dried with hot air-microwave heating. Food and Bioproducts Processing 89, 472−476.

El-Sayed, A.-F.M., 1990. Long-term evaluation of cotton seed meal as a protein source for Nile tilapia, *Oreochromis niloticus*. Aquaculture 84, 315−320.

El-Sayed, A.-F.M., 2013. On-farm feed management practices for Nile tilapia *(Oreochromis niloticus)* in Egypt. In: Hasan, M.R., New, M.B. (Eds.), On-farm Feeding and Feed Management in Aquaculture. FAO Fisheries and Aquaculture Technical Paper No. 583. FAO, Rome, pp. 101−129.

El-Sayed, A.-F.M., 2017. Social and economic performance of tilapia farming in Egypt. In: Cai, J., Quagrainie, K.K., Hishamunda, N. (Eds.), Social and Economic Performance of Tilapia Farming in Africa. FAO Fisheries and Aquaculture Circular No. 1130. FAO, Rome, pp. 1−48.

Emire, S.A., Gebremariam, M.M., 2010. Influence of frozen period on the proximate composition and microbiological quality of Nile tilapia fish (*Oreochromis niloticus*). Journal of Food Processing and Preservation 34, 743−757.

Enujiugha, V.N., Nwanna, L.C., 1998. The impacts of post harvest losses on supply and demand for *Clarias gariepinus* (Clariidae) and *Oreochromis niloticus* (Cichlidae) in Nigeria. In: Coetzee, L., Gon, J., Kulongowski, C. (Eds.), African Fishes and Fisheries diversity and Utilisation. International Conference for the Paradi Association and the Fisheries Society of Africa, FISA/Paradi, Grahamstown, South Africa, p. 111.

FAO (Food and Agriculture Organization of the United Nations), 2018. Fishery Commodities Global Production and Trade. http://www.fao.org/fishery/statistics/global-commodities-production/query/en.

Goes, E.S.R., Lara, J.A.F., Gasparino, E., Del Vesco, A.P., Goes, M.D., Filho, L.A., et al., 2015. Pre-slaughter stress affects ryanodine receptor protein gene expression and the water-holding capacity in fillets of the Nile tilapia. PLoS One 10 (6), e0129−145.

Guan, W.-L., Zhao, M.-M., Liu, T.-T., Fan, X., Chen, D.-W., 2017. Cooling combined with hyperoxic CO_2 anesthesia is effective in improving the air exposure duration of tilapia. Scientific Reports 7, 14016. https://doi.org/10.1038/s41598-017-14212-3.

Guerrero III., R.D., Guerrero, L.A., 2001. Domestic marketing of tilapia in Southeast Asia. In: Subasinghe, S., Singh, T. (Eds.), Tilapia: Production, Marketing and Technical Developments. Proceedings of the Tilapia 2001 International Technical and Trade Conference on Tilapia. Infofish, Kuala Lumpur, Malaysia, pp. 81−83.

Hargreaves, J.A., Behrends, L.L., 1997. Improving the economics of intensive tilapia aquaculture in the southeastern United States through integration: a conceptual assessment. In: Fitzsimmons, K. (Ed.), Proceedings from the Fourth International Symposium on Tilapia in Aquaculture. Northeast Regional Agriculture Engineering Service, Ithaca, New York, USA, pp. 642–649.

Hatch, U., Falck, J., 2001. Assessing Economic Risk in tilapia Production in Honduras. Aquaculture 2001- Book of Abstracts. World Aquaculture Society, Baton Rouge, Louisiana, USA, p. 281.

Head, W.D., Watanabe, W.O., 1995. Economic analysis of a commercial-scale, recirculating, brackishwater hatchery for Florida red tilapia. Journal of Applied Aquaculture 5, 1–24.

Head, W.D., Zerbi, A., Watanabe, W.O., 1996. Economic evaluation of commercial-scale, saltwater pond production of Florida red tilapia in Puerto Rico. Journal of the World Aquaculture Society 27, 275–289.

Hellin, J., Meijer, M., 2006. Guidelines for Value Chain Analysis. FAO, p. 24. http://www.fao.org/3/a-bq787e.pdf.

Hepher, B., Pruginin, Y., 1981. Commercial Fish Farming with Special Reference to Fish Culture in Israel. Wiley-Interscience, New York, USA, p. 261pp.

Irianto, G., Irianto, H.E., 1997. Post-harvest Technology of Nile Tilapia in Indonesia: A Review. FAO Fisheries Report, R563. FAO, Rome, pp. 71–83.

Jarding, S., Windmar, L., Paterson, R., Fjallsbak, J.P., 2000. Quality issues in commercial processing of tilapia (*Oreochromis niloticus*) in Zimbabwe. In: Fitzsimmons, K., Filho, J.C. (Eds.), Tilapia Culture in the 21st Century. Proceedings from the Fifth International Symposium on Tilapia Aquaculture. American Tilapia Association and ICLARM, Rio de Janeiro, Brazil, pp. 588–594.

Kaunda, E., Costa-Pierce, B.A., 1993. Catchability and selectivity of a low cost, traditional fishing gear in aquaculture ponds. Aquaculture and Fisheries Management 24, 783–789.

Kayan, A., Boontan, I., Jaturssitha, S., Wicke, M., Kreuzer, M., 2015. Effect of slaughter weight on meat quality of Nile tilapia (*Oreochromis niloticus*). Agriculture and Agricultural Science Procedia 5, 159–163.

Kituu, G.M., Shitanda, D., Kanali, C.L., Mailutha, J.T., Njoroge, C.K., Wainaina, J.K., et al., 2010. Thin layer drying model for simulating the drying of tilapia fish (*Oreochromis niloticus*) in a solar tunnel dryer. Journal of Food Engineering 98, 325–331.

Knud-Hansen, C.F., Lin, C.K., 1996. Strategies for stocking Nile tilapia (*Oreochromis niloticus*) in fertilized ponds. In: Pullin, R.S.V., Lazard, J., Legendre, M., Amon Kottias, J.B., Pauly, D. (Eds.), Proceedings of the Third International Symposium on Tilapia in Aquaculture. ICLARM Conference Proceedings No. 41. ICLARM, Penang, Malaysia, pp. 70–76.

Lambooij, E., Gerritzen, M.A., Reimert, H., Burggraaf, D., van de Vis, J.W., 2008. A humane protocol for electro-stunning and killing of Nile tilapia in fresh water. Aquaculture 275, 88–95.

Li, M., Wu, Y.-y., Guan, Z.-q., 2017. Effect of physical osmosis methods on quality of tilapia fillets processed by heat pump drying. Polish Journal of Food and Nutrition Sciences 67, 145–150.

Lines, J.A., Spence, J., 2014. Humane harvesting and slaughter of farmed fish. Revue Scientifique Et Technique De L Office International Des Epizooties 33, 255–264.

Liu, B., Cao, J., Feng, A., Liu, Y., Yu, Q., Li, C., et al., 2018. Effects of osmotic dehydration vacuum-microwave drying on the properties of tilapia fillets. Czech Journal of Food Sciences 36, 169–174.

Losordo, T.M., Westerman, P.W., 1994. An analysis of biological, economic, and engineering factors affecting the cost of fish production in recirculating aquaculture systems. Journal of the World Aquaculture Society 25, 193–203.

Macfadyen, G., Nasr-Alla, A.M., Kenawy, D.A., Fathi, M., Hebicha, H., Diab, A.M., et al., 2012. Value-chain analysis – an assessment methodology to estimate Egyptian aquaculture sector performance. Aquaculture 362–363, 18–27.

Mantilla, D., Kristinsson, H.G., Balaban, M.O., Otwell, W.S., Chapman, F.A., Raghavan, S., 2008. Carbon monoxide treatments to impart and retain muscle color in tilapia fillets. Journal of Food Sciences 73, 390–399.

McGinty, A.S., Alston, D.E., 1993. Multiple stocking and multiple harvesting of *Macrobrachium rosenbergii* and tilapia. In: Carrillo, M., Dahle, L., Morales, J., Sorgeloos, P., Svennevig, N., Wyban, J. (Eds.), From Discovery to Commercialization. European Aquaculture Society, Oostende (Belgium), p. 148. Special Publication No. 19.

Middendorp, A.J., Verreth, J.A.J., 1992. The feasibility of small-scale hapa culture of tilapia *Oreochromis niloticus* as an additional income source for rice farmers in northeast Thailand. Asian Fisheries Science 5, 303–314.

Monteiro, M.L.G., Mársico, E.T., Mano, S.B., da Silveira Alvares, T., Rosenthal, A., Lemos, M., et al., 2018. Combined effect of high hydrostatic pressure and ultraviolet radiation on quality parameters of refrigerated vacuum-packed tilapia (*Oreochromis niloticus*) fillets. Scientific Reports 8, 9524. https://doi.org/10.1038/s41598-018-27861-9.

Nakayama, T., Liu, D.-J., Ooi, A., 1992. Tension change of stressed and unstressed carp muscles in isometric rigor concentration and resolution. Nippon Suisan Gakkaishi 58, 1517–1522.

Naziri, D., 2011. Financial Services for SME Aquaculture Producers: Egypt Case Study. Project report funded by the German Agency for Technical Cooperation (GTZ) for the benefit of developing countries, p. 30.

Ndanga, L.Z.B., 2012. Value Chain Development for Tilapia and Catfish Products: Opportunities for Female Participation in Kenya (M.Sc. thesis). Purdue University.

Neira, I., Engle, C.R., Ngugi, C., 2009. Economic and risk analysis of tilapia production in Kenya. Journal of Applied Aquaculture 21, 73–95.

Nitithamyong, C., Chiayvareesajja, J., Chiayvareesajja, S., Wongwit, C., Tansakul, R., 1990. Production of Nile tilapia (*Oreochromis niloticus*) in different culture and harvesting systems. In: De Silva, S. (Ed.), Fish Nutrition Research in Asia. Proceedings of the Fourth Asian Fish Nutrition Workshop. Special Publication No. 5. Asian Fisheries Society, Manila, Philippines, pp. 169–174.

Oduro-Boateng, F., 1998. Tilapia cage culture in Ghana: studies on economic and technical viability. In: Coetzee, L., Gon, J., Kulongowski, C. (Eds.), African Fishes and Fisheries Diversity and Utilisation. International Conference for the Paradi Association and the Fisheries Society of Africa, Grahamstown, South Africa, p. 227.

Omondi, J.G., Gichuri, W.M., Veverica, K., 2001. A partial economic analysis for Nile tilapia *Oreochromis niloticus* L. and sharptoothed catfish *Clarias gariepinus* (Burchell 1822) polyculture in central Kenya. Aquaculture Research 32, 693–700.

Radwan, I.A., Leschen, W., 2011. Case Study on Developing Financially Viable Recirculation Aquaculture Systems (RAS) for Tilapia Production in Egypt: Technology Transfer from the Netherlands. EC FP7 Project, SARNISSA, p. 23.

Rajaratnam, S., Balasundaram, C., 2001. Qualitative and Quantitative Analysis of Fish and Prawn Maintained at Different Temperatures. The Sixth Asian Fisheries Forum- Book of Abstracts. Asian Fisheries Society, Quezon City, Philippines, p. 19.

Rodrigues, T.P., Freitas, M.Q., Mársico, E.T., Franco, R.M., Mello, S.C.R.P., Costa, I., et al., 2008. Assessing the quality of Nile tilapia (*Oreochromis niloticus*) cultured, eviscerated and stored on ice. Revista Brasileira de Medicina Veterinaria 15, 67–71.

Rothuis, A., van Duijn, A.P., Roem, A., Ouwehand, A., van der Pijl, W., Rurangwa, E., 2013. Aquaculture Business Opportunities in Egypt. Wageningen UR (University and Research Centre), Wageningen, p. 34. LEI Report 2013–039, IMARES Report C091/13.

Russell, D., Haanoomanjae, S., 2012. Manual on Value Chain Analysis and Promotion. Regional Training on Value Chain Analysis.. Project Ref. N° SA-4.1-B20 Pescares SRL Project Funded by the European Union, Italia.

Saiti, F., Jamu, D.M., Chisala, B., Kambewa, P., 2007. Simulation of optimal harvesting strategies for small-scale mixed-sex tilapia (*Oreochromis shiranus* Boulenger 1896) ponds using a bio-economic model. Aquaculture Research 38, 340–350.

Samonte, G.P., Agbayani, R.F., Tumaliuan, R.E., 1991. Economic feasibility of polyculture of tiger shrimp (*Penaeus monodon*) with Nile tilapia (*Oreochromis niloticus*) in brackishwater ponds. Asian Fisheries Science 4, 335–343.

Singh, T., Daud, W.J.W., 2001. Live handling and marketing of tilapia. In: Subasinghe, S., Singh, T. (Eds.), Tilapia: Production, Marketing and Technological Developments: Proceedings of the Tilapia 2001 International Technical and Trade Conference on Tilapia. Infofish, Kuala Lumpur, Malaysia, pp. 88–93.

Skibsted, L.H., 2011. Nitric oxide and quality and safety of muscle based foods. Nitric Oxide 24, 176–183.

Sneddon, L.U., 2003. The evidence for pain in fish: the use of morphine as analgesic. Applied Animal Behaviour Science 83, 153–162.

Snir, I.J., 2001. Value added tilapia products: deliberate policy or no other choice. In: Subasinghe, S., Singh, T. (Eds.), Tilapia: Production, Marketing and Technological Developments. Proceedings of the Tilapia 2001 International Technical and Trade Conference on Tilapia. Infofish, Kuala Lumpur, Malaysia, p. 84.

Souza, M.L.R., Macedo-Viegas, E.M., 2000. Effects of filleting on processing yield of Nile tilapia (*Oreochromis niloticus*). In: Fitzsimmons, K., Filho, J.C. (Eds.), Tilapia Culture in the 21st Century. Proceedings from the Fifth International Symposium on Tilapia Aquaculture. Rio de Janeiro, Brazil, pp. 451–457.

Souza, M.L.R., Marengoni, N.G., Pinto, A.A., Cacador, W.C., 2000. Processing yield of Nile tilapia (*Oreochromis niloticus*): head cut types and two weight classes. Acta Scientiarum 22, 701–706.

Stewart, J.A., 1993. The Economic Viability of Aquaculture in Malawi: A Short-Term Study for the Central and Northern Regions Fish Farming Project. Institute of Aquaculture, University of Stirling, Mzuzu, Malawi.

Van de Vis, H., Kestin, S., Robb, D., Oehlenschlager, J., Lambooij, B., Munkner, W., et al., 2003. Is humane slaughter of fish possible for industry? Aquaculture Research 34, 211–220.

Venturini, F.P., Baldi, S.C.V., Parisi, G., Costa, T.D., Rucinque, D.S., Melo, M.P., et al., 2018. Effects of different stunning methods on blood markers and enzymatic activity of stress responses of tilapia (*Oreochromis niloticus*). Italian Journal of Animal Science 17, 1094–1098.

Veverica, K.L., Liti, D., Were, E., Bowman, J., 2001. Fish yield and economic benefits of tilapia/*Clarias* polyculture in fertilized ponds receiving commercial feeds or pelleted agricultural by-products. In: Gupta, A., McElwee, K., Burke, D., Burright, J., Cummings, X., Egna, H. (Eds.), Eighteenth Annual Technical Report. Pond Dynamics/Aquaculture CRSP. Oregon State University, Corvallis, Oregon, pp. 27–29.

Viegas, E.M.M., de Carvalho, M.R.B., de Oliveira Filho, P.R.C., Kirschnik, P.G., Aiura, F.S., Vargas, S.C., 2013. Changes during chilled storage of whole tilapia and short-term frozen storage of tilapia fillets. Journal of Aquatic Food Product Technology 22, 192–200.

Wan Johari, W.D., Ismail, A.A., Wan Ismail, W.I., Tahir, S.M., 1999. Transportation of Live Red Tilapia (*Oreochromis niloticus*) under Minimal Water Condition. The Malaysian Agricultural Research and Development Institute (MARDI) Occasional Paper No. 10, p. 3.

Wang, Z.-C., Zhao, M.-M., Fang, Z., Chen, D.-W., 2017. Nitric oxide euthanasia: a potential procedure for improving animal welfare and fillet color of tilapia (*Oreochromis niloticus*). Aquaculture International 25, 1845–1856.

Wang, Z.-C., Yan, Y., Nisar, T., Sun, L., Su, P., Chen, D.-W., et al., 2018a. Influence of postmortem treatment with nitric oxide on the muscle color and color stability of tilapia (*Oreochromis niloticus*) fillets. Nitric Oxide 76, 122–128.

Wang, Z.-C., Yan, Y., Su, P., Zhao, M.-M., Xia, N., Chen, D.-W., 2018b. Treatments of tilapia (*Oreochromis niloticus*) using nitric oxide for quality improvement: establishing a potential method for large-scale processing of farmed fish. Nitric Oxide 77, 19–25.

Watanabe, W.O., Losordo, T.M., Fitzsimmons, K., Hanley, F., 2002. Tilapia production systems in the Americas: technological advances, trends, and challenges. Reviews in Fisheries Science 10, 465–498.

WorldFish, 2012. Value Chain Analysis: Shrimp, Prawn and Tilapia from the Southern Region of Bangladesh and Feasibility Analysis: Brackish Water Sea-Bass in the Southern Region in Bangladesh. Project Report. WorldFish, Penang, Malaysia, p. 80.

Yuan, Y., Yuan, Y., Dai, Y., Gong, Y., 2017. Economic profitability of tilapia farming in China. Aquaculture International 25, 1253–1264.

Zhi-qiang, G., Li-jing, Z., Min, L., Sheng-lan, G., 2012. Optimization of a combined heat pump–microwave drying process of tilapia fillets using a comprehensive weighted scoring method. Journal of Nutrition & Food Sciences 2, 168. https://doi.org/10.4172/2155-9600.1000168.

Zongli, Z., Yanan, Z., Feifan, L., Hui, Y., Yongming, Y., Xinhua, Y., 2017. Economic efficiency of small-scale tilapia farms in Guangxi, China. Aquaculture Economics and Management 21, 283–294.

Chapter 11

Tilapia trade and marketing

Chapter outline

11.1 Introduction

Tilapia culture is practiced mainly by small-scale farmers in rural areas in developing countries. Consequently, the fish are marketed in rural and local markets either fresh or iced. As expected, transportation, distribution and marketing channels in these areas are not well-managed due to the scattering of the farms in remote areas and the lack of technical and extension assistance. This situation is generally perpetuated by poor quality control, lack of corporate resources and limited market information (Young and Muir, 2000). The development of domestic and international tilapia marketing is, therefore, becoming of prime importance. Therefore, substantial amount of information has been gathered on tilapia trade and marketing, both domestically and internationally, during the past few years.

11.2 Domestic markets

Over 90% of farmed tilapia is destined for domestic markets, leaving little room for export to international markets. This is simply because tilapia is considered a low-priced fish, affordable by middle- and low-class communities in almost all tilapia producing countries, compared to high-valued seafoods. The African, American and Asian countries listed in Table 11.1 are the major tilapia producers. They produced about 98% of global farmed tilapia output in 2016, about 94.5% of which were directed to local markets. The only exception was Costa Rica, Ecuador, Honduras, China and Taiwan, where significant proportions of produced tilapia were exported (30.8%, 18.6%, 32.7%, 21.1% and 44%, respectively).

11.2.1 Asia

The early studies on tilapia economics and marketing potentials in the Philippines indicated that the substitution of Mozambique tilapia (*Oreochromis mossambicus*) with the introduced Nile tilapia (*Oreochromis niloticus*) has led to rapid development of tilapia culture in various parts of the country (Torres and Navera, 1985; Bimbao and Smith, 1988). This has narrowed the margins between wholesale and retail prices of farmed tilapia and resulted in more competition due to the increase in production. These studies suggested that the future market potential of farmed tilapia will depend on the future income and purchasing power of the consumers and the ability of producers to reduce production costs.

Today, the increased production of farmed tilapia, together with better income and increased purchasing power in many Southeast Asian countries have shifted the consumer preference from the traditional, small-sized, unprocessed, fresh tilapia to large-sized tilapia and other tilapia products. Guerrero and Guerrero (2001) reviewed

Tilapia Culture. https://doi.org/10.1016/B978-0-12-816541-6.00011-8
Copyright © 2020 Elsevier Inc. All rights reserved.

TABLE 11.1 Tilapia production and export by major producers in 2016.

			Domestic consumption	
Country	Production (t)	Export (t)	Amount (t)	Percent of total production
Africa				
Egypt	940,309	6,229	934,080	99.3
Ghana	50,900	0	50,900	100
Kenya	11,180	142	11,038	98.7
Nigeria	23,706	16	23,690	99.9
Uganda	74,654	1129	73,525	98.5
Zambia	30,085	83	30,002	99.7
Zimbabwe	10,000	2	9,998	100
The Americas				
Brazil	239,131	898	238,233	99.6
Colombia	61,800	5,007	56,793	91.9
Costa Rica	18,200	5,606	12,594	69.2
Ecuador	22,620	4,199	18,421	81.4
Guatemala	10,045	158	9,887	98.4
Honduras	30,100	9831	20,269	67.3
Mexico	58,191	3174	55,017	94.5
Asia				
Bangladesh	342,567	208	342,359	99.9
China	1,866,381	393,329	1,473,052	78.9
Indonesia	1,187,812	11,880	1,175,932	99.0
Malaysia	36,998	2,256	35,007	94.6
Myanmar	33,134	0	33,134	100
Philippines[a]	259,045	68	258,977	100
Taiwan	63,028	21,385	41,643	66.1
Thailand[b]	208,144	7,902	200,242	96.2
Vietnam	183,817	12,762	171,055	93.1
Total	5,761,847	486,181	5,275,848	94.5

[a]*Tilapia export was drastically reduced from 6176 t in 2013 to 68 t in 2016.*
[b]*Tilapia export was reduced by about 50% between 2014 and 2016.*
Source: FAO (2018).

tilapia domestic marketing practices in the Philippines, Thailand and Vietnam. They reported that tilapia is an important food commodity commercially produced in many Southeast Asian countries with Nile tilapia being the most important species marketed in the region. Consumer preference has been shifted to large-sized tilapia, which are generally sold fresh, chilled or frozen. Typically, tilapia producers sell their products to traders, who in turn sell them to wholesalers and/or retailers. As stated earlier, processed tilapia are also gaining increased marketing momentum in the region. However, Chinese domestic tilapia market is currently facing competition with growing imports of Asian catfish (*Pangasius*), which is getting more popular (Globefish, 2018). Some Chinese tilapia farmers are even switching to *Pangasius* farming due to the growing domestic demand as a result of its lower prices compared to tilapia.

A variety of market outlets for tilapia are now available in China, including local markets, processing manufacturers and the international market (Matlala et al., 2013). In local markets, most tilapia marketing is executed by the middlemen; but some famers sell their own product themselves directly to the local market or to tilapia processors. Farmers sometimes sell the entire crop of live tilapia to the middlemen, who distribute it according to the market outlet demand. Generally speaking, the marketing chains for tilapia and their products in China can be divided into two categories (Matlala et al., 2013):

1. A short marketing chain starting from the producer directly to domestic market, to the consumer, and
2. A longer chain, starting from producers to processors, then to domestic or international markets.

Southeast Asia and the Far East, namely mainland China, Indonesia, Bangladesh, the Philippines, Taiwan, Thailand and Vietnam, are the most important markets for tilapia, where 93%–100% of produced tilapia is consumed domestically (Ferdouse, 2001; FAO, 2018) (Table 11.1), except China and Taiwan where significant quantities of tilapia are exported (21% and 44% in 2016). Market acceptance is also sharply increasing in other Asian countries, such as Malaysia, Singapore, Hong Kong, Taiwan, Myanmar, Pakistan and India, especially in growing urban populations. The fish are sold fresh and/or chilled for household consumption in the cities. Ferdouse (2001) reported that the potential of local and regional tilapia marketing is very high due to the following:

1. Increased fish consumption in Asian countries
2. Availability and sustainability of supplying high-quality tilapia.
3. Better market opportunities within and outside Southeast Asia.
4. Consumer perspective towards healthy food.
5. Economic changes in the region since the mid-1990s.

The author stressed that tilapia is no longer considered a low-value species in Asian markets.

11.2.2 Africa

In Africa, tilapia marketing and distribution channels are very simple, with minimal interference from governmental authorities. In countries such as Egypt, Ghana, Kenya, Uganda and Nigeria, most of the tilapia produced from aquaculture or capture fisheries are directed to urban markets in large cities, in addition to the amounts which are consumed locally. The increased demand for tilapia in many African countries has increased the prices of these fishes. In Egypt, for example, the retail price of large-sized Nile tilapia (>200 g) grown in fish ponds is about US\$ 1.9 kg^{-1}, while the prices of small fish (100–<200 g) range from US\$ 1 to 1.5 kg^{-1} (El-Sayed, 2017). The prices also fluctuate from one season to another (higher in winter than in summer) and from one area to another.

The tilapia markets in sub-Saharan Africa (SSA) are diverse, ranging from local small-scale markets where the fish is sold mainly at farm gate and roadside to more commercial distribution channels, connected to large retail chains. However, small-scale and informal tilapia traders are currently an important activity in the tilapia distribution and marketing chain, leading to a significant improvement in the livelihood of households, especially among women traders. In addition, large-scale distribution and retail chains and supermarkets are expanding in urban areas in most SSA countries. These retailers generally sell both fresh and frozen products. Nonetheless, the high cost of tilapia production, processing and distribution remains a major challenge in SSA.

In Ghana, tilapia prices are much higher than those in Egypt. These prices are generally affected by the following factors:

- Market prices (Anane-Taabeah et al., 2016): since large commercial fish farms can dictate their farm-gate prices, on which traders have no control.
- Freshness: fresh tilapia cost at least twice as much as beef (Frimpong and Anane-Taabeah, 2017).
- Fish size: large-size tilapia is more expensive because it is preferred by consumers (Darko, 2011). Prices were 3.8, 4.1, 4.8 and 5.7 US\$ kg^{-1} in 2012 for a size range of 150–250 g, 250–400 g, 400–600 g and 600–1000 g, respectively (Frimpong and Anane-Taabeah, 2017).
- Source: wild-caught fresh tilapia is generally more expensive than farmed tilapia because of consumers' preference for wild fish (Kassam, 2013).
- Market location: prices in large urban areas are higher than in rural and remote areas.

In Kenya, the marketing channel for aquaculture products, including tilapia, is short and direct from producers to consumers or retailers with no organized marketing (Ngugi et al., 2017). Most tilapia are sold whole fresh in local markets, with little processing despite the fact that tilapia is processed into diverse products, such as fillet, portioned, cured, smoked or dried. Generally, wholesalers control both the entry of fish products into the markets and fish distribution and therefore determine fish prices. The prices of fish commodities, including tilapia, fluctuate considerably and are determined by supply and demand. A cartel of agents determines the prices of fish in large markets.

Similarly, most of the tilapia produced in Nigeria is used for domestic consumption. Tilapia is sold in different forms: fresh, smoked, fried, salted or cooked in different recipes. Value-added products such as fish fingers, fish cakes and other ready-to-serve fish are also produced, and their potential is increasing (Atanda and Fagbenro, 2017). The price of tilapia in Nigeria is determined mainly by consumer's preference. Nigerians prefer African catfish to tilapia, therefore the price of fresh catfish (4 US$ kg^{-1}) was almost twice as high as the price of farmed tilapia (2.3 US$ kg^{-1}) in May 2014 (Atanda and Fagbenro, 2017).

Uganda, like other SSA countries, produces tilapia for domestic consumption. These fish are sold directly to consumers at farm gate, or through a longer value chain, from farmers or farmer groups to intermediaries, processors, retailers and then to final consumers (Hyuha et al., 2017). Some fish farmers or traders process farmed fish by salting, sun drying or smoking to serve distant and bigger markets. The tilapia farm-gate price increased from 1.22 to 1.63 US$ kg^{-1} in 2009 to US$ 2.85 kg^{-1} in 2013. Consequently, the consumer preference had shifted from large-sized fish (500 g) to small-sized fish (<250 g) because they are more affordable (Hyuha et al., 2011).

11.2.3 Latin America

In South America, tilapia marketing is positively responsive to population growth and advertising, which are the two main factors affecting the consumer demand. Tilapia marketing in Costa Rica is an example of how advertising affects the demand for tilapia. There was a market resistance in the country to Mozambique tilapia because of its dark skin and the use of pig manure for pond fertilization. Nile tilapia was then introduced and given an attractive name 'St. Peter's fish' in order to convince consumers that this species was not tilapia. In this way, tilapia was successfully marketed and has gained increasing popularity. Similarly, the red tilapia (*Oreochromis* spp.) was introduced to the country in 1984 and was more acceptable because it resembles the colour of red snapper, which is a popular marine species.

Currently, Nile tilapia and tilapia hybrids are the major farmed tilapia groups in Latin America and the Caribbean. Most tilapia production in these regions is absorbed by domestic markets, while tilapia imports are relatively low. In 2016, about 93% (418,000 t) of tilapia produced were directed to domestic markets. In Mexico, 58,191 t of tilapia were produced in 2016, of which 46,100 t in live weight (79%) were destined for domestic market. In addition, 54,000 t of tilapia were imported to the country, exclusively in the form of frozen fillet. The main producing and consuming states in Mexico are Chiapas, Tabasco, Guerrero, Estado de México and Veracruz. In Brazil, the domestic market also absorbs almost all tilapia produced. In Honduras, the domestic consumption of tilapia was about 20,269 t in 2016, representing 67.3% of total tilapia production, while the rest of production was exported, mainly to the US market. Similarly, about 70% and 80% of tilapia produced in Costa Rica and Ecuador in 2016 was consumed locally (Table 11.1).

11.3 Global markets

Despite the fact that most of the produced tilapia is consumed in domestic markets in production areas, especially in rural Asia, Africa and South America, the demand for tilapia is growing in nontraditional, nonproducing countries. Therefore, global trade in tilapia products has witnessed an impressive flourishing in the last two decades and is expected to continue (Vannuccini, 2001; Liang et al., 2017; FAO, 2018). One of the major advantages of global tilapia marketing is their competitive prices, white flesh and easy processing that make them an important substitute for white fish species which face shortages in supply.

With increasing demand for processed fish in Western markets, the global demand for processed tilapia, especially frozen fillet and frozen whole fish, has been increasing (Fig. 11.1). It is no surprise, therefore, that tilapia is currently imported by over 130 countries worldwide. Among the 472,000 t of tilapia imported in 2015, about 55% (259,000 t) were frozen fillet and 33% (172,000 t) were frozen whole fish (Liang et al., 2017). The tilapia fish market is dominated by farmed Nile tilapia, while the contribution of wild-captured tilapia is limited. Global tilapia market includes the following two product categories:

1. Cheap, commoditized tilapia, with China being the main source of this category. The prices of this product are over 50% lower than the premium tilapia. The vast majority of tilapia is marketed under this category.
2. Premium tilapia, which is generally high-quality tilapia, is produced and marketed under restrict conditions and sold mostly fresh. There is generally a clear distinction between this tilapia and the cheaper category. Premium producers and marketers generally add more promotion differentiation and specifications to their products, such as eco-labelling, low-antibiotic production processes and convenience packaging (Globefish, 2018). Major producers of this category include Latin American countries, such as Ecuador, Colombia and Mexico, and Asian countries (e.g. Indonesia). Premium tilapia targets the growing middle-class, health-conscious urban societies, which may be willing to pay higher prices for higher-quality products.

11.4 Tilapia exports and imports

Tilapia export has witnessed a substantial increase during the past decade, increasing from 267,725 t in 2007 to 501,619 t in 2016, with an annual growth rate of 7.2%. However, tilapia export slightly declined during the past few years (2014–16) (Figs 11.2 and 11.3). This decline has been attributed partially to the occurrence of tilapia lake virus disease, which is a highly contagious disease,

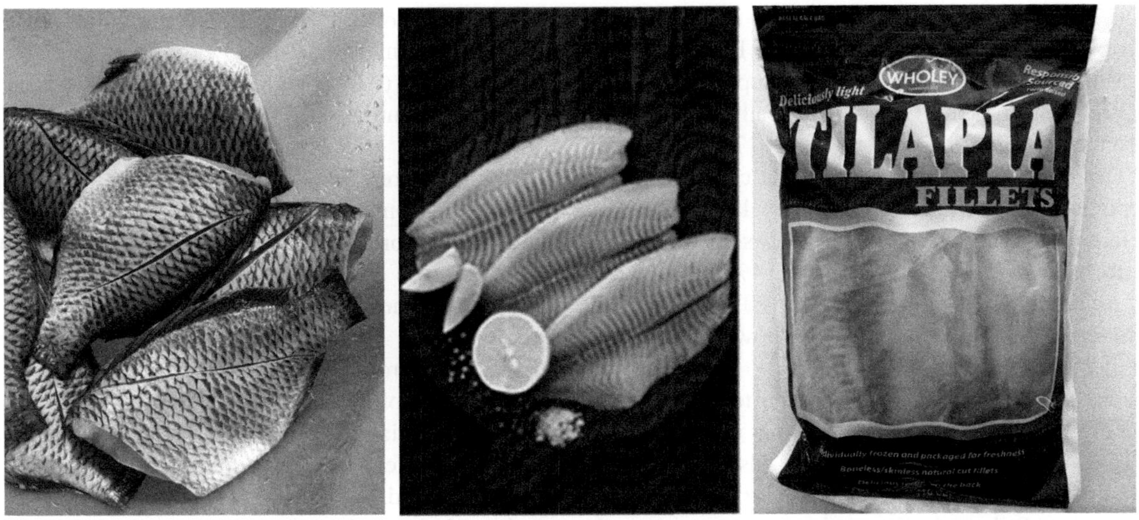

FIGURE 11.1 Tilapia fillets: fresh, skin on (left); fresh, skinned (middle) and frozen (right). *Left and middle photos from Shutterstock. Right photo provided by K. Vitzsimmons.*

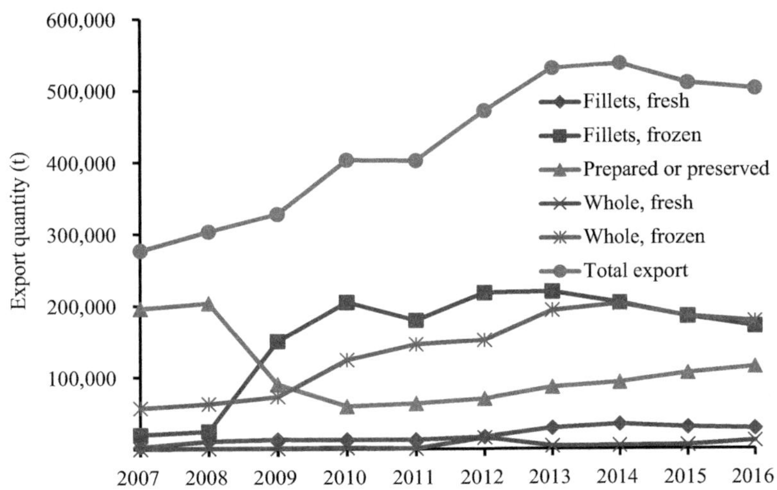

FIGURE 11.2 Global tilapia export during 2007–16. *Source: FAO (2018).*

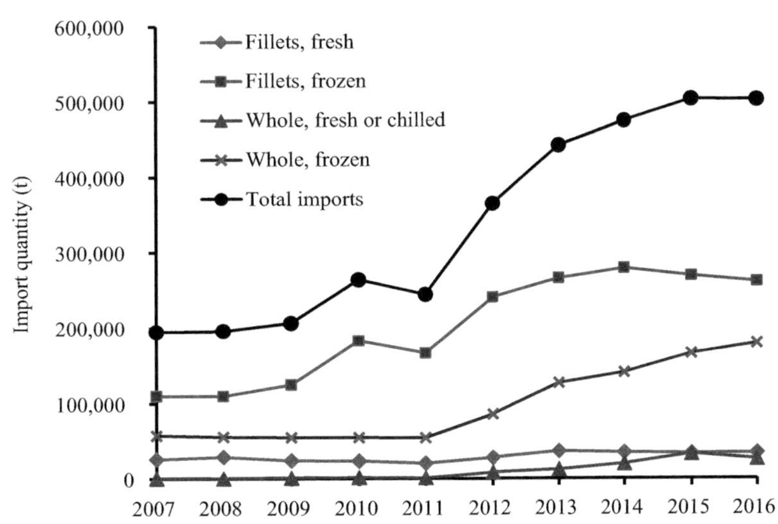

FIGURE 11.3 Global tilapia imports during 2007–16. *Source: FAO (2018).*

spreading among farmed and wild tilapia in many tilapia producing countries, including Colombia, Ecuador, Israel, Egypt, Malaysia, Thailand, and the Philippines (Ferguson et al., 2014; Bacharach et al., 2016; Fathi et al., 2017; Nicholson et al., 2017; Dong et al., 2017; Amal et al., 2018). This virus poses no public health concern but has been reported to cause devastating outbreaks with massive loss of farmed tilapia in these countries. As a result, tilapia export declined by 5.3% in 2015 and 1.4% in 2016. According to the FAO Globefish highlights 2017, tilapia trade in the international market was 10% lower in the first quarter of 2017 than that in 2016.

Asia is, by far, the largest tilapia exporter in the world; contributing 90%–95% of total tilapia export during 2007–16 (Table 11.2). The Americas also export large amounts of tilapia, mainly to the neighbouring US market. The popularity of tilapia in Europe is also increasing to the level that Europe currently exports over 10,000 t of tilapia annually, mainly as frozen fillet. Tilapia export in Europe is virtually through tilapia import (originally from China, Taiwan, Indonesia and Vietnam) and then re-export, mainly to other European countries. Despite the fact that tilapia export from Africa is still limited, it showed a significant increase from 2949 t in 2014 to 9886 t in 2016.

Large amounts of tilapia produced in Asia are exported to foreign markets, particularly to the United States, EU, Middle East and African markets (Table 11.3). China is the largest tilapia exporter in the world, contributing 50%–60% to the total export during 2010–16, with a total tilapia exports amounting to 393,000 t in 2016 (Globefish, 2018). Global tilapia export is dominated by frozen fillet and frozen whole fish, while fresh fish, either whole fish or fish fillets, are limited and almost stable. Chinese frozen fillet represented 82%–>90% of total global exports of frozen fillets (FAO, 2018). China exports frozen tilapia to over 50 countries, mainly to Africa and North America. About 64% of Chinese whole frozen tilapia went to African markets in 2016, presumably due to its relatively low prices compared with other tilapia exporters. The major African importers are Côte d'Ivoire, Kenya, Zambia and Cameroon.

The Chinese government realized the importance of tilapia as a major export commodity to international markets; therefore serious measures have been taken to promote tilapia export much further. Under the Agriculture Industrial Information System (AIIS), an early warning system on tilapia trade has been constructed for assessing and monitoring the status and trends of tilapia culture industry in China (Peng et al., 2013). The system uses economics, management science and information technology to analyze the status of tilapia industry, identify the major warning signals and, in turn, forecast its future trend. Thus, this system provides the necessary strategies that would facilitate the sustainable tilapia development in China.

According to the Vietnam Association of Seafood Exporters and Processors (VASEP) (seafood.vasep.com.vn), Vietnam tilapia exports also increased by 265% from 2012 to 2014. Tilapia importers from Vietnam also increased from 8 countries in 2005 to 68 countries in 2015. The positive growth of Vietnamese tilapia exports is expected to continue in the coming years. Major importers include the United States, Colombia, the Netherlands, Turkey, Italy, Belgium, Spain, Germany, South Korea and Saudi Arabia.

TABLE 11.2 Global tilapia export by continents during 2007–16.

Continent	2007	2008	2009	2010	2011	2012	2013	2014	2015	2016
Africa	0 -	0 -	0 -	0 -	0 -	581	1,796	2,966	5,098	9,965
The Americas	14,206	22,125	24,927	24,107	25,944	28,493	34,611	36,690	36,782	30,950
Asia	262,546	281,212	302,446	374,376	372,285	435,229	483,529	489,364	458,985	452,584
Europe	0 .	0 .	0 .	4,497	3,925	8,785	11,666	11,057	10,741	10,999
Oceania	0 .	0 .	0 .	0 .	0 .	30	58	28	28	26
Total export	276,752	303,337	327,373	402,980	402,154	473,118	531,660	540,105	511,634	504,524
Annual increase (%)		9.61	7.92	23.09	−0.21	17.65	12.37	1.59	−5.27	−1.39
Contribution of Asia to total export (%)	94.87	92.71	92.39	92.90	92.57	91.99	90.95	90.61	89.71	89.70

0 . denotes that data are not available; *0 -* denotes an actual null value.
Source: FAO (2018).

TABLE 11.3 Global tilapia import by continents during 2007–16.

Continent	2007	2008	2009	2010	2011	2012	2013	2014	2015	2016
Africa	628	1,244	1,672	224	1,105	15,189	30,431	48,684	76,142	91,009
The Americas	182,175	186,926	191,825	223,782	202,667	267,567	310,457	313,509	303,300	293,107
Asia	12,136	7,755	13,076	18,983	19,546	40,895	44,077	72,518	100,899	100,102
Europe	0 -	0 -	0 -	21,069	21,158	56,460	66,302	53,835	50,153	43,033
Oceania	0 .	0 .	0 .	0 .	0 .	1076	1270	1346	1298	1438
Total import	194,939	195,925	206,573	264,058	244,476	381,187	452,537	489,892	531,792	528,689
Annual increase (%)		0.50	5.43	27.83	−7.42	55.92	18.72	8.25	8.55	−0.58

0 . denotes that data are not available; 0 - denotes an actual null value.
Source: FAO (2018).

As mentioned earlier, and unlike China, Indonesia and Vietnam, all tilapia produced in Bangladesh are marketed domestically (Ahmed et al., 2012), using a traditional marketing system. Marketing chain includes primary, wholesale and retail markets.

In a comprehensive study by Liang et al. (2017), the status and trend of global tilapia markets in 2015 was examined. They analyzed the international markets of the major tilapia commodities (fresh whole, frozen whole, fresh fillet and frozen fillet) and their aggregates at the national, regional and global levels. The main findings of this study were the following:

- The total imports of frozen whole tilapia were 172,000 t, with a value of 345 million US$, and at least 133 countries imported frozen whole tilapia in 2015.
- African markets accounted for 51% of total frozen whole tilapia market in quantity, and 55% in value. However, the prices of frozen whole tilapia in most African markets are higher than the world average (2.0 US$ kg^{-1} in 2015).
- Imported frozen tilapia fillet amounted to 259,000 t in 2015, valuing 1090 million US$.
- Developed countries favour tilapia fillet, whereas developing regions prefer whole tilapia because their prices are more affordable. In developed regions, tilapia fillet represented 79% (mainly in frozen form) of total tilapia imports, while in developing regions, 63% of imported tilapia was in the form of frozen whole tilapia.
- Frozen whole tilapia markets in developed regions generally have more suppliers than those in developing regions. For example, the United States imported frozen whole tilapia from 17 countries, whereas over 50 developing countries imported the commodity from only one country, China).
- The main destination of fresh tilapia fillet is European market, with the Netherlands and Belgium being the largest markets and suppliers of this commodity.

11.5 Value-added tilapia products

The most common value added for tilapia product is the frozen form, either fillet or whole fish. These two forms contributed 69% to total tilapia exports in 2016. Most of the imported tilapia, especially in the United States and Europe, is consumed in the form of frozen fillet. However, in the early 2000s, prepared or preserved tilapia emerged in the global market as a new ready-to-eat product; with an increasing trend towards more ready-to-serve products. These products are more convenient for working households, where family members come home late from work and may not have time to clean and cook fish. Value-added products include breaded products, seasoned fillets in sauces, nuggets, fish fingers, fish cakes, smoked tilapia and other ready-to-eat products (Fig. 11.4).

The production of different forms of processed tilapia is gaining more attention in some producing countries (especially in Asia), with China being the most important producer. The export of prepared or preserved tilapia products amounted to 113,957 t in 2016, representing 23% of total tilapia exports. Chinese export of these products increased progressively from only 1000 t in 2002 to 203,687 t in 2008. However, a dramatic decline in prepared tilapia exports occurred in the following years. Nonetheless, the Chinese production and export of this commodity is slowly recovering. These processed tilapia products are advantageous to the producing

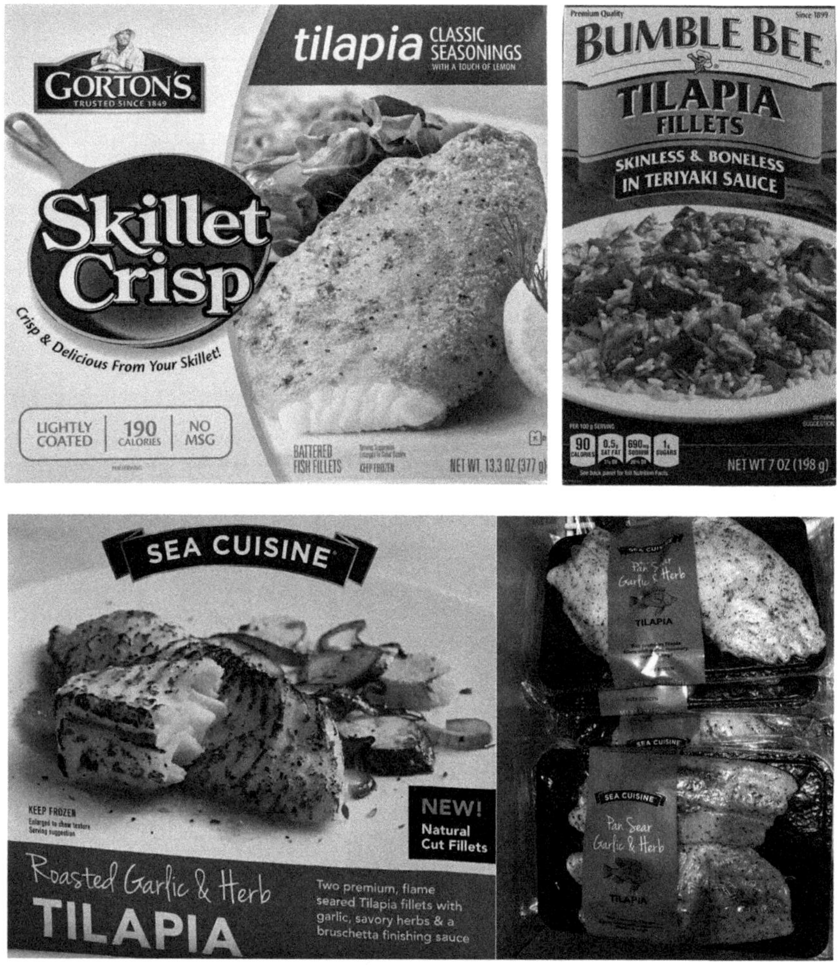

FIGURE 11.4 Different processed, ready-to-eat tilapia products. *Top photos from Shutterstock. Bottom photos provided by K. Fitzsimmons.*

country, since they are likely to create more jobs, generate more income and improve the standard of living, especially in rural areas.

11.6 The US market

Domestic production of tilapia in the United States has been about stable during the last two decades (1997–2016), with an annual production ranging between 8000 and 9000 t. This little production could not, by any means, meet the ever-increasing demand for tilapia in the US market. Among marketed finfish in the United States, tilapia was ranked first in terms of cumulative 5-year sales from 2006 to 2010. Tilapia also comes fourth among the top 10 list for per capita seafood consumption for 2016. As a result, substantial amounts of tilapia are imported annually, making the United States the largest market for tilapia import in the world, constituting about 70% of global tilapia market.

The US tilapia market is well developed, and the value chain is mature and well-articulated. Tilapia imports have been increasing during the last decade, and their share in retail markets has been rising to reach about 225,492 t in 2015, with a value of 982.7 million US$ (US Department of Commerce, 2018) (www.ers.usda.gov) (Figs. 11.5 and 11.6). However, tilapia imports declined by about 16% and 7.3% in 2016 and 2017, due to the significant decline in supplies of Chinese frozen tilapia fillets, which decreased by 22% (from 140,421 t in 2015 to 109,483 t in 2017). In terms of prices, the values of total tilapia import sharply declined from 1,114,381 US$ in 2014 to 674,463 US$ in 2017, with an average annual decline of 15.3%; while the average annual decline in the prices of frozen fillets was 17.8%, during the same period (Fig. 11.6). The volume of imported tilapia increased in all product categories; however, much of the increase has been attributed to the imports of frozen fillets, which represented about 60%–70% of total tilapia import, in terms of volume and value, during 2008–17. On the other hand, the imports of frozen whole fish and fresh fillets remained almost stable during the same period (Fig. 11.5).

The United States imported tilapia and tilapia products from over 38 countries during 2013–17 (Table 11.4).

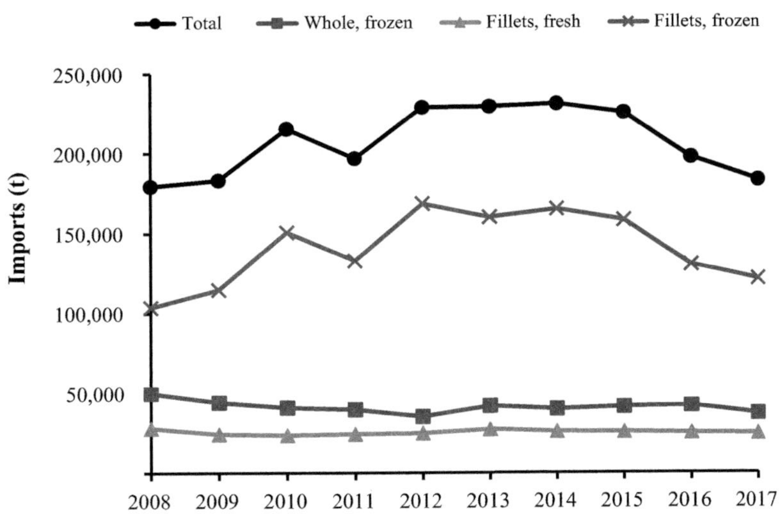

FIGURE 11.5 Tilapia imports to the US market during 2008–17. *Source: USDA (2018).*

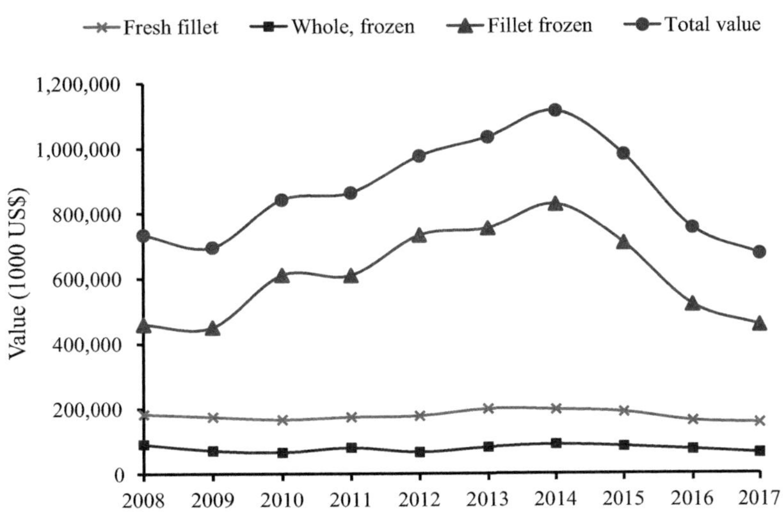

FIGURE 11.6 Value (1000 US$) of tilapia imports to the US market during 2008–17. *Source: USDA (2018).*

Surprisingly, some exporters are not traditionally tilapia producers, such as Japan, Canada, the United Kingdom and the United Arab Emirates. These countries may import tilapia from a third country and then re-export it to international markets, including the US market, mainly as fresh and/or frozen fillets.

Asia is the main tilapia exporter to the US market. Over 85% of imported tilapia in 2015–17 came from Asia. Mainland China is the biggest competitor in the US tilapia market and is now the dominant tilapia supplier, providing over 73% of total tilapia imports during 2015–17. More than 64% of tilapia imports from China in 2017 were in the form of frozen whole, while in fillet category, over 90% were frozen fillets. Other Asian countries, such as Indonesia, Thailand, Taiwan and Vietnam are also important tilapia exporters to the US market, especially frozen products.

While China remains the leading tilapia exporter to the United States, exports from South America to North America are increasing. The rising of production costs in China and the change in government policy with regard to product subsidies will make Chinese producers less competitive over time, leaving more room for other exporters, especially from neighbouring Central and South America. This may explain the increase in tilapia imports from North America, South America and the Caribbean regions in recent years. Thirteen countries from these regions are currently exporting tilapia and tilapia products to the US market. Honduras, Colombia, Costa Rica, Mexico and Ecuador, respectively, are the largest tilapia exporter, contributing 95% of total tilapia export from these regions to US market. The fresh tilapia market in the United States is dependent almost exclusively on these regions, since they contributed over 99.5% of total fresh fillet imported to

TABLE 11.4 Tilapia imports to the US market (t) during 2015–17.

Continent/	Whole, frozen			Fillet, fresh			Fillet, frozen			Total		
Country	2015	2016	2017	2015	2016	2017	2015	2016	2017	2015	2016	2017
Asia												
China	26,864.5	28,807.3	24,120.0	136.8	78.6	46.8	140,420.9	116,645.0	109,842.7	167,422.7	145,530.9	134,009.5
Indonesia	0.0	0.0	0.0	0.0	0.0	0.0	10,450.5	7752.7	7059.1	10,450.5	7752.7	7059.1
Malaysia	0.0	0.0	0.0	0.0	0.5	2.7	308.2	555.0	318.6	308.2	555.5	320.9
Hong Kong	0.0	20.0	1.8	0.0	0.0	0.0	22.3	45.9	117.7	22.3	65.9	119.5
Philippines	0.9	277.3	21.4	0.0	12.7	0.0	1.0	0.0	0.0	0.9	289.5	21.4
Taiwan	10,443.6	10,528.2	10,296.4		6.8	35.5	1983.6	1878.2	1990.0	12,427.3	12,413.2	12,321.8
Thailand	734.1	843.6	772.3		19.1	2.7	1155.9	871.4	327.3	1890.0	1734.1	1102.3
Vietnam	2967.3	1274.1	1730.0		56.4	107.3	353.6	222.7	305.0	3487.3	1553.2	2142.3
Myanmar (Burma)	7.7	26.8	23.6		668.2	852.3	76.4	0.0	0.0	596.4	695.0	875.9
Japan	0.0	0.0	0.0		0.0	0.0	0.0	0.0	2.3	0.0	0.0	2.3
Pakistan	0.0	0.0	10.0		71.8	25.9	0.0	0.0	0.0	146.4	71.8	25.9
Bangladesh	0.0	0.0	0.0		132.3	93.6	0.0	0.0	0.0	138.2	132.3	97.3
India	100.0	16.8	55.5		1.8	0.0	0.0	0.0	0.0	100.0	18.6	55.5
UAE	3.2	1.8	3.2		0.0	0.0	0.0	0.0	0.0	3.2	1.8	3.2
Subtotal	41,121.4	41,795.9	37,034.1	136.8	1048.2	1166.8	154,772.3	127,970.9	119,962.7	196,993.2	170,814.5	158,156.8

The Americas												
Argentina	0.0	9.5	18.2	0.0	0.0	18.2	0.0	0.0	0.0	0.0	0.0	18.2
Brazil	0.0	0.0	0.0	142.3	906.8	646.4	3.6	22.3	12.2	159.1	952.3	680.0
Canada	0.0	0.0	0.0	0.0	0.5	0.5	0.0	0.0	0.0	0.0	0.5	0.5
Chile	0.0	0.0	0.0	35.0	55.5	0.0	0.0	0.0	0.2	35.0	55.5	0.0
Colombia	0.9	0.0	8.6	5400.5	5469.1	6300.5	0.0	1.8	0.0	5401.4	5469.1	6309.1
Costa Rica	9.5	1.8	0.7	4933.2	4895.0	4835.9	0.0	1.0	1.1	5124.1	5063.6	4967.7
Ecuador	0.0	22.7	0.0	2848.6	2066.8	1272.3	63.4	123.5	84.7	2935.5	2119.5	1313.6
Honduras	0.0	0.0	0.0	8910.9	8934.1	7906.8	0.0	0.0	0.0	9899.5	9215.0	8223.2
Guatemala	7.3	25.0	0.0	135.5	97.7	209.1	12.5	8.7	8.2	142.3	124.5	209.1
Mexico	84.1	77.3	12.3	2044.5	1470.0	2309.1	0.0	0.0	0.0	4250.0	3315.9	2959.1
Nicaragua	2.3	3.2	0.0	1.7	0.4	1.3	7.7	11.2	3.8	2.3	3.2	0.0
Panama	153.2	100.0	80.5	26.8	0.0	11.8	0.0	21.9	18.9	235.5	181.4	157.7
Peru	0.0	0.0	0.0	131.4	104.1	27.3	0.0	0.0	0.0	299.5	187.3	127.3
Subtotal	257.3	239.5	120.3	24,610.4	24,000.0	23,539.0	87.2	190.4	129.2	28,484.1	26,687.7	24,965.5
Others[a]	10.0	21.8	0.0	4.5	0.0	0.0	0.0	23.2	14.1	14.5	45.0	14.1
Grand total	41,388.6	42,057.3	37,154.4	24,751.7	25,048.1	24,705.9	154,859.5	128,184.5	120,106.0	225,491.8	197,547.3	183,136.4

[a]*Include Ghana, Cocos Islands, Faroe Islands, Seychelles, Spain and the UK.*
Source: Economic Research Service, USDA (2018) (www.ers.usda.gov).

the US market during 2015–17. The switch in fresh fillet market in the United States from Asian sources to the Americas was mainly due to the following reasons:

- Their close location to the US market.
- Competitive labour costs.
- Meeting the prerequisites for successful exportation to the US market.
- Many of the top commercial South and Central American tilapia producers achieved high compliance standards.
- Many commercial operations in Central and South America are certified; branded high-quality fresh tilapia products are guaranteed.

11.7 Other international markets

11.7.1 Europe

The demand for tilapia is growing in many European countries, especially among particular ethnic groups such as in the African, Chinese and Asian communities in big cities. Thirty-seven European countries have recorded tilapia imports, mostly frozen fillet, during 2010–16. China is the main tilapia exporter, followed by Vietnam, Indonesia, Thailand and Taiwan (FAO, 2018). Tilapia imports to European market have been increasing steadily since 2010 to 2013 (from 21,069 to 65,423 t), but have been declining since then. The values of tilapia imports have also dramatically decreased by 43% during 2013–16 (from 218.9 to 123.7 million US$). This decline may be an indication of weakening demand in Europe, especially in the EU. The largest importers of frozen tilapia in Europe are Spain, Poland, the Netherlands and Germany; they accounted for more than 65% (€46 million) of the total value in 2014. On the other hand, France, the Netherlands, the United Kingdom and Belgium are the biggest importers of frozen whole tilapia, accounting for more than 75% of the value of total frozen whole tilapia import to Europe in 2014.

11.7.2 Middle East

Arab and Middle East countries also represent a huge market for tilapia imports. Despite the high tilapia production in some countries of the region (e.g. Egypt), local markets usually absorb that production, leaving little or no room for export. The region imports considerable quantities of tilapia, especially whole fresh (mainly to the Gulf States) and frozen fillets (to Israel and Iran) from China and Taiwan. Over 40,000 t were imported in 2016 to the Middle East region. The Arabian Gulf States are the major tilapia importer in the region, particularly for fresh or chilled tilapia, presumably due to the presence of large ethnic communities from Africa and Asia, where tilapia is a preferred fish for them. The Islamic Republic of Iran has recently emerged as an important market for tilapia. Tilapia imports to this country (mainly frozen fillet) increased from only 1550 t in 2012 to 15,900 t in 2016. Saudi Arabia and Israel are also major tilapia importers.

11.7.3 Sub-Saharan Africa

Despite the significant growth of tilapia culture in SSA in recent years, tilapia supplies from captured and farmed sources do not meet domestic demand, particularly in countries with notably increasing demand, such as Democratic Republic of Congo (DRC), Ghana, Malawi, Nigeria, Uganda and Zambia (INFOFISH International, 2015; www.infofish.org). Therefore, SSA will continue to present a strong marketing potential for tilapia producers, processers and traders. China has taken an advantage of this situation and begun exporting frozen tilapia products to over 50 African countries. However, the high cost of tilapia production, processing and distribution remains a major challenge in SSA compared to Asian and South American markets, making retail prices of tilapia and its various products very high. For example, tilapia prices in countries such as Angola, DRC, Equatorial Guinea, Ghana, Nigeria and Zambia are extremely high for domestic producers and importers.

11.8 Challenges facing tilapia trade and marketing

11.8.1 Misconception about eating tilapia

Despite the clearly recognized health benefits of tilapia consumption, these fishes and their products have been under severe negative criticism and attack from health, nutrition, cooking, seafood and environmental blogs. Several stories and articles have been written in unspecialized magazines, newspapers, blogs and other social media, warning consumers from eating tilapia. They claim that tilapia is not good for human health because it lacks essential nutrients, with a poor balance between omega-6 and omega-3 unsaturated fatty acids. They also keep insisting that farmed tilapia are genetically modified, are fed on dead animals and human and animal faeces and their flesh contains steroid hormones. Sarcastically, these fear-mongering groups do not cite any scientific references to support their false, extreme, unrealistic claims.

This misinformation and negative propaganda spread very quickly, creating misperception among consumers about the quality of farmed tilapia and causing a significant damage to this important global industry. Luckily, some tilapia lovers and tilapia industry people and researchers have fought back, providing evidences that tilapia is an excellent food fish, and it is consumed in more than 130 countries. The United States Food and Drug Administration (USFDA) included tilapia in its 2017 list of 'best choices' for seafood consumption by pregnant women and children, recommending two to three servings per week (FDA, 2017).

11.8.2 Farmed vs. wild tilapia: public perception

There is a common misperception among consumers about the quality of farmed tilapia (and other farmed aquatic animals). Many consumers believe that farmed fish, including tilapia, are inferior in quality to wild-caught fish, they are not flavoured and they have a muddy taste. Consumers also claim that tilapia feeds contain dead animals, animal wastes and hormones. Therefore, developing proper marketing strategies to change the general negative public perception of farmed tilapia is necessary. This may include promotional campaigns, organizing tasting days/panels, new recipes, new products, incentives, labelling and tractability, etc.

11.8.3 Labelling and traceability

Most international markets require that the basic information about specifications for fishery and aquaculture products be provided. Tilapia products should, therefore, comply with these requirements in order to gain more grounds, credibility and sustainability. These specifications include, but not necessarily restricted to, labelling and traceability, packaging and processing. Traceability has become a fundamental requirement for exporting aquaculture products. This means that all pre-packaged tilapia and tilapia products should be labelled with a name, components, validity (expiration date), storage conditions, producer's name, address, etc. Generally, labelling requirements apply to retail sales to the final consumer only, while traceability requirements target the whole distribution chain. Specific legislation is also required to regulate fishery and aquaculture products, including raw, iced and frozen fish and fish products. Tight inspections for the product quality and residues should be allowed for tilapia shipments. However, most tilapia traded in international markets lacks such labelling requirements. Only a few countries put specific labelling requirements for imported tilapia. For example, the European Union (EU) requires that the following information must be provided by the exporter, either on the labelling or packaging of fishery and aquaculture products or by specification document accompanying the products (CBI, 2015):

1. The name of the product: The commercial and scientific name of the species.
2. Production method: In the case of tilapia, it must be stated that it is a cultured product.
3. Origin: In the case of tilapia, there must be a reference to the country in which it is produced.
4. Presentation: It must be stated how the product is processed (for frozen whole fish or fillet products; for fresh gutted products, with or without head, filleted, thawed and others).
5. Net weight: The net weight must be stated on pre-packed products.
6. Date of minimum durability: Consisting of day, month and year, in that order and preceded by the words 'best before' or 'best before end' or the 'use by' date.
7. EU seller: The name or business name and address of the manufacturer, packager or seller established in the EU.
8. The package must contain an EU approval number.
9. The package must also contain a batch number.
10. Nutrition: Ingredients and nutrition must be stated.

11.9 Closing remarks

1. Tilapia is traditionally marketed as whole fresh and/or iced fish. Marketing of processed tilapia and tilapia products is now gaining great popularity in many parts of the world.
2. The production and global trade in tilapia and tilapia products have witnessed an impressive flourishing during the past two decades. Global markets for importing and exporting tilapia are also expanding.
3. Cooling (icing, refrigeration, freezing, etc.), filleting, radiation and industrial processing (drying, smoking, canning, fish balls, sausages, etc.) are commonly used for processing tilapia.
4. Frozen fillet and frozen whole fish are the most important forms of tilapia exports, contributing about 70% to total tilapia exports.
5. Asia is the largest tilapia exporter in the world, contributing more than 90% to total tilapia exports.
6. China is currently the largest tilapia exporter in the world; contributing over 50% to total tilapia exports. However, the rising of production costs in China and the change in government policy with regard to product subsidies will make Chinese producers less competitive in the international markets over time, leaving more room for other exporters.
7. The US market is the largest tilapia market in the world. A great variety of tilapia products, including live fish, fresh fish and frozen fillets, are currently marketed in the United States. Taiwan and mainland China are the major tilapia exporters to the US market.
8. Tilapia trade and marketing are faced by a number of challenges, including misconception about eating tilapia, misperception among consumers about the quality of farmed tilapia and lack of traceability and labelling. Extensive efforts should be spent to tackle these issues.

References

Ahmed, N., Young, J.A., Dey, M.M., Muir, J.F., 2012. From production to consumption: a case study of tilapia marketing systems in Bangladesh. Aquaculture International 20, 51–70.

Amal, M.N.A., Koh, C.B., Nurliyana, M., Suhaiba, M., Nor-Amalina, Z., Santha, S., et al., 2018. A case of natural co-infection of Tilapia Lake Virus and *Aeromonas veronii* in a Malaysian red hybrid tilapia (*Oreochromis niloticus* × *O . mossambicus*) farm experiencing high mortality. Aquaculture 485, 12–16.

Anane-Taabeah, G., Quagrainie, K., Amisah, S., 2016. Assessment of farmed tilapia value chain in Ghana. Aquaculture International 24, 903–919.

Atanda, A.N., Fagbenro, O.A., 2017. Social and economic performance of tilapia farming in Nigeria. In: Cai, J., Quagrainie, K.K., Hishamunda, N. (Eds.), Social and Economic Performance of Tilapia Farming in Africa. FAO Fisheries and Aquaculture Circular No. 1130. FAO, Rome, pp. 113–125.

Bacharach, E., Mishra, N., Briese, T., Zody, M.C., Tsofack, J.E.K., Zamostiano, R., et al., 2016. Characterization of a novel orthomyxo-like virus causing mass die-offs of tilapia. mBio 7, e00431–16.

Bimbao, M.P., Smith, I.R., 1988. Philippine tilapia economics: industry growth and potential. In: Pullin, R.S.V., Bhukaswan, T., Tonguthai, K., Maclean, J.L. (Eds.), Proceedings of the Second International Symposium on Tilapia in Aquaculture. ICLARM Conference Proceedings No. 15. Department of Fisheries, Bangkok, Thailand, and ICLARM, Manila, Philippines, pp. 539–551.

CBI, 2015. CBI Product Factsheet: Tilapia in Europe. CBI, Ministry of Foreign Affairs, the Netherlands, p. 9.

Darko, F.A., 2011. Consumer Preference for Farmed Fish in Ghana and Kenya: Opportunities for Domestic Demand-Driven Aquaculture. MSc. Thesis. Purdue University, West Lafayette, USA.

Dong, H.T., Siriroob, S., Meemetta, W., Santimanawong, W., Gangnonngiw, W., Pirarat, N., et al., 2017. Emergence of tilapia lake virus in Thailand and an alternative semi-nested RT-PCR for detection. Aquaculture 476, 111–118.

El-Sayed, A.-F.M., 2017. Social and economic performance of tilapia farming in Egypt. In: Cai, J., Quagrainie, K.K., Hishamunda, N. (Eds.), Social and Economic Performance of Tilapia Farming in Africa. FAO Fisheries and Aquaculture Circular No. 1130. FAO, Rome, pp. 1–48.

FAO, 2018. Fishery Commodities Global Production and Trade. http://www.fao.org/fishery/statistics/global-commodities-production/query/en.

Fathi, M., Dickson, C., Dickson, M., Leschen, W., Baily, J., Muir, F., et al., 2017. Identification of tilapia lake virus in Egypt in Nile tilapia affected by 'summer mortality' syndrome. Aquaculture 473, 430–432.

FDA (Food and Drug Administration), 2017. Eating Fish: What Pregnant Women and Parents Should Know. https://www.fda.gov/Food/ResourcesForYou/Consumers/ucm393070.htm.

Ferdouse, F., 2001. Tilapia in Asian Markets. Can we sell more? In: Subasinghe, S., Singh, T. (Eds.), Tilapia: Production, Marketing and Technical Developments. Proceedings of the Tilapia 2001 International Technical and Trade Conference on Tilapia. Infofish, Kuala Lumpur, Malaysia, pp. 71–74.

Ferguson, H.W., Kabuusu, R., Beltran, S., Reyes, E., Lince, J.A., Del Pozo, J., 2014. Syncytial hepatitis of farmed tilapia, *Oreochromis niloticus* (L.): a case report. Journal of Fish Diseases 37, 583–589.

Frimpong, E.A., Anane-Taabeah, G., 2017. Social and economic performance of tilapia farming in Ghana. In: Cai, J., Quagrainie, K.K., Hishamunda, N. (Eds.), Social and Economic Performance of Tilapia Farming in Africa. FAO Fisheries and Aquaculture Circular No. 1130. FAO, Rome, pp. 49–90.

Globefish, 2018. Analysis and Information on World Fish Trade. Tilapia Market Reports. http://www.fao.org/in-action/globefish/market-reports/tilapia/en/.

Guerrero III., R.D., Guerrero, L.A., 2001. Domestic marketing of tilapia in Southeast Asia. In: Subasinghe, S., Singh, T. (Eds.), Tilapia: Production, Marketing and Technical Developments. Proceedings of the Tilapia 2001 International Technical and Trade Conference on Tilapia. Infofish, Kuala Lumpur, Malaysia, pp. 81–83.

Hyuha, T.S., Bukenya, J.O., Twinamasiko, J., Molnar, J., 2011. Profitability analysis of small-scale aquaculture enterprise in Central Uganda. International Journal of Fisheries and Aquaculture 2, 271–278.

Hyuha, T.S., Ekere, W., Egna, H., Molnar, J.J., 2017. Social and economic performance of tilapia farming in Uganda. In: Cai, J., Quagrainie, K.K., Hishamunda, N. (Eds.), Social and Economic Performance of Tilapia Farming in Africa. FAO Fisheries and Aquaculture Circular No. 1130. FAO, Rome, pp. 127–144.

Kassam, L., 2013. Assessing the Contribution of Aquaculture to Poverty Reduction in Ghana. PhD Thesis. University of London, p. 404.

Liang, X., Wang, W., Cai, J., Shen, N., 2017. Assessment and monitoring of global tilapia markets. Paper Presented at the World Aquaculture Society Meeting, Cape Town, 26-30 June, 2017, p. 115.

Matlala, M.P., Kpundeh, M.D., Yongming, Y., 2013. Production and marketing systems of farmed tilapia in China. International Journal of Fisheries and Aquaculture 5, 12–18.

Ngugi, C.C., Nyandat, B., Manyala, J.O., Wagude, B., 2017. Social and economic performance of tilapia farming in Kenya. In: Cai, J., Quagrainie, K.K., Hishamunda, N. (Eds.), Social and Economic Performance of Tilapia Farming in Africa. FAO Fisheries and Aquaculture Circular No. 1130. FAO, Rome, pp. 91–111.

Nicholson, P., Fathi, M.A., Fischer, A., Mohan, C., Schieck, E., Mishra, N., et al., 2017. Detection of Tilapia Lake Virus in Egyptian fish farms experiencing high mortalities in 2015. Journal of Fish Diseases 40, 1925–1928.

Peng, Z., Yong-ming, Y., Didlyn, K.M., 2013. Establishment of indicators for early warning system on tilapia trade. African Journal of Business Management 7, 72–77.

Torres, E.B., Navera, E.R., 1985. Tilapia marketing in Central Luzon and Metro Manila, Philippines. In: Smith, I.R., Torres, E.B., Tan, E.O. (Eds.), Philippine Tilapia Economics. ICLARM Conference Proceedings No. 15. ICLARM, Manila, Philippines, pp. 181–191.

USDA (United States Department of Agriculture), 2018. Economic Research Service. https://www.ers.usda.gov/data-products/aquaculture-data/aquaculture-data/#Trade.

Vannuccini, S., 2001. Global markets for tilapia. In: Subasinghe, S., Singh, T. (Eds.), Tilapia: Production, Marketing and Technical Developments. Proceedings of the Tilapia 2001 International Technical and Trade Conference on Tilapia. Infofish, Kuala Lumpur, Malaysia, pp. 65–70.

Young, J.A., Muir, J.F., 2000. Economics and marketing. In: Beveridge, M.C.M., McAndrew, B.J. (Eds.), Tilapias: Biology and Exploitation. Kluwer Academic Publishers, Dordrecht, The Netherlands, pp. 447–487.

Chapter 12

The role of tilapia culture in rural development

Chapter outline

12.1 Introduction

The Sustainable Development Goals identified poverty eradication as one of the major global challenges facing the world today. Despite the continuous progress in addressing the needs of the world's poorest, over one billion people still live in extreme poverty. The improvement of food production systems has been recognized as a fundamental sector for the alleviation of extreme poverty, hunger and malnutrition in the developing and underdeveloped countries (CGIAR, 2015). Improved human health and well-being in these countries, particularly in rural areas, is also a major challenge. This means that rural development is a continuous process facilitated by governments, nongovernmental organizations (NGOs) and international donors to sustain the growth of rural economies, improve the livelihoods of rural communities and promote food security through the improvement of food supply, employment and income (Edwards et al., 2002; Halwart et al., 2003; CGIAR, 2015).

Aquaculture can play an important role in national economies in countries practicing aquaculture activities. This role includes increasing fish supply for domestic consumption, generating more foreign currency, raising producer's income and creating employment opportunities. As an agricultural subsector, aquaculture is also expected to play a core role in rural development, especially in developing countries in the tropical and subtropical regions of the world. It can contribute significantly to the alleviation of poverty and malnutrition and improving the welfare of rural households, due to the following main reasons:

1. Aquaculture is the fastest growing food-producing system in the world (Halwart et al., 2003; FAO, 2016).
2. More than 90% of the world aquaculture production comes from developing countries (including China; and about 40% if China is excluded).
3. Aquaculture is becoming an important component of rural livelihood and poverty alleviation in situations where the increasing population pressure, environmental degradation and/or loss of access will limit dependence on natural fisheries.

In rural areas, aquaculture is generally integrated with other farming activities and should not be examined in isolation from other sources of livelihood. This integration is generally more productive, sustainable and effective in

Tilapia Culture. https://doi.org/10.1016/B978-0-12-816541-6.00012-X
Copyright © 2020 Elsevier Inc. All rights reserved.

achieving food security in rural areas (Joffre et al., 2017). At the same time, it is important to understand the role of households not only as producers but also as consumers. Thus, to evaluate the role of aquaculture in rural development, one must consider the contribution of rural aquaculture to household economies, both in the case of smallholder fish farmers and subsistence farmers, and the interaction with the nonaquaculture economic activities of farmers, as well as the household's food/protein requirements and actual consumption levels.

Rural aquaculture is also a complex and diverse practice, including various aspects and interrelationships, such as technical aspects, environmental aspects, economic and socioeconomic aspects, extension services and policy issues. All these issues should be fully considered and integrated for sustainable rural aquaculture development. The benefits of aquaculture in the development of rural livelihood are also related to health, nutrition, employment, income, reduction of vulnerability and farm sustainability.

In small-farmer systems, aquaculture provides good quality animal protein and other nutrients, especially for nutritionally vulnerable groups, at low prices. It also provides jobs and "own enterprise" employment, including work for women and children generating additional income through harvesting and sale of their products (Fig. 12. 1). On larger farms, income can be increased through employment in seed supply networks, in market chains and through manufacture/repair functions. Indirect benefits include an increased availability of fish in local rural and urban markets and concomitant reduction in price, allowing savings to be spent on other income-generating farm products. Aquaculture can also offer benefit from the utilization of common resources, particularly for the landless, through cage culture, culture of molluscs and seaweeds and enhanced fisheries in communal water bodies.

One other important benefit of rural aquaculture is its relevance to integrated agriculture–aquaculture systems (IAAS), which increase farm efficiency and sustainability. Agricultural by-products, such as crop residues, livestock manures and green manures, can be used as feed/fertilizer inputs for small-scale commercial aquaculture systems. Similarly, farming fish in rice fields has several economic, biological and environmental benefits (discussed in Chapter 5).

In rural areas, aquaculture is likely to be more advantageous than other agricultural activities, such as cash crops and livestock production, due to:

1. It is being easily integrated into other agriculture and animal production activities,
2. The use of low-cost inputs and technologies by using locally available on-farm sources,
3. The limited investment needs,
4. The low levels of risk and
5. The low labour requirements.

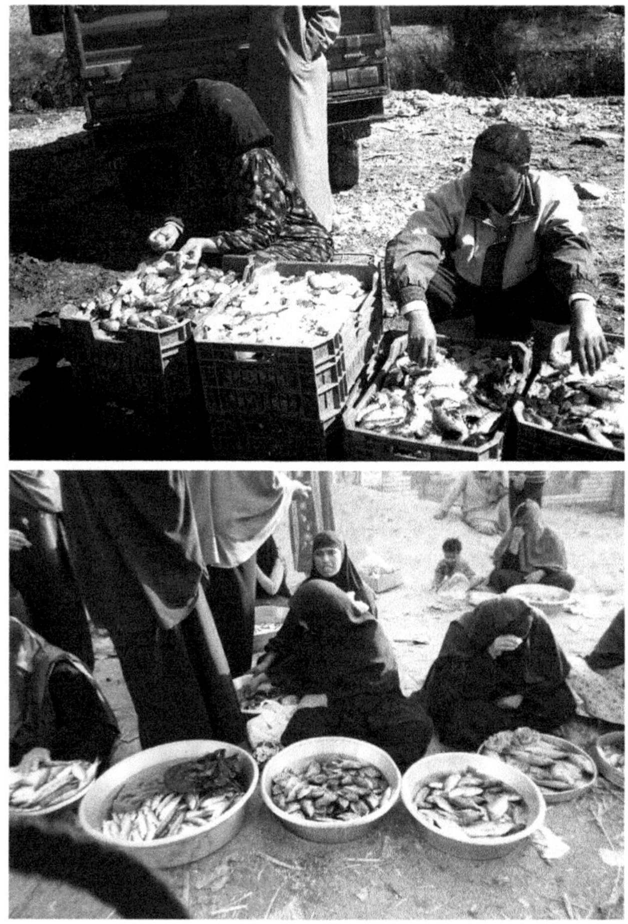

FIGURE 12.1 A rural woman and her son (top) and rural women (bottom) sell tilapia in a local fish market in Kafr El Sheikh, Egypt. *Photograph by A.-F.M. El-Sayed.*

As a result of the recognition and increasing role of aquaculture in rural development, both governments and governmental and nongovernmental organizations started paying more attention to the subject. Scientific conferences, workshops, training courses and extension services on rural aquaculture development are spreading worldwide. The scientific conference that was held in Thailand in 1998 on rural aquaculture, with emphasis on Asian experience, is just an example. The papers presented at the conference were published in a book entitled "Rural Aquaculture" by CAB International in 2002. Many FAO "*Technical Papers*" and "*Reports*" have also been published on the subject. A Training Handbook on Rural Aquaculture has been published by the Southeast Asian Fisheries Development Center (SEAFDEC) – Aquaculture Department in 2009 in the Philippines. A number of research projects on the contribution of small-scale aquaculture to sustainable aquaculture and rural livelihood development have also been carried out by different organizations (e.g., FAO, CGIAR, WorldFish) in different parts of the world (FAO,

2010). In addition, some methods/frameworks/case studies have assessed the impacts of small-scale rural aquaculture projects on poverty eradication and food security in developing countries.

Several other research studies have also considered the role of aquaculture in rural development. Ahmed and Lorica (2002) evaluated the role that aquaculture plays in attaining food security in Asian developing countries. They reported that pond culture along with cash crops and other on-farm activities contribute 5%–10% to total income in rural areas in Bangladesh. The effects of aquaculture adoption on household labour use and employment have also been significant (Ahmed et al., 1995). Aquaculture has been the most rapidly developing subsector within the agriculture sector in China during the past 3 decades and has played a significant role in boosting rural development, in terms of food security, income generation and employment opportunities (Li et al., 2011). In this regard, the government support, through technical extension service, policies and funding, has been a key player in rural aquaculture development. As a result, the contribution of aquaculture to total agricultural output increased from only 1.8% in 1985 to 10% in 2008. Currently, aquaculture produces one-third of China's total animal protein supply, playing an important role in food security in the country. The development of this subsector also improved the related industries such as processing, storage, transport, feed and veterinary supplies. This has led to a significant increase in the average income of fish farmers and other rural households engaged in aquaculture value chain.

Veerina et al. (1993) found that 71% of traditional crop farmers in Andra Pradesh, India, considered aquaculture as their primary activity, and about 49% of the farmers depended completely on aquaculture. Adeel and Safriel (2008) described the development of desert-based integrated aquaculture/agriculture, with accompanied longer-term storage of water, on the margins of the Cholistan Desert in Pakistan. They reported that this practice has provided a new source of income for the villagers, in addition to sustainable supply of a cheap protein source.

Rural aquaculture can also increase the consumption of aquatic food by both producers and domestic consumers by increasing fish availability in rural and urban areas. Per capita consumption of fish in various Asian countries has been reported to be significantly higher for fish-producing households in the rural areas, compared with both non-producers and the national average consumption (Dey et al., 2000; Ahmed and Lorica, 2002). Not only that, but there is a wide variation in per capita consumption and types of fish consumed among various economic and social strata. Consumer demand for major fish species, such as carp and tilapia, shows a price-elastic and income-elastic demand in India, Bangladesh, Thailand and the Philippines, but not in China (Dey, 2000). Price elasticity and income elasticity are the changes in consumer demand according to changes in fish price and consumers' income. This means that the degree by which consumers' demands will change because of the changes in fish price and consumer's income is lower in China than in the other four countries surveyed. Generally, low-value fishes, such as carp and tilapia, have lower price elasticity, whereas high-value products, such as crustaceans, sea bass and sea bream, have higher price elasticity. It has also been found that price elasticity of demand for big fish (e.g., carp) in Bangladesh is higher in the urban areas than in rural areas for all income groups, and the level of household income is inversely related to the income elasticity of demand for fish (Dey, 2000).

A considerable part of aquaculture production in rural areas is consumed on farm, especially when aquaculture becomes part of subsistence activities on the farm (Ahmed and Lorica, 2002). On-farm household consumption is directly related to pond production of low-price fish, such as tilapia and carp (Gupta et al., 1999). Increased on-farm fish availability reduces the dependence of household consumption on purchased fish (i.e., fish supply produced from family farms covers most of the needs of the household for fish). Consequently, as pond production increases in rural areas, a large proportion of this production is likely to be sold in local markets, in addition to the major amounts consumed by the households themselves (Karim et al., 2011). In the meantime, high-price fish crops are sent to the market and sold at higher prices (Ahmed and Lorica, 2002).

12.2 Tilapia and rural development

Tilapia have many attributes and advantages that make them an excellent candidate for aquaculture (see Chapter 1). As a result, tilapia culture has witnessed a rapid global expansion, during the past 3 decades, especially in developing countries, where the major bulk of farmed tilapia is produced. Moreover, tilapia culture is becoming more popular and well established in many small holders' ponds in rural areas, even in countries that do not have any history in tilapia culture and have traditionally relied on their native species, such as Vietnam, India, Pakistan, Bangladesh and Sri Lanka.

In Bangladesh, for example, where carps are considered the major cultured fishes while exotic fish culture is rare in Gazipur District (Ahmad et al., 1993), Barman et al. (2002) found that 56% of pond farmers in the Northwest Bangladesh raised tilapia either in monoculture systems or, more commonly, in polyculture systems with carps. Tilapia are also an important contributor to farmers' risk avoidance in riverine, flood-prone areas in the region. Farmers favour tilapia culture in these areas because tilapia do not need to be stocked or managed carefully and also require very low culture inputs, compared to carps, for which seeds are generally purchased. These advantages have led to relative popularity of tilapia culture in other areas of Bangladesh (Ahmed et al., 1996). The tendency to favour tilapia culture to reduce cash costs was also noticed in Northeast Thailand (Little et al., 1996). Similarly, despite tilapia not being endemic in Vietnam, and their introduction for aquaculture being relatively recent, tilapia culture is currently playing an important role in the food security of the local rural poor. It provides cheap, high-quality food both to farmers' households and local markets and generates cash incomes (Van Huong and Cuong, 2012).

Tilapia production systems are currently categorized into three distinctive categories: (1) smallholder, (2) commercial, and (3) industrial (Little, 1998). Little (1998) proposed a framework for categorizing factors affecting these production systems in relation to the market and the various beneficiaries (Table 12.1). It would be useful here to throw some lights on these production systems.

I. Smallholders' system

Smallholders' system is widely established in much of rural Asia, Africa and Latin America, where smallholders' ponds, ditches and rice fields, typically individually owned, are often used for tilapia culture. The farmers generally use very little inputs, if any (kitchen disposals, incidental fertilization), with poor management. Consequently, the yield of this system is generally low, but can still significantly improve the nutrition and livelihoods of rural households.

II. Commercial production system

Commercial production system is generally practiced semi-intensively, typically in densely populated peri-urban areas where culture inputs such as fertilizers and supplemental feed sources are available. These areas are also characterized by growing appreciation of the overall value

TABLE 12.1 Framework for the main types of tilapia production systems.

Category	Smallholder	Commercial	Industrial
Main descriptors	Rural, few/no inputs, organic spread, natural recruitment	Peri-urban fertilized pond, hatchery-supplied seed	Isolated, vertically integrated, seed production on-site
Inputs	None, fertile runoff, incidental fertilization	Wastes/fertilizers/supplementary feeds	Complete feeds
Systems	Small ponds, ditches, rice fields, community ponds	Large ponds	Raceways, cages, intensive ponds
Importance of self-sustained seed	XXX	XX	XXX
Importance of linkages with hatcheries by trading networks	X	XXX	X
Primary reasons for farmers self-sufficiency	Few options, minimal costs	Reduced costs	Assured supply, maintain and upgrade quality
Relevance of monosex	X	XX	XXX
Market	Poor, rural producers and consumers	Poor and middle-income, urban	Primarily export, domestic, urban better-off
Main beneficiaries	Producers, may be poorest within households, immediate community, local traders	Traders, land owners	Shareholders, processors, ice/equipment supplies, transporters, governments, grain farmers, importers, contract farmers
Other stakeholders	Fish seed traders	Transporters, harvest teams	Co-users of water resource/wastewater
Major constraints	Erratic seed supplies	Poor quality seed, land-related costs, nutrient availability	Off-flavours, water availability, cost of feed and labour

Notes: *X*, least important, *XX*, medium importance, *XXX*, most important
From Little, 1998, with permission.

and production profitability of tilapia culture. Culture inputs such as seeds, feeds, fertilization, harvesting, transportation, and marketing and overall management planning are generally higher than in smallholders' system.

III. Industrial production system

Industrial production system of tilapia is usually practiced by large companies that generally establish operation mechanisms to best suit the market needs. Extensive investments are usually pumped in this production system. This system also requires sophisticated production, marketing and overall management policies. In many Asian countries, tilapia produced by industrial production system are exported to foreign markets, particularly to the US market.

The following sections throw light on the role of tilapia culture in rural development in the major producing continents; namely, Asia, Africa and Latin America.

12.3 Tilapia and rural development in Asia

Developing countries in Asia are the world leaders in aquaculture production, with China alone producing over 57.5% of the total global production (64,358,481 t in 2017) and 62.5% of Asian aquaculture production (FAO, 2019). In addition, 7 out of the top 10 aquaculture producers in the world are Asian countries; 6 of them are developing countries (FAO, 2019). These figures reflect the importance of aquaculture in the developing countries in general and in rural areas in particular.

Asia is also the major producer of farmed tilapia, with a production of 4,140,896 t in 2017, contributing 70.4% to global tilapia production (FAO, 2019). Most of this production comes from small-scale, rural farms (Fig. 12.2). Therefore, small-scale, family-owned systems in much of Asia are becoming more competitive to large-scale, commercially managed tilapia farms (Little, 1998). However, little information is available on the importance of tilapia to households and their role in the overall economies in these rural areas. This gap is mainly because small-scale tilapia farms are scattered in remote and isolated areas that are difficult to approach. In the mean time, tilapia is cultured mainly in polyculture systems or in integrated systems with other plant/animal species and separate information and statistical data on their production, value, etc., is generally not available in many countries. Increasing attention has been given to the role of tilapia culture in rural development in some tilapia-producing countries in Asia.

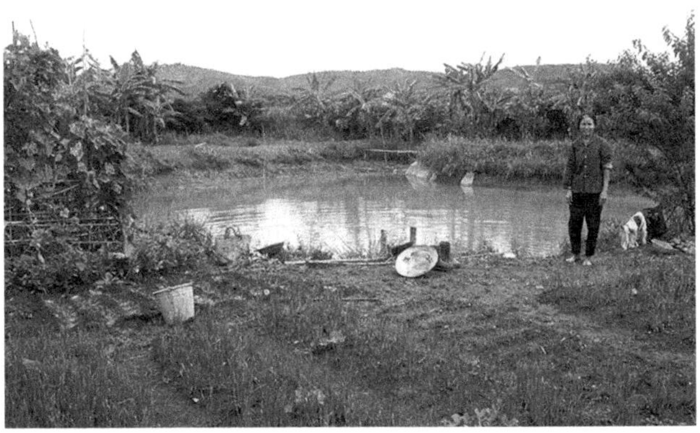

FIGURE 12.2 Tilapia culture in earthen ponds in rural areas in Vietnam *Photo provided by P. Edwards.*

Most cultured tilapia in Asia is produced in China, Indonesia, Bangladesh, the Philippines, Thailand and Vietnam. These six countries produced 89.6% of total farmed tilapia in Asia in 2017 (see Chapter 1). It would be appropriate to discuss the role that tilapia culture plays in rural development in these countries, taking into account that they are also among the most heavily populated countries in Asia. Considerable amount of information has also been gathered on the role of tilapia culture in rural development in these countries in recent years, especially in Bangladesh. The following section will be dedicated to Bangladesh, China, Indonesia, the Philippines and Thailand as examples of tilapia culture in rural Asia.

12.3.1 Bangladesh

As mentioned in Chapter 1, the story of tilapia culture in Bangladesh is amazing and could inspire other potential tilapia producers. Tilapia is not endemic to Bangladesh; Mozambique tilapia (*Oreochromis mossambicus*) and Nile tilapia (*O. niloticus*) were introduced into the country from Thailand in 1954 and 1974. Both species reproduced rapidly and were distributed in governmental and private fish farms throughout the whole country. Quickly they became widely accepted by the public, especially in rural areas, because they are considered a cheap protein source and low-cost operation with good financial returns. This incentive has encouraged poor rural farmers to culture these fishes (mainly Nile tilapia) in small seasonal ponds, ditches and micro-impoundments which are of little benefit.

The progressive expansion of tilapia culture in these rural areas has created an urgent need for technical and extension assistance on tilapia culture. Huge efforts and support from the government and regional and international organizations were provided during the past 3 decades. This assistance was essential because farmers in these remote areas generally lack the basic culture principals and adopt primitive methods, which lead to extremely low production. As a result, tilapia culture in Bangladesh has witnessed a breakthrough in recent years. Until 2008, no official tilapia production from Bangladesh was reported in

FAO records, whereas the reported production started in 2009, with only 16,237 t. Since then, tilapia production has been growing at an outstanding rate to reach 334,513 t in 2017, just in 9 years (FAO, 2019), with an exceptional average annual growth rate of 80%. Bangladesh is currently ranked third among the top tilapia producers in Asia (after China and Indonesia) and fourth in the world (after China, Indonesia and Egypt).

The role of tilapia culture in rural livelihood in Bangladesh is crucial, since these fish are produced exclusively in freshwater environments in rural areas. They are used mainly for subsistence and can be an economic source of food fish and additional income for households in rural areas in many parts of Bangladesh. Small-scale tilapia culture (especially Nile tilapia) in rural regions is simple, requiring very low inputs and labour and can be undertaken by women and even children. Selling a proportion of produced fish and fingerlings can meet the operational costs and sustain the operation. Gupta et al. (1992) reported that a pond of 169 m^2 yielded an average 23.6 kg of fish, with a return on investment of 343%, which is almost equivalent to the national annual consumption of low-income rural households with six family members. As expected, 70% of fish produced is consumed on-farm, improving the nutrition and health of farming families. It is clear that tilapia culture in this region is economically viable and 90% of the farmers are happy with this business and willing to expand their operations. Similarly, Gupta (2001) found that the culture of short-cycle species such as silver barb (*Puntius gonionotus*) or Nile tilapia (*O. niloticus*) in these seasonal ponds were profitable. In addition, landless farmers can benefit from this technology by culturing these fishes in common property roadside ditches.

Barman and Little (2006) evaluated the production of Nile tilapia seed in irrigated spring rice fields in a participatory approach in two poorer communities in Northwest Bangladesh. Each farmer was provided with 12 females and 6 males of mature Genetically Improved Farmed Tilapia (GIFT) Nile tilapia per trial plot (<0.15 ha). Management practices, production and sales of fish were monitored weekly during spring rice season (February–December). The majority of farmers succeeded in producing fingerlings in their plots, but seed production highly varied among households. Most fingerlings were sold (43%) and/or stocked for further fattening in their own grow-out systems (39%). In the meantime, 17% of produced fish were directly consumed by households. This clearly demonstrates the role that seed production can play in the livelihood of the rural poor. The same authors (Barman and Little, 2011) assessed the production of Nile tilapia seeds in nylon mesh net cages (hapas) in small-scale household food fish ponds in Northwest Bangladesh. GIFT tilapia broodfish (6 males and 12 females) were provided to each farmer to stock in a single spawning hapa (3 × 2 × 1 m) for breeding. Swim-up fry were collected from the hapas at 15-day intervals and stocked alternately in two nursing hapas (1.5 × 1 × 1 m). Most of the households produced tilapia fry from hapas for 4–5 months, in addition to the routine production of food fish/fingerlings in their ponds. The majority of produced fry (70%) were sold, while the remaining 30% were restocked for food fish production in the farmers' own ponds. Poorer households were more successful, and they preferred sale of fry over restocking in their own food fish ponds. Households engaged in fry trading and/or nursery businesses were also relatively successful. These results indicated clearly that local seed production has a significant impact on grow-out food fish production, since each hapa supplied seeds to 8 to 20 customers.

In another participatory trial, the effects of farming tilapia with existing integrated farming systems on pond-dike systems on the livelihoods and poverty reduction of households of varying socioeconomic levels in rural and peri-urban areas in Bangladesh were evaluated (Karim et al., 2011). The following findings were reported:

- Rural households benefit more than peri-urban households through enhanced direct consumption of fish and vegetables, whereas peri-urban households benefit more through trade of fish and vegetables.
- Households with access to ponds benefit equally selling and consuming fish and vegetables.
- Investment in fish production in integrated pond-dike farming systems is complementary, not competitive, to vegetable production.
- Further development of pond-dike systems is needed, which would improve livelihoods of both rural and peri-urban households.

The WorldFish Center initiated the genetic improvement programme of tilapia more than 25 years ago, which resulted in the production of the GIFT strain. The culture of GIFT has been tried in Bangladesh as a means of increasing tilapia production and economic return. Earlier studies indicated that GIFT yield was much higher than that of red tilapia and other existing strains, and this strain could substantially improve the livelihood of rural communities. Currently, there are more than 400 fish hatcheries in Bangladesh, using the GIFT strains, with a production of over four billion tilapia fry every year (Keus et al., 2017). However, many of these hatcheries lack the basics of proper management and misuse their broodstock by using the same parents repeatedly, without resting, rotations or adding new broodstock. This practice leads to inbreeding, which results in poor quality seeds, making the fish more susceptible to diseases and limiting the expansion of tilapia farming.

To tackle this problem, a United States Agency for International Development (USAID)-funded Aquaculture for Income and Nutrition (AIN) project was implemented by the WorldFish during 2011–15, within the framework of "Feed the Future (FTF)" strategy (Keus et al., 2017). The overall objective of the project was to increase income and nutrition in 18 of 20 FTF districts in southwest Bangladesh. To achieve this target, the project identified the following specific objectives:

- Increasing the productivity and profitability of fish and shrimp.
- Production and distribution of improved, high-quality tilapia seed to farmers, especially small- and medium-scale households.
- Building the technical capacity of public and private producers in hatchery and nursery techniques.
- Providing rural households with cheap, high-quality food.

Since 2012, the project has supplied the producers with GIFT seed from the improved 11th generation strain from Malaysia, which has a much higher growth rate than the existing local seed strains. A number of hatcheries were selected and technically supported to become tilapia breeding nuclei (TBNs) for tilapia seed production and dissemination. Selected TBNs received the necessary training on how to use selective and rotational breeding techniques in order to maintain high-quality broodstocks. The impact of this project on rural development in Bangladesh has been outstanding and can be summarized as follows (Keus et al., 2017):

1. Many tilapia hatcheries in the zone of influence currently use genetically improved broodfish and disseminate all-male tilapia seeds to neighbouring farmers at very good prices.
2. At the household level, the training provided by AIN-supported hatcheries and the access to improved seeds through TBNs have improved the productivity of pond-raised fishes, including tilapia.
3. In 2016, four TBNs produced 760,000 fry to be raised as improved broodstock, and four tilapia satellite hatcheries, which are specialized in multiplying and selling broodstock to regular hatcheries, supplied 1.2 million fry to regular hatcheries to be raised as improved broodstock. In 2015, 83 million tilapia fry were produced by 37 regular hatcheries, which make up 65% of all active hatcheries in the project area.
4. The evaluation of the project in 2016 indicated that GIFT strain grows about 30% faster than other tilapia strains used in the project region. Therefore, the introduction of improved GIFT tilapia increased the production by additional 15,000 t in the 2015–16 season.
5. In 2014, trained farmers generated 14,911 new jobs (25% for women) in their aquaculture farms.
6. Over 793,000 rural households in FTF's regions gained benefits from the project, including training, improvement of health status and production of quality fish and shrimp seed. A number of 43,000 children under five years in trained households have increased chances to consume good quality fish. In addition, out of the total of 138,000 t of fish, shrimp and vegetables produced in the project area in 2015, 2650 t of nutrient-rich food have been used by the beneficiary producer households.
7. By the end of the project period, the number of people living on less than US$ 1.25 day^{-1} in the project area was reduced by 39%, whereas 62% of the farmers increased their annual income by US$ 100.

In continuation with the above-mentioned effort, the Bangladeshi government in collaboration with the WorldFish and South Asia established a number of TBNs during 2012–16. This project was carried out under the Regional Fisheries and Livestock Development Component (RFLDC) of the Danish International Development Agency (DANIDA); the AIN and the Cereal Systems Initiative for South Asia–Bangladesh (CSISA-BD) projects using the 11th generation of the improved GIFT strain from the Jitra Station, Malaysia, and the Freshwater Station, BFRI, Bangladesh. Seven small-, medium- and large-scale TBNs have successfully been established and operated, adopting selective breeding and rotational breeding techniques to produce improved GIFT fry. In 2016, a number of 2,360,000 improved GIFT fry were produced by these TBNs and distributed/sold to 47 tilapia hatcheries scattered in different areas (Hussain et al., 2017). The production of more improved GIFT fry (3 million fry) was targeted in 2017 to be distributed among 70 multiplier tilapia hatcheries. These genuine efforts and attempts will certainly enhance the production of high-quality GIFT tilapia seeds and broodstock. It is expected that most of the commercial multiplier tilapia hatcheries in Bangladesh will be covered and supported by these TBNs between 2020 and 2022.

12.3.2 China

As mentioned earlier China is the leading country in aquaculture production in Asia and globally. Over 70% of aquaculture in China is pond-based, owned by private sector or community owned. Guangdong, Hainan, Guangxi, Fujian and Yunnan are the major tilapia producing provinces in China, contributing over 95% to national total tilapia production (Zongli et al., 2017). Small-scale and household-based tilapia farming is widely practiced in these provinces, making an important contribution to sustainable rural development. Contributions include food security, generating rural employment and income, efficient use of resources, diversifying livelihoods, utilizing family labour, fostering social harmony and empowering women (Bondad-Reantaso and Prein, 2009).

Guangxi province is the third largest tilapia producer in China, with a production of about 15% of total tilapia production in the country. Tilapia production is an important economic activity for small-scale tilapia farms in this province. Zongli et al. (2017) analyzed the economic efficiency of small-scale tilapia farms in Guangxi. They found that small-scale tilapia farms ($\leq$1 ha) have many advantages, including (1) low investment, (2) less vulnerability to risk and (3) easy management. The authors suggested that improving allocative efficiency is a key factor in economic success of small-scale tilapia farming in Guangxi. Overfeeding was considered as the major cause of the economic inefficiency in tilapia farming; and reducing the feed level is necessary to increase the efficiency.

A huge governmental support has been given to this sector; and one of the key factors in China's leadership is the very well-organized aquaculture extension system. Thousands of fisheries and aquaculture extension stations are distributed throughout the country, providing farmers and fishers with the necessary information, training and other extension services (APPG, 2018). A fascinating example in this regard is the amazing development of tilapia culture in Guangdong province, especially in the city of Maoming. The Maoming Fisheries Science and Technology Department provides comprehensive services and supervision for all tilapia industry stakeholders, including establishing breeding technology, disease prediction and treatment, improving farming technologies, funding, etc. As a result, tilapia culture was developed so rapidly in the city that it has become China's largest tilapia producer and was awarded the "Capital of China Tilapia" title in 2010. It is also currently the processing base in China for tilapia export.

Safina et al. (2017) analyzed the profitability of monosex tilapia production under three culture systems (monoculture, polyculture and integrated culture) in Guangdong, Guangxi, Hainan, Fujian and Yunnan in Southern China, and Hebei province in the Northern region. The study revealed that the culture systems had positive gross margins and net farm incomes. Polyculture and integrated culture, which are the major Chinese traditional farming systems, represent about 62% of total farming systems. In terms of profitability, tilapia production in monoculture system was more profitable and economically viable than the two other systems. However polyculture and integrated culture provided farmers with alternative options for production of quality fish and food, and better environmental conservation than monoculture. These two models are therefore adopted as development strategies for addressing household food security problems and poverty alleviation in rural areas. Farmers who are engaged within cooperatives have comparative advantages over individual farmers in terms of input (seed and feed) purchases and product marketing, due to higher bargaining power.

12.3.3 Indonesia

Despite carps having been the major cultured fish in freshwater systems in Indonesia for several years, tilapia have gradually overtaken carps as the dominant freshwater cultured species. This is partly due to consumers' demand, since tilapia have fewer bones in the muscle than carp. Initially, Mozambique tilapia was the main farmed tilapia species, until Nile tilapia was introduced into Indonesia in 1969. Since then, Nile tilapia has replaced Mozambique tilapia almost completely.

Freshwater aquaculture in Indonesia is practiced in earthen ponds mainly by small farmers and households. Small aquaculture enterprises currently comprise more than 80% of aquaculture farms in the country (Phillips et al., 2015). Based on the data from Indonesia Ministry of Fisheries and Marine Affairs in 2012, there are about 927,755 households practicing freshwater aquaculture in ponds; 65.8% of them have farm size less than 0.1 ha. Tilapia is currently representing about 34% of total inland freshwater aquaculture in Indonesia. Therefore, tilapia farming in ponds is the largest contributor to freshwater aquaculture sector and is expected to create more employment in the future (Phillips et al., 2015). This means that tilapia culture can play a substantial role in rural livelihood and welfare.

Despite Indonesia being currently the second largest tilapia producer in the world (after China) little information is available on the role of tilapia culture in rural development and livelihood since only a few studies have tackled this issue. Syandri et al. (2015) found that 73% of cage fish farmers in Lake Maninjau raise tilapia as a target species. This indicates that tilapia culture in floating net cages in the lake contributes significantly to the livelihood and food security of fish farmers. The Ministry of Marine Affairs and Fisheries (MMAF), through the Directorate General of Aquaculture (DGA) in cooperation with the FAO, has also implemented a pilot project on rice-fish farming (Fig. 12.3) in a number of villages in the District of Sleman (FAO, 2015). The rice-fish integration has increased the farmers' income, compared to rice monoculture, in addition to improving the land's productivity. It was projected that this practice will produce 1500 kg of red tilapia and 9000 kg of rice grains per ha, compared to 7000–8000 kg ha^{-1} of rice grains from rice farming alone. The farmer will receive around 4340 US\$ ha^{-1} in 3 months. This project is also a good example of all-sectors' synergy and cooperation to support food and nutrition sufficiency and improve the welfare of villagers as well.

The demand for Nile tilapia fingerlings to stock in grow-out systems, especially cages in reservoirs, is sharply

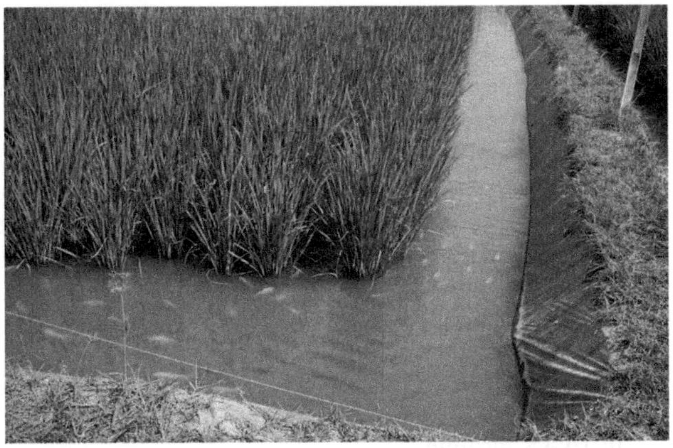

FIGURE 12.3 Red tilapia farming in rice fields in Indonesia. *Source: Shutterstock.*

increasing in Indonesia. Many small-scale farmers realized that it is not economic for them to continue to be involved in grow-out of low-value species (such as tilapia) if they want to make more profits. Thus, there has been a major shift of small-scale farmers from grow-out production to nursing business (Edwards, 2010). Four stages of tilapia nursing in West Java have been described by Edwards (2009), each undertaken by different groups of farmers. They are (1) spawning and fry harvest, (2) first-stage nursing to 2–3 cm total length (TL), (3) second-stage nursing to 3–5 cm TL and (4) third-stage nursing to 5–8 cm TL. After the fourth stage, tilapia fingerlings are sold for grow-out, mainly in cages in reservoirs (Edwards, 2009). It is evident that tilapia seed production and trade will be a major source of employment and profit in many rural regions in Indonesia.

12.3.4 Philippines

Among about 30 farmed aquatic species in the Philippines, carrageenophyte seaweeds and tilapia are the most important for livelihoods of rural poor, at regional and local levels (WorldFish, 2007). Tilapia serves as a cheap, high-quality food for consumers since it is generally cheaper and more affordable than red meat, chicken and even other freshwater fishes. As a result, the per capita consumption of tilapia by Filipinos has almost doubled during the past 2 decades, increasing from 1.6 kg $year^{-1}$ in the 1990s to about 3 kg $year^{-1}$ now (ADB, 2005a; PSA, 2018). Tilapia farming in the Philippines has also helped the fisheries sector in generating more income and employment opportunities (Aya, 2013). A cost and benefit survey of tilapia production was carried out by the Philippine's Bureau of Agricultural Statistics (PBAS) in 2011 in the major tilapia producing provinces in the Philippines (e.g., Pampanga, Batangas, Camarines Sur, Iloilo, South Cotabato and Sultan Kudarat). The results indicated that tilapia farming is the main practice, occupying 61% of farm operators (Aya, 2013).

However, tilapia culture industry in the Philippines has been constrained by a number of social, economic, technical and environmental factors (e.g., high input costs, fish mortality, water supply and typhoon damage), with limited supply of quality seeds at reasonable prices being a major constraint. To tackle this problem, the International Center for Living Aquatic Resources Management (ICLARM), (now known as the WorldFish Center), in cooperation with a number of partners launched the GIFT project in the Philippines in 1988. By 1993, three generations of GIFT were produced. After nine generations, the GIFT fish showed a 64% cumulative increase in growth over the original base population. After the GIFT project has been completed, the dissemination of the improved tilapia began by building the breeding capacity in neighbouring countries, in addition to the project's host country; the Philippines (ADB, 2005b).

GIFT fish were initially disseminated to farmers through government agencies. A wide, national distribution network for GIFT was created to take the lead through outreach stations and hatcheries. By 2003, GIFT strain and the GIFT-derived strain GET EXCEL accounted for 68% of total tilapia seed produced in the Philippines (ADB, 2004). GIFT tilapia and GIFT-derived seeds are currently used by the majority of tilapia farmers in the country, indicating that the impact of GIFT and GIFT-derived tilapia in the Philippines has been outstanding. Due to this technology, tilapia production has increased from only 13,214 t in 1980 to 267,735 t in 2017, representing 85% of freshwater aquaculture production and 33% of total aquaculture output (excluding aquatic plants) (FAO, 2019).

Over 60% of the country's hatcheries were dedicated to GIFT seed production (CGIAR, 2006). This switch significantly improved the livelihood of hatchery operators and fish farmers, especially poor, small-scale farmers. The net profits from GIFT tilapia production and trade are high because the GIFT technology has reduced production costs. In addition, the introduction and dissemination of GIFT strains have a significant contribution to rural employment and human nutrition, especially among the poor. Since many fish farmers are women, the use of GIFT strains has also empowered them, while providing local communities with affordable, high-quality protein and improving the nutrition and health status of rural households.

In continuation with improving tilapia strains through the adoption of GIFT technology, a "Strategy for Sustainable Aquaculture for Poverty Reduction in Philippines" has been approved by the Asian Development Bank. It was implemented in 2006–07 by the WorldFish Center, Malaysia, and the Pacific Rim Innovation and Management Exponents Inc. (PRIMEX) and Philippines, through the Philippine Department of Agriculture–Bureau of Fisheries and Aquatic Resources (DA-BFAR). The contribution of the strategy to poverty alleviation has been through the following (WorldFish Center, 2007):

(i) Increasing farm incomes through the use of viable production approaches in tilapia and seaweeds;
(ii) Promoting the investment in postharvest facilities, such as cold chains and farm-to-market roads to increase the income of farmers and
(iii) Improving capability of local government units to foster production and marketing partnerships with BFAR and the private sector.

The farm-level impact of GIFT and the way the GIFT technology has been disseminated and taken up were assessed by Pemsl et al. (2008) through surveying 780 tilapia producers in Luzon, the Philippines. The adoption of pure GIFT strains was very low (6%), while GIFT-derived strains were adopted by almost 50% of the farmers. However, over 27% of the farmers were uncertain about the genetic origin and purity of the strains they use. Meanwhile, most of the farmers reported that GIFT and GIFT-derived strains did not perform any better than other tilapia strains. This unexpected performance has been attributed to the poor management of improved strains rather than a shortcoming of the original GIFT technology (Pemsl et al., 2008).

12.3.5 Thailand

Thailand is currently the fifth top tilapia producer from aquaculture in Asia, after China, Indonesia, Bangladesh and the Philippines, with a production of 203,696 t in 2017 (FAO, 2019). Tilapia production comes exclusively from freshwater aquaculture, representing 53% of total freshwater aquaculture production in 2017 (FAO, 2019). It is no surprise, therefore, that tilapia production is at the top of freshwater fish culture in Thailand. Typically, tilapia is cultured in private/family-owned, small to moderate ponds (1–3 ha), in semi-intensive, polyculture systems with carps and silver barb (Pant et al., 2004; Belton, 2013). The vast majority of tilapia farms in Central Thailand are owned and managed by households. However, land renting for tilapia culture in more distant Central Region provinces is common (Belton, 2006).

Integrated agriculture-aquaculture systems (IAAS) (fish-chicken/duck-pig), in addition to fish-cum-rice, are very common in Thailand. Intensive monoculture of tilapia is also practiced at a very large scale. Integrated culture of tilapia can play a significant role in improving households livelihood, by providing them with high-quality, cheap protein source, generating additional income and rehabilitating the soil through better on-farm nutrient recycling (Pant et al., 2004; Belton, 2013). The prospects of IAAS farming for sustainability of agriculture development in the northeast region of Thailand have been evaluated by Pant et al. (2004). A survey of IAAS households with varying lengths of experience in four different agroecologies – one irrigated and three rain-fed ecologies (drought-prone, rain-fed lowland and rolling land) – was carried out. This survey collected an extensive amount of information on culture systems, fish species cultured, stocking densities, pond inputs, yield, gross return and the role of ponds in farming system diversification.

The main findings of the study were as follows:

1. The fish culture system of the IAAS varied with agroecology but not with the length of farmers' experience in IAAS farming.
2. The size of the pond holding in the rain-fed lowland was smaller than in the other three agroecologies.
3. The highest gross fish yield of 2.3 t ha^{-1} was recorded in the irrigated agroecologies and was significantly higher than in the rain-fed ecologies.
4. Over 75% of households raised tilapia and carp in a polyculture system, with nearly 90% in irrigated agroecology, compared with about 50% in the rain-fed lowland. In the drought-prone and rolling land agroecologies, about 75% of households practised tilapia/carp polyculture.
5. The average income of IAAS households from fish varied across agroecologies.
6. Farm ponds played a significant role in the diversification of farming systems in rain-fed areas.
7. Improved management practices and input supply are key factors for increasing fish production in IAAS.
8. Intensification of fish culture through pond fertilization with inorganic fertilizers can improve fish production in IAAS in the region.

It appears from that result that tilapia/carp polyculture has a significant contribution to the improvement of households' livelihood in Northeast Thailand. On the other hand, only about 10% of the households in the region raise tilapia in monoculture in IAAS. Tilapia/carp polyculture system appears appropriate and profitable in many parts of the region because pond inputs such as rice bran, crop byproducts, broken rice, cattle and buffalo manure are available, mostly on-farm, at low cost.

Tilapia culture in rice fields can play an essential role in the improvement of livelihood of rural communities, through food security assurance and profit generation. Earlier studies (Middendorp and Verreth, 1992) indicated that rice farmers may increase their household income by about 20% if they raise tilapia in hapas. Much more income has been reported from tilapia/rice farming in Southern Thailand (Pengseng, 2013). All-male Nile tilapia (15 g) were stocked in rice fields at a density of 1.25 fish m^{-2}, 30 days after sowing the rice seeds. Commercial organic fertilizer (625 kg ha^{-1}) and supplemental feed (25% cp, 2%

body weight d^{-1}) were applied. The fish and rice were harvested after 122 and 185 days, respectively. Rice monoculture provided a rice yield of 4288 kg ha^{-1}, with an average net return of 287.5 US\$ ha^{-1}. On the other hand, the rice–fish integration provided an average gross yield of 1350 kg of fish and 7013 kg rice ha^{-1}, respectively, with a net profit of 1227 US\$ ha^{-1}, more than 420% increase over rice monoculture. The study suggests that the adoption of this system will increase rice production, provide an additional good protein source and increase the farmers' income.

As tilapia production increases, the real sale value tends to decrease. This generally results in a decline in farmgate price and retail prices (Belton and Little, 2008) and rising consumers' demand, since demand for fish is highly price elastic (Dey et al., 2008). Therefore, small dead tilapia (300–400 g) are among the cheapest and most widely available products in Thailand. They are directed mainly to urban and peri-urban markets where they provide a good, healthy food for workers in the productive sectors (Belton et al., 2009). On the other hand, larger fish are sold to a different sector of customers. This means that tilapia contribute indirectly to the livelihoods and well-being of families of urban migrants from rural areas (Belton, 2013).

12.3.6 Other Asian countries

Tilapia culture has gained popularity in some other Asian countries and is expected to play a noticeable role in aquaculture development in these countries. Little et al. (2000) reported that semi-intensive aquaculture in Sri Lanka in on-farm ponds depends on hatchery-produced tilapia. Cage-based fattening of tilapia was also introduced as a means of poverty alleviation in some rural areas in Sri Lanka (Pollock and Little, 2002). The wide distribution and continuous improvement of GIFT tilapia in Sri Lanka has also significantly raised the standard of living among poor households and contributed to gender equality through increasing women employment in rural areas (Nguyen et al., 2011). Fish farming in backyard/home garden ponds was one of the components of a governmental, multisector programme on improving rural livelihoods and incomes in Sri Lanka during 2011–14 (Pushpalatha et al., 2016). A total number of 2109 ponds covering an area of 105.45 ha were established under this programme. A survey was carried out on culture practices, fish production and profitability of these ponds in the districts of Gampaha, Puttalam and Ampara. All-male or mixed-sex Nile Tilapia were the only farmed tilapia and were very profitable in all three districts, despite the sharp variations in stocking densities, inputs, fish production, operational costs and net returns among ponds.

In Vietnam, Pekar et al. (2002) reported that tilapia was the third most important fish species stocked in integrated systems in Mekong Delta (13%–21%), after silver barb (26%–34%) and common carp (19%–26%). Tilapias are also more attractive in Hanoi because they reach their marketable size faster than carps. Van Huong and Cuong (2012) investigated the contribution of small-scale tilapia culture to food security of rural households in Vietnam. They found that freshwater tilapia farming improved the food security of local rural poor through the provision of high-quality food and generation of cash incomes.

Tilapia culture is also spreading in many parts of India (Nandeesha, 2002). In Kolkata, for example, tilapia are the most demanded fish by both poor and rich consumers. Natarajan and Aravindan (2002) also reported that tilapia has been successfully cultured in sewage-fed ponds, rice fields and brackish water ponds in various parts of India. Tilapia culture also became well-established in bheries of West Bengal. In Lao People's Democratic Republic, tilapia farming in cages in reservoirs is gaining considerable attention. Most of the cages are restricted to Nam Ngum reservoir, the smaller Nam Souan and Nam Houm reservoirs, the mainstream Mekong and some major tributaries. The adoption of tilapia farming at Ban Keung significantly increased the income of rural farmers, who are mainly women.

12.4 Tilapia and rural development in Africa

Aquaculture practices in Africa are very limited, despite experimental trials having been conducted on fish farming in countries like Egypt in the early1930s. Except in Egypt, the contribution of aquaculture to food security, poverty alleviation and overall economic development in the continent is small. This is despite the high potential for aquatic genetic resources and water adequacy in many parts of Africa. About 56%–70% of Africa's lands have the highest production potential for warmwater fishes such as tilapias, carps and catfish (Aguilar-Manjarrez and Nath, 1998). The FAO has also reported that 37% of Sub-Saharan Africa (SSA) is suitable for small-scale fish farming (Aguilar-Manjarrez and Nath, 1998). However, freshwater resources in Sub-Saharan Africa (SSA) are abundant in some areas due to heavy rainfall, while drought is dominating in many other areas. Prolonged drought has resulted in a severe reduction in available freshwater resources during the last 20 years (UNECA, 2016; Satia, 2017).

There are several constraints that hamper the development of aquaculture in Africa. These constraints are listed as follows (Brummett and Williams, 2000; Satia, 2017):

- Limited access to land and water resources, and degradation of these sources.
- Competition for land and water resources by multiple users.
- Weather and climate change–related shocks.

- Increasing urbanization.
- The severe political instability in some African countries limits the development of agricultural sectors, including aquaculture. Such political problems also threaten the economic viability of aquaculture enterprises and security of investment.
- Poverty of consumers, leading to small local markets and reliance on external markets.
- The poor infrastructure, including poor storage, poor marketing channels and poor maintenance of farming facilities.
- Poor quality of governmental services such as extension.
- Sociocultural constraints.
- Shortage of good quality seeds and feeds.
- Shortage or lack of governmental budgets allocated for aquaculture.
- Lack of local expertise and technical experience, which may increase the risk of enterprise and limit technical options.

One other major constraint facing the development of rural aquaculture in Africa is its dependence, to a large extent, on external donations and technologies. In most cases, the farmers do not have the necessary experience and training in these new technologies, and the governments do not provide the necessary support (Moehl, 2002). The situation is getting worse because external funds have become very limited. As a result, the numbers of fish farms and farmers have increased dramatically, but production has not grown as progressively as planned for. Therefore, considerable attention has been paid to the aquaculture development in Africa from different regional and international organizations. Assistance has been provided by FAO and other development partners and donor organizations and investors, such as African Union-InterAfrican Bureau for Animal Resources (AU-IBAR), the World Bank, African Development Bank (AfDB), European Union (EU), USAID, Swedish International Development Cooperation (SIDA) and WorldFish (Satia, 2017). Several other initiatives and activities have been adopted to support African aquaculture development, including the 2005 AU/NEPAD Fish for All Summit in Abuja (Nigeria); the implementation of the FAO Special Programme for Aquaculture Development of Africa (SPADA); the NEPAD-FAO Fish Programme (NFFP); the Conference of African Ministers of Fisheries and Aquaculture (CAMFA) in Banjul (Gambia) in 2010 and Addis Ababa (Ethiopia) in 2014; and adoption of the Policy Framework and Reform Strategy for African Fisheries and Aquaculture (PFRS).

Small-scale African fish farmers have been better off, and better educated, than nonfish farmers (Sen et al., 1996). To alleviate the poverty of these rural fish farmers, appropriate extension and technology supports should be provided to them. The technology adopted and the level of extension services, rather than the financial situation or the level of formal education, are the driving forces for the success of small-scale tilapia culture in rural, poor Africa. For example, Van der Mheen-Sluijer (1991) found that small-scale aquaculture adopters in Eastern Province of Zambia had lower income than nonadopters. The author referred this to the extension service which had focussed on distributing aquaculture information to all small-scale farmers rather than better off farmers only.

Despite the constraints and difficulties facing rural aquaculture development, smallholder fish farms are increasing in many African countries and are integrated in the farmers' existing farming systems. These small-scale farms rely mainly on locally available inputs, with little investments; only in the form of land, water and labour (Brummett and Williams, 2000). They play an important role in increasing production efficiency, generating extra income, poverty alleviation, food security and improving overall household livelihoods in rural areas. It is estimated that more than 95% of African aquaculture production comes from these small-scale farms, with tilapia and/or African catfish being the dominant farmed species. Relatively large-scale, commercial farms are also raising tilapia as a cash crop in some African countries such as Egypt, Kenya, Nigeria, Zambia and Zimbabwe.

12.4.1 Tilapia and food security

Freshwater aquaculture dominates aquaculture systems in Africa, with tilapias, especially Nile tilapia, being the most important farmed fish group. They contribute over 55% of total aquaculture production in the continent. In SSA, tilapia is farmed almost exclusively in freshwater environment (99.6%), while in Egypt they are grown mostly in brackish water. Tilapia culture in small ponds (200–4200 m^2) remains the most common culture practice in Africa, contributing 40%–>90% of total tilapia production in many countries. Other farming systems, including tanks, cages and raceways, are also adopted in some areas, though at much smaller scales. Thus, tilapia farming has a great potential for improving the livelihoods in rural Africa.

As mentioned in Chapter 1, Egypt alone contributed 79.3% (967,301 t) to total production of farmed tilapia in Africa in 2017. Tilapia culture is also widely practiced in Uganda, Ghana, Nigeria and Zambia. These five countries contributed almost 90% to total tilapia production in Africa in 2017 (FAO, 2019). Therefore, it would be appropriate to throw light on the role of tilapia farming on rural livelihoods in these countries.

12.4.1.1 Egypt

Aquaculture in general, and tilapia culture in particular, have direct impact on the adopters, including improved food and nutrition security and increased household income. However, indirect impacts affecting nonadopters are more significant, including increased fish availability and reduced prices of fish for millions of Egyptians, especially in rural governorates. Because tilapia represent about 70% of total aquaculture production in Egypt, it is assumed that about 700 g from each kilogram of farmed fish consumed comes from farmed tilapia. Tilapia culture also greatly improves the livelihoods of the poor, mainly by generating thousands of employment opportunities through the whole value chain. The full-time equivalent (FTE) employment directly generated by tilapia farming (ponds, cages, tanks and rice fields) was estimated at 50,681 farmers and the FTE employment in the tilapia value chain are 84,265 persons (Macfadyen et al., 2011; El-Sayed, 2017).

Tilapia culture in rice fields has great potential in Egypt and can lead to substantial value addition in terms of extra income generation, improvement in rice crop production and part-time "own enterprise" employment, particularly during harvesting and selling of products. This practice can also play a significant role in poverty and malnutrition eradication of rural households, especially for nutritionally vulnerable groups, through providing good quality animal protein at low prices. The profitability of farming tilapia in rice fields in Egypt has been investigated by Salama (2009) in a number of major rice farming governorates (Dakahlia, Domiat, Faiyum, Kafr El Sheikh and Sharkia). The results indicate that an increase of 18%–40% in the net profits can be achieved when tilapia were raised in rice fields, depending on fish stocking density and size, rice strain and farming system applied.

Tilapia culture has made fish the most affordable source of animal protein in Egypt, especially for the poor. As a result, the annual per capita consumption of fish increased from 9.5 kg in 1995 to 20.6 kg in 2016, representing 45.5% of total animal protein consumption, while the consumption of poultry and red meat contributed 30.8% and 23.7%, respectively. Tilapia accounted for 61.4% of total fish production and 53% of total fish consumption in 2016, indicating that these fish are the most important single animal protein source for Egyptians. It should be emphasized also that almost all tilapia produced in Egypt are consumed domestically, while only a few tonnes are occasionally exported, exclusively to the Gulf region.

12.4.1.2 Ghana

Tilapia represent over 90% of total aquaculture production in Ghana and therefore appear to have a significant impact on Ghanaian livelihoods. Tilapia culture is practiced mostly in earthen ponds and, to a lesser extent, cages. Up to 90% of the ponds are small, ranging from 400 to 800 m^2 (300 m^2 in average), and each farmer owns one to two ponds (Fynn, 2014; Frimpong and Anane-Taabeah, 2017). Asmah (2008) reported that about 90% of households consume tilapia regularly or occasionally, and the average annual per capita consumption of tilapia ranged from 9.0 kg in the Ashanti Region to 20.5 kg in the Volta Region. This simply indicates that tilapia is becoming highly preferable by Ghanaians.

The actual and potential contribution of small- and medium-scale aquaculture to poverty reduction and food security in Ghana (Lake Volta, Eastern Region) has been assessed under the framework of the "Aquaculture for Food Security, Poverty Alleviation and Nutrition Project" (Kassam, 2013, 2014). The results suggest that aquaculture has direct impacts on the adopters, including increased on-farm income, enhanced food and nutrition security and increased farm sustainability through integrated agriculture–aquaculture practice. Indirect impacts affecting nonadopters include increased availability, and reduced prices, of fish for poor households, increased employment, wages and overall income of poor labourers. Small-scale pond aquaculture in the Ashanti Region does not have strong direct impacts on the poverty and livelihoods of poor households, despite they having been able to adopt aquaculture. On the other hand, small-scale aquaculture has positive direct impacts on the livelihoods of nonpoor fish-farming households who have been trained on better management practices (BMPs).

In a similar study, Kassam and Dorward (2017) reported that nonpoor, small-scale pond fish farmers who are trained and/or adopt BMPs have the highest indirect impact on poverty reduction through increasing economic growth. These impacts are higher than the direct impacts on poor, small-scale fish farmers and the indirect impacts from small and medium enterprises (SMEs). Asmah (2009) also recounted several benefits of tilapia cage farm workers, including regular incomes, free meals at work, informal interest-free loans provided by their employers, employer contributions to social security and health care coverage, and the education and experience gained through their employment. Traders can also gain income and employ temporary labour to clean fish for selling.

12.4.1.3 Kenya

In Kenya, Nile tilapia comprises about 73% of total farmed fish. However, tilapia culture development is still a real challenge among resource-limited rural households. Limited adoption of improved technologies and management practices, lack of capital and operational resources and poor marketing are the main constraints limiting tilapia culture industry (Kaliba et al., 2007). It has also been reported that little or no farmed fish is available in Nairobi markets. Fish farmers normally sell their fish to traders at the farm gate, which is destined fresh directly to local town markets. Farmed fish is also becoming less affordable to rural communities because of the low and inconsistent supplies (KMAP, 2016). Therefore, changes in marking strategies are needed to increase the availability of fish in both rural and urban markets. It should also be emphasized that small-scale aquaculture in Kenya is no longer a subsistence production activity for household consumption. It has rather become a major livelihood source for smallholder households through commercial practices as well as a major contributor of fish products to national markets (Ngugi et al., 2017).

Raising tilapia in rice fields is a potential alternative for food security in Kenya. Rasowo and Auma (2006) reported that farming Nile tilapia in rice fields can be profitable and can contribute to food security in Kenya. Due to the smaller size of harvested fish from rice fields, they are readily consumed by the farmers' families. Small-sized fish could be an asset to the households' nutrition. However, Rasowo and Auma (2006) suggested that the growing period should be extended to about 6 months to attain the required marketable size.

12.4.1.4 Zambia

Zambia is the biggest producer of tilapia in the South African Development Community (SADC). Tilapia production represents 99% of total aquaculture production and is a highly preferable food for most Zambians. The pond-based, small-scale sector produces mainly for household consumption and local sales. There are about 12,000 registered small-scale farmers in the country; most of them are relatively resource poor. About 40% of fish farming households use all of the harvest for family consumption, while about 57% sell their harvest in local markets (Musuka and Musonda, 2013; Genschick et al., 2017; Kaminski et al., 2018). This means that tilapia contributes directly to food security and indirectly to income generation through fish retail and job creation. According to a World Bank report (Krishnan and Peterburs, 2017), about 13,000 jobs are engaged in aquaculture sector in Zambia, primarily on-farm jobs, such as pond digging and construction, farm labour, farm operation, feed and seed production and trade, and fish processing.

In a comprehensive assessment of small-scale aquaculture profitability in selected areas in Zambia, Namonje-Kapembwa and Samboko (2017) listed the following findings:

1. More than 80% of fish ponds owned by small-scale fish farmers are small earthen ponds (about 500 m^2), with an average production of 475 kg per cycle.
2. The estimated initial fixed and operational costs for 500-m^2 pond for fish farming are about 10,469 US$.
3. The internal rate of return was 42.38% measured at the discount rate of 15%, and the benefit—cost ratio was 1.2 at the 15% discount rate. These values mean that small-scale aquaculture enterprises are feasible and profitable.
4. Aquaculture production in Zambia is sensitive to changes in the price of fish. For example, a 10% reduction in the price of fish resulted in a 59% decrease in the estimated net present value holding other factors constant.
5. The main farming constraints include animal and bird predators, high cost of feed, lack of finance, nonavailability of quality seeds, limited and inconsistent water supply and limited access to extension services.

12.4.1.5 Uganda

In Uganda, farmed tilapia is the most important species, representing 67% of total aquaculture production in 2017 (FAO, 2019), and most tilapia farmers are small farmers. Bukenya et al. (2013) found that 82% of small-scale fish farmers in Central Uganda reported activities in tilapia farming. This means that tilapia contribute significantly to food security and poverty reduction and resistance of children to diseases (Hyuha et al., 2017), especially among rural societies. Tilapia culture also generates employment opportunities along the entire value chain, including pond diggers and constructors, farm labourers, operators and managers, seed production and selling, harvesting and product marketing. However, Hyuha et al. (2011) found that despite the potential profitability of small-scale aquaculture enterprises in Central Uganda, the profit margins were relatively small. The authors identified several factors behind the low profitability, including limited farming experience, low fish price, poor record keeping, high feed cost and small volume of fish harvested. The key factors limiting aquaculture development in the region include unavailability of credit facilities, predators, expensive feeds and poor-quality seeds.

12.4.1.6 Nigeria

Most of the tilapia produced in Nigeria are used for domestic consumption in different forms (fresh, smoked, fried, salted or cooked), while export markets do not exist. Therefore, tilapia play a significant role in the livelihood and sustenance of many Nigerians in terms of nutrition and health status, and employment opportunities along the whole value chain (construction of ponds, tanks or cages, seed and feed production and trade, fish processing and selling, etc.) (Atanda and Fagbenro, 2017). More women are involved in tilapia processing, value addition and marketing in most parts of Nigeria, except for northern

Nigeria, than men. In the south, more than 70% of fish processors are women. Local restaurants serving fresh, smoked or grilled tilapia, and tilapia added to stews and pepper soup, are also run mainly by women (Atanda and Fagbenro, 2017).

12.4.1.7 Other African countries

The role of tilapia farming in food security has also been documented in other African regions. In the Ruvuma Region, Tanzania, fish farming has rapidly grown to the extent that it was ranked as the third most important source of income by farmers with fish ponds (Seki and Maly, 1994). Similarly, Vincke and Schmidt (1991) suggested that economic return from tilapia farming was higher than that generated from coffee, dairy or poultry. Under Rwandan conditions, and similar conditions in other African countries, tilapia are better farmed as a cash crop, whereas the cash generated from their sale can be used for buying the necessary commodities, including cheaper protein sources (Hishamunda and Jolly, 1998). Fish farming is also a strong competitor with horticulture for land fertilization in Rwanda. Enterprise analyses indicated that fish farming yielded the highest net return to land, labour and management compared to land crops (sweet potatoes and soybean). The management practices, yield, marketing and production constraints of Nile tilapia farming in earthen ponds owned by small-scale farmers in Mvomero and Mbarali districts in Tanzania were assessed (Chenyambuga et al., 2014). The results indicated that most farmers owned one (54.2%) to two ponds (37.5%) and the average pond size ranged from 345 to 631 m^2. About 38% of the harvest in Mbarali and 46.6% in Mvomero were consumed by farmers' households and the remaining portions were sold mostly fresh to their neighbours. Once again, these results clearly demonstrate the major role that tilapia can play in the livelihood and income generation of rural households in Tanzania.

12.4.2 Aquaculture/agriculture integration

For small-scale tilapia culture to be sustainable and profitable, it should be integrated with broader rural development initiatives, especially with agricultural farming activities. This type of integration can also lead to a significant improvement in the cash income of farmers' households in Africa. If properly integrated, tilapia culture can lead to more fish production, better diversification and enhancement of the farming systems and retaining environmental and social sustainability (Brummett and Williams, 2000). Research in Malawi (Brummett and Noble, 1995; Brummett, 2002) has shown that fish ponds integrated into farm activities, such as rice–fish integration, in such a way that they recycle wastes from other agricultural and household enterprises, can increase production and profitability. Fish ponds integrated with vegetable gardens in Malawi significantly increased fish and vegetable productivity (Brummett and Noble, 1995). Vegetable by-products are generally used as pond inputs, whereas pond water is used for irrigating garden vegetables. With continuous practice and appreciation of the system, farmers become able to further improve productivity and profitability. The success of small-scale integrated system generally encourages other farmers to adopt it. This generally leads to a rapid spread of this system from farmer to farmer. Switching from smallholder tilapia production (i.e., production for subsistence) to a more commercial practice requires additional inputs and new technologies for the storage and/or processing of feed ingredients. This will add more operating costs, but can still be highly profitable. In Malawi, for example, when commercial production systems in rural areas are properly conducted, fish production can be more profitable than most other cash crops (Chimatiro and Janke, 1994).

Although it can be highly profitable, small-scale aquaculture/agriculture integration is faced with many constraints that may render the system unable to achieve its objectives (Aganyira, 2005). This is mainly because integrated livestock–fish aquaculture is practiced mainly in remote villages by few poor farmers with little knowledge and experience (Aganyira, 2005). Farmers are also generally unable to innovate their choice of economic strategies. Moreover, the socioeconomic constraints of the farmers were totally unknown, and the internal economic system of the rural development projects often fail to propose production units that could be accessible to the farmers.

Despite these constraints, a number of research projects have considered the integration of fish culture with other agriculture activities in Malawi (discussed above), Ghana (Ruddle, 1996), Kenya (van Dam et al., 2006), Tanzania (Shoko et al., 2011) and Uganda (Aganyira, 2005). These studies have shown that rural aquaculture integrated with agriculture, and the use of agricultural wastes as pond inputs was highly profitable. Liti et al. (2002) evaluated the growth performance and economic efficiency of Nile tilapia/African catfish raised in polyculture in fertilized ponds in Kenya for 80 days. Feed inputs included commercial peg finisher pellets (12.5% cp), rice bran (6.5% cp) or a test diet (12.5% cp). Rice bran exhibited the poorest growth and lowest production. But the cost/benefit analyses indicated that rice bran had the lowest break-even price and the least investment cost, and in turn, was economically better than the other diets. Fertilization of nurseries and grow-out ponds with cow dung is also a common practice in Kenya, and fresh cow dung from two cows is sufficient to fertilize 1 ha of pond area. Reports on integrated livestock–tilapia culture on the Kenyan side of the Lake Victoria Basin indicated that a 200-m^2 pond fertilized with cow dung can provide an additional per capita fish supply of 3.4 kg to a household of 7 people and an average production of about 200 kg ha^{-1} per year (van Dam et al., 2006).

A comparison of growth performance, yield and net profit of integrated tilapia pond, fertilized with chicken manure and fed with 35% cp supplementary feed, and nonintegrated culture of tilapia was conducted in Tanzania (Shoko et al., 2011). Fish cultured under the integrated system showed higher growth rates, yield and net profit than those in nonintegrated systems. Similarly, Mlelwa (2016) evaluated the growth performance and economic benefit of Nile tilapia and Chinese cabbage under integrated system. Fish raised in fertilized ponds and received supplemental feed had much higher growth rates, yield and net profit than those received feed or manure only. Cabbage plots irrigated from fish ponds had significantly higher leave diameter, length, number of leaves and yield compared to those irrigated with stream water.

An interesting approach regarding reconsidering rural fish farming development in Africa and how tilapia culture can be well integrated in smallholder farming systems has been described by Oswald et al. (1997). These authors reported that the process which aimed at improving fish farming efficiency in the early 1990s has failed and the productivity of smallholders who had adopted fish farming was lower than that of smallholders who had not attempted such diversification. After communication with fish farmers, they realized that the stocking density of Nile tilapia must be decreased, since the quality requirements of the market could only be met at low fish densities. This finding has imposed a new pond planning model "pond-dam" and an initiation of a new innovation process. The pond-dam model was well adapted to the local economy and integrated with spontaneous swamp rice cultivation in fish ponds. It is clear from this particular example that fish farming methods should be compatible with the local agricultural development processes.

12.5 Tilapia and rural development in Latin America and the Caribbean

Latin America and the Caribbean region have a wide variety of ecosystems with strong potential for developing aquaculture activities. The inland and coastal waters of Brazil and Mexico are by far the largest and most promising ecosystems for aquaculture development. Thus, the potential for aquaculture in the region is high.

Studies that analyzed the contribution of rural aquaculture to household economies in Latin America and the Caribbean are scarce (Charles et al., 1997). Only general estimates, based on gross figures of total production or employment (by species or production system), were found. The impact of aquaculture on rural livelihoods is rarely evaluated. Meanwhile, the impacts of aquaculture on other nonaquaculture economic activities are generally made in terms of effects on specific factors, such as water and soil quality, sedimentation and diseases (Molnar et al., 1996).

According to Martinez Espinosa (1995), rural aquaculture in Latin America can be divided into two categories: (1) the "poorest of the poor" aquaculture, which is characterized by very low input and cost and very low output as well and (2) the "less poor" aquaculture, characterized by low/medium inputs and low/medium outputs. The second type of aquaculture is believed to have an excellent potential for rural development. This category has already received assistance from governments and international organizations such as FAO for the formulation of general plans for the development of rural aquaculture in the region. Martinez Espinosa (1994) evaluated the possibilities of the development of aquaculture in the rural environment, in the framework of the "Support to regional aquaculture activities in Latin America and the Caribbean project" (AQUILA II). Two pilot cases were selected for the proposed study; one in Barrancabermeja in Colombia and the other in San Cristobal in Venezuela. Various strategies for the formulation of a plan of development were put and discussed. The results indicated that small-scale farmers were present with adequate characteristics to carry out this type of aquaculture. It was also concluded that rural aquaculture is highly potential if technical, economic and financial support is provided.

Among all fish species suggested for rural aquaculture in the Latin America and the Caribbean, the semi-intensive culture of tilapia seems to be the most profitable. Alceste et al. (2001) reported that small-scale as well as commercial, large-scale tilapia culture is currently practiced in many Latin American countries. Tilapia appears very advantageous in countries like Costa Rica, Brazil and Venezuela. Mixed-sex Nile tilapia have been cultured in family- and communally managed fish ponds in Panama and Guatemala since the 1980s, for family consumption and as a cash crop (Lovshin, 2000). Tilapia culture systems were originally designed to allow farmers without any experience in fish culture to produce their own fish from "egg to market size" using cheap and locally available inputs such as household by-product and animal manure.

In semiarid regions of Brazil, reservoirs were created primarily for drinking water and for agricultural activities and are currently used for cage aquaculture, especially for Nile tilapia. The culture of tilapia in floating cages has become an important means of alternative livelihoods for resource-poor rural households, leading to improving poverty indices and food security levels in these Brazilian regions, which are generally characterized by harsh environmental conditions and low social development (Gunkel et al., 2015; Lopes et al., 2018).

The "dry corridor", which is an ecoregion in Central America characterized by dry tropical forests, has limited infrastructure and natural resources to secure the livelihoods for the population, particularly in rural areas (FAO, 2017). FAO has promoted rural development programmes in the region, with the participation of all stakeholders. Tilapia culture was a major contributor to this development in a number of countries in the region. For example, Nile tilapia farming resulted in a significant improvement in the livelihoods of a large number of households in rural areas in Guatemala (FAO, 2017). In this regard, two strategic approaches were adopted: (1) production of food for family consumption and (2) promotion of the standard of living and economy of rural families by selling surplus tilapia production. Farmers' households consumed 40% of total tilapia production, while the remaining 60% were distributed among the local schools, thus improving nutrition among school children. In addition, farmers earned 0.26 US$ for each US dollar invested. Small-scale tilapia farmers raise tilapia using low-quality nutrient inputs, including agricultural and food wastes, organic and chemical fertilizers that are commonly used. This type of culture is very profitable for rural families. Many fish farms are integrated with chicken broilers or layers. A 100-m^2 pond with 48 broilers can produce 38 kg of fish in 6 months, while 17 layers can produce 29 kg during the same period (Popma et al., 1995). Popma et al. (1995) also reported that annual fish production from a typical 120-m^2 pond was 48 kg of fish, of which 20 kg were sold and 23 kg were consumed by the producer's family. As a result, the average annual per capita consumption of fish among producers' families increased from 0.5 to 3.3 kg yr^{-1}. On-farm income has also increased by 18% as a result of selling farmed fish, despite fish ponds occupying only 2% of total land.

A similar rural development programme is being implemented in El Salvador with assistance from FAO, to promote polyculture of tilapia and whiteleg shrimp (*Penaeus vannamei*) as a means of optimizing the use of natural resources, food production and income generation (FAO, 2017). Programme reports revealed that the average farmers' income increased by up to 28%, mainly due to the high value of shrimps in the local markets. The prices of shrimp are more resilient than that of tilapia because large amounts of tilapia are imported from Honduras and often saturate the local market. Nonetheless, this system is economically attractive, as it improves the incomes for farming households.

As a result of the continuous national and international efforts, small-scale production of tilapia in some other Latin American countries such as Chile, Costa Rica and Honduras have recorded a significant increase, generated by a small number of aquaculture producers (ECLAC, FAO, IICA, 2017). This may have resulted in an increase in production efficiency from a microeconomic perspective, leading to increased rural employment. According to Poot-López et al. (2010), Yucatan State has one of the highest marginalization indices in Mexico, indicating poor social situation in terms of access to education, housing quality and financial income. In response to this situation, the Yucatan State Secretariat of Social Development (Secretaría de Desarrollo Social – SDS) initiated a rural development programme in the state, including building of 116 concrete tanks in 2002, for integrating tilapia culture into the existing agricultural activities. However, only a few studies have evaluated the role of integrated tilapia culture in rural development in Yucatan, and other Mexican states, since then.

Ponce-Marbán et al. (2006) evaluated the economic viability of farming Nile tilapia with Australian redclaw crayfish in a polyculture system also in Yucatan, Mexico. They found that this approach resulted in a significant improvement in profitability, particularly over a 5-year period. Nile tilapia with Australian redclaw crayfish polyculture shortened investment return time and buffered risk related to changes in tilapia sale price. This finding clearly indicated that polyculture of tilapia with other more commercially valuable species provides an opportunity to substantially improve the economic yields of rural producers. Poot-López et al. (2010) also found that the use of tree spinach leaves in tilapia diets as a part of IAAS in Yucatan significantly improved feed management efficiency and resulted in a significant reduction in feed cost and increase in net profit.

12.6 Closing remarks

1. Rural aquaculture is a multidisciplinary practice, including technical, economic and socioeconomic aspects, extension services and policy aspects. It is necessary that all these factors be considered for efficient and sustainable development of rural aquaculture.
2. If the existing aquaculture technologies are not efficiently used, improving their efficiency becomes more cost-effective than introducing new technologies.
3. Rural aquaculture development should fully consider the social factors such as family context, social status and habits.
4. The introduction of any new technology into rural areas should consider the age and education background of the selected candidates who would apply this technology. Capacity building and continuous training and extension services should be provided to farmers and/or farm operators.
5. Asia is the most important tilapia producer with a contribution of 70.4% to global tilapia production in 2017. Most of this production comes from small-scale, rural farms and therefore, has a significant impact on rural development, especially in the major producing countries; namely, China, Indonesia, Bangladesh, the Philippines, Thailand and Vietnam.
6. Except in Egypt, rural aquaculture development in Africa relied mainly on external donations and

technologies, with little local experience and/or governmental assistance. Tilapia culture has made fish the most affordable source of animal protein in Egypt, especially for the poor. The annual per capita consumption of fish reached 20.6 kg in 2016, of which 54% came from tilapia. Indirect impacts of tilapia culture include increased fish availability, reduced fish prices, especially in rural governorates, and job creations for thousands of Egyptians.

7. Although the development of small-scale tilapia culture in rural, poor African regions is affected by many economic and social factors, such as family context, social status and habits, it seems that the technology adopted and the level of extension services play a crucial role in the success or failure of rural aquaculture in these regions. Considerable attention has recently been paid to aquaculture development in Africa, particularly in Sub-Saharan countries, by different regional and international organizations.
8. Tilapia culture in rural areas is practiced mainly for subsistence. Increased use of commercial inputs may not be realistic because of the subsistence nature of tilapia farms and the limited resources available for these rural small-scale farmers.

References

ADB (Asian Development Bank), 2004. Special Evaluation Study on Small-Scale Freshwater Rural Aquaculture Development for Poverty Reduction. A report, Manila, the Philippines, p. 55.

ADB (Asian Development Bank), 2005a. An Evaluation of Small-Scale Freshwater Rural Aquaculture Development for Poverty Alleviation. Asian Development Bank, Manila, p. 163.

ADB (Asian Development Bank), 2005b. An Impact Evaluation of the Development of Genetically Improved Farmed Tilapia and Their Dissemination in Selected Countries. Manila, Philippines, p. 124.

Adeel, Z., Safriel, U., 2008. Achieving sustainability by introducing alternative livelihoods. Sustainability Science 3, 125–133.

Aganyira, K., 2005. Aquaculture: a tool for sustainable development in Uganda. MSc. Thesis. In: A Case Study of Kigoowa Catholic Women's Development Association in Kampala District. Norwegian University of Science and Technology, Trondheim-Norway.

Aguilar-Manjarrez, J., Nath, S.S., 1998. A Strategic Reassessment of Fish Farming Potential in Africa. FAO, Rome, p. 170. FAO Technical Paper, No. 32.

Ahmed, M., Abdur Rab, M., Bimbao, M.A.P., 1993. Household Socioeconomics, Resource Use and Fish Marketing in Two Thanas of Bangladesh. ICLARM Technical Report No. 40, Manila, Philippines, p. 82.

Ahmed, M., Rab, M.A., Gupta, M.V., 1995. Impact of improved aquaculture technologies: results of an extension program on the farming systems of Bangladesh. Asian Fisheries Science 8, 27–39.

Ahmed, M., Bimbao, M.P., Gupta, M.V., 1996. Economics of tilapia aquaculture in small water bodies in Bangladesh. In: Pullin, R.S.V., Lazard, J., Legendre, M., Amon Kottias, J.B., Pauly, D. (Eds.), Proceedings of the Third International Symposium on Tilapia in Aquaculture. ICLARM Conference Proceedings No. 41. ICLARM, Penang, Malaysia, pp. 471–475.

Ahmed, M., Lorica, M.H., 2002. Improving developing country food security through aquaculture development-lessons from Asia. Food Policy 27, 125–141.

Alceste, C.C., Illingworth, J.A., Jory, D.E., 2001. Tilapia farming industry in Ecuador. Aquaculture Magazine 27, 77–82.

APPG (All-Party Parliamentary Group), 2018. Aquaculture for Smallholder Farmers. http://www.appg-agdev.co.uk/images/APPG_Aquaculture.pdf.

Asmah, R., 2008. Development Potential and Financial Viability of Fish Farming in Ghana. PhD Thesis. Institute of Aquaculture, University of Sterling, UK.

Asmah, R., 2009. Social and Economic Benefits of Commercial Aquaculture in Rural Communities: A Case Study of Two Commercial Cage Culture Farms in Ghana. Aquaculture Compendium Report.

Atanda, A.N., Fagbenro, O.A., 2017. Social and economic performance of tilapia farming in Nigeria. In: Cai, J., Quagrainie, K.K., Hishamunda, N. (Eds.), Social and Economic Performance of Tilapia Farming in Africa. FAO Fisheries and Aquaculture Circular No. 1130. FAO, Rome, pp. 113–125.

Aya, F.A., 2013. Small-scale Aquaculture Development: Experiences from the Philippines on Giant Freshwater Prawn, Milkfish and tilapia. Network of Aquaculture Centres in Asia-Pacific (NACA)/The Aquaculture Department of the Southeast Asian Fisheries Development Center (SEAFDEC/AQD). https://enaca.org/?id=197.

Barman, B.K., Little, D., Edwards, P., 2002. Small-scale fish culture in Northwest Bangladesh: a participatory appraisal focussing on the role of tilapia. In: Edwards, P., Little, D., Demaine, H. (Eds.), Rural Aquaculture. CABI Publishing, CAB International, Wallingford, Oxon, UK, pp. 227–244.

Barman, B.K., Little, D.C., 2006. Nile tilapia (*Oreochromis niloticus*) seed production in irrigated rice-fields in Northwest Bangladesh—an approach appropriate for poorer farmers? Aquaculture 261, 72–79.

Barman, B.K., Little, D.C., 2011. Use of hapas to produce Nile tilapia (*Oreochromis niloticus* L.) seed in household foodfish ponds: a participatory trial with small-scale farming households in Northwest Bangladesh. Aquaculture 317, 214–222.

Belton, B., 2006. An assessment of the sustainability of Tilapia culture in Central Thailand. In: Production in Aquatic Peri-Urban Systems in Southeast Asia Project Report. University of Sterling, Scotland, p. 63.

Belton, B., Little, D., 2008. The development of aquaculture in Central Thailand: domestic demand versus export-led production. Journal of Agrarian Change 8, 123–143.

Belton, B., Little, D., Grady, K., 2009. Is responsible aquaculture sustainable aquaculture? WWF and the eco-certification of tilapia. Society & Natural Resources 22, 840–855.

Belton, B., 2013. Small-scale aquaculture, development and poverty: a reassessment. In: Bondad-Reantaso, M.G., Subasinghe, R.P. (Eds.), Enhancing the Contribution of Smallscale Aquaculture to Food Security, Poverty Alleviation and Socio-Economic Development. FAO Fisheries and Aquaculture Proceedings, No. 31. FAO, Rome, pp. 93–108.

Bondad-Reantaso, M.G., Prein, M. (Eds.), 2009. Measuring the Contribution of Small-Scale Aquaculture: An Assessment. FAO Fisheries and Aquaculture Technical Paper. No. 534. FAO, Rome, p. 179.

Brummett, R.E., Williams, M.J., 2000. The evolution of aquaculture in African rural and economic development. Ecological Economics 33, 193–203.

Brummett, R.E., 2002. Seasonality, labour and integration of aquaculture into southern African smallhold farming systems. Naga: The ICLARM Quarterly 25, 23–27.

Brummett, R.E., Noble, R.P., 1995. Aquaculture for African Smallholders. In: ICLARM Technical Report, vol. 46. ICLARM, Manila, Philippines, p. 69.

Bukenya, J.O., Hyuha, T.S., Molnar, J., Twinamasiko, J., 2013. Efficiency of resource use among pond fish farmers in central Uganda: a stochastic frontier production function approach. Aquaculture Economics and Management 17 (2), 148–170.

CGIAR (Consultative Group for International Agricultural Research), 2006. Improved Tilapia Benefits Asia. Science Council/Standing Panel on Impact Assessment Brief Number 6. Rome. http://www.fao.org/docs/eims/upload/232128/06(WF)-Final_l-r.pdf.

CGIAR (Consultative Group for International Agricultural Research), 2015. CGIAR Strategy and Results Framework 2016–2030, p. 52.

Charles, A.T., Agbayani, R.F., Agbayani, E.C., Agüero, M., Belleza, E.T., González, E., et al., 1997. Aquaculture Economics in Developing Countries: Regional Assessments and an Annotated Bibliography. FAO Fisheries Circular No. 932. FAO, Rome, p. 401.

Chenyambuga, S.W., Mwandya, A., Lamtane, H.A., Madalla, N.A., 2014. Productivity and marketing of Nile tilapia (*Oreochromis niloticus*) cultured in ponds of small-scale farmers in Mvomero and Mbarali districts, Tanzania. Livestock Research for Rural Development 26, 3. http://www.lrrd.org/lrrd26/3/chen26043.htm.

Chimatiro, S.K., Janke, A., 1994. Socioeconomic assessment of smallholder aquaculture: a case study of smallholder farmers in Mwanza and Zomba Districts. In: Brummett, R.E. (Ed.), Aquaculture Policy Options for Integrated Resource Management in Sub Saharan Africa. ICLARM Conference Proceedings (Extended Abstracts) No. 46 GTZ/ICLARM, Manila, Philippines, p. 38.

Dey, M.M., 2000. The impact of genetically improved farmed Nile tilapia in Asia. Aquaculture Economics and Management 4, 107–124.

Dey, M.M., Paraguas, F.J., Bimbao, G.B., Regaspi, P.B., 2000. Technical efficiency of tilapia growout pond operations in the Philippines. Aquaculture Economics and Management 4, 33–47.

Dey, M.M., Garcia, Y.T., Kumar, P., Piusombum, S., Haque, M.S., Li, L., et al., 2008. Demand for fish in Asia: a cross-country analysis. The Australian Journal of Agricultural and Resource Economics 52, 321–338.

ECLAC, FAO, IICA, 2017. The Outlook for Agriculture and Rural Development in the Americas: A Perspective on Latin America and the Caribbean 2017–2018. ECLAC, FAO, IICA, San Jose, p. 252. C.R.: IICA.

Edwards, P., Little, D., Demaine, H., 2002. Issues in rural aquaculture. In: Edwards, P., Little, D., Demaine, H. (Eds.), Rural Aquaculture. CABI Publishing, CAB International, Oxon, Wallingford, UK and New York, USA, pp. 323–340.

Edwards, P., 2009. Changes in traditional inland aquaculture in West Java, Indonesia. Aquaculture Asia 14, 3–8.

Edwards, P., 2010. The development of 'modern' aquaculture in Java, Indonesia. Aquaculture Asia Magazine XV (1), 3–9.

El-Sayed, A.-F.M., 2017. Social and economic performance of tilapia farming in Egypt. In: Cai, J., Quagrainie, K.K., Hishamunda, N. (Eds.), Social and Economic Performance of Tilapia Farming in Africa. FAO Fisheries and Aquaculture Circular No. 1130. FAO, Rome, pp. 1–48.

FAO (Food and Agriculture Organization of the United Nations), 2010. Report of FAO Expert Workshop on Assessing the Contribution of Small-Scale Aquaculture to Sustainable Rural Development. Tagaytay City, the Philippines, 6–8 August 2009. In: FAO Fisheries and Aquaculture Report. No. 952. FAO, Rome, p. 34.

FAO (Food and Agriculture Organization of the United Nations), 2016. The State of World Fisheries and Aquaculture 2016- Contributing to Food Security and Nutrition for All. FAO, Rome, p. 200.

FAO (Food and Agriculture Organization of the United Nations), 2015. Ricefish-farming increases farmers' income. FAO Indonesia on news, (http://www.fao.org/indonesia/news/detail-events/en/c/409216/).

FAO (Food and Agriculture Organization of the United Nations), 2017. Aquaculture Newsletter, No. 56, p. 62.

FAO (Food and Agriculture Organization of theUnited Nations), 2019. Global Aquaculture Production 1950–2017. http://www.fao.org/fishery/statistics/global-aquaculture-production/query/en.

Frimpong, E.A., Anane-Taabeah, G., 2017. Social and economic performance of tilapia farming in Ghana. In: Cai, J., Quagrainie, K.K., Hishamunda, N. (Eds.), Social and Economic Performance of Tilapia Farming in Africa. FAO Fisheries and Aquaculture Circular No. 1130. FAO, Rome, pp. 49–90.

Fynn, I.E.M., 2014. Pond Aquaculture Spatial Distribution, Production and Productivity Determinants in Ghana. MSc Thesis. Virginia Polytechnic Institute and State University, Blacksburg, USA.

Genschick, S., Kaminski, A.M., Kefi, A.S., Cole, S.M., 2017. Aquaculture in Zambia: an overview and evaluation of the sector's responsiveness to the needs of the poor. Penang, Malaysia. In: CGIAR Research Program on Fish Agri-Food Systems and Lusaka. Department of Fisheries, Zambia, p. 31. Working Paper: FISH-2017-08.

Gunkel, G., Lima, D., Selge, F., Sobral, M., Calado, S., 2015. Aquatic ecosystem services of reservoirs in semiarid areas: sustainability and reservoir management. WIT Transactions on Ecology and the Environment 197, 187–200.

Gupta, M.V., Ahmed, M., Bimbao, M.A.P., Lightfoot, C., 1992. report-Socioeconomic Impact and Farmers' Assessment of Nile tilapia (*Oreochromis niloticus*) Culture in Bangladesh. ICLARM Technical Reports, No. 35, Manila, Philippines, p. 50.

Gupta, M.V., Mazid, M.A., Islam, M.S., Rahman, M., Hussain, M.G., 1999. Integration of Aquaculture into the Farming Systems of the Floodprone Ecosystems of Bangladesh: An Evaluation of Adoption and Impact. ICLARM Technical Reports, No. 56. ICLARM, Manila, Philippines, p. 32.

Gupta, M.V., 2001. Culture of short-cycle species in seasonal ponds and ditches in Bangladesh. FAO Fisheries Technical Paper 407. In: Integrated Agriculture-Aquaculture: A primer. FAO, Rome, pp. 40–42.

Halwart, M., Funge-Smith, S., Moehl, J., 2003. The role of aquaculture in rural development. In: Review of the State of World Aquaculture. FAO Fisheries Circular, No. 886, Revision 2. FAO, Rome, pp. 47–58.

Hishamunda, N., Jolly, C., 1998. Evaluation of small-scale aquaculture with intra-rural household trade as an alternative enterprise for limited-resource farmers: the case of Rwanda. Food Policy 23, 143–154.

Hussain, G., Kohinoor, A., Rahman, Mr M., Rahman, Z., Nguyen, N.H., 2017. Bangladesh's tilapia aquaculture industry shows resilience. Global Aquaculture Advocate. https://www.aquaculturealliance.org/advocate/bangladesh-tilapia/.

Hyuha, T.S., Bukenya, J.O., Twinamasiko, J., Molnar, J., 2011. Profitability analysis of small scale aquaculture enterprise in Central Uganda. International Journal of Fisheries and Aquaculture 2, 271–278.

Hyuha, T.S., Ekere, W., Egna, H., Molnar, J.J., 2017. Social and economic performance of tilapia farming in Uganda. In: Cai, J.,

Quagrainie, K.K., Hishamunda, N. (Eds.), Social and Economic Performance of Tilapia Farming in Africa. FAO Fisheries and Aquaculture Circular No. 1130. FAO, Rome, pp. 127–144.

Joffre, O.M., Castine, S.A., Phillips, M.J., Sellamuttu, S.S., Chandrabalan, D., Cohen, P., 2017. Increasing productivity and improving livelihoods in aquatic agricultural systems: a review of interventions. Food Security 9, 39–60.

Kaliba, A.R., Ngugi, C.C., Mackambo, J., Quagrainie, K.K., 2007. Economic profitability of Nile tilapia (*Oreochromis niloticus* L.) production in Kenya. Aquaculture Research 38, 1129–1136.

Kaminski, A.M., Genschick, S., Kefi, A.S., Kruijssen, F., 2018. Commercialization and upgrading in the aquaculture value chain in Zambia. Aquaculture 493, 355–364.

Karim, M., Little, D.C., Kabir, M.d. S., Verdegem, M.J.C., Telfer, T., Abdul Wahab, M.d., 2011. Enhancing benefits from polycultures including tilapia (*Oreochromis niloticus*) within integrated pond-dike systems: a participatory trial with households of varying socio-economic level in rural and peri-urban areas of Bangladesh. Aquaculture 314, 225–235.

Kassam, L., 2013. Assessing the Contribution of Aquaculture to Poverty Reduction in Ghana. PhD Thesis. University of London, UK.

Kassam, L., 2014. Aquaculture and Food Security, Poverty Alleviation and Nutrition in Ghana: Case Study Prepared for the Aquaculture for Food Security, Poverty Alleviation and Nutrition Project. Project Report: 2014-48. WorldFish, penang, Malaysia, p. 46.

Kassam, L., Dorward, A., 2017. A comparative assessment of the poverty impacts of pond and cage aquaculture in Ghana. Aquaculture 470, 110–122.

Keus, E.H.J., Subasinghe, R., Aleem, N.A., Sarwer, R.H., Islam, M.M., Hossain, M.Z., 2017. Aquaculture for Income and Nutrition: Final Report. WorldFish, Penang, Malaysia, pp. 2017–2030. Program Report.

KMAP (Kenya Market-Led Aquaculture Programme), 2016. Gender impact study of the Kenya Market-led Aquaculture Program (KMAP). In: A Report Submitted by ETC East Africa to Farm Africa, p. 71.

Krishnan, S.B., Peterburs, T., 2017. Zambia Jobs in Value Chains: Opportunities in Agribusiness. Jobs Series; no. 6. World Bank Group, Washington, D.C., p. 42

Li, X., Li, J., Wang, Y., Fu, L., Fu, Y., Li, B., et al., 2011. Aquaculture industry in China: current state, challenges, and outlook. Reviews in Fisheries Science 19, 187–200.

Liti, D.M., Mac'Were, O.E., Veverica, K.L., 2002. Growth performance and economic benefits of *Oreochromis niloticus/Clarias gariepinus* polyculture fed on three supplementary feeds in fertilized tropical ponds. In: McElwee, K., Lewis, K., Nidiffer, M., Buitrago, P. (Eds.), Nineteenth Annual Technical Report. Pond Dynamics/Aquaculture CRSP. Oregon State University, Corvallis, Oregon, USA, pp. 11–16.

Little, D.C., Surentaraseree, P., Innes-Taylor, N.L., 1996. Review: fish culture in rainfed ricefields of Northeast Thailand. Aquaculture 140, 295–321.

Little, D.C., July/August, 1998. Options in the development of the "aquatic chicken". Fish Farmer 35–37.

Little, D.C., Coward, K., Bhujel, R.C., Pham, T.A., Bromage, N.R., 2000. Effect of broodfish exchange strategy on the spawning performance and sex steroid hormone levels of *Oreochromis niloticus* broodfish in hapas. Aquaculture 186, 77–88.

Lopes, P.F.M., Carvalho, A.R., Villasante, S., Henry-Silva, G.G., 2018. Fisheries or aquaculture? Unravelling key determinants of livelihoods in the Brazilian semi-arid region. Aquaculture Research 49, 232–242.

Lovshin, L.L., 2000. Evaluation of tilapia culture by resource-limited farmers in Panama and Guatemala. In: Fitzsimmons, K., Filho, J.C. (Eds.), Tilapia Culture in the 21st Century. Proceedings from the Fifth International Symposium on Tilapia Aquaculture. American Tilapia Association and ICLARM, Rio de Janeiro, Brazil, pp. 633–638.

Macfadyen, G., Nasr-Allah, A., Kenawy, D.A., Ahmed, M.F.M., Hebicha, H., Diab, A.S., et al., 2011. Value-chain Analysis of Egyptian Aquaculture. Project Report 2011-54. WorldFish, Penang, Malaysia, 84 pp.

Martinez Espinosa, M., 1994. Between the Aquaculture of the "more Poor" and that of the "less Poor". A Methodologic Proposal for the Development of Type 2 Rural Aquaculture: Two Pilot Cases in Venezuela and Colombia. FAO, Mexico City (Mexico).

Martinez Espinosa, M., 1995. Development of Type 2 Rural Aquaculture in Latin America. FAO Aquaculture Newsletter, Rome, pp. 6–10. No. 11.

Middendorp, A.J., Verreth, J.A.J., 1992. The feasibility of small-scale hapa culture of tilapia *Oreochromis niloticus* as an additional income source for rice farmers in northeast Thailand. Asian Fisheries Science 5, 303–314.

Mlelwa, T., 2016. Growth Performance and Economic Benefit of Nile tilapia (*Oreochromis niloticus*) and Chinese Cabbage (Brassica Rapachinensis) in Aquaculture Integration. MSc Thesis. Sokoine University of Agriculture, Morogoro, Tanzania.

Moehl, J.F., 2002. Aquaculture Development as a National Strategy for Poverty Alleviation and Improved Food Security in Africa. World Aquaculture 2002 – Book of Abstracts. World Aquaculture Society, Baton Rouge, Louisiana, USA, p. 513.

Molnar, J.J., Hanson, T.R., Lovshin, L.L., 1996. Social, Economic, and Institutional Impacts of Aquacultural Research on tilapia: The PD/ACRSP in Rwanda, Honduras, the Philippines, and Thailand. Research and Development Series No. 40. Auburn, Alabama, USA. International Centre for Aquaculture and Aquatic Environments, Auburn University, Alabama, USA, 72 pp.

Musuka, C.G., Musonda, F.F., 2013. Contribution of small water bodies and smallholder aquaculture towards poverty alleviation and enhancing household food security in Zambia. International Journal of Fisheries and Aquaculture 5, 295–302.

Namonje-Kapembwa, T., Samboko, P., 2017. Assessing the Profitability of Small -Scale Aquaculture Fish Production in Zambia. Working Paper 123. Indaba Agricultural Policy Research Institute (IAPRI), Lusaka, Zambia, 24 pp.

Nandeesha, M.C., 2002. Contribution of Aquaculture to Poverty Alleviation and Food Security in India. World Aquaculture 2002 – Book of Abstracts. World Aquaculture Society, Baton Rouge, Louisiana, USA, p. 535.

Natarajan, P., Aravindan, C.M., 2002. Status of tilapia farming and its prospects in India. In: Guerrero III, R.D., Guerrero-del Castillo, M.R. (Eds.), Tilapia Farming in the 21st Century. Proceedings of the International Forum on Tilapia Farming in the 21st Century (Tilapia Forum 2002). The Philippine Fisheries Association, Inc., Los Banos, Laguna, Philippines, pp. 78–86.

Ngugi, C.C., Nyandat, B., Manyala, J.O., Wagude, B., 2017. Social and economic performance of tilapia farming in Kenya. In: Cai, J., Quagrainie, K.K., Hishamunda, N. (Eds.), Social and Economic Performance of Tilapia Farming in Africa. FAO Fisheries and Aquaculture Circular No. 1130. FAO, Rome, pp. 91–111.

Nguyen, N.H., Ponzoni, R.W., Chandrasoma, J., Wathurawadu, K., 2011. GIFT tilapia raise culture efficiency in Sri Lanka. Global Aquaculture Advocate 32–33. November/December.

Oswald, M., Glasser, F., Sanchez, F., Bamba, V., 1997. Reconsidering rural fish farming in Africa. In: Fitzsimmons, K. (Ed.), Proceedings from the Fourth International Symposium on Tilapia in Aquaculture. Northeast Regional Agriculture Engineering Service, Ithaca, New York, USA, pp. 499–511.

Pant, J., Demaine, H., Edwards, P., 2004. Assessment of the aquaculture subsystem in integrated agriculture-aquaculture systems in Northeast Thailand. Aquaculture Research 35, 289–298.

Pekar, F., Be, N.V., Long, D.N., Cong, N.V., Dung, D.T., Olah, J., 2002. Eco-technological analysis of fish farming households in the Mekong Delta of Vietnam. In: Edwards, P., Little, D., Demaine, H. (Eds.), Rural Aquaculture. CABI Publishing, CAB International, Wallingford, Oxon, UK, pp. 77–95.

Pemsl, D.E., Chen, O.L., Tongruksawatta, S., Garcia, Y., Vera-Cruz, E., Abella, T., et al., 2008. Adoption and farm-level impact of genetically improved farmed tilapia (GIFT) in the Philippines. In: Proceedings of the Fourteenth Biennial Conference of the International Institute of Fisheries Economics & Trade. July 22–25, 2008, Nha Trang, Vietnam. Compiled by Ann L. Shriver. International Institute of Fisheries Economics & Trade, Corvallis, Oregon, USA, 2008. CD ROM. ISBN 0-9763432-5-8.

Pengseng, P., 2013. On farm trial with rice fish cultivation in Nakhon Si Thammarat Southern Thailand. Walailak Journal of Science and Technology 10, 67–75.

Phillips, M., Henriksson, P.J.G., Tran, N., Chan, C.Y., Mohan, C.V., Rodriguez, U.-P., et al., 2015. Exploring Indonesian Aquaculture Futures. WorldFish, Penang, Malaysia, p. 15. Program Report 2015–39.

Pollock, L.J., Little, D., 2002. The Nature of Participation of the Rural Poor in Poverty-Focused Aquaculture Research: Empirical Finding from Process Monitoring and Livelihoods Studies with Inland Fishing Communities in Sri Lanka. World Aquaculture 2002 – Book of Abstracts. World Aquaculture Society, Baton Rouge Louisiana, p. 610.

Ponce-Marbán, D., Hernández, J.M., Gasca-Leyva, E., 2006. Simulating the economic viability of Nile tilapia and Australian redclaw crayfish polyculture in Yucatan, Mexico. Aquaculture 261, 151–159.

Poot-López, G.R., Hernández, J.M., Eucario Gasca-Leyva, E., 2010. Input management in integrated agriculture–aquaculture systems in Yucatan: tree spinach leaves as a dietary supplement in tilapia culture. Agricultural Systems 103, 98–104.

Popma, T.J., Phelps, R.P., Castillo, S., Hatch, L.U., Hanson, T.R., 1995. Family-scale fish farming in Guatemala, Part 1: outreach strategies and production practices. Journal of Aquaculture in the Tropics 10, 43–56.

PSA (Philippine Statistics Authority), 2018. Selected Statistics on Agriculture 2018, 58 pp.

Pushpalatha, K.B.C., Chandrasoma, J., Liyanage, H.S.W.A., Fernando, W.A.J.R., Jayabahu, J.M., 2016. Farming of Nile tilapia (*Oreochromis niloticus*) in backyard ponds in Sri Lanka: culture practices, fish production and profitability. Sri Lanka Journal of Aquatic Sciences 21, 27–34.

Rasowo, J., Auma, E.O., 2006. On-farm trials with rice-fish cultivation in the West Kano rice irrigation scheme, Kenya. NAGA, WorldFish Center Quarterly 29 (1 & 2), 36–41.

Ruddle, K., 1996. The potential role of integrated management of natural resources in improving the nutritional and economic status of resource-poor farm households in Ghana. In: Prein, M., Ofori, J.K., Lightfoot, C. (Eds.), Research for the Future Development of Aquaculture in Ghana. ICLARM Conference Proceedings No. 42. ICLARM, Manila, Philippines, pp. 57–85.

Safina, N., Yongming, Y., Andrew, S., Pei, S., Yuan, Y., Yunyun, D., 2017. Profitability analysis of monosex tilapia production under three culture models in Hebei and Southern Coastal Provinces of China. Israeli Journal of Aquaculture – Bamidgeh 69, 1405–1409.

Salama, A., 2009. Economic study of fish farming systems in rice fields in Egypt. Special Issue for Global Fisheries and Aquaculture Research Conference, Cairo International Convention Center, 24–26 October 2009 Abbassa International Journal for Aquaculture 135–153. In Arabic, with English abstract.

Satia, B.P., 2017. Regional Review on Status and Trends in Aquaculture Development in Sub-Saharan Africa – 2015. In: FAO Fisheries and Aquaculture Circular No. 1135/4. FAO, Rome, p. 29.

Seki, E., Maly, R., 1994. A Pilot Socio-Economic Survey of Aquaculture in Ruvuma Region, Tanzania. ALCOM Field Document No. 20. FAO, Harare, Zimbabwe, p. 107.

Sen, S., van der Mheen, H., van der Mheen-Sluijer, J., 1996. The place of aquaculture in rural development. In: Expert Consultation on Small-Scale Rural Aquaculture. FAO, Rome, pp. 91–118. FAO Fisheries Technical Report No. 548.

Shoko, A.P., Getabu, A., Mwayuli, G., Mgaya, Y.D., 2011. Growth performance, yields and economic benefits of Nile tilapia *Oreochromis niloticus* and kales *Brassica oleracea* cultured under vegetable-fish culture integration. Tanzania Journal of Science 37, 37–48.

Syandri, H., Elfiondri, J., Azrita, 2015. Social status of the fish-farmers of floating-net-cages in Lake Maninjau, Indonesia. Journal of Aquaculture Research and Development 6, 391. https://doi.org/10.4172/2155-9546.1000391.

UNECA (United Nations Economic Commission for Africa), 2016. Economic Report on Africa 2016: Greening Africa's Industrialization. UNECA, Addis Ababa, Ethiopia, p. 254.

van Dam, A.A., Kaggwa, R.C., Kipkemboi, J., 2006. Integrated pond aquaculture in Lake Victoria wetlands. In: Halwart, M., van Dam, A.A. (Eds.), Integrated Irrigation and Aquaculture in West Africa: Concepts, Practices and Potential. FAO, Rome, pp. 129–134.

Van der Mheen-Sluijer, J., 1991. Adoption of Fish Farming: Promoting and Inhibiting Factors in Eastern Province, Zambia. FAO, Harare, Zimbabwe. Field Document GCP/INT/436/SWE.13, 41 pp.

Van Huong, N., Cuong, T.H., 2012. Freshwater aquaculture's contribution to food security in Vietnam: a case study of freshwater tilapia aquaculture in Hai Duong province. Journal of the International Society of Southeast Asian Agricultural Sciences 18, 6–17.

Veerina, S.S., Nandeesha, M.C., Gopal Roa, K., 1993. Status and Technology of Indian Major Carp Farming in Andra Pradesh. Asian Fishery Society, Special Publication No. 9, India.

Vincke, M.M.J., Schmidt, U.W., 1991. Report on the Mid-term Evaluation of the Central and Northern Regions Fish Farming Projects, 17/3-28/4/91. EEC/Government of Malawi, p. 67.

WorldFish Center, 2007. Strategy for Sustainable Aquaculture Development for Poverty Reduction Project, Philippines (Adta 4708-phi). Final Report, 58 pp.

Zongli, Z., Yanan, Z., Feifan, L., Hui, Y., Yongming, Y., Xinhua, Y., 2017. Economic efficiency of small-scale tilapia farms in Guangxi, China. Aquaculture Economics and Management 21, 283–294.

Chapter 13

Technological innovations

Chapter outline

13.1 Introduction

Tilapia culture is globally expanding at a very high rate, with a 9.8% average annual increase in production during the past 10 years (2007–16). Currently, tilapia is cultured in more than 130 countries worldwide. As a result, aquaculture in general, and tilapia culture in developing countries in particular, is expected to face many challenges over the coming years, in order to meet the increasing demand of growing populations. Improvement in tilapia broodstock, reproductive performance and seed production, hatchery and grow-out technologies, stress and disease control, water quality management, and nutrition and feeding mechanisms will be the major challenge facing tilapia farmers, researchers and farm managers.

Modern technologies, particularly biotechnology, will play the core role in confronting these challenges. Biotechnology can be used for growth enhancement, improvement of reproduction and early development of farmed organisms, enhancement of ecological sustainability, satisfying new markets for farmed products and conserving aquatic biodiversity. The recent technologies in molecular biology and genetics have already been involved and will continue to be highly involved, in tilapia culture development, with an ultimate goal of food security, poverty alleviation, and income generation in developing countries. This chapter throws some light on the recent technological innovations in tilapia culture, with emphasis on the following areas: genetics and reproduction including transgenesis and selective breeding, disease management, feed and feeding and farming systems.

Tilapia Culture. https://doi.org/10.1016/B978-0-12-816541-6.00013-1
Copyright © 2020 Elsevier Inc. All rights reserved.

13.2 Genetic improvement

13.2.1 Selective breeding

The tilapia production systems have been focussing on enhancing production through improving growth rate and reducing age at harvest. Therefore, most of tilapia breeding programs have used production traits (e.g. body weight and daily weight gain) as the main selection criterion (Thodesen et al., 2011; Bentsen et al., 2012, 2017; Hamzah et al., 2014, 2016; Zak et al., 2014). Improvement of other traits of economic importance, such as fillet weight, fat content and yield has also gained considerable attention (Nguyen et al., 2010a; 2010b; Gjerde et al., 2012; Thodesen (Ma) et al., 2012).

Garcia et al. (2017) estimated genetic parameters for fillet weight, yield and fat content in 'Aquaamerica' tilapia strain. The heritability estimates for fillet yield and fat content were moderate (0.2−0.32) and slightly higher for body weight at slaughter (0.41). The genetic correlation between fillet yield and fillet fat content was significant (0.6). This study suggests that changes in fillet yield and fat content may not occur when using growth performance as a selection criterion; and indirect changes may occur in fat content if selecting for higher fillet yield. Zak et al. (2014) obtained genetic parameters and selection responses for harvest body weight of blue tilapia (*O. aureus*) over three generations of selection. The genetic correlation between harvest body weight and survival was 0.22, while the total selection response for harvest body weight was 17.7%. These results demonstrated the high potential for the genetic improvement of harvest body weight in blue tilapia.

Selective breeding programmes for red tilapia (*Oreochromis* spp.) have also achieved considerable genetic improvement for a wide range of commercially important traits in this species, as demonstrated by Hamzah et al. (2017). These authors found that the estimates of heritability for body traits studied (body weight, standard length, body width, body depth, body colour, early sexual maturation and survival) after three generations of selection were moderate to high (0.13−0.45). The cumulative improvement for harvest body weight of red tilapia (*Oreochromis* spp.) was 12.5% per generation after three generations of selection. Genetic correlations among body traits and survival were highly positive. These results suggest also that the large genetic variation in body colour and survival in this species indicate that there is a wide room for future improvement of these traits, taking into account that this species is the most commonly produced and consumed fish among tilapias and other freshwater fish species (Hamzah et al., 2017).

13.2.2 Transgenesis

The application of genetic principles in aquaculture for increasing the production of farmed aquatic animals lags far behind its application in the plant and livestock sectors. Very little attention has been paid to genetic improvement of most farmed aquatic species despite the great potential of biotechnology in this field. However, tilapia are one of few fish groups that have been subject to reproduction and genetic improvements during recent years. Extensive research has been carried out on genetic development of farmed tilapia in many parts of the world during the past two decades. Transgenesis is a modern genetic biotechnology which has received a great attention in recent years.

Transgenesis is the introduction of any foreign gene of interest into the genome of plants and animals by gene transfer technology. When the introduced gene is integrated, inherited and expressed, the transgenic organisms acquire new genotypes and phenotypes, depending on the nature of the gene introduced, and the specificity and strength of the promoters driving the expression (Hew and Fletcher, 2001). Transgenic technology is one of the most promising technologies for generating rapid genetic improvements. This technology is expected to become more beneficial to aquaculture in developing new fish strains than traditional breeding programmes. Transgenesis is also expected to witness a continuous improvement and development in order to produce less costly and more affordable fish and will be applicable in the developing countries. According to Hew and Fletcher (2001), transgenesis in aquaculture can be used for the following:

1. Enhancement of growth, feed conversion ratios (FCRs) and survival.
2. Increasing disease resistance against pathogens.
3. Controlling sexual maturation, sterility and sex differentiation.
4. Improving fish adaptability to extreme environmental conditions, such as cold resistance.
5. Altering the biochemical characteristics of the flesh to enhance its nutritional qualities.
6. Altering the biochemical or metabolic pathways to improve food utilization.

In addition, transgenic tilapia can be used as biofactories for producing pharmaceutical products. Growth enhancement and cold resistance of farmed transgenic tilapia have received more attention than the other uses.

13.2.2.1 Growth enhancement

The improvement of growth and feed conversion efficiency of farmed fishes has been the principal objective of transgenic studies. Transgenic fishes, including tilapia (Rahman et al., 2001), containing exogenous growth hormone (GH) gene construct exhibited better growth and feed efficiency than their nontransgenic siblings. The increase in the growth rates of transgenic fishes ranges from 20% to 1000%, compared to nontransgenic controls (Rahman et al., 2001).

Tilapia have many attributes that make them ideal candidates for transgenic studies. These include (1) frequent, aseasonal reproduction (i.e. eggs are constantly available for research studies), (2) short generation time (5–8 months), (3) easy reproduction in captivity, (4) embryos and fry can be easily reared, (5) embryos are semi-transparent, so that some reporter genes can be detected without sectioning or sacrifice and (6) eggs can be fairly easily injected via micropyle. Therefore, extensive research has been carried out on transgenic tilapia over the past two decades. As a result, some of the lines of growth-enhanced tilapia have been commercially marketed (de la Fuente et al., 1999).

Rahman and Maclean (1999) studied the growth performance of transgenic tilapia containing a Chinook salmon GH gene construct spliced into the ocean pout antifreeze gene regulatory sequence. The initial transmission rate from generation G0 to G1 was less than 10%, with mosaic distribution of the transgene in the germ cells, but transmission rates from G1 to G2 followed expected Mendelian ratio. Meanwhile, transgenic tilapia lines exhibited dramatic growth enhancement. The average weight of the G1 and G2 transgenic fish was three times heavier than that of their nontransgenic siblings. Long-term and short-term evaluation of growth and feed efficiency of transgenic Nile tilapia containing an exogenous fish GH gene have also been investigated by Rahman et al. (2001). In a long-term trial, the authors found that transgenic tilapia showed a 2.5-fold increase in growth compared with nontransgenic siblings. After a rearing period of 7 months, the average weight of transgenic tilapia was 653 g compared with 260 g for nontransgenic fish. Feed conversion efficiency was also more than 20% greater in the transgenic fish. In a shorter-term trial (4 weeks), the growth rate of transgenic fish was about four times higher than nontransgenic siblings. Furthermore, apparent protein and energy digestibility were higher in the transgenic fish. This means that transgenic tilapia utilized the feed more efficiently than nontransgenic fish. Similar growth enhancement of transgenic tilapia has been reported by Maclean et al. (2002). These authors emphasized that farmed transgenic fish should be sterile. Sterility can be achieved through triploidy, gene knockout of crucial hormone encoding genes via homologous recombination and knock down of the function of the same genes via ribozyme or antisense technologies.

Growth enhancement and feed efficiency in transgenic tilapia (*Oreochromis* sp.) carrying a single copy of a homologous cDNA growth hormone (GH cDNA) have also been evaluated by Martinez et al. (2000). Transgenic tilapia consumed about 3.6-fold less feed than nontransgenic siblings. Subsequently, the feed conversion efficiency was 290% higher in transgenic tilapia than in the control group. Growth efficiency, synthesis retention, anabolic stimulation and average protein synthesis were also higher in transgenic than in nontransgenic tilapia. Clear metabolic differences were also found in transgenic juvenile tilapia, including differences in hepatic glucose and in the level of enzymatic activities in target organs. The authors concluded that GH-transgenic juvenile tilapia showed altered physiological and metabolic conditions and are biologically more efficient than the control fish.

The GHs of different animals have been used for induction of transgenesis in tilapia. Hernandez et al. (1997) characterized transgenic tilapia lines with different ectopic expression of tilapia GH (tiGH) cDNA. The tilapia GH was used to construct chimeric genes expressing different levels of tiGH in vitro and in vivo. These constructs were, in turn, used to generate different lines of transgenic tilapia. Various patterns and levels of ectopic expression of tiGH were, therefore, detected in transgenic tilapia. The lines with lower ectopic tiGH mRNA levels were the only ones that showed growth acceleration. This result suggested that the expression of ectopic tiGH promoted growth only at low expression levels. Another technique used for producing transgenic tilapia was the expression of recombinant common carp GH (rcGH) in the yeast (*Pichia pastoris*) (Li et al., 2003). The growth of juvenile tilapia injected with purified rcGH was 24.5% and 53.1% higher than the control at a dose of 0.1 and 1.0 μg g^{-1} body weight $week^{-1}$. However, the chemical composition of fish muscles was not significantly affected by the rcGH treatment.

Lu et al. (2009) found that the growth rate of GH-transgenic tilapia (GHTi) was 80%–160% higher than their nontransgenic siblings. The same authors reported also that GHTi reached market size 69 days earlier, and their feed efficiency was 37.3% higher than their nontransgenic strain. Moreover, the total nitrogen (N) and phosphorus (P) discharge loads from GHTi were 50.1% and 61.1% lower, respectively, than those of the control fish. However, body compositions of market-size GHTi were significantly lower, due to the high moisture content. Commercial use of such strains could significantly reduce the environmental impact of tilapia culture and reduce the cost for waste treatment. Incomplete bone mineralization was also observed in early adult GHTi, whereas skeletal abnormalities were observed in late adult GHTi. The authors suggest that optimal feeds should be developed to meet the altered nutritional requirements of GH-transgenic tilapia.

As mentioned earlier, GH increases fish growth, protein retention and absorption; therefore, it is expected to reduce ammonia excretion. This assumption was tested by

Kobayashi et al. (2007), who produced transgenic Nile tilapia that overexpressed the GH gene in their bodies. They found that feed utilization efficiency of the transgenic fish was 35% higher than that of their nontransgenic siblings. Total ammonium–nitrogen excretion by the transgenic fish was about 31% lower than that excreted by nontransgenic fish. Thus, transgenic fish have a high potential to reduce nitrogenous pollution in aquaculture, and therefore, can be a step forward to 'environmentally friendly' aquaculture. Liñán-Cabello et al. (2013) treated Nile tilapia with either 17α-methyltestosterone (17-MT) or GH or combination of both. Intramuscular injection of GH resulted in a significant increase in weight gain of fish in the presence or absence of 17-MT. However, fish treated with both the GH and 17-MT showed the highest weight gain, suggesting a possible interaction between 17-MT and injected GH.

Costa et al. (2016) investigated the presence of daily rhythms in the somatotropic axis of Nile tilapia fed at midlight (ML) or middark (MD) and the influence of the time of day of GH administration on the response of this axis. Two GH injection times were tested; 3 h after lights on (ZT 3) and 3 h after lights off (ZT 15). The results revealed daily rhythms in liver and muscle GH receptors (ghr1 and ghr2) and liver insulin-like growth factors (igf2a) only in fish fed at ML. The acrophases were also located in the light phase (ZT 3:30, 3:31 and 7:38 h, respectively). In the muscle, ghr1 displayed a significant rhythm in both groups and ghr2 in ML-fed fish (acrophases at ZT 5:29, 7:14 and 9:23 h). The time of both feeding and GH administration significantly affected the response of the fish to GH injection. The ML-fed fish injected with GH at ZT 15 h showed a significant increase in liver igf1, igf2a and ghr2 and ghr2 expression in the muscles. This study demonstrated a presence of daily rhythms in the somatotropic axis of tilapia, and its time depends on GH administration.

MicroRNAs (miRNAs) are endogenous, noncoding small RNA molecules that could participate in growth and development of organisms through regulating the expression of target genes. GH-inducible transmembrane protein (ghitm) plays an important role in such growth and development processes. However, miR-1338-5p expression may be negatively correlated with ghitm expression (Qiang et al., 2017). These authors injected genetically improved farmed tilapia (GIFT) juveniles with miR-1338-5p antagomir, to analyze the regulatory function of the miR-1338-5p-ghitm pair. The results showed that ghitm can interfere with GH-ghr-igf signalling pathway by competing with the ghr1 for combination with GH, leading to growth reduction of GIFT. This study suggests that miR-1338-5p participates in the growth and development of GIFT through the regulation of ghitm.

Ghrelin, which is also known as lenomorelin or the 'hunger hormone', is a 28-amino-acid peptide hormone produced in the animal gut. It plays a key role in stimulating GH release from the pituitary and has been implicated as a hunger signal, stimulating food intake in mammals and fish, including tilapia (Fox, 2005; Peddu et al., 2009). Taking an advantage of these features, Fox (2005) evaluated the effects of intraperitoneal (IP) injection of ghrelin-C10 on stimulating GH and prolactin release in Mozambique tilapia (*Oreochromis mossambicus*). Ghrelin injection stimulated GH release after 5 and 10 h following injection, while insulin-like growth factor-I (igf-I) increased only after l0 h. The stimulatory effect of ghrelin on GH release was abolished by the growth hormone secretagogue (GHS)-receptor antagonist [D-Ly ~ 3]-GHRP-6, indicating that GHS-receptor acts as a mediator of ghrelin's actions. Riley et al. (2005) found also that treating tilapia with ghrelin-C10 for 21 days (via osmotic pumps) resulted in a sharp increase in food intake and growth rate, presumably due to the induction of adiposity in liver and muscle tissues by ghrelin-C10, while ghrelin-C8 had no effect.

13.2.2.2 Cold resistance

Despite that tilapia are tropical fishes, well adapted to warm water environments, they are sensitive to cold stress. Mass mortalities of farmed tilapia have been reported in different countries due to severe drop in water temperature in winter, leading to economic losses. Mortality has been attributed mainly to the sensitivity of fish cell membranes to cold stress. Cell membranes sensitivity makes them a potential target of chill and freeze damage (Cao-Hoang et al., 2010). In addition, cold stress leads to reduction or loss of active transport across cell membranes, causing severe impacts on water and ion homoeostasis (Overgaard and MacMillan, 2017). Therefore, improving tilapia tolerance to low temperature is highly demanded to prolong their growth period, reduce mortality during winter and avoid economic loss (Charo-Karisa et al., 2005). The administration of antifreeze proteins (AFPs) could be an ideal solution to avoid cold stress and freeze damage.

Several cold-water marine and freshwater fishes inhabiting ice-laden environments are well adapted to freezing water. To avoid freezing, these fishes are able to produce a unique group of proteins known as 'the antifreeze proteins' (AFPs) or 'the antifreeze glycoproteins' which can interact with ice crystals and effectively lower the freezing temperature (Ewart et al., 1999). The administration of AFPs in temperate and tropical fish species may improve their cold resistance during cold seasons (e.g. during overwintering). This assumption has been tested by Wu et al. (1998) who studied the effect of AFP on cold tolerance in juvenile Mozambique tilapia and milkfish (*Chanos chanos*) exposed to low temperature. The AFP was administered via anal injection or by feeding at 0 (control) or 20 μg AFP g^{-1} body weight every 2 d for six doses. The fish were later subjected to cold-tolerance test. In the injection trial, the mortality of tilapia, 24 h after the transfer from 26°C to 13°C, was 53.3% in the control and only 14.3% in the AFP-treated group. In the feeding trial, the AFP was included in the feed at 0 (control), 100, or 1000 μg AFP g^{-1} body weight, and fed to tilapia juveniles at a rate of 20% body weight d^{-1} for 12 days. The mortality at 24 h after the transfer to 13°C was 60% in the control, 41.9% in the 100 μg g^{-1} AFP group and 3.4% in the 1000 μg g^{-1} AFP group. Milkfish juveniles were given the AFP via anal injection of 100 μg AFP g^{-1} body weight, 100 μg bovine serum albumin (BSA) g^{-1} body weight or saline every 2 d for six doses. After injections, milkfish were treated by gradually decreasing temperature within 4–5 days from 26°C to 16 or 13°C. The mortality of milkfish was 66.7%–100% in the controls and 13.3%–33.3% in the AFP group. These results clearly demonstrated that AFP is able to enhance the tolerance of tilapia and milkfish juveniles to low temperatures.

The effect of thermal stress in winter (December, temperature 14°C) and summer (August, temperature 36 °C) on the expression of type IV antifreeze gene (ANF IV) and some immune-related genes in Nile tilapia has recently been investigated (Ammar et al., 2018). A significant upregulation of mRNA transcript levels occurred in the intestine, gills, skin, spleen, liver, and brain in winter. Upregulation in the gene was also observed in summer, but at lower levels, in the liver, gills, skin, intestine and brain. The expression of immune-related genes was significantly higher in winter than in summer. Cc-chemokine gene expression was the most affected in both winter and summer.

13.2.2.3 Producing pharmaceutical products

There is a great possibility that transgenic tilapia can be used as biofactories for producing valuable pharmaceutical products. For example, Wright and Pohajdak (2001) developed transgenic tilapia containing a humanized insulin gene. Humanized insulin encodes human insulin α and/or β chains while using fish-preferred codons and regulatory sequences. Because tilapia and human insulins are different in certain amino acids, the authors cloned, sequenced, and modified the tilapia insulin gene by site-directed mutagenesis resulting in a tilapia insulin gene that codes for humanized insulin, while still maintaining the tilapia regulatory (noncoding) sequences. These humanized genes are expressible in fish islet cells, providing transgenic fish with islet cells containing, and capable of expressing, humanized insulin genes. These islet cells can be harvested, encapsulated and transplanted into diabetic patients. By this way, normoglycaemia can be achieved into these recipient organisms.

In continuation with this line, Pohajdak et al. (2004) produced transgenic tilapia carrying and expressing a humanized tilapia insulin gene. A male founder was mated to wild females and the F1 offspring were tested for the presence of the transgene. Three copies of the humanized gene were found in the genome of all tested fish, suggesting that these copies were integrated in the same chromosomal locus. Also, Hrytsenko et al. (2010) reported production of phenotypically normal, fertile, homozygous transgenic tilapia (species not provided) carrying a humanized insulin transgene. The over-expression of humanized insulin did not have any impact on fish health, survival and behaviour (swimming, feeding, aggression, territoriality, mating, etc.) compared to wild tilapia.

13.2.2.4 Risk assessment

It appears from the previous discussion that transgenesis would offer several advantages for tilapia culture (high growth rates, cold resistance, etc.). However, the rate of genetic change in transgenic tilapia is such that their phenotypic and behavioural properties cannot easily be predicted (Mair, 2002). Marketing of these fish also faces many constraints. Consumer response to such genetically modified fish is negative in many countries, to the extent that their culture could be an economic risk. At the same time, they may have adverse ecological effects when they are introduced into new environments. Therefore, food safety assessment is necessary before consuming these fish on a commercial scale (de la Fuente et al., 1999). The environmental impacts and risks associated with the adoption of transgenic tilapia for aquaculture activities should also be adequately and carefully assessed. Necessary protective measures must also be taken before introducing these fish into national aquaculture programmes (see Chapter 14 for details).

In this regard, Guillen et al. (1999) evaluated the behaviour of transgenic tilapia in comparison with wild tilapia as a way of assessing their environmental impact in Cuba. They also evaluated the safety of consuming transgenic tilapia as food. Transgenic tilapia had a lower feeding motivation and dominance status than wild tilapia. Food safety assessment indicated that GH contained in transgenic fish has no biological activity when administered to nonhuman primates. No effects were detected in human volunteers after the consumption of transgenic tilapia. It would appear from these results that transgenic tilapia have no environmental impacts, and they are also safe for human consumption. However, more long-term work is needed along this line before a final conclusion can be drawn regarding the impacts of transgenic tilapia on human health and on the aquatic environment.

13.2.2.5 Sex control

Hormonal sex reversal has been the most widely used technique for producing monosex progeny for aquaculture purposes. However, hormone treatments have been under increasing public criticism due to their possible health and environmental impacts. As a result, the use of hormones for sex reversal of tilapia is either licenced (in United States) or banned (in Europe) (Penman and McAndrew, 2000).

The establishment of sex control alternatives based on a nonhazardous approach represents a major challenge for aquaculture. In this regard, genetic control is probably the best way to obtain monosex populations. For example, components of the transforming growth factor beta (TGF-β) signalling pathway, including gonadal soma-derived factor (*gsdf*) and Y-linked duplicate of the anti-Müllerian hormone (*amhy*), have been engaged in sex determination and differentiation in teleost fishes (Kaneko et al., 2015; Li et al., 2015). Kaneko et al. (2015) screened novel genes that were predominantly expressed in either XY or XX undifferentiated Nile tilapia gonads during differentiation into ovaries or testes using microarray screening, with a focus on #9475 gonadal soma-derived factor (*gsdf*). *gsdf* was microinjected into XX-fertilized eggs at the one-cell stage. *gsdf*-transgenic XX tilapia showed normal testis development. This finding suggests that #9475/*gsdf* can play an important role in male determination and/or differentiation in tilapia. In addition, Li et al. (2015) found that XX Nile tilapia with *amhy* transgene were sex reversed into males with functional testis. Therefore, crossing *gsdf* and *amhy* transgenic male with normal XX female could be an effective technique for producing all-male tilapia.

In addition, Nile tilapia females with differentiated ovaries were masculinized by long-term treatment with fadrozole (an aromatase inhibitor) into functional testes with fertile sperms (Sun et al., 2014). Longer sex differentiation time requires longer treatment time for successful sex reversal. In the meantime, sex-reversed males were successfully reversed into females again by exogenous 17β-oestradiol supplementation. In this particular process, ovarian transdifferentiation requires downregulation of endogenous oestrogen, which leads to suppression of female pathway genes, and in turn, upregulates endogenous androgen and activates male pathway genes.

13.2.2.6 Genome-editing technology

Genome editing, or engineering, is a technology through which the living organism is genetically engineered by DNA insertion, deletion, modification or replacement in specific locations of the genome. In this technique, editing is directed to specific engineered nucleases at desired locations in the genome. Targeted nuclease technologies have been rapidly developed in recent years, including zinc finger nucleases, transcription activator-like effector nucleases and clustered, regularly interspaced, short palindromic repeats (CRISPR)-associated systems (CRISPR/Cas9) (see Chen et al., 2018; for review). These technologies can be used for targeted genome editing or knockouts.

Genome-editing technology (genome engineering) can be a breakthrough in producing monosex, fast-growing tilapia. The CRISPR/Cas9 system was applied, for the first time, to genetic engineering in Nile tilapia in 2014 (Li et al., 2014). *gsdf* was mutated via CRISPR/Cas9; and the disruption of *gsdf* in YY tilapia resulted in complete reversal to functional females (Chen et al., 2018). Crossing fertile $YY^{gsdf-/-}$ (♀) pseudofemales with YY males is a potential protocol to produce all YY tilapia; but the fertility of these mutant males remains unknown. In addition, Zhang et al. (2017) found that mutation of *foxl2* or *cyp19a1a* led to female-to-male sex reversal. Therefore, crossing $XX^{cyp19a1a-/-}$ (♂) or $XX^{foxl2-/-}$ (♂) pseudomales with XX females may produce all XX female populations.

13.3 Genetically improved farmed tilapia

One of the most recent technological developments in tilapia culture is the production of 'genetically improved farmed tilapia (GIFT)' through a selective breeding project. The GIFT project was a multidisciplinary research and development program implemented by the International Centre for Living Aquatic Resources Management (ICLARM) (now known as the WorldFish Center) and co-partners (such as UNDP) to develop a selective breeding programme for Nile tilapia (Eknath and Acosta, 1998). It was one of the longest international research projects, since it started in 1988 and ended in 1997. The project was based in the Philippines using a combined selection methodology on a synthetic base population developed from tilapia populations newly introduced from Africa and domesticated in Asia. The three main specific targets of project were the following:

1. To develop improved breeds of Nile tilapia and disseminate them to the fish farmers;
2. To strengthen national institutions in aquaculture genetics research and
3. To establish a mechanism for exchange and evaluation of improved breeds and research methods among international institutions (Eknath et al., 1998).

To date, many selective breeding programs for Nile tilapia have been well established and implemented, particularly in Asia (Table 13.1). These include GIFT (Eknath et al., 1993; Eknath and Acosta, 1998), GET EXCEL (Tayamen, 2004), FaST (Bolivar, 1998), ProGift Hainan (Thodesen et al., 2011) and GenoMar Supreme Tilapia (GST) (Zimmermann and Natividad, 2004). Several tilapia strains have also been developed in Indonesia (see Table 13.1). In Africa, the 'Akosombo

TABLE 13.1 Examples of improved tilapia strains in different countries.

Strain	Country	References
GIFT	Malaysia, Bangladesh	Fitzsimmons (2015)
FaST	Philippines	Bolivar (1998)
GET EXCEL	Philippines	Tayamen (2004)
Molobicus	Philippines	Fitzsimmons (2015)
TabTim	Thailand	Fitzsimmons (2015)
Chitralada	Thailand	Fitzsimmons (2015)
ProGift	China (Hainan)	Thodesen et al. (2011)
GenoMar Supreme Tilapia (GST)	Brazil, Norway, Philippines	Zimmermann and Natividad (2004)
Akosombo tilapia strain	Ghana	CGIAR (2013)
Genetically Improved Abbassa Nile Tilapia (GIANT)	Egypt	H. Charo-Karisa (Personal communication, 2019)
Aquaamerica Strain	Brazil	Garcia et al. (2017)
BEST	Indonesia	Widiarti (2015)
GESIT		
LARASATI		
SRIKANDI		
NIRWANA		
JATIMBLAN		
ANJANI		
SULTANA		
SALINA		

tilapia strain' is another example of applying the GIFT methodology in Ghana in collaboration with the World-Fish Center in 2003 (CGIAR, 2013). In Egypt, the WorldFish has also been running a selective breeding program for faster-growing strain of Nile tilapia since 2002, using the GIFT technology. The program has resulted in the development of a new strain known as 'Genetically Improved Abbassa Nile Tilapia (GIANT) (Charo-Karisa; personal communication, 2019)', which is currently disseminated to several tilapia farmers across the country. Aquaamerica strain (Garcia et al., 2017) is also widely used in Latin America.

The GIFT project focused on growth studies of tilapia, in addition to studying the genetic parameters of other important traits such as size at maturity, survival, disease resistance, skin colour, body conformation and cold tolerance. The following sections discuss the studies conducted on some of these traits.

13.3.1 Growth, survival and fillet yield

The genetic gain of GIFT has been documented by a number of authors. An estimated heritability of 0.24 for growth in Nile tilapia has been reported by Eknath et al. (1993). Further investigations on genetic gains of Nile tilapia over successive generations have also been reported (Eknath and Acosta, 1998). These investigations revealed that GIFT achieved 13% genetic gains over five generations, providing estimated accumulative increase of 85% in growth rate compared to the base population from which they were selected. An average sustained genetic gains across six generations of selection using a combined selection was 10%–15% per generation (Ponzoni et al., 2011). By 2003, GIFT strain and the GIFT-derived strain GET EXCEL accounted for 68% of total tilapia seed produced in the Philippines (ADB, 2005). GIFT tilapia and GIFT-derived seeds are currently used by the majority of tilapia farmers in the country; indicating that the impact of GIFT and GIFT-derived tilapia in the Philippines has been outstanding. By 2013, 16 generations of GIFT strain have been produced by the Department of Fisheries, Malaysia (Hamzah et al., 2014; Nguyen, 2016). However, there is still a room for further selective breeding to achieve additional increases in body weight.

As a result of their outstanding performance, the GIFT strains have been distributed for aquaculture in 9 Asia—Pacific countries (Bangladesh, China, Indonesia, Malaysia, the Philippines, Papua New Guinea, Sri Lanka, Thailand and Vietnam) and four Latin American countries (Brazil, Costa Rica, Ecuador and Mexico). These fish have performed extremely well in these countries in different farming systems and environments. For example, the body weight at harvest of GIFT strain in Sri Lanka was 112% higher than the local tilapia strains when raised in experimental ponds, commercial earthen ponds or seasonal tanks. The survival rates of GIFT were also 8.2%—23.8% higher than local stocks (Nguyen et al., 2011). Substantial improvement in growth rates of the GIFT strain has also been achieved over the course of 10 generations of selection, with an average gain of 10% per generation (Hamzah et al., 2014) (Table 13.2). This means that the average body weight was more than doubled over 10 generations of selection, when compared with the control, nonselected strains. The response to five generations of selection for increased body weight at harvest in GIFT strain was assessed by Bentsen et al. (2017). The results indicated that the average response to selection per generation was 13.6%, leading to an accumulated response of 88% relative to the base population over the five generations. However, the authors suggested an accumulated response of 67% after the termination of the project, based on best linear unbiased prediction analysis.

In a comprehensive study, Bentsen et al. (2012) estimated the phenotypic and genetic parameters for harvest body weight within and across multiple farming environments during five consecutive generations of GIFT population. The farming environments included earthen ponds (fertilized with inorganic fertilizer, organic manure or on-farm agricultural residues), cage culture, rice—fish, and ponds at test stations located in different agro-climatic regions. The average heritability estimates for harvest body weight within test environments and generation was 0.31; but was higher in cage environments. When heterogeneous variances of harvest body weight across generations, test environments and sexes were adjusted, the average estimates across tested environments within generations were $h^2 = 0.23$ and $c^2 = 0.03$ over the five generations, while the estimate across all test environments and generations was $h^2 = 0.16$ and $c^2 = 0.10$. The genetic correlations between harvest body weights of sibs in the different environments were generally high, ranging from 0.53 to 0.99, with an average of 0.89 for all environments (except for cage culture), indicating that the genotype by environment ($G \times E$) interactions is minor. The genetic correlations involving the cage culture environment were lower (0.08—0.43), suggesting that $G \times E$ interactions may occur in widely different test environments. It is proposed that this $G \times E$ interaction may involve the effects of sexual maturation on growth in pond environments. Similarly, when GIFT strains and hybrid red tilapia were grown in periphyton-based system in integration with prawn culture in Bangladesh, the GIFT tilapia strain showed significantly higher survival, gross and net yields and economic return than the hybrid red tilapia (Haque et al., 2016).

The genetic correlations between body weight and fillet weight of GIFT tilapia is very high (up to 0.96), indicating that improvement can enhance both growth and carcass performance in the same time (Nguyen et al., 2010a). However, the genetic correlations between fillet yield and body traits were generally low (0.35—0.44), suggesting that harvest weight should be selected as a criterion to improve both growth and fillet weight in breeding programs (Ponzoni et al., 2011). Much higher fillet yields were reported in GIFT tilapia (31.0%—>38.0%), depending on whether the fillet is skinned or with skin compared with other Nile

TABLE 13.2 Weight gain per generation of different improved tilapia strains across different generations.

Tilapia strain	Average gain (%) per generation	References
GIFT base to G6	10—15	Ponzoni et al. (2011)
GIFT base to G5	13.6	Bentsen et al. (2017)
GIFT G6—G14	13.2—>5.3[a]	Thodesen et al. (2011)
FaST G0—G12	12.9	Bolivar and Newkirk (2002)
GIFT base to G10	10	Hamzah et al. (2014)
Red tilapia (*Oreochromis* sp.) G0—G3	12.5	Hamzah et al. (2017)

[a]*Reduction due to decreased selection intensity in later generations.*

tilapia strains (Rutten et al., 2005; Nguyen et al., 2010a). Similarly, multitrait selective breeding of GIFT Nile tilapia strain in China has led to a significant genetic improvement in growth and fillet weight, while improvements in fillet yield were much slower (Thodesen et al., 2012).

The genetic improvement of uniformity of harvest weight and body size traits (length, depth and width) has also been investigated in GIFT strain (Marjanovic et al., 2016). The results revealed substantial genetic variation in uniformity of all analyzed traits. Genetic correlation between trait level and variance was strongly positive for harvest weight (0.60), moderate and positive for body depth (0.37), but not significantly different from 0 for body length and width. This study indicates that the potential for genetic improvement of uniformity in the GIFT strain is high.

13.3.2 Early and late maturation

One of the disadvantages of tilapia culture is their early maturation and reproduction at small sizes. Generally, uncontrolled reproduction leads to overpopulation, stunting and poor growth rates. However, tilapia show great plasticity in growth and maturation. Some tilapia species can grow to a large size, and both males and females grow to, and mature at, similar sizes (Longalong et al., 1999). Under certain conditions (e.g. trapping in lagoons), these fish become very small and mature at small size, but the females are much smaller than males at first maturity. Females which do not mature at an early age follow the growth trends of the males (Bolivar et al., 1993). Therefore, delaying of the onset of sexual maturation in tilapia females by selection can be an effective tool for reproduction management of these fishes.

The possibility of delaying the onset of sexual maturation in Nile tilapia has been investigated in the laboratory using a breeding base population of 35 full-sib families (Hörstgen-Schwark and Langholz, 1998). Gonad weight, gonadosomatic index (GSI) and the stage of gonadal development were used as indicators of sexual maturation. The heaviest individuals within each selected family were used as spawners for the next generation. After two generations, males of the selected line exhibited lower states of maturity (i.e. lower gonad weights) as compared to the control group, whereas the values of the GSI were lower in the females of the selected lines than in the control females. These selection responses indicated the possibility of delaying sexual maturity in Nile tilapia to a later stage without affecting their growth rates. A similar degree of genetic variability for maturation indices has been achieved when the reference strain was tested under field conditions (Oldorf et al., 1989).

The selection for early maturation of Nile tilapia was also investigated several years ago. Fish selected for early maturation matured 11−14 days earlier after one generation of selection, but inconsistent results were obtained in the second generation. The response to bidirectional selection for frequency of early maturation in Nile tilapia females was evaluated in 42 full-sib families within 21 randomly chosen half-sib families of Nile tilapia, among the families representing the third generation of selection for improved growth performance in the GIFT project (Longalong et al., 1999). Sex, body weight and sexual maturity in the females were recorded at 2, 3 or 4 weeks after the first swim-up fry were observed in the earthen ponds holding the communally families. The broodstock was selected from full-sib families with a high (>75%) or a low (<20%) frequency of mature females. The fry of 16 pairs of high selected early maturity (83%) and 9 pairs of low early maturity (0) were collected, and each pair was reared separately until they reached a size of 3−5 g. The response to selection was highly significant, and there was a positive correlation between early maturity and fish size (i.e. early maturing fish were the fastest growing).

13.3.3 Red body colour

Body colour is an important trait in some cultured tilapia, with respect to market demand. In some countries, fish consumers prefer the red morph to the common black morph. The market price of red fish is expected to be higher than that of black fish in these countries. Some progress has been achieved in the efforts to select for homogeneity of colour in red tilapia.

A number of 'red' tilapia strains/hybrids have been developed and commercially produced, generating high market acceptance for tilapia, especially in the United States, Europe and Asia. This indicates that the improvement of 'colour quality' in tilapia is an important approach for the development of tilapia culture. In accordance, a number of studies have considered mass selection for red colour in tilapia with promising results. Mather et al. (2001) evaluated the mass selection of Fijian hybrid tilapia (*Oreochromis niloticus* × *O. mossambicus*) in order to improve their red body colour by reducing the amount of black spots on the red phenotypes. The responses of two selection intensities (low-selection line, top 50%) and (high-selection line, top 30%) were compared with that of a control line (no selection). After three generations, about 100% improvement in colour quality (i.e. reduction in black spots on the red phenotype) was achieved. These authors suggested that red phenotype can be improved significantly by applying mass selection, without adversely affecting fish growth.

Mass selection for red colour in Nile tilapia has been investigated in Mexico (Granduño-Lugo et al., 2004). The selection was applied using the Stirling strain of Nile tilapia to obtain red-coloured homozygous dominant population from a base population containing wild fish and red fish with black blotches. After five selection generations, red colour proportion increased from 5.6% in the first generation to 100% in the fifth generation. All the fry produced were red coloured, indicating that the population was homozygous dominant for that trait. The fecundity and fry production of red tilapia were similar to those of wild fish. Again, these results clearly indicate that mass selection for red colour is very appropriate and unlikely to cause any adverse effects on growth and reproduction performances. Red tilapia were introduced in Jamaica because the people were used to marine fish and preferred the silver or red colour of these fish (R. Stickney, Texas, USA, 2004; personal communication). The red tilapia were sold at a premium price, but once consumers did a side-by-side taste comparison, they realized that the normal coloured tilapia were just as good, and the red ones were no longer able to demand a higher price.

In their selective breeding programs on red tilapia (*Oreochromis* spp.) in China, Thodesen et al. (2013) recorded significant genetic improvements of external colour traits after four generations of multitrait selection. Basavaraja and Raghavendra (2017) also found that when *O. mossambicus* were mated with red hybrid tilapia (*O. niloticus* × *O. mossambicus*) in India, the produced F1 progeny had brown colour, an intermediate colour between the two parental body colours. When F1 hybrids were interbred, the three phenotypes got separated in the F2 generation with a phenotypic ratio of 1:2:1 black:-brown:red, as expected of a single autosomal gene with incomplete dominant gene action.

13.3.4 Cold resistance

As mentioned in Chapter 4, tilapia feeding is sharply reduced below 20°C, and the fish stop feeding at about 16°C, while severe mortality occurs at 12°C. Tilapia can also tolerate temperatures as low as 4–10°C, but only for short time, depending on tilapia species and size and strains. It is therefore essential to produce tilapia strains that can tolerate cold weather, especially during winter seasons in temperate regions. This problem has been tackled through mass selection for cold tolerance (Behrends et al., 1996). Based on data derived from bidirectional selection for cold tolerance, the heritability estimates of Nile tilapia, blue tilapia and their hybrids were calculated according to the ratio response: selection differential. After one generation of selection, estimates for up-selected populations (most cold tolerant) were blue tilapia (0.33), Nile tilapia (−0.05) and tilapia hybrids (0.31). Estimates for two down-selected populations (least cold tolerant) were blue tilapia (0.04) and Nile tilapia (0.42). In addition, fingerlings from up-selected populations grew faster than those obtained from down-selected populations at temperatures ranging from 17.2 to 21.2°C. Under low temperature regimes, blue tilapia grew significantly better than Nile tilapia, irrespective of selection criteria. These results demonstrated the possibility of increasing cold tolerance in blue tilapia and related hybrids through directed selection.

The genetic basis of cold tolerance of Mozambique and blue tilapia and their F1 and F2 hybrids was also studied by Cnaani et al. (2000). Groups of fish of similar age and grown under similar conditions were housed in net enclosures in a controlled water system. Water temperature was gradually decreased and survival time was observed. There was no correlation between cold tolerance and fish size (within the range of 2.3–10.5 cm standard length), and the distribution for the trait was not normal. Mozambique tilapia were the most cold-sensitive fish, followed by F2, and F1 groups, which were similar to blue tilapia. The authors concluded that genetic variation in cold tolerance seems to have a large dominance component, based on the similarity of the F1 hybrid to the blue tilapia parent.

13.3.5 GenoMar supreme tilapia and GET EXCEL tilapia

The success made with the GIFT programme has encouraged researchers to further develop breeding programmes in order to maximize the genetic gain for the traits of interest. As a result, new tilapia strains characterized with tremendous genetic gains have been developed, and the GenoMar Supreme Tilapia (GST) strain is an example of such innovation. This strain is a continuation of the GIFT breeding programme, with some changes. The two major changes were to:

1. apply DNA fingerprinting as an identification tool and
2. change to a revolving mating scheme in order to complete the generation after nine monthly batches (Gjøen, 2004).

DNA fingerprinting makes it much easier and faster to produce the strains with the desired characteristics. DNA fingerprinting also provides many advantages, such as increased selection intensity and shorter generation intervals, in addition to other operational benefits. Among the genetic traits contained in GenoMar Supreme Tilapia are salt tolerance, growth rate, feed conversion efficiency, disease resistance and fillet yield. Gjøen (2004) estimated the genetic gain of GST by testing generations 10 and 11 (G10/G11) as a base, against generation 13 (G13). The selection was adequately successful, with an average genetic gain of about 20% per generation compared to conventional schemes. The survival rate also increased to about 11% per generation, leading to a total average survival of more than 80% in G13. The average FCR was also less than 1.1.

GET EXCEL tilapia is another new breed developed by the government of the Philippines by combining improved breed of Nile tilapia using within-family selection and a rotational mating scheme (Tayamen, 2004). Consequently, the Bureau of Fisheries and Aquatic Resources-National Freshwater Fisheries Technology Centre (BFAR-NFFTC) has sustained the development of a fast-growing fish known as GET EXCEL 2002 through the use of genetically improved tilapia. GET EXCEL 2002 is therefore a product of a selection programme combining strain crosses and within-family selection, with rotational mating using the four parent lines:

- Generation 8 (G8) of GIFT strain-developed by crossing the best performing genetic groups from eight Nile tilapia strains and their crosses.
- Generation 13 (G13) FAC (Freshwater Aquaculture Centre) selected tilapia (FaST) — a product of within-family selection of Nile tilapia in a rotational mating scheme.
- Egypt strain.
- Kenya strain.

The term EXCEL implies for **EX**cellent strain that has **C**omparable advantage with other tilapia strains for **E**ntrepreneurial **L**ivelihood projects in support to aquaculture for rural development (Tayamen, 2004). Preliminary evaluation of GET EXCEL tilapia indicated that the strain grew much faster, with better survival than the other improved commercial Nile tilapia strains. This breed has a great potential for increasing the yield and profitability for tilapia farmers. Therefore, the government of the Philippines has initiated a flagship project known as 'Nationwide Dissemination of GET EXCEL tilapia' with an ultimate goal of replacing the old tilapia breed, currently in use, with the latest improved breed, in order to approach the targeted incremental production and participate in global market for value-added products.

13.4 Gynogenesis, androgenesis and cloning

Gynogenesis and androgenesis are forms of uniparental inheritance, induced by fertilizing one gamete with another, in which the DNA has been denatured by irradiation. Gynogenesis is therefore the production of progeny with only a maternal genome, while androgenesis produces diploid organisms the nuclear DNA of which is wholly of paternal origin. This process produces a haploid zygote that can be diploidized by application of physical shock such as temperature or pressure (Mair, 2002). The resulting individuals are completely homozygous and 100% inbred. The induction and survival rate of these homozygous fish are very low (Müller-Belecke and Hörstgen-Schwark, 2000), but the lethal or deleterious genes, in the homozygous state, are selected out during the process. Genetically identical individuals or homozygous clones are produced in the second generation of androgenesis or gynogenesis (Mair, 2002). Meanwhile, crosses between these homozygous fish produce heterozygous clones.

Androgenesis is more difficult to accomplish than gynogenesis (Scheerer et al., 1986), since diploidy can only be induced in androgens at first cell division, a difficult time to manipulate the embryo. Androgens are also totally homozygous, and their mortality rates are very high due to the presence of lethal or deleterious genes (Scheerer et al., 1986). The production of diploid androgenic organisms depends on the following: (1) the denucleation of 'host' eggs using UV irradiation and (2) the inhibition of the first mitotic division in order to double the haploid sperm chromosome complement following fertilization of host eggs.

Myers et al. (1995) succeeded in producing diploid Nile tilapia androgens by denucleation of their eggs by UV irradiation. A total dose of 450–720 J m^{-2} for 5–8 min produced an acceptable 22.9% denucleated eggs, as estimated by the survival of haploid androgenetic fish to 48 h post fertilization. Successful mitotic inhibition was accomplished using a heat shock of 42.5°C for 3–4 min, applied at 2.5-min intervals, 22.5–30 min post fertilization. The mean survival of androgenetic diploid fish to yolk-sac absorption varied from 0.4% to 5.3%, compared to the controls. A survival peak of 1.6% in androgenic diploid Nile tilapia and 0.9% in hybrid Nile tilapia x blue tilapia at a dose of 5940–6930 erg mm^{-2} have also been reported by Marengoni and Onoue (1998). These results demonstrated the possibility of producing androgenetic tilapia and indicated that the application of this technique may be useful in quantitative and conservation genetics.

The external egg fertilization and embryonic development in fishes make the development of homozygous clones by the use of induced gynogenetic or androgenetic reproduction techniques much easier and more successful than with farm animals such as pigs and poultry (Müller-Belecke and Hörstgen-Schwark, 2000). The probability of producing homozygous genotypes free from expression of harmful genes is also higher in fishes due to their high fecundity. Therefore, clones have been developed within many commercial fish species, including tilapia (Müller-Belecke and Hörstgen-Schwark, 1995; Hussain et al., 1998).

Cloning can be very useful as a pure 'gene pool' for genetic studies such as cell and tissue culture, genetic fingerprinting, immunology, disease resistance, heritability and sex differentiation studies, in addition to the development of breeding schemes based on the exploitation of heterosis. However, little information is available on the production, reproduction and performance of homozygous and heterozygous clones as compared to normal heterozygous tilapia. Hussain et al. (1998) produced heterozygous and homozygous clones of Nile tilapia. An outbred clonal line (OCL) was produced by cross-breeding between a viable mitotic gynogenetic female and male (recessive mutation in a sex-determining gene). In addition, an inbred clonal line (ICL) was produced by gynogenetic reproduction (retention of second polar body) using pressure/heat-shock techniques. The ICL showed very poor viability and high levels of abnormality, presumably due to inbreeding or the increased sensitivity of the eggs to the pressure/heat shocks. The OCL clone had higher survival (25%–40%) to first feeding and low levels of abnormality. The authors related the superior viability of OCL to ICL to the effect of heterosis. They further suggested that hybrid or heterozygous clonal lines can be utilized for fixing superior genes desirable for selective breeding and genetic improvement of tilapia.

It should be emphasized here that the development and reproduction of ICL and OCL are difficult and expensive. It is also too early to conclude whether the development and continuation of clonal lines in tilapia is worthwhile for practical applications in breeding programmes, especially in developing countries, where funds for this type of research may not be available.

13.5 Triploidy

Under aquaculture conditions, tilapia generally mature at small sizes, and are also characterized by multiple annual spawning, if environmental conditions are favourable. This reproduction pattern usually leads to overpopulation and stunting of cultured fish. Therefore, controlling reproduction has been a major challenge in tilapia culture for many years. The culture of monosex tilapia is probably the most common method of tackling the problem. Traditionally, monosex tilapia are produced by (1) manual sorting, (2) hormonal sex reversal and (3) interspecific hybridization. These methods have been addressed in details in Chapter 8. In addition, triploidy can be used as a useful tool to induce sexually sterile tilapia (Hussain et al., 1991, 1995). The use of sterile fish has several applications, including controlling reproduction, preventing backcrosses of hybrids with their parents and improving growth of farmed species because more energy is saved for somatic growth and less for reproduction (Rottmann et al., 1991).

The induction of triploidy occurs after ovulation and sperm entrance into the egg. The cells of triploid individuals have three sets of chromosomes (3n), whereas diploid individuals have two sets (2n). Triploidy is produced by preventing the second meiotic division, after the sperm enters the egg. This process results in two sets of chromosomes from the female and one set from the male. Heat, cold and pressure shocks are commonly used for triploid induction in fish.

Successful induction of triploidy in different tilapia species has been reported. Hussain et al. (1991) investigated triploidy induction in Nile tilapia using pressure, heat and cold shocks. The best results were obtained at a pressure of 8000 psi, applied for 2 min, 9 min post fertilization (pf); heat of 41°C applied for 3.5 min, 5 min pf and cold of 9°C applied for 30 min, 7 min pf. Pressure and heat shocks produced better triploid yields than cold shocks. A similar study was conducted by El Gamal et al. (1999) where heat shock, cold shock, hydrostatic pressure and/or a chemical (cytochalasin) were applied to induce triploidy and tetraploidy in Nile tilapia. Heat shock, 10 min after fertilization, induced triploidy at an incubation temperature of 42°C but not at 31°C. Up to 100% triploidy was induced using heat shock of 40–41°C, 4–6 min pf, with hatchability similar to controls. Cold shock at 13°C for 45 min, 5 min pf induced 85%–100% triploids.

Heat shock and multiple heat shocking were the most effective treatments for the induction of tetraploidy in Nile tilapia (El Gamal et al., 1999). When two heat treatments of 41°C were applied at 65 and 80 min pf, for 5 min, each of them induced about 80% tetraploidy. The use of cytochalasin was ineffective in inducing triploidy or tetraploidy in the fish.

The aquaculture potential of triploid tilapia has been investigated (Bramick et al., 1995). Diploid and triploid tilapia were reared in earthen ponds and fed with rice bran as a supplemental feed, in addition to weekly fertilization, for 285 days. No differences in growth between triploid and diploid fish were observed at the age of maturation. However, the final weights of triploids were significantly heavier than diploids. Triploid males were 66% heavier, whereas triploid females were 95% heavier than diploid fish. As expected, gonad weights were lower and gonadal development was retarded in triploid fish, but about 15% of triploid females had extremely high gonadosomatic indices. Stocking the ponds with triploid tilapia also prevented fish overproduction and stunting. Chang et al. (1996) found also that the growth of diploid and triploid blue tilapia did not differ significantly, but the triploids were of more uniform size than the diploids. The genital papillae of triploid fish showed no development compared with diploids at 18 weeks of age. Mean gonad weights of females and males were similar for diploids, but different for triploids. Some triploid testes developed well with high numbers of sperms of variable shapes accumulating in the lobular lumina. Yolk accumulation was pronounced in the oocytes of diploids, but the threadlike triploid ovaries contained mainly oogonia with only a few yolky oocytes.

On the other hand, Puckhaber and Hörstgen-Schwak (1996) reported that the growth and gonadal development of triploid Nile tilapia were poorer than diploids. Triploids were also incapable of producing viable progenies. The survival and growth of diploid blue tilapia reared in tanks and fed with pelleted feeds or in fertilized ponds were also better than triploids (Byamungu et al., 2001), but the performance of both lines was better in tanks than in ponds. It is clear that induced triploidy can be an effective tool for controlling excessive reproduction of farmed tilapia. But the contradictory results over survival and growth performance make it difficult to conclude whether triploid tilapia can be used for growth enhancement. Once again, more research is needed on the growth and feed efficiency of triploid tilapia as compared with their diploid counterparts.

As mentioned in Section 13.2.2, transgenesis can enhance tilapia growth. Triploidy may also have a promising potential in tilapia culture (see above). One may ask: would it be possible to induce triploidy in transgenic fish, and what would be the expected results?. These questions have been addressed by Razak et al. (1999) who evaluated growth performance and gonadal development of growth-enhanced transgenic Nile tilapia following heat shock-induced triploidy. The authors found that the red blood cells of triploid fish were 1.5 times larger than those in diploids. Growth performance and gonadal development were compared between diploids and triploids from both transgenic and nontransgenic full siblings. The growth of transgenic diploids was superior, followed by transgenic triploids, nontransgenic diploids and nontransgenic triploids, respectively. The testes of transgenic triploids were smaller than nontransgenic triploids and nontransgenic diploids. However, some triploid testes contained some spermatozoa, indicating reproductive functionality, while the ovaries of triploid fish were completely nonfunctional. The authors suggested that triploid transgenic females could be a good option for tilapia culture, due to their sterility and superior growth over the normal wild tilapia. At the same time, they emphasized that careful monitoring of potential gene flow is required prior to commercial use of the technology.

13.6 Production of genetically male Nile tilapia

It is well accepted that tilapia males grow much faster than females, and therefore, tilapia farmers prefer male tilapia to female fish for culture. The culture of tilapia males also overcomes the problem of massive recruitment resulting from excessive reproduction. The traditional methods of producing all-male tilapia have been addressed in details in Chapter 8. An alternative is the use of genetically male tilapia (GMT) technology for producing all-male tilapia populations. The production of GMT, which is also known as YY male or supermale has been developed through the use of YY chromosome male fish. These YY males are the offspring of a breeding between normal male and a female produced by hormonal sex reversal of a genetic male. Twenty-five percent of the offspring from such a mating will have a YY configuration of their sex chromosomes, instead of the normal XY. When a YY male is crossed with a normal XX female, it produces a high percentage of XY (male) offspring (Fig. 13.1).

In fact, the production of YY-*O. mossambicus* was reported many years ago, using the endocrine sex reversal technique with selective breeding or gynogenetic technique, but the numbers of produced YY males were relatively low (Varadaraj and Pandian, 1989). The adoption of endocrine and gynogenetic techniques increased the production of YY males from 25% to 50% and reduced the time cost of production from 22 months to only 8 months.

For Nile tilapia, Mair et al. (1995) reported that up to 100% GMT can be produced using YY technology. Under controlled conditions, GMT have a sex ratio of over 95% males, whereas in commercial production systems, this ratio is variable due to genetic contamination (Mair et al., 2002). The performance of GMT was also compared with hormonally sex-reversed Nile tilapia and mixed-sex Nile tilapia, both on station and on farm (Mair et al., 1995). The growth rates, feed utilization efficiency, harvest weight, total yield and market income were superior in GMT to the other two groups. Farm trials in the Philippines demonstrated also that GMT culture was 100% more profitable than the culture of mixed-sex tilapia. As a result, GMT are currently being cultured in many countries worldwide, with reasonable success. The YY male technology is also being disseminated through the provision of YY male and normal female broodstocks to hatcheries in many regions of the world, particularly in Asia.

Müller-Belecke and Hörstgen-Schwark (2007) developed a YY-male Nile tilapia strain from an exceptional mitotic gynogenetic male, by mating the YY males with YY females. However, when the new YY females were treated with diethylstilbestrol (DES) administration, a maximum of 5% phenotypically female fish were produced. This weak response to DES treatment represented a limitation in the production of YY females, which is a necessary step for the continuation of the strain and for sustainable production of YY-male fish. The same authors (Müller-Belecke and Hörstgen-Schwark, 2007) evaluated the growth performance of the developed YY-male progenies in comparison with the traditional mixed-sex Nile tilapia. The all-male fish were 14.5% larger than the whole mixed-sex groups and their weights were comparable to the males within the mixed-sex groups.

However, the identification of XY females (for YY male production) is difficult because they are indistinguishable from normal XX females (Alcántar-Vázquez et al., 2014). 'Atypical fish' may provide a rapid and precise alternative for identification of XY females. Atypical fish may have abnormal papillae or, sometimes, have

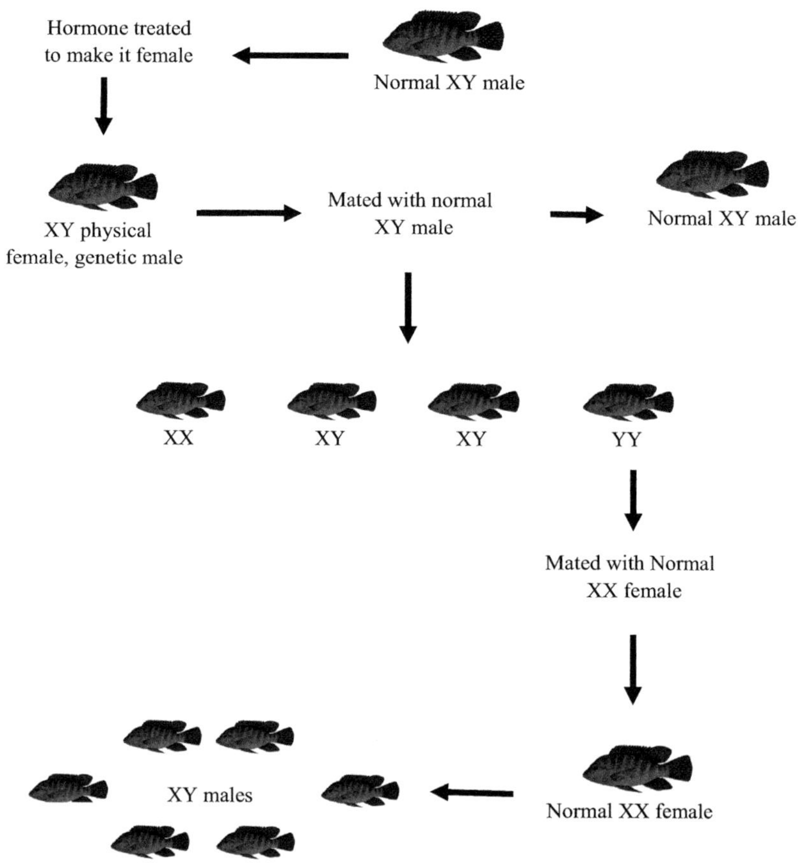

FIGURE 13.1 Production of genetically male tilapia via YY chromosome males. *Modified from Subasinghe et al. (2003).*

ovaries but a male papilla. These fish generally lack a functional oviduct, and therefore, may not be sexually functional. Alcántar-Vázquez et al. (2014) also reported that selected atypical fish were functional and able to produce a viable number of fry with a high survival rate. They evaluated the ability of atypical Nile tilapia (sex reversed by oestradiol (E_2) treatment) to produce YY males. Normal males and atypical females were stocked at a sex ratio of 2:1 and left to spawn. Produced larvae were reared for 120 days and their sex was differentiated by examining the genital papilla structure. The authors found that 66% of the atypical fish showed a 3:1 male:female ratio. They suggested that atypical fish could help reduce the time and effort spent to identify XY females during the initial stages of YY-male technology.

13.7 Nonsurgical spermatogonial transplantation

Unlike mammals, spermatogenesis in teleost fish occurs synchronously within cysts and is maintained by self-regeneration and differentiation of the spermatogonial stem cells to produce spermatozoa (Schulz et al., 2010). Therefore, understanding spermatogonial stem cell biology is necessary for the development of biotechnologies applied to teleost fishes. In this regard, Lacerda et al. (2010) described a new and fast nonsurgical technique for efficient spermatogonial transplantation from a donor tilapia strain into the testes of recipient adult Nile tilapia, in which endogenous spermatogenesis had been depleted using cytostatic drug busulfan. The recipient fish received the donor germ cells through the spermatic duct using a glass micropipette (70 μm outside diameter) under a stereomicroscope. Recipient tilapia were capable of producing functional fertile spermatozoa and generate progeny with the donor genotype. After cryopreservation, tilapia spermatogonial cells were able to differentiate to spermatozoa in the testes of recipient fish. This technique can lead to a number of applications, including the following:

1. Fast generation of donor spermatogenesis and offspring using transgenic spermatogonia.
2. The improvement of the production of commercially valuable fish.
3. Generation of transgenic fish.
4. Preservation and propagation of endangered fish species.

5. Adult spermatogonia are able to generate both spermatozoa and oocytes (Okutsu et al., 2006).

13.8 Disease management

Tilapia culture has witnessed a huge expansion in recent decades, concomitant with a rapid intensification. These developments in tilapia culture have made them more vulnerable to stress and disease outbreaks, leading to severe economic losses. Also, the wide introduction of tilapia into many countries worldwide, mainly for aquaculture and fisheries purposes, has increased the spreading potential of pathogens and parasites. As a result, disease management of farmed tilapia has received considerable attention in recent years. Full details on tilapia stress and diseases are provided in Chapter 9 (Stress and Diseases).

Infectious diseases cause considerable loss in aquaculture, especially on shrimp farms, in many parts of the world. Conventional protective and treatment methods (such as antibiotics and disinfection) may be ineffective, particularly with pathogens such as viruses. Also, it may not be possible to export the product to some countries if it contains antibiotic residues. Thus, unconventional methods of disease management have received great attention in recent years. Molecular techniques, such as DNA- or RNA-based probes and in vitro tissue culture, have great potentials for disease detection, and in turn, for enhancing protective measurements. These techniques have been very successful with shrimp aquaculture (Subasinghe et al., 2003). The production of specific pathogen-free (SPF) and specific pathogen-resistant populations has also been successful with shrimp broodstocks. SPF shrimp are produced by selecting animals free of specific pathogens, using them as broodstock and raising their offspring under controlled sanitary conditions.

13.8.1 Selective breeding

Selective breeding can provide an efficient way for improving fish resistance against bacterial diseases as has been reported in Atlantic salmon (Storset et al., 2007), rainbow trout (Leeds et al., 2010) and white shrimp (Huang et al., 2012). This approach has also been tested in tilapia by many authors. Cai et al. (2004) investigated the resistance of Nile tilapia, blue tilapia and their hybrids (♀ Nile tilapia x ♂ blue tilapia) to disease caused by the bacteria *Aeromonas sobria*. Based on nonspecific immunity functions, significant differences occurred between interspecific hybrids and their parental species to *A. sobria*, where the hybrids have the highest resistance, while blue tilapia have the lowest resistance. These results suggest that specific variations exist in immunity against a specific pathogen and pointed out the potential for genetic improvement of disease resistance in tilapia.

Substantial additive genetic variation in resistance of Nile tilapia to *Streptococcus iniae* has also been demonstrated by LaFrentz et al. (2016). Nile tilapia families were challenged for estimation of genetic parameters for resistance to *S. iniae*. Fish were challenged by IP injection with *S. iniae* and were utilized as shedder fish to transfer the bacterium to another cohabitated fish group, reared in the same tank. Accumulated mortality was 60% for the fish challenged by injection and 6.4% for fish challenged by cohabitation. The estimated heritability of post-challenge survival in the injected fish was 0.42 on the observed binary scale and 0.58 on the underlying liability scale. This result demonstrates the potential of additive genetic variation in resistance to *S. iniae* and suggests that genetic improvement of Nile tilapia for resistance to *S. iniae* through selective breeding is promising. The heritability of *S. iniae* resistance in Nile tilapia was also demonstrated by Shoemaker et al. (2017). These authors confirmed the additive genetic variation in resistance of Nile tilapia to *S. iniae* and suggested that genetic gain for survival to *S. iniae* is possible. Similar results have been reported by Wonmongkol et al. (2018) who estimated quantitative genetic parameters for resistance against columnaris bacteria (*Flavobacterium columnare*) in the Chitralada strain of Nile tilapia. Fish fry from 43 full-sib families were initially subjected to bath challenge with *F. columnare* for 14 days, and disease resistance was estimated. The results revealed that selective breeding can increase disease resistance of Nile tilapia to *F. columnare*.

The lipopolysaccharide-binding protein (*LBP*) gene is an important immune-related gene, mediating the inflammatory reaction. Fu et al. (2014) investigated the response of the *LBP* gene in tilapia to bacterial pathogen (*Streptococcus agalactiae* and *Aeromonas hydrophila*) infections and examined whether single nucleotide polymorphism (SNP) markers in the gene were associated with the resistance to these pathogens. The gene was significantly upregulated in kidney and spleen post infection with *S. agalactiae* and *A. hydrophila*, respectively; suggesting that the *LBP* gene is involved in the acute-phase immunologic response to the bacterial infections. The two SNPs associated with the resistance, particularly to *A. hydrophila*, could be useful in the selection of tilapia resistance to *A. hydrophila*.

13.8.2 Vaccination

Extensive research has been carried out during the last decade on developing protective vaccines in aquaculture using different strategies. Replicative vaccines (comprising live attenuated, heterologous live vector and DNA vaccines) and nonreplicative vaccines (including the inactivated whole cell, subunit and extracellular vaccines) have been developed and tested, especially against *Streptococcus* infection. Among the various vaccine types, inactivated whole-cell vaccines appear superior in protection efficiency to live attenuated, recombinant and DNA vaccines, especially against *S. agalactiae* (Liu et al., 2016).

The injection of tilapia with extracellular products (ECP) of certain bacteria and various adjuvants seems to induce nonspecific immune response. When Nile tilapia were injected with ECP of *Mycobacterium* spp. and various adjuvants, the level of lysozyme activity detected in the serum of fish 4 days after being immunized with ECP from various *Mycobacterium* spp. was significantly higher than that found in the serum of the control fish (Chen et al., 1998). Sukenda et al. (2018) evaluated the effect of *S. agalactiae* vaccine preparations on tilapia broodstock (species not provided) and their progenies. A whole-cell vaccine, an ECP vaccine and a combination of the two with a ratio of 1:1 were administered through IP injections. The results showed that vaccination of tilapia broodstock with a combination of whole-cell/ECP, 2 and 3 weeks before spawning, increased specific and nonspecific immunity in the broodstock and protect the larvae they produced from *S. agalactiae* infection.

Vaccination of tilapia is done through injection, oral administration, spray administration or bath immersion (Evans et al., 2004; Pasnik et al., 2005; Noraini et al., 2013; Liu et al., 2016; Munang'andu et al., 2016). However, injecting the vaccine into tilapia provided the most effective immunoprotection. The vaccine efficacy is also influenced by other factors, such as fish species and size, immunization duration and number of vaccine doses (Liu et al., 2016). The protective effect of anti-*S. iniae* whole sera (ASI), heat-inactivated anti-*S. iniae* whole sera (HIASI) and normal whole sera (NWS) intraperitoneally injected into the fish has been examined (Shelby et al., 2002). Significantly higher mortality was noted in tilapia passively immunized with NWS than in fish passively immunized with ASI or HIASI, 14 days after *S. iniae* infection. The immunity induced by ASI and HIASI injection against *S. iniae* infection was related to antibodies against *S. iniae*. In other words, *S. iniae* infection stimulates protective antibodies against these bacteria, indicating that ASI antibody plays a primary role in immunity to *S. iniae*.

Oral administration of DNA vaccines has been suggested as an easy way of vaccination, compared to IP injection. The effect of oral vaccination by two immune routes (gavage and mixed fodder administration) using a recombinant DNA vaccine SL7207-pVAX1-sip against *S. agalactiae* in Nile tilapia was evaluated (Zhu et al., 2017). After vaccine administration, various innate immune responses, including total serum protein, superoxide dismutase activity, lysozyme activity, serum antibacterial activity, interleukin 1b and tumour necrosis factor-a, were all significantly enhanced. Vaccinated fish also had higher survival rates, 10 weeks following *S. agalactiae* infection. The results suggested that the DNA vaccine SL7207-pVAX1-sip against *S. agalactiae* when administered with mixed fodder may produce more effective protection.

Nile tilapia were also vaccinated intraperitoneally with formalin-killed *A. hydrophila* bacterin and challenged with *A. hydrophila* (Aly et al., 2015). Vaccination enhanced the resistance of tilapia against *A. hydrophila* infection and improved the survival and economic outcome of tilapia culture. Similarly, LaFrentz and Shoemaker (2015) determined the role of antibodies specific for *Vibrio vulnificus* in protection by passive immunization and identified the components of the bacterium which the antibodies recognize. Antiserum was produced by vaccinating hybrid tilapia (*O. niloticus* × *O. aureus*) with formalin-killed *V. vulnificus* ARS-1-Br-09 bacterin by IP injection. The fish were then challenged with homologous *V. vulnificus* 24 h post immunization. The survival rates were extremely high (86%–90%) following the challenge with nonheated and heat-inactivated antiserum. This result supports the role of specific antibodies in the protection of tilapia against *V. vulnificus*.

The effect of feed-based vaccine on naturally occurring streptococcosis in a red tilapia farm in Malaysia was evaluated at different time intervals (on days 0 and 14 or 0, 14 and 42) (Ismail et al., 2017). Vaccination of caged fish was done by oral administration of bacterin vaccine with the feed. Vaccination resulted in a significant increase in the antibody levels in all vaccinated fish from week 1 and reached a peak at week 3 before declining gradually until week 6. The third vaccination (on day 42) significantly increased the antibody level that remained high until the end of the 4-month trial. Vaccination also increased the survival rate, which was higher in the group which received three doses (75.1%) than those received two doses (65.35%), while the survival of unvaccinated group was 45.2%. This field study clearly demonstrated that feed-based vaccination can significantly improve the survival rate of farmed tilapia and therefore reduce the economic loss.

13.9 Feed and feeding

Feed represents more than 50% of total operating costs of intensive aquaculture enterprises, while protein itself represents about 50% of feed costs. It is no surprise that a great deal of attention has been paid to tilapia nutrition and feeding management, with the ultimate goal being to develop commercial, cost-effective tilapia feeds, using locally available, cheap and unconventional resources.

As stated in Chapter 7, fish meal (FM) has been traditionally used as the main protein source in the aquafeed industry. The increased demand for FM, coupled with a significant shortage in global FM production has created sharp competition for its use by the animal feed industry.

As a result, FM has become the most expensive protein commodity in aquaculture feeds. Many developing countries have realized that, in the long-run, they will be unable to afford FM as a major protein source in tilapia feeds. Therefore, extensive research has been carried out to partially or totally replace FM with less expensive, locally available protein sources. Remarkable progress was achieved in this area, where FM-free (or FM-low) tilapia diets are now commercially available in many parts of the world.

13.9.1 Unconventional protein sources

A wide variety of unconventional protein sources, including animal proteins, plant proteins, single-cell proteins and industrial and agricultural wastes have been evaluated with respect to their utility in farmed tilapia feeds. These sources have been reviewed by El-Sayed and Teshima (1991), Jauncey (1998), El-Sayed (1999) and Shiau (2002). However, the herbivorous/omnivorous nature of tilapia has directed the research on protein nutrition of tilapia toward plant protein sources. Biotechnology plays a great role in enhancing plant protein production, improving processing techniques (to destroy anti-nutritional compounds) and enhancing efficacy of feed storage and delivery and feeding efficiency. Full details on these sources are provided in Chapter 7.

13.9.1.1 Insect and worm meals

Considerable research has also been carried out on different animal protein sources which could partially replace FM in tilapia feeds. These sources are also described in Chapter 7. However, it is worth throwing the light here on insect-based proteins as a protein source for tilapia. Insect meals have recently been recognized as an efficient and cheap alternative to FM and soybean in aquaculture feeds. The nutritional values of insects such as housefly (*Musca domestica*), black soldier fly (BSF) (*Hermetia illucens*), blowfly (*Chrysomya megacephala*) and mealworm beetle (*Tenebrio molitor*) are reasonably good. They contain high protein (up to 55%) and lipid (up to 35%) levels (Sing et al., 2014; Muin et al., 2017; Wang et al., 2017). These insects have been evaluated as alternative protein sources in tilapia diets with promising results.

Significant attention has been directed to housefly (*M. domestica*) maggot meal (MM) (Ogunji et al., 2008; Wang et al., 2017) and blowfly (*C. megacephala*) MM (Sing et al., 2014) which can replace 75%−100% of FM as a protein source for farmed tilapia. The BSF is also a nonpest tropical insect, with a huge potential as a protein source in animal feed industry. The BSF larvae grow very quickly; with a grow-out cycle taking about 2 weeks to reach a weight of 0.25 g per larva (Maquart et al., 2018). They can also feed on a wide range of substrates, including manures and food wastes. The larvae contain 28%−48% crude protein, with an excellent amino acid profile and 12%−42% lipid, depending on the substrate on which they were bred (Maquart et al., 2018). This high nutritional value makes BSF an ideal FM replacer in commercial tilapia feed (Devic et al., 2018). The yellow mealworm (*T. molitor*) (TM) and mopane worm (*Imbrasia belina*) meal also have a good potential as a FM replacer in tilapia feeds (Sánchez-Muros et al., 2016; Rapatsa and Moyo, 2017).

13.9.2 Amino acid versus mineral supplementation

Many of the protein sources used in tilapia feeds are deficient in certain essential amino acids (EAAs). The supplementation of these EAAs into the diet has been a common practice. However, it was found that the utilization of many protein sources in tilapia feeds may be limited by dietary minerals (such as phosphorus and zinc), rather than the deficient EAAs. This means that the inclusion of dietary EAA may not be necessary if the deficient mineral(s) in the protein source is added to the diet. In other words, the incorporation of deficient mineral(s) in the diet may meet the requirement for deficient EAA. For example, the inclusion of dietary phosphorus source such as dicalcium phosphate (DCP) to soybean meal (SBM)-based diets may meet the requirement for methionine, which is essential for tilapia, but deficient in SBM. Viola et al. (1986, 1988) reported that the noninclusion of the deficient EAA to SBM-based diets did not result in growth retardation, while SBM supplemented with 3% DCP and oil completely replaced FM without any adverse effects on fish growth. The nonnecessity of the EAA (lysine) supplementation has also been reported with sesame seeds, if they are supplemented with zinc (El-Sayed, 1987). The adoption of this approach may therefore improve feed protein quality and reduce the cost of the diet. However, this assumption should not be generalized, at least for now, until it is further supported by laboratory and field experiments on other feed ingredients deficient in various EAAs and/or minerals.

13.9.3 Phytase supplementation

Many plant protein sources contain high levels of phytic acid, which binds with divalent minerals such as Ca, P, Zn, Mn, Mg and Fe to form water-insoluble salts, rendering the minerals unavailable. Traditionally, higher supplementary mineral levels are added when these plants are used as the primary source of protein in aquaculture feeds. The inclusion of bacterial phytase in tilapia diets is a new and effective tool used to reduce phytic acid activity and improve the quality of these plant protein sources.

The supplementation of phytase into tilapia diets has been reported to improve growth rates, digestibility and utilization of dietary protein and phosphorous (Riche et al., 2001; Liebert and Portz, 2005; Li et al., 2019; Rachmawati et al., 2018). These studies demonstrated that about 500–1000 phytase units kg^{-1} feed were required for optimum performance, depending on dietary plant protein/animal protein ratios and mineral contents of the diets. In addition, phytase supplementation to Nile tilapia fed low dietary phosphorus improved immune response and reduced the pathological lesions of liver, spleen, stomach and intestines (Abo Norag et al., 2018). On the other hand, Hu et al. (2016) found that supplemental microbial phytase did not improve growth rates and FCR of hybrid tilapia (*O. niloticus* ♀ × *O. aureus* ♂). Moreover, microbial phytase stimulated intestinal inflammation and stress status, as indicated by the upregulation of intestinal expressions of the cytokine genes (tnf-α and tgf-β) and HSP70. This means that dietary microbial phytase may exhibit mixed effects on farmed tilapia. Therefore, phytases should be carefully selected as aquafeed additives, and these that may induce intestinal inflammation should be avoided.

13.9.4 Essential fatty acid requirements

Early studies on essential fatty acid (EFA) requirements of tilapia revealed that these fishes require n-6 EFA rather than n-3 EFA. However, a number of studies demonstrated that they require both n-6 and n-3 highly unsaturated fatty acids (HUFAs) (Chou and Shiau, 1999). El-Sayed et al. (2005) found that Nile tilapia broodstock reared in brackish water required n-3 HUFA for optimum spawning performance, while the reproductive performance of fish reared in freshwater was not affected by dietary oil source. It is evident that the requirements of tilapias for EFA are species-specific, and more work is needed to quantify the requirements of different tilapias for these EFAs under different culture conditions.

13.9.5 Probiotics

The term probiotic was derived from the Greek words 'Pro' and 'bios' meaning 'for life'. Probiotics are defined by the Food and Agriculture Organization of the United Nations and the World Health Organization (FAO/WHO, 2006) as 'live microorganisms that, when administered in adequate amounts, confer a health benefit on the host'. According to FAO Aquaculture Glossary, a probiotic is defined as 'a preparation of viable microorganisms which are added to the diet of humans to control the growth of undesirable/less desirable microorganisms in the gastrointestinal tract'. During the last 30 years, considerable research has been conducted on probiotics, and significant advances have been achieved on characterization and production of different specific probiotics and evaluation of their effects on the health of different animals.

Different microorganisms, especially Gram-negative and Gram-positive bacteria, have been widely used as probiotics in aquaculture, including *Lactobacillus*, *Bacillus*, *Lactococcus*, *Leuconostoc*, *Enterococcus*, *Carnobacterium*, *Shewanella*, *Aeromonas*, *Vibrio*, *Enterobacter*, *Pseudomonas*, *Clostridium* and *Saccharomyces* species (Nayak, 2010). On the other hand, prebiotics are indigestible food ingredients (mainly indigestible fibres) that enhance beneficial commensally gut bacteria resulting in improved growth, health and immunity of the host. Prebiotics generally act as immunosaccharides (such as fructooligosaccharide, mannanooligosaccharide, inulin or β-glucan) and directly enhance the innate immune system of the target organism.

A wide variety of probiotics and prebiotics are extensively applied in aquaculture, both commercially or experimentally, for the following goals:

- Combating diseases,
- Improving growth performance, feed digestibility and utilization, and fish production,
- Stimulating immunity response of the host,
- Acting as alternative antimicrobial components, and
- Improving water quality in aquaculture systems.

Extensive research has been directed to the use of probiotics for many farmed fish and shellfish species (see Akhter et al., 2015; Hai, 2015; Wang et al., 2019 for review).

Many studies have evaluated the effects of probiotics, mainly as an alternative strategy to antibiotics, on tilapia culture worldwide, with Nile tilapia receiving most of the attention (Hai, 2015). Lactic acid bacteria (*Lactobacillus* and *Bacillus*) are the most widely employed probiotics in tilapia culture. For example, *Lactobacillus acidophilus* (Aly et al., 2008), *Lactobacillus brevis* (Liu et al., 2013), *Lactobacillus plantarum* (Ren et al., 2013; Hamdan et al., 2016), *Bacillus subtilis* (Addo et al., 2017a, 2017b), *Bacillus cereus* (Wang et al., 2017) and *Bacillus amyloliquefaciens* have been used as growth promoters and immune enhancers for tilapia. These bacteria significantly improved fish growth, survival, feed digestibility and utilization and enhanced innate immune responses, and disease resistance.

Some other novel bacterial strains have also been tested as probiotics for tilapia. Makled et al. (2017) evaluated the efficacy of marine *Psychrobacter namhaensis* (cold-adapted bacteria that can thrive at/or below 0°C) on growth performance and immune response of Nile tilapia. Growth rates and feed utilization efficiency, blood parameters, immunoglobulin M (IgM), alternative complement haemolysis (ACH50), phagocytic and lysozyme activities significantly increased following dietary *P. namhaensis* supplementation at 0.5% level compared to the control group. The expression of IL-4 and IL-12 genes was also significantly upregulated in *P. namhaensis* groups. Increasing bacterial concentration above 0.5% resulted in a significant retardation in these parameters. Similarly, oral supplementation of *Pediococcus acidilactici* has a protective action on the intestinal mucosal cells, modulating intestinal microbial communities in Nile tilapia and also stimulating the nonspecific immune response, without impairing growth performance (Ferguson et al., 2010; Standen et al., 2013).

Several commercial bacterial products are now available under different names and widely applied in aquaculture. For example, supplemental baker's yeast *Saccharomyces cerevisiae* reduced mortality in Nile tilapia after IP injection with pathogenic *A. hydrophila* (Abdel-Tawwab et al., 2008) and also improved the resistance against the waterborne Cu toxicity in Galilee tilapia *Sarotherodon galilaeus* (Abdel-Tawwab et al., 2010). He et al. (2009) also evaluated the effects of dietary *S. cerevisiae* fermentation product (DVAQUA) on growth performance, intestinal autochthonous bacterial community and nonspecific immunity of hybrid tilapia (*O. niloticus* ♀ × *O. aureus* ♂). Despite the fact that supplemental DVAQUA did not affect growth performance or survival rate, it significantly affected the autochthonous gut bacterial community. Many beneficial bacteria were stimulated and nonspecific immunity improved, while potentially harmful species were depressed, by dietary DVAQUA supplementation. Similarly, Elsabagh et al. (2018) found that a commercial probiotic blend of *Bacillus* strains (*B. subtilis*, *Bacillus licheniformis* and *Bacillus pumilus*) (Sanolife PRO-F) improved water quality, growth performance, haemato-biochemical parameters and intestinal morphometry of Nile tilapia raised in earthen ponds in Egypt. Ridha and Azad (2012) also reported that the use of an autochthonous *B. subtilis* isolated from the gut of cultured tilapia together with a mixture of commercial *Lactobacillus* resulted in a significant enhancement of growth, immunity and disease resistance in tilapia than the commercial products alone. Also, Giorgia et al. (2018) evaluated the effects of a new probiotic preparation Lactogen 13 (*Lactobacillus rhamnosus* IMC 501 encapsulated with vegetable oil matrices by spray chilling and then used as probiotic microgranules) on growth and appetite during larval development of Nile tilapia. Results indicated that these microgranules were able to colonize in the gastrointestinal tract and modulate the microbial communities by increasing *Lactobacillus* proportion and reducing the potentially harmful pathogens. Growth rates were also significantly increased following probiotic administration, as supported by the modulation of genes belonging to the insulin-like growth factors (igfs) system and genes involved in myogenesis.

13.9.6 Organic acids

The use of antibiotics in animal production has been under continuous criticism, which has led to their ban by many countries. Organic acids and/or their respective salts have emerged as a potential alternative to antibiotics for growth promotion in aquaculture, especially in aquafeed industry. Dietary organic acids have been the focus of extensive research and development as feed additives in commercial aquafeeds in recent years. They have a wide range of benefits for cultured fish and shellfish, including enhanced growth rates, nutrient utilization, mineral availability, gut beneficial microbiota and disease resistance (see Ng and Koh, 2017 for details).

A number of studies have considered the use of dietary organic acids, especially formic acid and its salts in tilapia culture, with controversial results. For example, graded levels of dietary potassium diformate (KDF) ((Ng et al., 2009; Abu Elala and Ragaa, 2015) and sodium diformate (Liebert et al., 2010) improved growth rates, feed utilization efficiency and nutrient digestibility. In contrast, Zhou et al. (2009) reported that supplemental KDF did not significantly affect growth performance of hybrid tilapia (*O. niloticus* × *O. aureus*). In addition, dietary sodium formate, sodium propionate, sodium acetate or sodium butyrate had no effect on the performance of hybrid tilapia (*Oreochromis* sp.) (Ebrahimi et al., 2017). These contradictions may be due, in part, to the variation in farming systems, fish species/strains, form and dose of the organic acid administered.

Dietary citric acid increased the activities of protease and amylase (but not lipase activities) in digestive tract of hybrid tilapia (Li et al., 2009). On the other hand, Romano et al. (2016) found that dietary sodium citrate improved oxidative stability in red hybrid tilapia (*Oreochromis* sp.) but reduced growth, health status, intestinal short chain fatty acids and induced liver damage. The authors concluded that sodium citrate is toxic to tilapia at the levels tested (1%, 2% and 4%) and is not recommended as a feed additive for tilapia. It is noteworthy that dietary citric acid and its salts improved the growth and feed utilization of other farmed fishes, including rainbow trout (Hernández et al., 2012), yellowtail (*Seriola quinqueradiata*) (Sarker et al., 2012) and yellow catfish (*Pelteobagrus fulvidraco*) (Zhu et al., 2015). It appears from this discussion that dietary effects of supplemental organic acids are species-specific. More research is also needed before we could come to a concrete conclusion about whether these acids are beneficial to farmed tilapia, and which acids or salts are more effective and at what concentrations.

13.9.7 Extruded feeds

Steam-pelleted or compressed (sinking) feeds have traditionally been used for feeding farmed tilapia for several years. These feeds are relatively inexpensive because their production technology is simple and the energy expended in their manufacture is also low. In recent years, a more advanced, extruded aquafeed technology has been introduced to aquaculture feed industry and has become a breakthrough in aquaculture development. Extrusion is a process through which feed ingredients are plasticized and cooked in the extruder barrel by a combination of pressure, heat and friction, in the presence of moisture. Cooking the raw materials breaks down polysaccharides and makes them more digestible by the fish. Temperature inside the barrel ranges from 90 to 150°C and is generated from friction in the extruder. The superheated mixture is then forced through dies (varying in diameter, but mainly 3−8 mm) located at the end of the extruder barrel, which shape the pellets.

Extruded feeds are more preferable to compressed sinking feeds due to:

- The complete gelatinization of polysaccharides;
- Their better stability and digestibility;
- Better FCR and
- Complete removal of anti-nutritional factors during heat processing.

Therefore, extruded feeds, especially floating feeds, are currently widely used in tilapia culture worldwide. For example, most tilapia farms in Egypt are currently using extruded feeds (both floating and sinking forms) because they are more efficient than conventionally pelleted feeds. FCR of extruded feeds ranges from 1.0 to 1.5:1, compared to 1.5:>2.0 of pelleted feeds (El-Sayed, 2017). Other studies indicated that feed digestibility, growth rates and feed utilization were better in tilapia fed extruded diets than those offered pelleted feeds (Ma et al., 2015, 2016).

13.9.8 Feeding regimes

Many other nutritional innovations with respect to diet form, feeding frequency and feeding methods on tilapia farms have been achieved (see Chapter 6 for details). These innovations include the development of low-protein, high-energy supplemental feeds for semi-intensive culture. The adoption of the best timing of supplemental feeding in well-fertilized ponds has also received considerable attention (see Chapter 5), aiming at delaying supplemental feeding as long as the natural food, provided through pond fertilization, supports good fish growth. This approach is very likely to result in a great reduction in operating costs, without significantly affecting fish growth and yield (Diana et al., 1996; Abdelghany et al., 2002). Studies of Lin and Yi (2003) and Yi et al. (2004) indicated that when Nile tilapia and red tilapia were fed supplemental diets at only 50% satiation, they produced comparable yields to 75%, and 100% satiation levels. At the 50% satiation level, 50% of feed costs were saved, in addition to significant reduction in nutrient loading.

13.10 Innovations in farming systems

A full description of tilapia culture systems is provided in Chapters 5 and 6. These culture systems have undergone notable technology-based developments in many parts of the world. The intensification of tilapia production in indoor closed-recirculation systems is probably among the most highly developed technologies. These technologies include the use of liquid oxygen, the development and use of microscreens and fluidized bead biofilters and the adoption of extremely high stocking densities. Significant expansion of these technology-based systems has occurred in the United States. For example, Rosati et al. (1993) raised Nile tilapia in recirculating systems under commercial conditions at high stocking densities of 263.2 fish m^{-3}, using vertical screen biofilters and particle filters. The final yield was 65.6 kg m^{-3}, which is considered extremely high. In another closed system consisting of six raceways with a total capacity of 160 m^3, the annual yield of Nile tilapia was 11.33 t (70.8 kg m^{-3}) with an average weight of 560 g $fish^{-1}$. However, it should be emphasized that these systems are complicated, difficult to manage and costly. It is hoped that the recent innovations would lead to the reduction in the costs and enable small-scale tilapia farmers, especially in developing countries, to adopt these systems.

13.10.1 Effluent treatment and management

There has been a switch from the traditional, semi-intensive tilapia culture systems to more intensive systems. This jump was accompanied by a substantial development in the inputs to intensive culture systems. The developments in treatment and management of culture effluents in recirculating systems focused mainly on (1) waste settlement and removal and (2) water discharge and replacement (see Chapter 6 for details).

13.10.1.1 Waste settlement and removal

The removal of solids from culture water is an essential process in closed-recirculating systems. This procedure maintains the quality of water and improves fish performance and yield. As indicated in Chapter 6, traditional biofiltration such as water exchange, back-flushing and fixed film media is inconvenient for small-scale tilapia culture enterprises because of occasional system failure and high costs. A number of unconventional biofiltration methods have been developed to tackle this problem. Most of these methods are simple, cheap and efficient and can be easily applied using locally available inputs. For example, the addition of carbon-rich agricultural by-products, such as rice hulls, to fish tanks have been successfully used as primary media for solids removal from recirculating tilapia culture systems (Scott et al., 1998).

Different biofiltration media such as polypropylene plastic chips and polyethylene blocks have been developed for ammonia removal in recirculating tilapia culture systems. Different types of bead filters (such as the bubble-washed bead filter) are also widely used for nitrification and clarification of culture water and capturing solid wastes. Slow-sand filters have also been developed for the treatment of effluents within recycle aquaculture systems. These filters are simple, cheap, easy to construct and operate and effective in removing suspended solids.

13.10.1.2 Water discharge

Recirculating systems are generally adopted in areas having limited freshwater sources and rough weather conditions. Economic use of these water sources becomes a necessity, and waste water discharge may not be a good idea. Instead, water recycling and reuse is highly recommended under these conditions. Extensive research has been carried out to minimize, or even eliminate, water discharge from tilapia recycle systems. This approach has been tried in greenhouses (Shnel et al., 2002) where a zero water discharge from tilapia recirculating system was applied. Neither water nor organic matter was discharged, while sludge was biologically digested and nitrate was reduced to nitrogen gas. This system was very successful in maintaining water quality within acceptable levels for tilapia and removing metabolic wastes. Total tilapia yield was also reasonably high, reaching 81.1 kg m^{-3} at a maximum stocking density of 61.8 kg m^{-3}.

Water exchange may also be sharply reduced without any adverse effect on the performance of tilapia reared intensively in earthen ponds if sufficient aeration is provided. The addition of carbon source (wheat bran, rice bran, etc.) on water surface can also be used as a surface for the growth of bacteria which reduces ammonia accumulation, while tilapia consume bacteria produced in the system as natural food. Applying this technology can reduce dietary protein by about 10% and the overall cost can be reduced by up to 50% (Chamberlain and Hopkins, 1994).

Active sedimentation and resuspension can also be applied to reduce water exchange in intensive pond culture. This process is based on the resuspension of solid particles from pond sediments into the water column by continuous aeration, mixing, stirring and turbulence. Resuspension favours the aerobic decomposition of organic matter. Suspended particles and bacterial blooms can be used as natural food for tilapia, leading to additional savings in operational and feed costs.

13.10.2 Tilapia production in aquaponic systems

Aquaponics is the integration of hydroponics with aquaculture in a recirculating system, where the wastes and metabolites produced by cultured fish are removed by nitrification and taken up by the plants (Fig. 13.2). The bacteria living in the gravel and in association with the plant roots play a critical role in nutrient removal. Aquaponics is a simple, promising and sustainable food production technology, especially in developing countries and arid zones, where resources are limited, freshwater is scare and populations are increasing.

The first report on tilapia culture in aquaponic systems was published almost four decades ago (Rakocy and Alison, 1981). Since then, considerable development and innovation in the system have been going on (see Chapter 6, section 6.9 for details). The production of tilapia and vegetables in aquaponics systems appears very promising and profitable. The break-even prices of tilapia and vegetables could be even lower if production costs are reduced and if the proper crops are selected.

A number of recent research studies have evaluated the productivity, cost-effectiveness and environmental impacts in innovated aquaponics system. English (2015) found that when tilapia, basil and lettuce were grown in aquaponic system, only lettuce and basil were profitable within the system, while tilapia production was not. However, the production of tilapia in combination with these vegetables resulted in net profit; with tilapia and basil being more profitable than tilapia and lettuce production. The use of aquaponics system to improve sustainability and productivity and, in the same time, lower

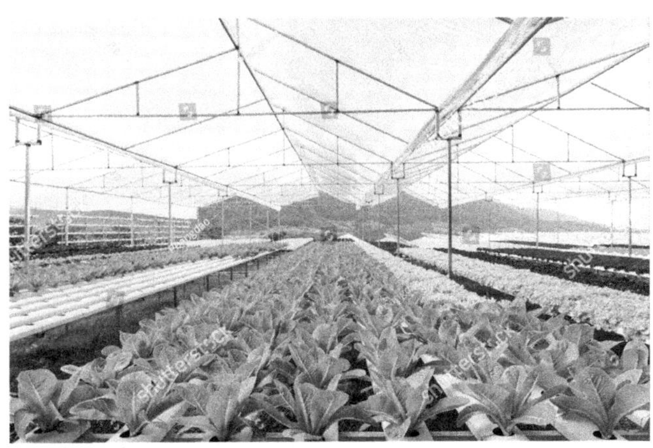

FIGURE 13.2 Growing vegetables with fish in an aquaponic system. *Source: Shutterstock.*

environmental emissions has been evaluated by Kloas et al. (2015). The authors used innovated, double recirculation aquaponic system (DRAPS) for (nearly) emission-free tomato and tilapia production (ASTAF-PRO) in greenhouses. The use of DRAPS increased productivity and prevented adverse interactions between fish and plant units. This finding indicated that ASTAF-PRO can improve sustainability and productivity, and lower environmental emissions. Silva et al. (2017) investigated whether biological filters (BFs) are necessary in aquaponics systems. They evaluated water quality of semi-intensive, small-scale Nile tilapia-pak choi (*Brassica chinensis*) aquaponics system, with (BF) and without a bacterial biofilter (NBF). They found that there is no need for BF, since aquaponics plants can act as a biofilter. This result suggests that NBF aquaponics system could be used for small-scale farmers in the tropics. This system is less costly and easier to manage and more ecologically sustainable than BF aquaponics system.

13.10.3 Biofloc technology

Biofloc technology (BT) is defined as 'the use of aggregates of bacteria, algae, or protozoa, held together in a matrix along with particulate organic matter for the purpose of improving water quality, waste treatment and disease prevention in intensive aquaculture systems'. In other words, biofloc is a symbiotic process that includes confined aquatic animals, heterotrophic bacteria and other microbial species in the water. Consumption of bioflocs also provides nutritional value to cultured aquatic species. This simply means that BT can be an ideal option for sustainable and environmentally friendly aquaculture (Crab et al., 2009, 2012). Generally speaking, BT can lead to many benefits, including the following:

1. Prevention of the introduction of disease to fish farms from incoming water.
2. Improvement of biosecurity.
3. Improvement of feed conversion.
4. Improvement of water quality.
5. Improvement of water-use efficiency.
6. Increasing land-use efficiency.
7. Reduction of sensitivity to light fluctuations.

BT can be applied in tilapia farming, both in semi-intensive and intensive pond systems and intensive tank and RAS culture systems. Extensive research has been carried out on tilapia culture in biofloc systems under experimental and commercial conditions, with encouraging results (see Chapter 6, Section 6.10 for more details). Tilapia is currently among the most common species farmed in biofloc systems, since they are able to take up bioflocs as an additional protein source, resulting in a considerable reduction in production inputs (Crab et al., 2009, 2012).

13.10.4 In-pond raceway system

The 'in-pond raceway system (IPRS)' has emerged as an excellent means for increasing fish productivity in existing fish ponds, particularly of subtropical fish species such as tilapia. IPRS is simply an aquaculture system in which farmed fish or shrimp are raised in raceways (cells) built inside ponds or enclosed water space with continuous aerated flowing water from one end and removing fish wastes and uneaten feeds from the opposite end. A waste

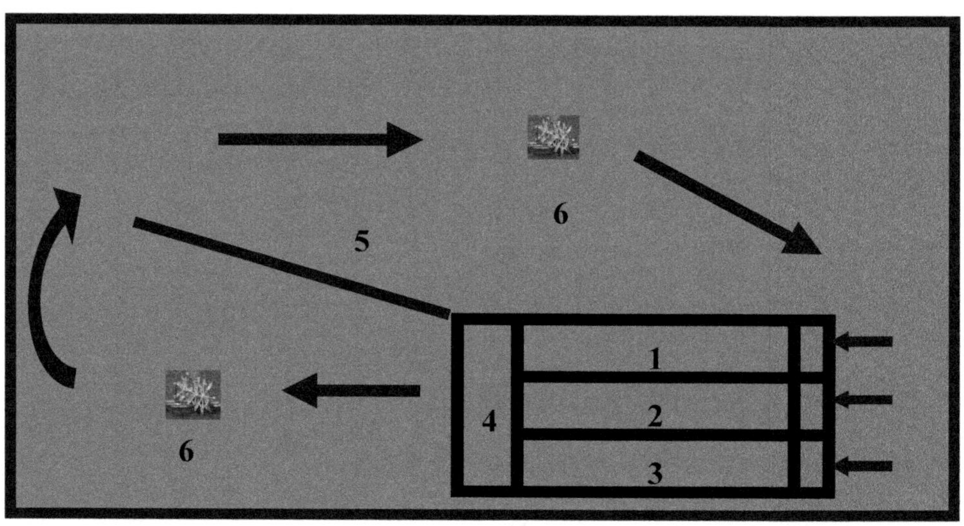

FIGURE 13.3 Layout of in-pond raceway system. The idea is to keep the water continuously mixed and aerated. 1, 2 and 3, fish raceways; 4, waste settlement area; 5, baffle or dyke to force the water to take a long course around the pond before returning to the raceways; 6, paddle wheel for aeration. *Arrows* indicate the water current direction through the pond.

settling area is built at the raceway output end for waste trapping and settlement. Solid wastes are collected two to three times a day by a vacuum pump. The raceway area is generally about 3%–5% of pond size, but it can be larger (up to 10%), depending on water quality and feed quality, stocked fish, level of management, etc. The raceway system is generally constructed of a number of rectangular concrete cells (generally 2-3 per pond) parallel to each other (Fig. 13.3).

The IPRS technology was first developed in Alabama, USA. It has many advantages, over the traditional pond culture, including:

- Higher growth rates, and net yield
- Better feed utilization and, in turn, reduction of feed costs
- Better quality products
- Reduced disease and mortality chances
- Better water remediation
- Lower environmental impacts
- Water conservation through pond water recycling and reusing

However, the following conditions are required for operational optimization of IPRS:

- Stocked fish must be healthy and clean.
- Top-grade feeds should be used.
- Pond water should be kept well mixed.
- Solid wastes should be removed continuously.
- Equipment should be maintained.

A number of studies have been carried out to evaluate the use of IPRS for growing fish (Brown et al., 2011, 2014; Enhua et al., 2013). Brown et al. (2011) found that IPRS was efficient of producing both channel catfish and hybrid catfish along with the co-culture of other species compared to traditional catfish culture in earthen ponds. Fish survival, FCR and production improved in IPRS as compared to traditional production techniques.

Just recently, farming tilapia in IPRS has attracted the attention in some countries. In Egypt, for example, an experimental IPRS unit was installed at the WorldFish Center at Abbassa, Sharkya Governorate, and used for tilapia culture (Nasr-Allah et al., 2018). The unit consisted of two production raceways (12 × 3 × 1.5 m) installed in a 4000-m^2 pond (0.40 ha) (Fig. 13.4). The cells were used as fish containment units, while the rest of the open area was used for water treatment. Each cell was equipped with an airlift unit to create water current inside the cell in one direction and to push the solid wastes to the settlement area. A plastic baffle (fence) was fixed in the open part of the pond to force the water to circulate around the pond before returning to the raceways.

A feeding trial was carried out in this IPRS in 2018 (Nasr-Allah et al., 2018). The first cell was stocked with

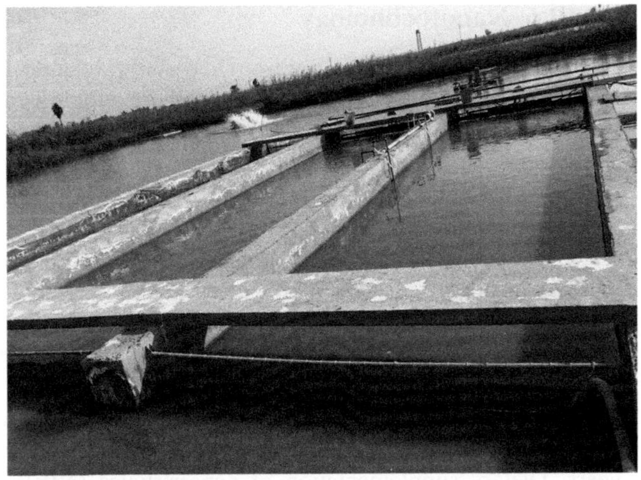

FIGURE 13.4 Tilapia culture in-pond raceway system at the Worldfish Center, Abbassa, Sharkya Governorate, Egypt. *Photograph by A.-F.M. El-Sayed.*

10,000 Nile tilapia (60 g average weight), while the second cell was stocked with the same number of fish at an average weight of 18 g. The fish were fed with a 32%–35% cp floating feeds for 81 and 113 days for the first and second cell, respectively. At the end of the trial, the gross yield reached 3.25 t (72.2 kg m^{-3}) and 2.69 t (59.8 kg m^{-3}) from cell 1 and cell 2, respectively. Returns on investment were 29% and 5%, respectively. The total production of these two cells (5.94 t) was much higher than the production obtained from the same pond when traditional tilapia culture is adopted (about 3 t per cycle). This study also indicates the importance of initial fish size in order to reach market size in shorter time.

13.10.5 Dual cage culture

A dual cage culture system (locally known as 'lapis dua') has been developed and applied in reservoirs Saguling, Cirata and Jatiuhur in West Java, Indonesia, since the mid-1990s (Abery et al., 2005; De Silva and Phillips, 2007). Common carp is raised in the inner cage and tilapia in the outer cage. Inner cage is 7 × 7 × 3 m, with bamboo frames, while the depth of the outer cages ranges from 5 to 7 m, depending on the depth of the reservoirs. Cages are generally stocked with fish fingerlings (7–8 cm) at a density of 100 kg each of carp and tilapia. Commercial pelleted feed (26%–28% cp) is provided only for common carp in the inner cage, whereas tilapia in the outer cage are not fed but depend on the fall out of excess feed provided to common carp and also on available natural foods. Tilapia and carp are harvested at a size of 330–500 and 250 g, respectively. The system was initially used for livelihood of local communities. But it is currently used as a commercial enterprise, resulting in more investment and high returns relatively quickly.

13.10.6 Nanotechnology

According to Cambridge English Dictionary, 'nanotechnology is an area of science that deals with developing and producing extremely small tools and machines by controlling the arrangement of separate atoms'. In other words, nanotechnology is the study and applications of extremely small materials in a wide range of scientific fields. Nanomaterials have unique physical or chemical properties, due to their small size, shape, surface area or conductivity. These materials have a wide range of applications in different fields, including biology, medicine, agriculture, physics, materials science, engineering and electronics.

The application of nanotechnology in aquaculture has attracted the attention of a number of authors in recent years. Dietary supplementation of nanoparticles (NPs) of minerals and products such selenium, iron, zinc and chitosan could improve growth performance, feed utilization, reproductive performance and many other physiological functions. It is suggested that dietary NPs may be absorbed into the cells more readily than the large particles, leading to better growth and feed efficiency (Huang et al., 2015). Nanotechnology can also be used for water treatment.

However, only a few studies have considered NPs as growth and health promoters in tilapia aquaculture. A couple of studies investigated the effects of chitosan nanoparticles (CNPs) on growth and immune response of tilapia with promising results. Chitosan is a linear homopolymer of β-(1,4)-2-amino-2-deoxy-D-glucose, produced by alkaline deacetylation of chitin (Abdel-Tawwab et al., 2019.). It has attracted the attention as a feed additive in aquaculture, as a growth promoter and immune stimulant. Abdel-Tawwab et al. (2019) investigated the effect of dietary CNPs on growth performance, antioxidant activity and innate immunity of Nile tilapia. Juvenile fish (20 g) were fed on diets containing 0.0, 0.25, 0.5, 1.0 and 2.0 g CNP kg^{-1} feed diet for 45 days. Fish growth and feed efficiency and antioxidant-stimulated activity improved with increasing CNP levels up to 1.0 g CNP kg^{-1}. CNP also enhanced the activities of catalase, superoxide dismutase, lysozyme and respiratory burst in a dose-dependent manner. The authors concluded that dietary CNP has a strong immunostimulatory effect and can significantly improve the performance and health status of farmed Nile tilapia, with an optimum level of about 1.0 g kg^{-1} feed. Similarly, Wang and Li (2011) found that dietary CNP (5 g kg^{-1}) significantly improved the growth rates, FCR and meat quality of Nile tilapia, compared to conventional chitosan.

The effects of nano-selenium on growth rates of Nile tilapia were not significant at low concentration (0.1 mg kg^{-1}) (Deng and Chen, 2003). At higher concentration (2.5 mg kg^{-1}), fish performance was significantly promoted. Tawfik et al. (2017) evaluated the effects of dietary nano zinc oxide (nZnO) (15, 30, 45 and 60 mg kg^{-1} of the feed) on growth and immune stimulation of Nile tilapia, compared to conventional zinc oxide (ZnO). nZnO significantly improved fish growth, even at lower levels compared to normal ZnO. The highest growth rates were achieved at 60 mg kg^{-1} nZnO. Supplemental nZnO also upregulated interleukin (IL1-β) gene. Additionally, dietary nZnO resulted in higher muscle Zn concentration than conventional ZnO.

It should be mentioned, however, that despite the necessity of Zn for aquatic organism, it could pose significant risks to these organisms, including tilapia. For example, Kaya et al. (2015) found that colloidal suspensions of ZnO NPs induced elevated oxidative stress and toxic effects on Nile tilapia compared to the larger NPs. When the fish were exposed to small (10−30 nm) and large (100 nm) NPs, both small and large ZnO NPs accumulated in fish tissues; however, the accumulation level of the small ZnO NPs was significantly higher than that of larger NPs. Lipid peroxidation was also higher in tilapia groups exposed to small ZnO NPs than that of large ZnO NPs and controls.

13.11 Closing remarks

1. The modern technology has played a significant role in tilapia culture and is expected to be more pronounced in the future.
2. Transgenesis and selective breeding have received considerable attention as important tools for genetic enhancement and growth improvements of farmed tilapia.
3. The application of sex-specific markers to increase the efficiency of sex control breeding programmes (such as the YY male technology) aiming at increasing the sex ratio to 100% males has been very successful.
4. Several genetically improved tilapia strains, with better growth, survival, yield, feed utilization, disease resistance and product quality, have been developed in many countries.
5. GIFT has been commercially distributed to many countries, especially in Southeast Asia, making a remarkable development in tilapia culture industry in these countries, particularly in rural areas.
6. The incorporation of cloned tilapia genes into the production of new strains of transgenic tilapia is expected to attract more attention in the future.
7. The production of tilapia with desirable characteristics such as salinity and cold tolerance, disease resistance, colour and enhanced growth will be of prime priority.
8. There has been a significant improvement in the quality of fish meal replacers in tilapia feeds, especially plant proteins. Insect meals have also emerged as a potential fish meal replacer in aquafeed industry. In

addition, extruded feed has been a breakthrough in tilapia culture. The role of dietary probiotic and organic acids in tilapia production is also expected to be more pronounced in the future.

9. The shortage in fresh water concomitant with the competition for it with other agricultural and urban activities dictates the intensification of tilapia production. Tilapia culture in closed-recirculation systems, aquaponic systems, biofloc systems and in-pond raceway systems is very likely to witness significant global expansion, accompanied with improvements in aeration (e.g. liquid oxygen), biological and mechanical filtration techniques, waste settlement and removal, water reuse, increased fish density and feed quality and on-farm feeding management.
10. Nanotechnology is expected to play a role in tilapia culture development. However, extensive research is needed in this area.

References

Abdelghany, A.E., Ayyat, M.-S., Ahmad, M.H., 2002. Appropriate timing of supplemental feeding for production of Nile tilapia, silver carp, and common carp in fertilized polyculture ponds. Journal of the World Aquaculture Society 33, 307–315.

Abdel-Tawwab, M., Abdel-Rahman, A.M., Ismael, N.E.M., 2008. Evaluation of commercial live bakers' yeast, *Saccharomyces cerevisiae* as a growth and immunity promoter for Fry Nile tilapia, *Oreochromis niloticus* (L.) challenged in situ with *Aeromonas hydrophila*. Aquaculture 280, 185–189.

Abdel-Tawwab, M., Mousa, M.A.A., Mohammed, M.A., 2010. Use of live baker's yeast, *Saccharomyces cerevisiae*, in practical diet to enhance the growth performance of Galilee tilapia, *Sarotherodon galilaeus* (L.), and its resistance to environmental copper toxicity. Journal of the World Aquaculture Society 41, 214–223.

Abdel-Tawwab, M., Abdel Razek, N, and Abdel-Rahman, A.M. (2019). Immunostimulatory effect of dietary chitosan nanoparticles on growth performance of Nile tilapia, Oreochromis niloticus (L.). Fish and Shellfish Immunology, 88, 2019, 254–258.

Abery, N.W., Sukadi, F., Budhiman, A.A., Kartamihardja, E.S., Koeshendrajana, S., Buddhiman, et al., 2005. Fisheries and cage culture of three reservoirs in West Java, Indonesia; a case study of ambitious developments and resulting interactions. Fisheries Management and Ecology 12, 315–330.

Abo Norag, M.A., El-Shenawy, A.M., Fadl, S.E., Abdo, W.S., Gad, D.M., Rashed, M.A., et al., 2018. Effect of phytase enzyme on growth performance, serum biochemical alteration, immune response and gene expression in Nile tilapia. Fish and Shellfish Immunology 80, 97–108.

Abu Elala, N.M., Ragaa, N.M., 2015. Eubiotic effect of a dietary acidifier (potassium diformate) on the health status of cultured *Oreochromis niloticus*. Journal of Advanced Research 6, 621–629.

ADB (Asian Development Bank), 2005. An Impact Evaluation of the Development of Genetically Improved Farmed Tilapia and Their Dissemination in Selected Countries. Operations Evaluation Department, ADB, 124 pp. http://www.adb.org/Publications.

Addo, S., Carrias, A.A., Williams, M.A., Liles, M.R., Terhune, J.S., Davis, D.A., 2017a. Effects of *Bacillus subtilis* strains on growth, immune parameters, and *Streptococcus iniae* susceptibility in Nile Tilapia, *Oreochromis niloticus*. Journal of the World Aquaculture Society 48, 257–267.

Addo, S., Carrias, A.A., Williams, M.A., Liles, M.R., Terhune, J.S., Davis, D.A., 2017b. Effects of *Bacillus subtilis* strains and the prebiotic Previda on growth, immune parameters and susceptibility to *Aeromonas hydrophila* infection in Nile tilapia, *Oreochromis niloticus*. Aquaculture Research 48, 4798–4810.

Akhter, N., Wu, B., Memon, A.M., Mohsin, M., 2015. Probiotics and prebiotics associated with aquaculture: a review. Fish and Shellfish Immunology 45, 733–741.

Alcántar-Vázquez, J.P., Moreno-de la Torre, P., Calzada-Ruíz, D., Antonio-Estrada, C., 2014. Production of YY-male of nile tilapia *Oreochromis niloticus* (Linnaeus, 1758) from atypical fish. Latin American Journal of Aquatic Research 42, 644–648.

Aly, S.M., Abdel-Galil, A.Y., Abdel-Aziz, G.A., Mohamed, M.F., 2008. Studies on *Bacillus subtilis* and *Lactobacillus acidophilus*, as potential probiotics, on the immune response and resistance of *Tilapia nilotica* (*Oreochromis niloticus*) to challenge infections. Fish and Shellfish Immunology 25, 128–136.

Aly, S.M., Albutti, A.S., Rahmani, A.H., Abdel Atti, N.M., 2015. The response of new-season Nile tilapia to *Aeromonas hydrophila* vaccine. International Journal of Clinical and Experimental Medicine 8, 4508–4514.

Ammar, A.Y., El Nahas, A.F., Mahmoud, S., Barakat, M.E., Hassan, A.M., 2018. Characterization of type IV antifreeze gene in Nile tilapia (*Oreochromis niloticus*) and influence of cold and hot weather on its expression and some immune-related genes. Fish Physiology and Biochemistry 44, 515–525.

Basavaraja, N., Raghavendra, C.H., 2017. Hormonal sex reversal in red tilapia (*Oreochromis niloticus* and *Oreochromis mossambicus*) and inheritance of body colour in *O. mossambicus* and red tilapia: implications for commercial farming. Aquaculture International 25, 1317–1331.

Behrends, L.L., Kingsley, J.B., Bulls, M.J., 1996. Cold tolerance in maternal mouthbrooding tilapias: heritability estimates and correlated growth responses at suboptimal temperatures. In: Pullin, R.S.V., Lazard, J., Legendre, M., Amon Kottias, J.B., Pauly, D. (Eds.), Proceedings of the Third International Symposium on Tilapia in Aquaculture. ICLARM Conference Proceedings No. 41. ICLARM, Penang, Malaysia, pp. 257–265.

Bentsen, H.B., Gjerde, B., Nguyen, N.H., Rye, M., Ponzoni, R.W., de Vera, M.S.P., et al., 2012. Genetic improvement of farmed tilapias: genetic parameters for body weight at harvest in Nile tilapia (*Oreochromis niloticus*) during five generations of testing in multiple environments. Aquaculture 338–341, 56–65.

Bentsen, H.B., Gjerde, B., Eknath, A.E., de Vera, M.S.P., Velasco, R.R., Danting, J.C., et al., 2017. Genetic improvement of farmed tilapias: response to five generations of selection for increased body weight at harvest in *Oreochromis niloticus* and the further impact of the project. Aquaculture 468, 206–217.

Bolivar, R.B., 1998. Estimation of Response to Within-Family Selection for Growth in Nile Tilapia (*O. niloticus*) (Ph.D. dissertation). Dalhousie University, Halifax, Canada.

Bolivar, R.B., Eknath, A.E., Bolivar, H.L., Abella, T.A., 1993. Growth and reproduction of individually tagged Nile tilapia (*Oreochromis niloticus*) of different strains. Aquaculture 111, 159–169.

Bolivar, R.B., Newkirk, G.F., 2002. Response to within family selection for body weight in Nile tilapia (*Oreochromis niloticus*) using a single-trait animal model. Aquaculture 204, 371–381.

Bramick, U., Puckhaber, B., Langholz, H.-J., Hörstgen-Schwark, G., 1995. Testing of triploid tilapia (*Oreochromis niloticus*) under tropical pond conditions. Aquaculture 137, 343–353.

Brown, T.W., Chappell, J.A., Boyd, C.E., 2011. A commercial-scale, in-pond raceway system for Ictalurid catfish production. Aquacultural Engineering 44, 72–79.

Brown, T.W., Hanson, T.R., Chappell, J.A., Boyd, C.E., 2014. Economic feasibility of an in-pond raceway system for commercial catfish production in West Alabama. North American Journal of Aquaculture 76, 79–89.

Byamungu, N., Darras, V.M., Kühn, E.R., 2001. Growth of heat-shock induced triploids of blue tilapia, *O. aureus*, reared in tanks and in ponds in eastern Congo: feeding regimes and compensatory growth response of triploid females. Aquaculture 198, 109–122.

Cai, W.-Q., Li, S-f., Ma, J-y., 2004. Disease resistance of Nile tilapia (*Oreochromis niloticus*), blue tilapia (*O. aureus*) and their hybrid (female Nile tilapia x male blue tilapia) to *Aeromonas sobria*. Aquaculture 229, 79–87.

Cao-Hoang, L., Dumont, F., Marechal, P.-A., Gervais, P., 2010. Inactivation of *Escherichia coli* and *Lactobacillus plantarum* in relation to membrane permeabilization due to rapid chilling followed by cold storage. Archives of Microbiology 192, 299–305.

CGIAR (Consultative Group on International Agricultural Research), 2013. Ex-ante Impact Evaluation: Case Studies From Malawi, Bangladesh and Ghana. CGIAR Research Program on Aquatic Agricultural Systems. Penang, Malaysia. Working Paper: AAS-2013-05, 38 pp.

Chamberlain, G.W., Hopkins, J.S., 1994. Reducing water use and feed cost in intensive ponds. World Aquaculture 25 (3), 29–32.

Chang, S.L., Chang, C.F., Liao, I.C., 1996. Studies on the growth performance and gonadal development of triploid tilapia *O. aureus*. In: Pullin, R.S.V., Lazard, J., Legendre, M., Amon Kottias, J.B., Pauly, D. (Eds.), Proceedings of the Third International Symposium on Tilapia in Aquaculture. ICLARM Conference Proceedings No. 41. ICLARM, Penang, Malaysia, p. 539.

Charo-Karisa, H., Rezk, M.A., Bovenhuis, H., Komen, H., 2005. Heritability of cold tolerance in Nile tilapia (*Oreochromis niloticus*) juveniles. Aquaculture 249, 115–123.

Chen, J., Fan, Z., Tan, D., Jiang, D., Wang, D., 2018. A review of genetic advances related to sex control and manipulation in tilapia. Journal of the World Aquaculture Society 49, 277–291.

Chen, S.-C., Yoshida, T., Adams, A., Thompson, K.D., Richards, R.H., 1998. Non-specific immune response of Nile tilapia, *Oreochromis nilotica,* to the extracellular products of *Mycobacterium* spp. and to various adjuvants. Journal of Fish Diseases 21, 39–46.

Chou, B.S., Shiau, S.-Y., 1999. Both n-6 and n-3 fatty acids are required for maximum growth of juvenile hybrid tilapia, *Oreochromis niloticus* × *O. aureus*. North American Journal of Aquaculture 61, 13–20.

Cnaani, A., Gall, G.A.E., Hulata, G., 2000. Cold tolerance of tilapia species and hybrids. Aquaculture International 8, 289–298.

Costa, L.S., Rosa, P.V., Fortes-Silva, R., Sánchez-Vázquez, F.J., López-Olmeda, J.F., 2016. Daily rhythms of the expression of genes from the somatotropic axis: the influence on tilapia (*Oreochromis niloticus*) of feeding and growth hormone administration at different times. Comparative Biochemistry and Physiology A, Part C 181–182, 27–34.

Crab, R., Kochva, M., Verstraete, W., Avnimelech, Y., 2009. Bio-flocs technology application in over-wintering of tilapia. Aquacultural Engineering 40, 105–112.

Crab, R., Defoird, T., Bossier, P., Verstraete, W., 2012. Biofloc technology in aquaculture: beneficial effects and future challenges. Aquaculture 356–357, 351–356.

de la Fuente, J., Guillen, I., Martinez, R., Estrada, M.P., 1999. Growth regulation and enhancement in tilapia: basic research findings and their applications. Genetic Analysis: Biomolecular Engineering 15, 85–90.

De Silva, S.S., Phillips, M.J., 2007. A review of cage aquaculture: Asia (excluding China). FAO Fisheries Technical Paper No. 498. In: Halwart, M., Soto, D., Arthur, J.R. (Eds.), Cage Aquaculture – Regional Reviews and Global Overview. FAO, Rome, pp. 18–48.

Deng, Y.S., Chen, Q.J., 2003. Affects of nano-selenium on the growth of Nile tilapia (*Oreochromis niloticus*). Inland Aquatic Products 6, 28–30 (in Chinese).

Devic, E., Leschen, W., Murray, F., Little, D.C., 2018. Growth performance, feed utilization and body composition of advanced nursing Nile tilapia (*Oreochromis niloticus*) fed diets containing black soldier fly (*Hermetia illucens*) larvae meal. Aquaculture Nutrition 24, 416–423.

Diana, J.S., Lin, C.K., Yi, Y., 1996. Timing of supplemental feeding for tilapia production. Journal of the World Aquaculture Society 27, 410–419.

Ebrahimi, M., Daeman, N.H., Chong, C.M., Karami, A., Kumar, V., Hoseinifar, S.H., et al., 2017. Comparing the effects of different dietary organic acids on the growth, intestinal short-chain fatty acids, and liver histopathology of red hybrid tilapia (*Oreochromis* sp.) and potential use of these as preservatives. Fish Physiology and Biochemistry 43, 1195–1207.

Eknath, A.E., Acosta, B.O., 1998. Genetic Improvement of Farmed Tilapias (GIFT) Project: Final Report, March 1988 to December 1997. ICLARM, Manila, Philippines, 75 pp.

Eknath, A.E., Dey, M.M., Rye, M., Gjerde, B., Abella, T.A., Sevilleja, R., et al., 1998. Selective breeding of nile tilapia for Asia. In: Proceedings of the 6th World Congress on Genetics Applied to Livestock Production, 11–16 January, vol. 27. University of New England, Armidale, Australia, pp. 89–96.

Eknath, A.E., Tayamen, M.M., Palada-de Vera, M.S., Danting, J.C., Reyes, R.A., Dionisio, E.E., et al., 1993. Genetic improvement of farmed tilapias: the growth performance of eight strains of *Oreochromis niloticus* tested in different farm environments. Aquaculture 111, 171–188.

El Gamal, A.-R., Davis, K.B., Jenkins, J.A., Torrans, E.L., 1999. Induction of triploidy and tetraploidy in Nile tilapia, *Oreochromis niloticus* (L.). Journal of the World Aquaculture Society 30, 269–275.

Elsabagh, M., Mohamed, R., Moustafa, E.M., Hamza, A., Farrag, F., Decamp, O., et al., 2018. Assessing the impact of *Bacillus* strains mixture probiotic on water quality, growth performance, blood profile and intestinal morphology of Nile tilapia, *Oreochromis niloticus*. Aquaculture Nutrition 24, 1613−1622.

El-Sayed, A.-F.M., 1987. Protein and Energy Requirements of *Tilapia zillii* (Ph.D. thesis). Michigan State University, East Lansing, MI, USA.

El-Sayed, A.-F.M., Teshima, S., 1991. Tilapia nutrition in aquaculture. Reviews in Aquatic Sciences 5, 247−265.

El-Sayed, A.-F.M., 1999. Alternative dietary protein sources for farmed tilapia spp. Aquaculture 179, 149−168.

El-Sayed, A.-F.M., Mansour, C.R., Ezzat, A.A., 2005. Effects of dietary lipid source on spawning performance of Nile tilapia (*Oreochromis niloticus*) broodstock reared at different water salinities. Aquaculture 248, 187−196.

El-Sayed, A.-F.M., 2017. Social and economic performance of tilapia farming in Egypt. In: Cai, J., Quagrainie, K.K., Hishamunda, N. (Eds.), Social and Economic Performance of Tilapia Farming in Africa. FAO Fisheries and Aquaculture Circular No. 1130. FAO, Rome, pp. 1−48.

English, L.A., 2015. Economic Feasibility of Aquaponics in Arkansas (M.Sc. thesis). University of Arkansas, Fayetteville, 85 pp.

Enhua Z., Jian Z., Cremer M.C., 2013. In-pond Raceway Aquaculture (IPA) Technology Successfully Demonstrated in China- Results of USSEC/China. Freshwater Aquaculture Feeding Demonstration, Project U13CXNA006, U.S. Soybean Export Council, Beijing, China.

Evans, J.J., Klesius, P.H., Shoemaker, C.A., 2004. Efficacy of *Streptococcus agalactiae* (group B) vaccine in tilapia (*Oreochromis niloticus*) by intraperitoneal and bath immersion administration. Vaccine 22, 3769−3773.

Ewart, K.V., Lin, Q., Hew, C.L., 1999. Structure, function and evolution of antifreeze proteins. Cellular and Molecular Life Sciences 55, 271−283.

FAO/WHO, 2006. Probiotics in Food: Health and Nutritional Properties and Guidelines for Evaluation. Joint FAO/WHO Expert Consultation on Evaluation of Health and Nutritional Properties of Probiotics in Food Including Powder Milk with Live Lactic Acid Bacteria. Cordoba, Argentina, 1−4 October 2001. FAO Food and Nutrition Paper No. 85, 48 pp.

Ferguson, R.M.W., Merrifield, D.L., Harper, G.M., Rawling, M.D., Mustafa, S., Picchietti, S., et al., 2010. The effect of *Pediococcus acidilactici* on the gut microbiota and immune status of on-growing red tilapia (*Oreochromis niloticus*). Journal of Applied Microbiology 109, 851−862.

Fitzsimmons, K., 2015. Market Stability: Why tilapia Supply and Demand Have Avoided the Boom and Bust of Other Commodities. Paper Presented at 4th International Trade and Technical Conference and Exposition on Tilapia, 2-4 April 2015, Kuala Lumpur.

Fox, B.K., 2005. Ghrelin Stimulates Growth Hormone and Prolactin Release in the Tilapia, *Oreochromis mossambicus* (M.Sc. thesis). University of Hawai'i.

Fu, G.H., Liu, F., Xia, J.H., Yue, G.H., 2014. The *LBP* gene and its association with resistance to *Aeromonas hydrophila* in tilapia. International Journal of Molecular Sciences 15, 22028−22041.

Garcia, A.L.S., de Oliveira, C.A.L., Karim, H.M., Sary, C., Todesco, H., Ribeiro, R.P., 2017. Genetic parameters for growth performance, fillet traits, and fat percentage of male Nile tilapia (*Oreochromis niloticus*). Journal of Applied Genetics 58, 527−533.

Giorgia, G., Elia, C., Andrea, P., Cinzia, C., Stefania, S., Ana, R., et al., 2018. Effects of Lactogen 13, a new probiotic preparation, on gut microbiota and endocrine signals controlling growth and appetite of *Oreochromis niloticus* juveniles. Microbial Ecology 76, 1063−1074.

Gjerde, B., Mengistu, S.B., Ødegård, J., Johansen, H., Altamirano, D.S., 2012. Quantitative genetics of body weight, fillet weight and fillet yield in Nile tilapia (*Oreochromis niloticus*). Aquaculture 342−343, 117−124.

Gjøen, H.M., 2004. A new era: the merging of quantitative and molecular genetics- prospects for tilapia breeding programs. In: Bolivar, R.B., Mair, G.C., Fitzsimmons, K. (Eds.), Proceedings of the Sixth International Symposium on Tilapia in Aquaculture. Manila, Philippines, pp. 53−59.

Granduño-Lugo, M., Muñoz-Córdova, G., Olvera-Novoa, M.Ă., 2004. Mass selection for red colour in *Oreochromis niloticus* (Linnaeus 1758). Aquaculture Research 35, 340−344.

Guillen, I., Berlanga, J., Valenzuela, C.M., Morales, A., Toledo, J., Estrada, M.P., et al., 1999. Safety evaluation of transgenic tilapia with accelerated growth. Marine Biotechnology 1, 2−14.

Hai, N.V., 2015. Research findings from the use of probiotics in tilapia aquaculture: a review. Fish and Shellfish Immunology 45, 592−597.

Hamdan, A.M., El-Sayed, A.-F.M., Mahmoud, M.M., 2016. Effects of a novel marine probiotic, *Lactobacillus plantarum* AH 78, on growth performance and immune response of Nile tilapia (*Oreochromis niloticus*). Journal of Applied Microbiology 120, 1061−1073.

Hamzah, A., Ponzoni, R.W., Nguyen, N.H., Khaw, H.L., Yee, H.Y., Nor, S.A.M., 2014. Genetic evaluation of the genetically improved farmed tilapia (GIFT) strain over ten generations of selection in Malaysia. Journal of Tropical Agricultural Science 37, 411−429.

Hamzah, A., Nguyen, N.H., Mekkawy, W., Ponzoni, R.W., Khaw, H.L., Yee, H.Y., et al., 2016. Flesh characteristics: estimation of genetic parameters and correlated responses to selection for growth rate in the GIFT strain. Aquaculture Research 47, 2139−2149.

Hamzah, A., Thoa, N.P., Nguyen, N.H., 2017. Genetic analysis of a red tilapia (*Oreochromis* spp.) population undergoing three generations of selection for increased body weight at harvest. Journal of Applied Genetics 58, 509−519.

Haque, M.R., Islam, M.A., Abdul Wahab, M., Hoq, E., Md, Rahman, M.M., Azim, M.E., 2016. Evaluation of production performance and profitability of hybrid red tilapia and genetically improved farmed tilapia (GIFT) strains in the carbon/nitrogen controlled periphyton-based (C/N-CP) on-farm prawn culture system in Bangladesh. Aquaculture Reports 4, 101−111.

He, S., Zhou, Z., Liu, Y., Shi, P., Yao, B., Ringø, E., et al., 2009. Effects of dietary *Saccharomyces cerevisiae* fermentation product (DVAQUA®) on growth performance, intestinal autochthonous bacterial community and non-specific immunity of hybrid tilapia (*Oreochromis niloticus* ♀ × *O. aureus* ♂) cultured in cages. Aquaculture 294, 99−107.

Hernández, A.J., Satoh, S., Kiron, V., 2012. Supplementation of citric acid and amino acid chelated trace elements in low-fish meal diet for rainbow trout affect growth and phosphorous utilization. Journal of the World Aquaculture Society 43, 688−696.

Hernandez, O., Guillen, I., Estrada, M.P., Cabrera, E., Pimentel, R., Pina, J.C., et al., 1997. Characterization of transgenic tilapia lines with different ectopic expression of tilapia growth hormone. Molecular Marine Biology and Biotechnology 6, 364–375.

Hew, C.L., Fletcher, G.L., 2001. The role of aquatic biotechnology in aquaculture. Aquaculture 197, 191–204.

Hörstgen-Schwark, G., Langholz, H.-J., 1998. Prospects of selecting for late maturity in tilapia (*Oreochromis niloticus*): III. A selection experiment under laboratory conditions. Aquaculture 167, 123–133.

Hrytsenko, O., Pohajdak, B., Wright Jr., J.R., 2010. Production of transgenic tilapia homozygous for a humanized insulin gene. Transgenic Research 19, 305–306.

Hu, J., Ran, C., He, S., Cao, Y., Yao, B., Ye, Y., et al., 2016. Dietary microbial phytase exerts mixed effects on the gut health of tilapia: a possible reason for the null effect on growth promotion. British Journal of Nutrition 115, 1958–1966.

Huang, S., Wang, L., Liu, L., Hou, Y., Li, L., 2015. Nanotechnology in agriculture, livestock, and aquaculture in China. A review. Agronomy for Sustainable Development 35, 369–400.

Huang, Y., Yin, Z., Weng, S., He, J., Li, S., 2012. Selective breeding and preliminary commercial performance of *Penaeus vannamei* for resistance to white spot syndrome virus (WSSV). Aquaculture 364–365, 111–117.

Hussain, M.G., Chatterji, A., McAndrew, B.J., Johnstone, R., 1991. Triploidy induction in Nile tilapia, *Oreochromis niloticus* L. using pressure, heat and cold shocks. Theoretical and Applied Genetics 81, 6–12.

Hussain, M.G., Rao, G.P.S., Humayun, N.M., Randall, C.F., Penman, D.J., Kime, D., et al., 1995. Comparative performance of growth, biochemical composition and endocrine profiles in diploid and triploid tilapia *Oreochromis niloticus* L. Aquaculture 138, 87–97.

Hussain, M.G., Penman, D.J., McAndrew, B.J., 1998. Production of heterozygous and homozygous clones in Nile tilapia. Aquaculture International 6, 197–205.

Ismail, M.S., Syafiq, M.R., Siti-Zahrah, A., Fahmi, S., Shahidan, H., Hanan, Y., et al., 2017. The effect of feed-based vaccination on tilapia farm endemic for streptococcosis. Fish and Shellfish Immunology 60, 21–24.

Jauncey, K., 1998. Tilapia Feeds and Feeding. Pisces Press Ltd, Stirling, Scotland, 241 pp.

Kaneko, H., Ijiri, S., Kobayashi, T., Izumi, H., Kuramochi, Y., Wang, D.S., et al., 2015. Gonadal soma-derived factor (gsdf), a TGF-beta superfamily gene, induces testis differentiation in the teleost fish *Oreochromis niloticus*. Molecular and Cellular Endocrinology 415, 87–99.

Kaya, H., Aydın, F., Gürkan, M., Yılmaz, S., Ates, M., Demir, V., et al., 2015. Effects of zinc oxide nanoparticles on bioaccumulation and oxidative stress in different organs of tilapia (*Oreochromis niloticus*). Environmental Toxicology and Pharmacology 40, 936–947.

Kloas, W., Groß, R., Baganz, D., Graupner, J., Monsees, H., Schmidt, U., et al., 2015. A new concept for aquaponic systems to improve sustainability, increase productivity, and reduce environmental impacts. Aquaculture Environment Interactions 7, 179–192.

Kobayashi, S.-I., Alimuddin Morita, T., Miwa, M., Lu, J., Endo, M., et al., 2007. Transgenic Nile tilapia (*Oreochromis niloticus*) over-expressing growth hormone show reduced ammonia excretion. Aquaculture 270, 427–435.

Lacerda, S.M.S.N., Batlouni, S.R., Costa, G.M.J., Segatelli, T.M., Quirino, B.R., Queiroz, B.M., et al., 2010. A new and fast technique to generate offspring after germ cells transplantation in adult fish: the Nile tilapia (*Oreochromis niloticus*) model. PLoS One 5 (5), e10740. https://doi.org/10.1371/journal.pone.0010740.

LaFrentz, B.R., Shoemaker, C.A., 2015. Passive transfer of serum from tilapia vaccinated with a *Vibrio vulnificus* vaccine provides protection from specific pathogen challenge. Aquaculture 442, 16–20.

LaFrentz, B.R., Lozano, C.A., Shoemaker, C.A., García, J.C., Xu, D.-H., Løvoll, M., et al., 2016. Controlled challenge experiment demonstrates substantial additive genetic variation in resistance of Nile tilapia (*Oreochromis niloticus*) to *Streptococcus iniae*. Aquaculture 458, 134–139.

Leeds, T.D., Silverstein, J.T., Weber, G.M., Vallejo, R.L., Palti, Y., Rexroad III, C.E., et al., 2010. Response for selection to bacterial cold water disease resistance in rainbow trout. Journal of Animal Science 88, 1936–1946.

Li, J.S., Li, J.L., Wu, T.T., 2009. Effects of non-starch polysaccharides enzyme, phytase and citric acid on activities of endogenous digestive enzymes of tilapia (*Oreochromis niloticus* × *O. aureus*). Aquaculture Nutrition 15, 415–420.

Li, M., Yang, H., Zhao, J., Fang, L., Shi, H., Li, M., et al., 2014. Efficient and heritable gene targeting in tilapia by CRISPR/Cas9. Genetics 197, 591–599.

Li, M., Sun, Y., Zhao, J., Shi, H., Zeng, S., Ye, K., et al., 2015. A tandem duplicate of anti-mullerian hormone with a missense SNP on the Y chromosome is essential for male sex determination in Nile tilapia, *Oreochromis niloticus*. PLoS Genetics 11 (11), e1005678.

Li, X.-Q., Zhang, X.-Q., Chowdhury, M.A.K., Zhang, Y., Leng, X.-J., 2019. Dietary phytase and protease improved growth and nutrient utilization in tilapia (*Oreochromis niloticus* × *O. aureus*) fed low phosphorus and fishmeal-free diets. Aquaculture Nutrition 25, 46–55.

Li, Y., Bai, J., Jian, Q., Ye, X., Lao, H., Li, X., et al., 2003. Expression of common carp growth hormone in the yeast *Pichia pastoris* and growth stimulation of juvenile tilapia (*Oreochromis niloticus*). Aquaculture 216, 329–341.

Liebert, F., Portz, L., 2005. Nutrient utilization of Nile tilapia *Oreochromis niloticus* fed plant-based low phosphorus diets supplemented with graded levels of different sources of microbial phytase. Aquaculture 248, 111–119.

Liebert, F., Mohamed, K., Lückstädt, C., 2010. Effects of diformates on growth and feed utilization of all male Nile tilapia fingerlings (*Oreochromis niloticus*) reared in tank culture. In: Proceedings of the Fourteenth International Symposium on Fish Nutrition and Feeding, 31 May–4 Jun 2010, Qingdao, China, p. 190.

Lin, C.K., Yi, Y., 2003. Minimizing environmental impacts of freshwater aquaculture and reuse of pond effluents and mud. Aquaculture 226, 57–68.

Liñán-Cabello, M.A., Robles-Basto, C.M., Mena-Herrera, A., 2013. Somatic growth effects of intramuscular injection of growth hormone in androgen-treated juvenile Nile tilapia, *Oreochromis niloticus* (Perciformes: Cichlidae). Revista de Biologia Tropical 61, 203–212.

Liu, G., Zhu, J., Chen, K., Gao, T., Yao, H., Liu, Y., et al., 2016. Development of *Streptococcus agalactiae* vaccines for tilapia. Diseases of Aquatic Organisms 122, 163–170.

Liu, W., Ren, P., He, S., Xu, L., Yang, Y., Gu, Z., et al., 2013. Comparison of adhesive gut bacteria composition, immunity, and disease resistance in juvenile hybrid tilapia fed two different *Lactobacillus* strains. Fish and Shellfish Immunology 35, 54–62.

Longalong, F.M., Eknath, A.E., Bentsen, H.B., 1999. Response to bi-directional selection for frequency of early maturing females in Nile tilapia (*Oreochromis niloticus*). Aquaculture 178, 13–25.

Lu, J., Ji, L., Furuya, Y., Yoshizaki, G., Sun, H., Endo, M., et al., 2009. Efficient productivity and lowered nitrogen and phosphorus discharge load from GH-transgenic tilapia (*Oreochromis niloticus*) under visual satiation feeding. Aquaculture 293, 241–247.

Ma, F., Li, X., Li, B., Leng, X., 2015. Effects of extruded and pelleted diets with differing protein levels on growth and nutrient retention of tilapia, *Oreochromis niloticus* × *O. aureus*. Aquaculture International 23, 1341–1356.

Ma, F., Li, X.Q., Li, B.A., Leng, X.J., 2016. Effects of extruded and pelleted diets with differing lipid levels on growth, nutrient retention and serum biochemical indices of tilapia (*O. aureus* × *Tilapia nilotica*). Aquaculture Nutrition 22, 61–71.

Maclean, N., Rahman, M.A., Sohm, F., Hwang, G., Iyengar, A., Ayad, H., et al., 2002. Transgenic tilapia and the tilapia genome. Gene 295, 265–277.

Mair, G.C., Abucay, J.S., Beardmore, J.A., Skibinski, D.O.F., 1995. Growth performance trials of genetically male tilapia (GMT) derived from "YY" males in *Oreochromis niloticus* L.: on-station comparisons with mixed sex and sex reversed male populations. Aquaculture 137, 313–322.

Mair, G.C., 2002. Tilapia genetics and breeding in Asia. In: Guerrero III, R.D., Guerrero-del Castillo, M.R. (Eds.), Tilapia Farming in the 21st Century. Proceeding of the International Forum on Tilapia Farming in the 21st Century (Tilapia Forum 2002). Philippines Fisheries Association Inc., Los Banos, Laguna, Philippines, pp. 100–123.

Mair, G.C., Clarke, G.J.C., Morales, E.J., Sevilleja, R.C., 2002. Genetic technologies focused on poverty? A case study of genetically improved tilapia (GMT) in the Philippines. In: Edwards, P., Little, D.C., Demaine, H. (Eds.), Rural Aquaculture. CABI Publishing, CAB International, Wallingford, Oxon, UK, pp. 197–225.

Makled, S.O., Hamdan, A.M., El-Sayed, A.-F.M., Hafez, E.E., 2017. Evaluation of marine psychrophile, *Psychrobacter namhaensis* SO89, as a probiotic in Nile tilapia (*Oreochromis niloticus*) diets. Fish and Shellfish Immunology 61, 194–200.

Maquart, P.O., Murray, F., Leschen, W., Netwon, R., Little, D., 2018. Black soldier fly- A future for tilapia feed? International Aquafeed 20–22.

Marengoni, N.G., Onoue, Y., 1998. Ultraviolet-induced androgenesis in Nile tilapia, *Oreochromis niloticus* (L.) and hybrid Nile x blue tilapia, *O. aureus* (Steindachner). Aquaculture Research 29, 359–366.

Marjanovic, J., Mulder, H.A., Khaw, H.L., Bijma, P., 2016. Genetic parameters for uniformity of harvest weight and body size traits in the GIFT strain of Nile tilapia. Genetics Selection Evolution 48, 41. https://doi.org/10.1186/s12711-016-0218-9.

Martinez, R., Juncal, J., Zaldivar, C., Arenal, A., Guillen, I., Morera, V., et al., 2000. Growth efficiency in transgenic tilapia (*Oreochromis* sp.) carrying a single copy of an homologous cDNA growth hormone. Biochemical and Biophysical Research Communications 267, 466–472.

Mather, P.B., Lal, S.N., Wilson, J., 2001. Experimental evaluation of mass selection to improve red body colour in Fijian hybrid tilapia (*Oreochromis niloticus* × *Oreochromis mossambicus*). Aquaculture Research 32, 329–336.

Muin, H., Taufek, N.M., Kamarudin, M.S., Razak, S.A., 2017. Growth performance, feed utilization and body composition of Nile tilapia, *Oreochromis niloticus* (Linnaeus, 1758) fed with different levels of black soldier fly, *Hermetia illucens (*Linnaeus, 1758) maggot meal diet. Iranian Journal of Fisheries Sciences 16, 567–577.

Müller-Belecke, A., Hörstgen-Schwark, G., 1995. Sex determination in tilapia *Oreochromis niloticus.* Sex ratios in homozygous gynogenetic progeny and their offspring. Aquaculture 137, 57–65.

Müller-Belecke, A., Hörstgen-Schwark, G., 2000. Performance testing of clonal *Oreochromis niloticus* lines. Aquaculture 184, 67–76.

Müller-Belecke, A., Hörstgen-Schwark, G., 2007. A YY-male *Oreochromis niloticus* strain developed from an exceptional mitotic gynogenetic male and growth performance testing of genetically all-male progenies. Aquaculture Research 38, 773–775.

Munang'andu, H.M., Paul, J., Evensen, Ø., 2016. An overview of vaccination strategies and antigen delivery systems for *Streptococcus agalactiae* vaccines in Nile tilapia (*Oreochromis niloticus*). Vaccines 4, 48. https://doi.org/10.3390/vaccines4040048.

Myers, J.M., Penman, D.J., Basavaraju, Y., Powell, S.F., Baoprasertkul, P., Rana, K.J., et al., 1995. Induction of diploid androgenetic and mitotic gynogenetic Nile tilapia (*Oreochromis niloticus* L.). Theoretical and Applied Genetics 90, 205–210.

Nasr-Allah, A., Shaban, A., Charo-Karisa, H., 2018. Low Cost In-Pond Raceway Production System. Project Report. WorldFish.

Nayak, S.K., 2010. Review: probiotics and immunity: a fish perspective. Fish and Shellfish Immunology 29, 2–14.

Ng, W.K., Koh, C.B., Sudesh, K., Siti-Zahrah, A., 2009. Effects of dietary organic acids on growth, nutrient digestibility and gut microflora of red hybrid tilapia, *Oreochromis* sp., and subsequent survival during a challenge test with *Streptococcus agalactiae*. Aquaculture Research 40, 1490–1500.

Ng, W.-K., Koh, C.-B., 2017. The utilization and mode of action of organic acids in the feeds of cultured aquatic animals. Reviews in Aquaculture 9, 342–368.

Nguyen, N.H., Ponzoni, R.W., Abu-Bakar, K.R., Hamzah, A., Khaw, H.L., Yee, H.Y., 2010a. Correlated responses in fillet weight and yield to selection for high growth in genetically improved farmed tilapia (gift strain) *Oreochromis niloticus*. Aquaculture 305, 1–5.

Nguyen, N.H., Ponzoni, R.W., Yee, H.Y., Abu-Bakar, K.R., Hamzah, A., Khaw, H.L., 2010b. Quantitative genetic basis of fatty acid composition in the GIFT strain of Nile tilapia (*Oreochromis niloticus*) selected for high growth. Aquaculture 309, 66–74.

Nguyen, N.H., Ponzoni, R.W., Chandrasoma, J., Herath, H.M.V.K.P.B., Wathurawadu, K., 2011. GIFT tilapia raise culture efficiency in Sri Lanka. Global Aquaculture Advocate 11/12, 32–33.

Nguyen, N.H., 2016. Genetic improvement for important farmed aquaculture species with a reference to carp, tilapia and prawns in Asia: achievements, lessons and challenges. Fish and Fisheries 17, 483–506.

Noraini, O., Sabri, M.Y., Siti-Zahrah, A., 2013. Efficacy of spray administration of formalin-killed *Streptococcus agalactiae* in hybrid red tilapia. Journal of Aquatic Animal Health 25, 142–148.

Ogunji, J.O., Kloas, W., Wirth, M., Schulz, C., Rennert, B., 2008. Housefly maggot meal (magmeal) as a protein source for *Oreochromis niloticus* (Linn.). Asian Fisheries Science 21, 319–331.

Okutsu, T., Suzuki, K., Takeuchi, Y., Takeuchi, T., Yoshizaki, G., 2006. Testicular germ cells can colonize sexually undifferentiated embryonic gonad and produce functional eggs in fish. Proceedings of the National Academy of Sciences 103, 2725–2729.

Oldorf, W., Kronert, U., Balarin, J., Haller, R., Hörstgen-Schwark, G., Langholz, H.J., 1989. Prospects of selecting for late maturity in tilapia *Oreochromis niloticus*: II. Strain comparison under laboratory and field conditions. Aquaculture 77, 123–133.

Overgaard, J., MacMillan, H.A., 2017. The integrative physiology of insect chill tolerance. Annual Review of Physiology 79, 187–208.

Pasnik, D.J., Evans, J.J., Klesius, P.H., 2005. Duration of protective antibodies and correlation with survival in Nile tilapia *Oreochromis niloticus* following *Streptococcus agalactiae* vaccination. Diseases of Aquatic Organisms 66, 129–134.

Peddu, S.C., Breves, J.P., Kaiya, H., Grau, E.G., Riley Jr., L.G., 2009. Pre- and postprandial effects on ghrelin signaling in the brain and on the GH/IGF-I axis in the Mozambique tilapia (*Oreochromis mossambicus*). General and Comparative Endocrinology 161, 412–418.

Penman, D.J., McAndrew, B.J., 2000. Genetics for the management and improvement of cultured tilapia. In: Beveridge, M.C.M., McAndrew, B.J. (Eds.), Tilapias: Biology and Exploitation. Kluwer Academic Publishers, Dordrecht/Boston/London, pp. 227–266.

Pohajdak, B., Mansour, M., Hrytsenko, O., Conlon, J.M., Dymond, C., Wright Jr., J.R., 2004. Production of transgenic tilapia with Brockmann bodies secreting [desThrB30] human insulin. Transgenic Research 13, 313–323.

Ponzoni, R.W., Nguyen, N.H., Khaw, H.L., Hamzah, A., Abu Bakar, K.R., Yee, H.Y., 2011. Genetic improvement of Nile tilapia (*Oreochromis niloticus*) with special reference to the work conducted by the WorldFish Center with the GIFT strain. Reviews in Aquaculture 3, 27–41.

Puckhaber, B., Hörstgen-Schwak, G., 1996. Growth and gonadal development of triploid tilapia (*Oreochromis niloticus*). In: Pullin, R.S.V., Lazard, J., Legendre, M., Amon Kottias, J.B., Pauly, D. (Eds.), Proceedings of the Third International Symposium on Tilapia in Aquaculture. ICLARM Conference Proceedings No. 41. ICLARM, Penang, Malaysia, pp. 377–382.

Qiang, J., Bao, J.W., Li, H.X., Chen, D.J., He, J., Tao, Y.F., et al., 2017. miR-1338-5p modulates growth hormone secretion and glucose utilization by regulating ghitm in genetically improved farmed tilapia (GIFT, *Oreochromis niloticus*). Frontiers in Physiology 8, 998. https://doi.org/10.3389/fphys.2017.00998.

Rachmawati, D., Samidjan, I., Elfitasari, T., 2018. Effect of the phytase enzyme addition in the artificial feed on digestibility of feed, feed conversion ratio and growth of GIFT tilapia saline fish (*Oreochromis niloticus*). Nursery Stadia I. In: Third International Conference on Tropical and Coastal Region Eco Development 2017. IOP Conference Series: Earth and Environmental Science, vol. 116, 012009.

Rahman, M.A., Maclean, N., 1999. Growth performance of transgenic tilapia containing an exogenous piscine growth hormone gene. Aquaculture 173, 333–346.

Rahman, M.A., Ronyai, A., Engidaw, B.Z., Jauncey, K., Hwang, G., Smith, A., et al., 2001. Growth and nutritional trials on transgenic Nile tilapia containing an exogenous fish growth hormone gene. Journal of Fish Biology 59, 62–78.

Rakocy, J.E., Allison, R., 1981. Evaluation of a closed recirculating system for the culture of tilapia and aquatic macrophytes. In: Allen, L.J., Kinney, E.C. (Eds.), Proceedings of the Bio-Engineering Symposium for Fish Culture. American Fisheries Society, Bethesda, MD, pp. 296–307.

Rapatsa, M.M., Moyo, N.A.G., 2017. Evaluation of *Imbrasia belina* meal as a fishmeal substitute in *Oreochromis mossambicus* diets: growth performance, histological analysis and enzyme activity. Aquaculture Reports 5, 18–26.

Razak, S.A., Hwang, G.-L., Rahman, M.A., Maclean, N., 1999. Growth performance and gonadal development of growth-enhanced transgenic tilapia *Oreochromis niloticus* (L.) following heat-shock-induced triploidy. Marine Biotechnology 1, 533–544.

Ren, P., Xu, L., Yang, Y., He, S., Liu, W., Ringø, E., Zhou, Z., 2013. *Lactobacillus planarum subsp. plantarum* JCM 1149 vs. *Aeromonas hydrophila* NJ-1 in the anterior intestine and posterior intestine of hybrid tilapia *Oreochromis niloticus* ♀x *Oreochromis aureus* ♂: An ex vivo study. Fish and Shellfish Immunology 35, 146–153.

Riche, M., Trottier, N.L., Ku, P.K., Garling, D.L., 2001. Apparent digestibility of crude protein and apparent availability of individual amino acids in tilapia (*Oreochromis niloticus*) fed phytase pretreated soybean meal diets. Fish Physiology and Biochemistry 25, 181–194.

Ridha, M.T., Azad, I.S., 2012. Preliminary evaluation of growth performance and immune response of Nile tilapia *Oreochromis niloticus* supplemented with two putative probiotic bacteria. Aquaculture Research 43, 843–852.

Riley, L.G., Fox, B.K., Kaiya, H., Hirano, T., Grau, E.G., 2005. Long-term treatment of ghrelin stimulates feeding, fat deposition, and alters the GH/IGF- I axis in the tilapia, *Oreochromis mossambicus*. General and Comparative Endocrinology 142, 234–240.

Romano, N., Simon, W., Ebrahimi, M., Fadel, A.H.I., Chong, C.M., Kamarudin, M.S., 2016. Dietary sodium citrate improved oxidative stability in red hybrid tilapia (*Oreochromis* sp.) but reduced growth, health status, intestinal short chain fatty acids and induced liver damage. Aquaculture 458, 170–176.

Rosati, R., O'Rourke, P.D., Tudor, K., Henry, R.D., 1993. Performance of a raceway and vertical screen filter while growing *Tilapia niloticus* under commercial conditions. In: Wang, J.-K. (Ed.), Techniques for Modern Aquaculture. American Society of Agricultural Engineers, St. Joseph, MI, USA, pp. 303–314.

Rottmann, R.W., Shireman, J.V., Chapman, F.A., 1991. Induction and Verification of Triploidy in Fish. Southern Regional Aquaculture Centre Publication No, p. 427.

Rutten, M.J.M., Bovenhuis, H., Komen, H., 2005. Genetic parameters for fillet traits and body measurements in Nile tilapia (*Oreochromis niloticus* L.). Aquaculture 246, 101–113.

Sánchez-Muros, M.J., De Haro, C., Sanz, A., Trenzado, C.E., Villareces, S., Barroso, F.G., 2016. Nutritional evaluation of *Tenebrio molitor* meal as fish meal substitute for tilapia (*Oreochromis niloticus*) diet. Aquaculture Nutrition 22, 943–955.

Sarker, M.S.A., Satoh, S., Kamata, K., Haga, Y., Yamamoto, Y., 2012. Supplementation effect(s) of organic acids and/or lipid to plant protein-based diets on juvenile yellowtail, *Seriola quinqueradiata* Temminck et Schlegel 1845, growth and, nitrogen and phosphorus excretion. Aquaculture Research 43, 538–545.

Scheerer, P.D., Thorgaard, G.H., Allendorf, F.W., Knudsen, K.L., 1986. Androgenetic rainbow trout production from inbred and outbred sperm sources show similar survival. Aquaculture 57, 289–298.

Schulz, R.W., França, L.R., Lareyre, J.J., LeGac, F., Chiarini-Garcia, H., Nobrega, R.H., et al., 2010. Spermatogenesis in fish. General and Comparative Endocrinology 165, 390–411.

Scott, J.T., Scott, D.M., Lawson, T.B., 1998. Rice hulls as solids removal media for aquaculture. In: Aquaculture'98 - Book of Abstracts. World Aquaculture Society, Baton Rouge, LA, USA, p. 480.

Shelby, R.A., Klesius, P.H., Shoemaker, C.A., Evans, J.J., 2002. Passive immunization of tilapia, *Oreochromis niloticus* (L.), with anti-*Streptococcus iniae* whole sera. Journal of Fish Diseases 25, 1–6.

Shiau, S.-Y., 2002. Tilapia, *Oreochromis* spp. In: Webster, C.D., Lim, C. (Eds.), Nutrient Requirements and Feeding of Finfish for Aquaculture. CABI Publishing, CAB International, Wallingford, Oxon, UK, pp. 273–293.

Shnel, N., Barak, Y., Ezer, T., Dafni, Z., Rijn, J.V., 2002. Design and performance of a Zero-discharge tilapia recirculating system. Aquacultural Engineering 26, 191–203.

Shoemaker, C.A., Lozano, C.A., LaFrentz, B.R., García, J.C., Soto, E., Xu, D.-H., et al., 2017. Additive genetic variation in resistance of Nile tilapia (*Oreochromis niloticus*) to *Streptococcus iniae* and *S. agalactiae* capsular type Ib: is genetic resistance correlated? Aquaculture 468, 193–198.

Silva, L., Escalante, E., Valdés-Lozano, D., Hernández, M., Gasca-Leyva, E., 2017. Evaluation of a semi-intensive aquaponics system, with and without bacterial biofilter in a tropical location. Sustainability 9, 592–605.

Sing, K., Kamarudin, M., Wilson, J., Azirun, M., 2014. Evaluation of blowfly (*Chrysomya megacephala*) maggot meal as an effective, sustainable replacement for fishmeal in the diet of farmed juvenile red tilapia (*Oreochromis* sp.). Pakistan Veterinary Journal 34, 288–292.

Standen, B.T., Rawling, M.D., Davies, S.J., Castex, M., Foey, A., Gioacchini, G., et al., 2013. Probiotic *Pediococcus acidilactici* modulates both localised intestinal and peripheral-immunity in tilapia (*Oreochromis niloticus*). Fish and Shellfish Immunology 35, 1097–1104.

Storset, A., Strand, C., Wetten, M., Kjøglum, S., Ramstad, A., 2007. Response to selection for resistance against infectious pancreatic necrosis in Atlantic salmon (*Salmo salar* L.). Aquaculture 272, S62–S68.

Subasinghe, R.P., Curry, D., McGladdery, S.E., Bartley, D., 2003. Recent technological innovations in aquaculture. Revision 2. In: Review of the State of World Aquaculture. FAO Fisheries Circular 882. FAO, Rome, pp. 59–74.

Sukenda, S., Rahman, R., Nisaa, K., Hidayatullah, D., Vinasyiam, A., 2018. The efficacy of *Streptococcus agalactiae* vaccine preparations, administered to tilapia broodstock, in preventing streptococcosis in their offspring, via transfer of maternal immunity. Aquaculture International 26, 785–798.

Sun, L.-N., Jiang, X.-L., Xie, Q.-P., Yuan, J., Huang, B.-F., Tao, W.-J., et al., 2014. Transdifferentiation of differentiated ovary into functional testis by long-term treatment of aromatase inhibitor in Nile tilapia. Endocrinology 155, 1476–1488.

Tawfik, M.M., Moustafa, M.M., Abumourad, I.M.K., El-Meliegy, E.M., Refai, M.K., 2017. Evaluation of nano zinc oxide feed additive on tilapia growth and immunity. In: Proceedings of the 15th International Conference on Environmental Science and Technology. Rhodes, Greece, 31 August to 2 September 2017, 01342.

Tayamen, M.M., 2004. Nationwide dissemination of GET EXCEL tilapia in the Philippines. In: Bolivar, R.B., Mair, G.C., Fitzsimmons, K. (Eds.), Proceedings of the Sixth International Symposium on Tilapia in Aquaculture. Manila, Philippines, pp. 74–85.

Thodesen, J., Rye, M., Wang, Y.X., Yang, K.S., Bentsen, H.B., Gjedrem, T., 2011. Genetic improvement of tilapias in China: genetic parameters and selection responses in growth of Nile tilapia (*Oreochromis niloticus*) after six generations of multi-trait selection for growth and fillet yield. Aquaculture 322–323, 51–64.

Thodesen, J. (Ma, D.Y.), Rye, M., Wang, Y.-X., Bentsen, H.B., Gjedrem, T., 2012. Genetic improvement of tilapias in China: genetic parameters and selection responses in fillet traits of Nile tilapia (*Oreochromis niloticus*) after six generations of multi-trait selection for growth and fillet yield. Aquaculture 366–367, 67–75.

Thodesen, J. (Ma, D.Y.), Rye, M., Wang, Y.X., Li, S.-J., Bentsen, H.B., Yazdi, M.H., et al., 2013. Genetic improvement of tilapias in China: genetic parameters and selection responses in growth, survival and external color traits of red tilapia (*Oreochromis* spp.) after four generations of multi-trait selection. Aquaculture 416–417, 354–366.

Varadaraj, K., Pandian, T.J., 1989. First report on production of supermale tilapia by integrating endocrine sex reversal with gynogenetic technique. Current Science 58, 434–441.

Viola, S., Zohar, G., Arieli, Y., 1986. Phosphorus requirements and its availability from different sources for intensive pond culture species in Israel. Part 1. Tilapia. Bamidgeh 38, 3–12.

Viola, S., Arieli, Y., Zohar, G., 1988. Animal-protein-free feeds for hybrid tilapia (*Oreochromis niloticus* x *O. aureus*) in intensive culture. Aquaculture 75, 115–125.

Wang, A., Ran, C., Wang, Y., Zhang, Z., Ding, Q., Yang, Y., et al., 2019. Use of probiotics in aquaculture of China – a review of the past decade. Fish and Shellfish Immunology 86, 734–755.

Wang, L., Li, J., Jin, J.N., Zhu, F., Roffeis, M., Zhang, X.Z., 2017. A comprehensive evaluation of replacing fishmeal with housefly (*Musca domestica*) maggot meal in the diet of Nile tilapia (*Oreochromis niloticus*): growth performance, flesh quality, innate immunity and water environment. Aquaculture Nutrition 23, 983–993.

Wang, M., Liu, G., Lu, M., Ke, X., Liu, Z., Gao, F., et al., 2017. Effect of *Bacillus cereus* as a water or feed additive on the gut microbiota and immunological parameters of Nile tilapia. Aquaculture Research 48, 3163–3173.

Wang, Y., Li, J., 2011. Effects of chitosan nanoparticles on survival, growth and meat quality of tilapia, *Oreochromis nilotica*. Nanotoxicology 5, 425–431.

Widiarti, A., 2015. Indonesia tilapia production and trade. In: Paper Presented at 4th International Trade and Technical Conference and Exposition on Tilapia, 2–4 April 2015, Kuala Lumpur.

Wonmongkol, P., Sukhavachana, S., Ampolsak, K., Srisapoome, P., Suwanasopee, T., Poompuang, S., 2018. Genetic parameters for resistance against *Flavobacterium columnare* in nile tilapia *Oreochromis niloticus* (Linnaeus, 1758). Journal of Fish Diseases 41, 321–328.

Wright Jr., J.R., Pohajdak, B., 2001. Cell therapy for diabetes using piscine islet tissue. Cell Transplantation 10, 125–143.

Wu, S.-M., Hwang, P.-P., Hew, C.-L., Wu, J.-L., 1998. Effect of antifreeze protein on cold tolerance in juvenile tilapia (*Oreochromis mossambicus* Peters) and milkfish (*Chanos chanos* Forsskal). Zoological Studies 37, 39–44.

Yi, Y., Diana, J.S., Lin, C.K., 2004. Supplemental feeding for red tilapia culture in brackishwater. In: Bolivar, R., Mair, G., Fitzsimmons, K. (Eds.), Proceedings of the Sixth International Symposium on Tilapia in Aquaculture. Manila, Philippines, pp. 451–462.

Zak, T., Deshev, R., Benet-Perlberg, A., Naor, A., Magen, I., Shapira, Y., et al., 2014. Genetic improvement of Israeli blue (Jordan) tilapia, *O. aureus* (Steindachner), through selective breeding for harvest weight. Aquaculture Research 45, 546–557.

Zhang, X., Li, M., Ma, H., Liu, X., Shi, H., Li, M., et al., 2017. Mutation of *foxl2* or *cyp19a1a* results in female to male sex reversal in XX Nile tilapia. Endocrinology 158, 1–14.

Zhou, Z., Liu, Y., He, S., Shi, P., Gao, X., Yao, B., et al., 2009. Effects of dietary potassium diformate (KDF) on growth performance, feed conversion and intestinal bacterial community of hybrid tilapia (*Oreochromis niloticus* ♀ × *O. aureus* ♂). Aquaculture 291, 89–94.

Zhu, L., Yang, Q., Huang, L., Wang, K., Wang, X., Chen, D., et al., 2017. Effectivity of oral recombinant DNA vaccine against *Streptococcus agalactiae* in Nile tilapia. Developmental & Comparative Immunology 77, 77–87.

Zhu, Y., Ding, Q., Chan, J., Chen, P., Wang, C., 2015. The effects of concurrent supplementation of dietary phytase, citric acid and vitamin D3 on growth and mineral utilization in juvenile yellow catfish *Pelteobagrus fulvidraco*. Aquaculture 436, 143–150.

Zimmermann, S., Natividad, J.M., 2004. Comparative pond performance evaluation of GenoMar Supreme TilapiaTM GST1 and GST3 groups. In: Bolivar, R.B., Mair, G.C., Fitzsimmons, K. (Eds.), New Dimensions of Farmed Tilapia, Proceedings of the Sixth International Symposium on Tilapia in Aquaculture, 12–16 September, Manila, The Philippines, p. 89.

Chapter 14

Environmental impacts

Chapter outline

14.1 Introduction

The aquaculture industry is expanding worldwide at an outstanding rate during the last two decades. As a result, aquaculture production has sharply increased more than 160%, from 41,724,570 t in 2000, representing 30.62% of global fish production (136,284,859 t) to 111,948,623 t in 2017, comprising 54.5% of the fish production (205,582,364 t) (FAO, 2019). This rapid expansion of aquaculture has caused several ecological, human health and socioeconomic impacts.

Traditionally, small-scale, semi-intensive aquaculture has been sustainable in many countries, especially in rural areas, with minimum adverse effects on surrounding environments. In recent years, however, there has been a growing trend towards tilapia intensification, which is usually driven by market forces and competitive use of the resources. The use of artificial culture inputs such as prepared feed, drugs, additives, hormones, fuels, etc., has become inevitable in intensive culture practices. This may pose serious environmental and socioeconomic threats. It is also very likely that the high intensity of farmed species will lead to enrichment of aquatic environments. According to Joint Group of Experts on the Scientific Aspects of Marine Pollution (GESAMP) (1991), the environmental impacts of coastal aquaculture are listed as follows:

1. Ecological impacts: These include enrichment, interaction with food web, oxygen consumption, disturbance of wildlife, habitat destruction, interaction between escaped farmed stock and wild species, introductions and transfers and bioactive compounds (including pesticides and antibiotics, chemicals introduced via construction materials, hormones and growth promoters).
2. Implications for human health: These include outbreaks of diseases associated with the consumption of shellfish; typhoid fever; infectious hepatitis and other viral diseases; survival of enteric viruses in the marine environment; cholera; influence of fish pathogens on human health, phycotoxins and depuration.
3. Socioeconomic considerations: As mentioned in Chapter 1, tilapia culture is expanding at a very high rate, so that it is now ranked second in terms of global production, only after carps. Tilapia are currently cultured in more than 120 countries around the world. The traditional, small-scale, semi-intensive system of tilapia culture, especially in Asia, is now being replaced with more intensive, large-scale farming systems.

Tilapia Culture. https://doi.org/10.1016/B978-0-12-816541-6.00014-3
Copyright © 2020 Elsevier Inc. All rights reserved.

Intensive tilapia culture can thus pose a possible threat to the environment. This chapter discusses the major environmental impacts of tilapia culture, with emphases on the following impacts: (1) transfers and introductions, (2) farm effluents, (3) bioactive compounds and hormones, (4) human health risks and (5) reducing environmental impacts.

14.2 Transfers and introductions

Transfers of aquatic species are movements of that species within its geographical range. Transfers generally take place to support stressed populations, enhance genetic characteristics or re-establish a species that has failed locally (GESAMP, 1991). Introductions are the movements of a species beyond its present geographical range. Introductions are intended to establish new taxa into the flora and fauna of an environment. Transfers and introductions can pose a wide variety of risks to the integrity of ecosystems, existing species, human health, agriculture, aquaculture and related primary industries. In other words, transfers and introductions may change the biodiversity of the receiving ecosystem through interbreeding, predation, competition for food and space and habitat destruction.

Tilapia have been introduced as alien species into more than 100 countries worldwide. They are known to thrive and reproduce in most of their new habitats. The introductions of tilapia can be unsuccessful, successful, or successful but with high environmental costs ranging from habitat destruction, hybridization with endemic species, to disappearance of native species. Therefore, a full chapter (Chapter 3) is dedicated to tilapia transfers and introductions. Chapter 3 provides full details on the distribution of tilapia in their natural habitats and the factors affecting this distribution. It also covers the introductions of tilapia into the different geographical regions of the world. The negative impacts, including ecological impacts and genetic pollution of introduced tilapia were also highlighted. The current chapter will, therefore, be dedicated to the following environmental issues.

14.3 Farm effluents and organic enrichments

Considerable amounts of uneaten feed along with wastes, including organic matter, nutrients such as phosphorus and nitrogen and suspended solids are released from intensive, land-based, tilapia farms into the water. For example, David et al. (2015) reported that the estimated emission of phosphorus per ton of Nile tilapia produced in cage aquaculture in a large hydroelectrical reservoir in south-eastern Brazil was 14.8 kg, based on farming data of feed composition, whole body composition and feed conversion ratio. These compounds are generally toxic to fish and other aquatic animals. They may also have varying degrees of environmental impacts, depending on the intensity of the culture operations. In fish ponds, part of these wastes settle to the pond bottom, while the remainder is discharged with farm effluents into the environment. If not removed or treated, they may be subject to oxidation, leading to oxygen depletion and, in turn, producing anaerobic conditions that may stress and/or kill the fish, both in the ponds and in receiving waters.

The global expansion of tilapia culture in floating cages is also very likely to pose severe environmental and socioeconomic impacts. The assimilation of wastes and nutrients accumulated underneath the cages requires a very large area of the aquatic system. Berg et al. (1996) reported that the production of *Tilapia rendalli*, *Oreochromis mossambicus* and *Oreochromis niloticus* in 1 m^2 of intensively managed lacustrine cages required an ecosystem area of 115 and 160 m^2 for phosphorus assimilation and oxygen production. This simply means that the production of tilapia in large cages, which are currently widely used, would require a tremendous ecosystem area for the assimilation of wastes resulting from the cages.

Tilapia culture in floating cages in Sampaloc Lake (Philippines) is a good example of the catastrophic environmental and socioeconomic impacts of unmanaged culture practices. Tilapia cage culture in the lake was introduced in 1976 and has been expanding since then, with overuse of commercial feeds. It was reported that about 6000 mt of feed are wasted through the cages and settled on the sediments annually, in addition to the accumulation of fish faeces and other organic wastes underneath the cages. This situation has created severe anoxic conditions and toxic waters, resulting in the progressive depletion of dissolved oxygen (DO), a high biological oxygen demand load and extremely high concentrations of ammonia and total sulphides. In 1990, the operators were warned about the possibility of a fish kill due to the huge volume of anoxic and toxic waters underneath the cages and were also advised to harvest their stocks. The warning was ignored, and, as expected, a massive fish kill of market-size tilapia occurred, causing the farmers to lose their investment (Santiago and Arcilla, 1993; Santiago, 1994). A number of fish kills due to eutrophication caused by cage culture have also been reported in Lake Taal in the Philippines (ADB, 2005). Upwelling of deep deoxygenated and hydrogen sulphide-containing water from the anaerobic degradation of fish wastes generally leads to fish kill in the lake. In addition, about 64% of the nitrogen and 81% of phosphorous of the feed provided to caged fishes is released to the environment causing severe eutrophication (ADB, 2005). Farm wastes can also be a major cause of changes in the structure of benthic communities because uneaten feed may favour certain aquatic species over others. Sedentary animals may also suffer from mass mortality when the water is depleted of oxygen, while the mobile population may migrate to other areas.

Nile tilapia cage culture has also been widely practiced in many natural freshwater masses (rivers, canals, reservoirs, etc.) in Thailand over the past decade. This has led to a rapid increase in the number of tilapia cages and has also created many social, economic and environmental problems. The FAO (2018) listed the following impacts as a sequence of expanding tilapia cage culture in Thailand:

1. High investment cost especially for feed;
2. High risk of declining profitability because of increased fish mortality and low growth rate of fish;
3. Climate change (air and water temperature) which makes fish more susceptible to disease;
4. Change in water level and quality, especially during the dry season;
5. Increased water pollution;
6. Limited number of waterbodies for operating tilapia cage culture and
7. Carrying capacity of tilapia cage culture in natural waterbodies being exceeded.

These impacts indicated the urgent need for environmental carrying capacity assessment (ECCA) tool for tilapia planning in Thailand. This assessment will help to establish the number of cages that would allow the most sustainable farming practice, with highest performance and lowest adverse impacts.

In Egypt, cage culture of tilapia in the Nile River, particularly in Damietta and Rosetta branches, has expanded at outstanding rats during the past few years (Fig. 14.1). This has increased public awareness and created a debate among governmental authorities, the academics and environmental protection bodies, with respect to the environmental impacts of these cages. The Egyptian authority removed the cages from the Nile branches by force, after warning the farmers several times, taking into account that most of these cage farms were not licenced. This situation has divided the public opinion into two mainstreams. Those in favour of tilapia cage culture suspect that the cages pollute the Nile and claim that this culture system is practiced all over the globe. They suggest that removing the cages is not the solution, whereas proper management, such as limiting the number of cages km^{-2}, use of high-quality feed with optimum feeding strategies, proper selection of cage sites, farming other fish species such as silver carp with tilapia and continuous governmental monitoring and inspections, would certainly minimize the effects of the cages. Researchers, academics and farmers are in favour of this opinion. On the other side, environmental protection authority and governorate administration claim that cage culture is deteriorating the quality of the Nile and is very likely to cause health hazard, and therefore, removing these cages is the only solution. Unfortunately, removing the cages has caused a catastrophic loss to the farmers.

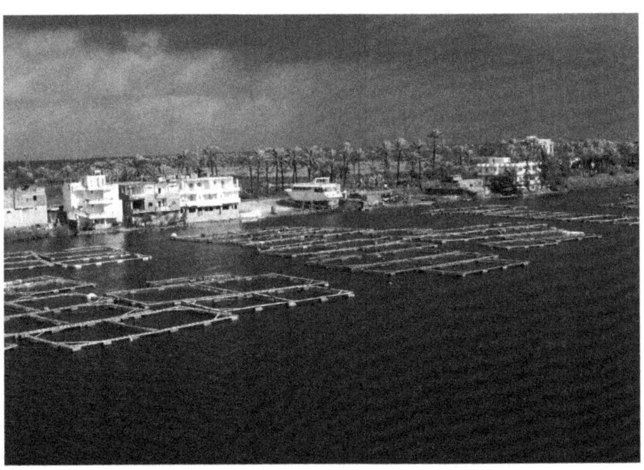

FIGURE 14.1 Several long arrays of tilapia cages in the Nile River (Egypt) may pose a threat to the environment. *Photograph by A.-F.M El-Sayed.*

Troell and Berg (1997) suggested that intensive tilapia farming in cages in the tropics can generate severe eutrophication. They found that average flux of particulate nutrients (ammonium and phosphates) under tilapia cages in Lake Kariba (Zimbabwe) was up to 22 times greater than in control areas. The release of the nutrients usually stimulates phytoplankton production and other algal blooms, which may further increase oxygen consumption during the decomposition of uneaten food and organic wastes. These algal blooms may also be toxic. Moreover, when the algae die, they settle to the bottom, decompose and further deplete the oxygen in the water, making the already eutrophic conditions worse.

The status of tilapia cage culture in Lake Victoria (Kenya) was evaluated in 2016 and 2017 using geographical information system (GIS), standard water quality monitoring procedures and stakeholder questionnaires and interviews (Aura et al., 2018; Njiru et al., 2018). In addition to the remarkable benefits gained from cage culture, significant adverse impacts were recorded. Dissolved oxygen (DO) was much lower inside the cages than outside them. Ammonia concentration around the cages was also much higher than in cage-free areas, due to the protein in uneaten feed and fish waste that had been broken down into ammonia and nitrite. Waste feed increased eutrophication, decreased DO, enhanced blooming of algae and water hyacinth in the lake and led to a number of fish kills. Frequent occurrence of fish disease was also reported and attributed to poor management practices among cage farmers.

On the other hand, no consistent environmental changes were reported in the Tanzanian part of Lake Victoria, as a result of tilapia cage culture (Kashindye et al., 2015).

However, a significant increase in total nutrient (phosphorus and nitrogen) concentrations was observed in the cage locations after the set of cages, compared to offshore areas. An increase in phytoplankton, bivalves and gastropods communities was also observed after stocking of fish in cages. Regular fish kills due to eutrophication caused by intensive tilapia cage culture have also been recorded in Cirata Reservoir, Indonesia (Abery et al., 2005). Similarly, mass mortalities of tilapia farmed in cages in different rivers in Thailand due to illegal release of untreated effluents from different factories, especially in the Chao Phraya River, has also been reported (Edwards, 2015).

14.4 Bioactive compounds

Bioactive compounds, including pesticides, antibiotics and other therapeutic drugs are used in aquaculture for various reasons, including disease control, fertilization, liming, disinfection, oxidation, coagulation, pesticides and adsorption. They are generally added to feed and/or culture water. Some of these compounds, especially drugs, pesticides, and antibiotics may be toxic to aquatic animals and/or may accumulate in the environment. Aquaculture effluents containing these compounds may therefore produce adverse ecological impacts, in addition to the possible contamination of the flesh of aquatic animals which could pose a hazard to consumers.

Rico et al. (2014) found that the maximum concentrations of the most commonly used antibiotics, oxytetracycline and enrofloxacin, in the Tha Chin River (Thailand), in which tilapia cage culture is widely practiced, was much higher than the concentrations recorded in other Asian aquatic environments receiving aquaculture effluents. The peak antibiotic concentrations in the river water occurred during antibiotic administration in the tilapia cages, presumably due to the leaching of antibiotics from fish pelleted feed. Antibiotics accumulated mainly underneath or next to the tilapia cages, suggesting that water-sediment sorption, fish waste and wasted feed are responsible for the transport of antibiotics to the sediment. Accumulated antibiotics were widely distributed in the river and were found to remain in the river sediments for several weeks. These results clearly indicated that tilapia cage aquaculture is an important source of antibiotic pollution.

14.5 Hormones

As mentioned in Chapter 8 (Section 8.8.2), steroid hormones are widely used for producing monosex tilapia. Hormones are generally incorporated either with larval feeds or through the immersion of fertilized eggs or sac fry. However, the use of hormones for sex reversal has been under increasing public criticism due to their potential health and environmental impacts. The hormone residues and metabolites can be a potential environmental contaminant. For example, feeding tilapia with 17-α methyltestosterone (MT)-treated feed has resulted in considerable 'leakage' of MT into pond water and sediments (Contreras-Sánchez et al., 2001, 2002). MT has been detected in the water during MT treatment, accumulated and remained in the sediments of the ponds for up to 8 weeks. Hormone traces pose a risk of hatchery workers and also of other nontarget aquatic organisms. MT traces remained at 2.8–2.9 ng g^{-1} in soils for 3 months and in water at 3.6 $\mu g\ L^{-1}$ for 2 weeks, before returning to the base level (up to 0.02 $\mu g\ L^{-1}$), which has been reported in tilapia masculinization ponds (Homklin et al., 2009, 2012; Megbowon and Mojekwu, 2014). MT leakage to the environment can also disrupt the normal sex ratio in wild fish populations. The human food safety and environmental hazards associated with the use of MT and other steroids in production of sex-reversed tilapia have been comprehensively reviewed by Mlalila et al. (2015).

Many tilapia farmers and hatchery operators in Egypt use higher amounts of MT hormones than they really need (A.-F.M. El-Sayed, personal survey, 2017), leading to accumulation of hormone residues in the environment. This practice may lead to adverse ecological and human health impacts. For example, the sex ratio of Nile tilapia in the canals and drains adjacent to fish farms and hatcheries in Kafr El-Shaikh Governorate (Egypt) has dramatically changed in favour of males (A.-F.M. El-Sayed, 2018; personal observation). Catching wild females, as broodstock for breeding, from these waterbodies becomes very difficult, since most of the catch is males.

The above finding supports the argument that the exposure of untargeted organisms to steroid hormones can result in biased sex ratios. In support, significant masculinization occurred in common carp exposed to water used in MT-impregnated feeding trials (Gomelsky et al., 1994). Abucay et al. (1997) also reported high rates of masculinization and feminization in sexually undifferentiated Nile tilapia fry reared in aquarium water previously used for oral application of hormones used for sex reversal. Also, high proportions of males were found in Nile tilapia fry fed with normal feed in cages adjacent to cages containing MT-incorporated feed (Abucay et al., 1997). These findings clearly demonstrate that hormone (or hormone metabolites) leaching from uneaten food can induce sex reversal in exposed untargeted organisms.

14.6 Human health risks

As mentioned earlier, many contaminants from land-based run-offs and anthropogenic activities, including organic pesticides, heavy metals, polychlorinated biphenyls, hormones, etc., end up in the aquatic environments, causing a wide range of environmental impacts. Farming tilapia in these environments may also pose human health risks, depending on the source, exposure time and concentration of the contaminant. For example, Ling et al. (2009) assessed the heavy metals (arsenic, As; chromium, Cr; copper, Cu; manganese, Mn; nickel, Ni; lead, Pb; selenium, Se and zinc, Zn) in tilapia collected from farms located in industrialized (polluted) areas in Taiwan, compared with samples collected from unpolluted areas. They found that the concentrations of almost all of these heavy metals were higher in the body tissue of tilapia farmed in the polluted areas than in fish grown in relatively clean areas. These results indicated that heavy metals in tilapia muscles may pose a significant risk to residents in the vicinity of industrial zones. Excess lifetime cancer risk and hazard quotients for residents consuming contaminated tilapia located in the vicinity of industrial zones were also higher than those for residents consuming tilapia farmed at the uncontaminated areas. Similarly, the concentrations of heavy metals in Mozambique tilapia (*O. mossambicus*) collected from ponds receiving domestic effluents in Malaysia were significantly higher than in fish collected from uncontaminated ponds (Yap et al., 2015). However, health risk assessments and the amount of fish required to reach the provisional tolerable weekly intake, estimated daily intake and target hazard quotient revealed that no health risks were associated with heavy metals intake via consumption of tilapia collected from ponds receiving domestic effluents.

In addition to their potential environmental impacts, steroid hormones applied in aquaculture may also pose human health risks. However, the effects of these steroids depend mainly on their type, doses, exposure time, pharmacokinetic characteristics and genetic susceptibility. There has been a long debate among societal and scientific communities on whether the MT-treated fish are safe for human consumption. The fish carcass, viscera, blood, and muscle of treated fish have been investigated for MT and its metabolites. Available information and argument concluded that MT-treated fish are safe for human consumption. Pandian and Kirankumar (2003) reported that the estimated residual steroids are less than 5 ng g^{-1} fish, which is too low to cause any human health risks. In support, Green and Teichert-Coddington (2000) demonstrated that the levels of MT and metabolites in tilapia carcass were less than 100 pg g^{-1} after 8–40 days of withdrawal, and less than 10 pg g^{-1} after 6–50 days of withdrawal. Once again, it is very unlikely that these low hormone levels can cause any health problems to humans. In addition, no cases of pharmaceutically active MT and its metabolites from aquaculture effluents to surrounding environments have been reported (Mlalila et al., 2015).

14.7 Reducing environmental impacts

14.7.1 Effluent management

The treatment and management of tilapia culture effluents have been described in details in Chapter 6 (Section 6.8). Boyd (2003) listed the following best aquaculture management practices (BAMPs) for minimizing nutrient loads in aquaculture effluents:

1. Use fertilizers only as needed to maintain phytoplankton blooms.
2. Select stocking and feeding rates that do not exceed the assimilation capacity of ponds.
3. Feeds should be of high quality, water stable and contain no more nitrogen and phosphorus than necessary.
4. Apply feeds conservatively to avoid overfeeding and to assure that as much of the feed is consumed as possible.
5. Do not use water exchange or reduce water exchange rates as much as possible.
6. In intensive aquaculture, apply enough mechanical aeration to prevent chronically low DO concentration and to promote nitrification and other aerobic, natural water purification processes.
7. Provide storage volume for heavy rainfall to minimize storm overflow.
8. Deep water release structures should not be installed in ponds, for they discharge lower-quality water from near pond bottoms.
9. Where possible, seine-harvested fish without partially or completely draining ponds.
10. Where possible, discharge pond draining effluent through a settling basin or a vegetated ditch.
11. Reuse water where possible.

While these practices are valid for reducing nutrient loads in tilapia culture, there are certain practices that have been exceptionally successful in effluent management at the farm level. Extensive research was conducted at the Asian Institute of Technology (AIT) in Thailand to mitigate the environmental impact of tilapia culture through reducing nutrient loading in pond culture of Nile tilapia. Special attention was given to (1) optimization of feeding regimes; (2) maximizing nutrient utilization through integration and recycling systems and (3) minimizing waste loading from effluents through appropriate draining techniques during harvest. Lin and Yi (2003) described the results of these practices. It would be useful here to throw light on these results.

14.7.1.1 Optimization of feeding regimes

When Nile tilapia reared in fertilized ponds were fed supplemental diets at 50%, 75%, and 100% satiation, they produced comparable yields (Lin and Yi, 2003). However, considerable reduction in nutrient loading was achieved at the 50% level. This means that about 50% of the feed can be saved, since the fish are able to supplement their diets with natural food available in the pond. This also indicates that an optimal feeding regime may reduce both feed costs and nutrient loading in the ponds.

14.7.1.2 Reducing effluent impact with a cage-cum-pond integrated system

Tilapia culture in a cage-cum-pond integrated system has been described in details in Chapter 5 (Section 5.6.3) and Chapter 6 (Section 6.4.5). The system involves rearing hybrid catfish (*Clarias macrocephalus* × *Clarias gariepinus*) in cages in ponds and feeding them with formulated feeds, whereas their wastes are used as a natural food for tilapia reared in open pond. This system yields considerable production of catfish and tilapia and also reduces nutrient loading through the use of fish wastes for pond fertilization and natural food production.

14.7.1.3 Effluent management during harvest

Seining fish ponds with nets, despite being most common, stirs bottom sediments, leading to the deterioration of water quality and its effluents. Appropriate harvest methods and draining treatments can significantly reduce pollutants from Nile tilapia ponds. In a novel study, Lin et al. (2001) evaluated four treatments to determine the efficiency of fish harvest and effectiveness in reducing nutrient loading in the effluents. The treatments were (1) treating the ponds with tea seed cake (10 ppm) to partially anaesthetize Nile tilapia 1.5 h prior to harvest by seining, (2) liming the ponds (75 g m^{-3} of calcium hydroxide) 24 h prior to harvest to precipitate phosphorus and organic matter, followed by sequential complete draining with a pump, and Nile tilapia collected from a harvesting pit, (3) draining the ponds by sequential complete draining with a pump and Nile tilapia collected from a harvesting pit and (4) ponds drawn down from 100 to 50 cm with a pump and Nile tilapia harvested by seining twice, followed by complete draining and collection of the remaining Nile tilapia from a harvesting pit. The results of that study revealed that liming the pond 24 h before draining and gradually draining ponds to a 25-cm depth during harvest were most effective.

14.7.2 Reducing nutrient loading through green water tank culture

Green water tank culture system can be an efficient method for reducing nutrient loading in fish tanks. In this system, fish wastes and other metabolites are treated in such a way to increase natural food production in the tanks. This process involves the oxidation of toxic ammonia (NH_3) and nitrite (NO_2) into relatively nontoxic nitrate (NO_3) through nitrifying bacteria grown on suspended organic matter. The bacteria remove the organic matter from the tanks and use it as food, while the bacteria are used as natural food for filter-feeding fishes such as tilapia and carp. However, in green water systems, solid wastes should be removed continuously, and both biofiltration and aeration should be provided. Vigorous aeration is also necessary to support the suspension of the microbial community, maximize contact between bacteria and waste products and, in turn, increase phytoplankton productivity. This system has been successfully used for tilapia culture in various parts of the world, particularly in the Virgin Islands (Fig. 14.2). The advantages of green water culture are summarized in Chapter 6 (Section 6.6).

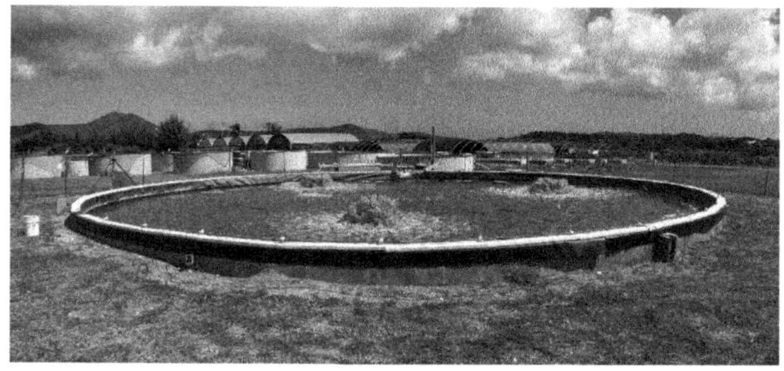

FIGURE 14.2 Growing tilapia in green water system in Virgin Islands, USA. *Photo provided by J. Rakocy.*

14.7.3 Removing nutrients through planting rooted plants

In semi-intensive tilapia culture, about 80% of the nitrogen and phosphorus added in fertilizers settles to the pond mud (Lin and Yi, 2003). The removal (de-sludging) of pond mud is tedious and labour-demanding. Planting rooted aquatic plants in fish ponds can be an effective way of extracting nutrients from the mud. This approach has been tested with lotus (*Nelumbo mucifera*) seedlings planted in Nile tilapia ponds fertilized weekly with urea and triple superphosphate at a rate of 4 kg N and 1 kg P ha^{-1} d^{-1} (Yi et al., 2002). Lotus effectively removed nutrients from pond mud. The annual nutrient losses from the mud were 2.4 t N and 1 t P ha^{-1}, about 300 kg N and 43 kg of which were taken by lotus.

In temperate zones, water temperature drops during winter times and becomes unsuitable for tilapia culture. Generally, tilapia farmers in these regions harvest their fish during September—November. During winter season, these ponds are dried and become useless. Growing land winter crops, such as wheat and alfalfa, in these ponds can be an effective method of removing nutrients from pond muds in addition to generating an additional income to the farmer.

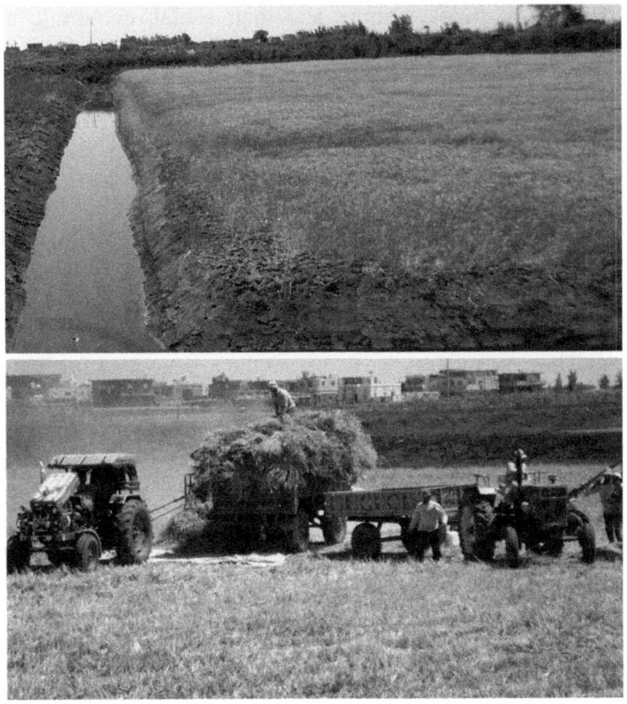

FIGURE 14.3 Growing (*top*) and harvesting and threshing (*bottom*) a wheat crop in tilapia ponds in Kafr El-Shaikh Governorate, Egypt. *Photograph by A.-F.M. El-Sayed.*

This approach has been tested in some areas in Egypt, where alfalfa and wheat have been grown in tilapia ponds during the winter, with promising results (El-Sayed, 2017) (Fig. 14.3).

14.7.4 Removing nutrients through aquaponic systems

Aquaponics is the integration of hydroponics with aquaculture in a recirculating system. The wastes and metabolites produced by cultured fish are removed by nitrification and taken up by the plants, while the bacteria living in the gravel and in association with the plant roots play a critical role in nutrient removal (Fig. 14.4). This means that the plants act as a biological filter by removing fish wastes and improving the quality of culture water. Many studies have been conducted on aquaponic systems at the University of Virgin Islands Agricultural Experimental Station and also in other geographical regions, using tilapia and various vegetables, with considerable success. The results of these studies are discussed in Chapter 6 (Section 6.9).

14.7.5 Removing nutrients through integrated multitrophic aquaculture systems

Integrated multitrophic aquaculture (IMTA) systems are designed mainly for efficient use of resources. IMTA

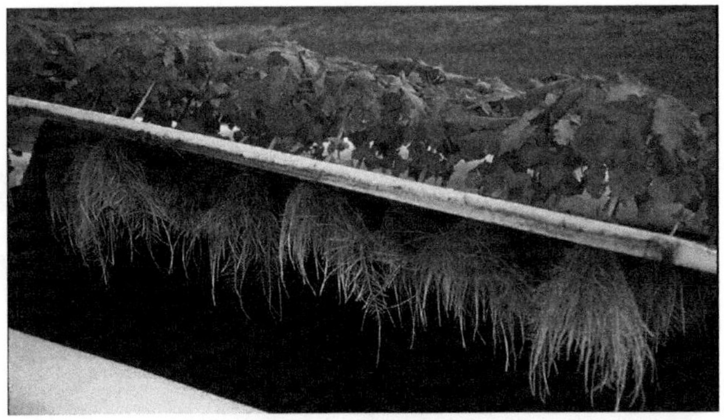

FIGURE 14.4 Growing plants with tilapia in an aquaponic system is an effective way of removing nutrients from culture water. *Photo provided by J. Rakocy.*

systems combine species of different feeding habits and trophic levels in the same aquaculture system. In this combination, the biological and chemical processes are balanced because the waste from one species can be used as food for the other(s). For example, farming tilapia and prawns in polyculture system can be an efficient way of nutrient removal and improving water quality. They have different feeding habits and special distribution and thus can behave synergistically. In a polyculture system, tilapia consume artificial feed and natural foods, while prawns can eat tilapia wastes and unused tilapia feed. In addition, prawn bioturbation at the pond bottom brings the nutrients back to the water column and enhances phytoplankton production, which in turn increases natural food availability for tilapia. In this regard, David et al. (2017a) found that the levels of phosphorus retained from tilapia/prawn IMTA system were higher (20%–28%) than in tilapia and prawn monocultures (10%–20% and 10%–13%, respectively). The same authors (David et al., 2017b) suggested that the integration of Nile tilapia and Amazon River prawn in stagnant ponds may remove significant amounts of nitrogen from nutrient-rich water and could be considered as a mitigation tool. These results clearly indicate that IMTA systems can be used in mitigation programs for aquatic environments receiving high levels of nutrients, especially phosphorus and nitrogen.

In-pond raceway system (IPRS) (Fig. 14.5) can be an excellent model for nutrient removal or recovery. In this system, one fish species is raised in raceways installed inside an earthen pond and fed with high-quality feed. Another species (or more) is stocked in the rest of the pond, mainly for water quality improvement, since it depends on the wastes of the raceways for feeding (see Chapter 13, Section 13.10.4 for more details on IPRS). Brown et al. (2012) raised channel catfish (*Ictalurus punctatus*) in in-pond raceways, while Nile tilapia and paddlefish (*Polyodon spathula*) were co-cultured in the pond where the raceways were installed. The harvest of Nile tilapia and

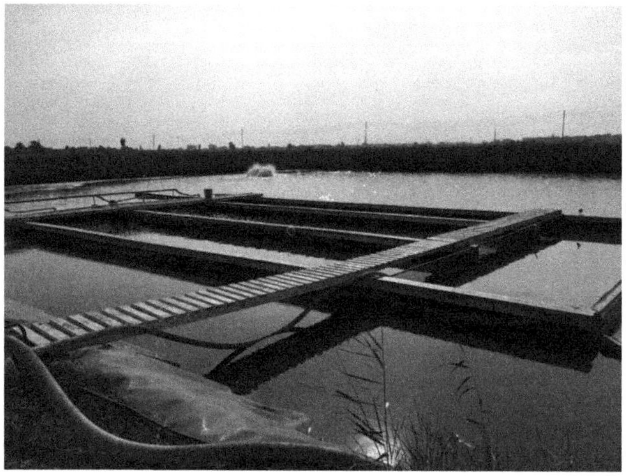

FIGURE 14.5 Growing Nile tilapia in in-pond raceways at the World-Fish Center, Abbassa, Sharkya Governorate, Egypt. *Photograph by A.-F.M. El-Sayed.*

paddlefish increased phosphorus and nitrogen recovery/removal by 47.5% and 40%.

14.7.6 Reducing environmental impacts through best aquaculture management practices

In addition to the technical and practical measures that should be adopted to reduce the adverse impacts of aquaculture, the BAMPs can play a significant role in preventing these adverse effects. BAMPs in aquaculture can be defined as 'the application of good management practices to support sustainable aquaculture growth, with minimum risks to the environment, through the adoption of cost-effective and continually assessed management measures' (White et al., 2018). A number of recent documents have been published on the effects of BAMPs on aquaculture performance (tilapia included) including the following:

- Better management practices for tilapia aquaculture (WWF, 2011);
- *On-farm Feeding and Feed Management in Aquaculture* (Hasan and New, 3013). This publication included 6 case studies/reviews on 'On-farm feed management practices for Nile tilapia (*Oreochromis niloticus*)' in six countries (China, Egypt, Ghana, Malaysia, the Philippines and Thailand).
- Pilot application of selected aquaculture planning and management tools in Indonesia, Thailand and Vietnam (FAO, 2018);
- Better management practices for feed production and management of Nile tilapia and milkfish in the Philippines (White et al., 2018).

This is in addition to several papers published in different specialized journals on the best management practices (BMPs) of tilapia culture and their social, economic and environmental effects.

A number of examples are provided on the adoption of the BAMPs in tilapia culture and their effects on environmental performance and disease reduction. In Thailand, for example, cage culture of Nile tilapia has been widely practised in many natural freshwater environments over the past decade. This practice has led to a rapid increase in the number of tilapia cages and has also created many social, economic and environmental problems. These problems are listed in Section 14.3.

These sequences demonstrate the urgent need for ECCA tool for tilapia planning as a means for BMPs for tilapia cage culture in Thailand. This assessment tool will help to establish the correct number of cages that would allow the most sustainable farming practice, with highest performance and lowest adverse impacts.

Another interesting example, also in Thailand, is the spreading of diseases due to the expansion of tilapia cage culture in Chainat Province and the role of BAMPs in reducing their risk impacts. Several irrigation projects have recently been developed in this province for agricultural development, and aquaculture as well, especially cage culture in the Noi River. As a result, the number of tilapia cage farms has rapidly increased, leading to significant adverse impacts, including disease occurrence due to the changes in the environment, water quality, high fish density, inappropriate farm management and the lack of control of fish disease/pathogens (FAO, 2018). To face this problem, a farm biosecurity plan has been developed and put in place to describe the measures and actions that should be followed to protect farms from diseases. These measures should be able to reduce the risks and impacts of disease outbreaks and prevent health issues emerging within the cage farms. To maximize its benefits, the farm-level biosecurity plan should be piloted and disseminated to fish farmers, hatcheries and other concerned stakeholders.

A field implementation of the farm-level biosecurity plan tool included the following: (1) providing training for 25 selected farmers; (2) the biosecurity plan for each farm was adopted; (3) the biosecurity plan was adopted by 25 selected cage tilapia farms; (4) on-farm implementation of the biosecurity plan was strictly monitored for 3 months, with continuous data collection and (5) a national evaluation was conducted. The results showed that trained farmers had a better understanding about fish diseases and their prevention. Farmers are now able to check cages and collect dead fish from cages daily and no longer throw the dead fish into the river. They also record the necessary farm information such as date, fish size and number at stocking, the daily amount of feed provided and fish mortality. This would certainly lead to a reduction of overfeeding and minimizing the accumulation of feed waste and losses.

The adoption of best on-farm feed and feeding management would certainly lead to a reduction in wasted feed and fish waste, better growth and feed utilization, lower organic and inorganic loads in aquaculture effluents and in turn, lower environmental impacts. The following feed and feeding practices should be adopted to improve feed efficiency and reduce the amount of waste entering the environment (see Hasan and New, 2013; White et al., 2018 for details):

- Relevant practical knowledge and skills in feed and feeding should be gained.
- The best available ingredients should be used for feed production.
- Species-specific feeds containing the correct nutrient requirements should be developed, with good pellet integrity, shape, density and water stability.
- The most appropriate feed type (floating vs. sinking pellets), feeding methods (manual feeding, demand feeder, automatic feeder), feeding levels (percent body weight, ad libitum, satiation) and feeding frequencies should be used.
- Farmers, farm managers, hatchery operators and feeding staff should be trained on the most appropriate on-farm feed handling, storage and use.
- Water quality should be monitored continuously.
- Appropriate initial fish stocking number and size should be used.

14.8 Closing remarks

1. The introductions and/or transfers of tilapia can be unsuccessful, successful or successful but with environmental impacts ranging from habitat destruction, hybridization with endemic species, to disappearance of native species. Full details on the environmental impacts of tilapia introductions are provided in Chapter 3.
2. Varying amounts of uneaten feed, fish wastes, organic matter, nutrients such as phosphorus and nitrogen, hormones and bioactive compounds are released from land-based and cage culture of tilapia. If these wastes are not removed or treated, they will adversely affect the environmental impacts, produce anaerobic conditions that stress and/or kill the fish.
3. The public criticism concerning the use of steroid hormones for sex reversal in tilapia is increasing because hormone residues and metabolites can pose health and environmental impacts.
4. Various techniques, including effluent management, green water tank culture, planting rooted plants, aquaponic systems and IMTA systems have been successfully used for reducing environmental impacts of tilapia culture.
5. The BAMPs should be adopted for minimizing nutrient loads in tilapia effluents and reducing their environmental impacts. The adoption of best feed and feeding management will lead to a reduction in wasted feed and fish waste, better growth and feed utilization, lower organic and inorganic loads in aquaculture effluents and, in turn, will lower the overall environmental impacts.

References

Abery, N.W., Sukadi, F., Budhiman, A.A., Kartamihardja, E.S., Koeshendrajana, S., Buddhiman, et al., 2005. Fisheries and cage culture of three reservoirs in West Java, Indonesia; a case study of ambitious development and resulting interactions. Fisheries Management and Ecology 12, 315–330.

Abucay, J.S., Mair, G.C., Skibinski, D.O.F., Beardmore, J.A., 1997. The occurrence of incidental sex reversal in *Oreochromis niloticus* L. In: Fitzsimmons, K. (Ed.), Tilapia Aquaculture, Proceedings from the Fourth International Symposium on Tilapia in Aquaculture. Orlando, FL, USA, pp. 729–738.

ADB (Asian Development Bank), 2005. An Evaluation of Small-Scale Freshwater Rural Aquaculture Development for Poverty Reduction. Operations Evaluation Department, Asian Development Bank, Manila, Philippines, pp. 164.

Aura, C.M., Musa, S., Yongo, E., Okechi, J.K., Njiru, J.M., Ogari, Z., et al., 2018. Integration of mapping and socio-economic status of cage culture: towards balancing lake-use and culture fisheries in Lake Victoria, Kenya. Aquaculture Research 49, 532–545.

Berg, H., Michélsen, P., Troell, M., Folke, C., Kautsky, N., 1996. Managing aquaculture for sustainability in tropical Lake Kariba, Zimbabwe. Ecological Economics 18, 141–159.

Boyd, C.E., 2003. Guidelines for aquaculture effluent management at the farm level. Aquaculture 226, 101–112.

Brown, T.W., Boyd, C.E., Chappell, J.A., 2012. Approximate water and chemical budgets for an experimental, in-pond raceway system. Journal of the World Aquaculture Society 43, 526–537.

Contreras-Sánchez, W.M., Fitzpatrick, M.S., Schreck, C.B., 2001. Fate of methyltestosterone in the pond environment: detection of MT in pond soil from a CRSP site. In: Gupta, A., McElwee, K., Burke, D., Burright, J., Cummings, X., Egna, H. (Eds.), Eighteenth Annual Technical Report. Pond Dynamics/Aquaculture CRSP, Oregon State University, Corvallis, OR, USA, pp. 79–82.

Contreras-Sánchez, W.M., Couturrier, G.M., Schreck, C.B., 2002. Fate of methyltestosterone in the pond environment: use of MT in earthen ponds with no record of hormone usage. In: McElwee, K., Lewis, K., Nidiffer, M., Buitrago, P. (Eds.), Nineteenth Annual Technical Report. Pond Dynamics/Aquaculture CRSP, Oregon State University, Corvallis, Oregon, USA, pp. 103–106.

David, G.S., Carvalho, E.D., Lemos, D., Silveira, A.N., Dall'Aglio-Sobrinho, M., 2015. Ecological carrying capacity for intensive tilapia (*Oreochromis niloticus*) cage aquaculture in a large hydroelectrical reservoir in Southeastern Brazil. Aquacultural Engineering 66, 30–40.

David, F.S., Proença, D.C., Valenti, W.C., 2017a. Phosphorus budget in integrated multitrophic aquaculture systems with Nile tilapia,

Oreochromis niloticus, and Amazon River prawn, *Macrobrachium amazonicum*. Journal of the World Aquaculture Society 48, 402–414.

David, F.S., Proença, D.C., Valenti, W.C., 2017b. Nitrogen budget in integrated aquaculture systems with Nile tilapia and Amazon River prawn. Aquaculture International 25, 1733–1746.

Edwards, P., 2015. Aquaculture environment interactions: past, present and likely future trends. Aquaculture 447, 2–14.

El-Sayed, A.-F.M., 2017. Social and economic performance of tilapia farming in Egypt. In: Cai, J., Quagrainie, K.K., Hishamunda, N. (Eds.), Social and Economic Performance of Tilapia Farming in Africa. FAO Fisheries and Aquaculture Circular No. 1130. FAO, Rome, pp. 1–48.

FAO (Food and Agriculture Organization of the United Nations), 2018. Pilot Application of Selected Aquaculture Planning and Management Tools in Indonesia, Thailand and Viet Nam. Bangkok. pp. 121 Licence: CC BY-NC-SA 3.0 IGO.

FAO (Food and Agriculture Organization of the United Nations), 2019. Global Aquaculture Production, pp. 1950–2017. http://www.fao.org/fishery/statistics/global-aquaculture-production/query/en.

GESAMP (IMO/FAO/Unesco/WMO/WHO/IAEA/UN/UNEP (Joint Group of Experts on the Scientific Aspects of Marine Pollution, 1991. Reducing Environmental Impacts of Coastal Aquaculture. Reports and Studies No. 47. GESAMP, Rome, Italy, pp. 35.

Gomelsky, B., Cherfas, N.B., Peretz, Y., Ben-Dom, N., Hulata, G., 1994. Hormonal sex inversion in the common carp (*Cyprinus carpio* L.). Aquaculture 126, 265–270.

Green, B.W., Teichert-Coddington, D.R., 2000. Human food safety and environmental assessment of the use of 17α-methyltestosterone to produce male tilapia in the United States. Journal of the World Aquaculture Society 31, 337–357.

Hasan, M.R., New, M.B., 2013. On-farm Feeding and Feed Management in Aquaculture. In: FAO Fisheries and Aquaculture Technical Paper No. 583. FAO, Rome, pp. 585.

Homklin, S., Wattanodorn, T., Ong, S.K., Limpiyakorn, T., 2009. Biodegradation of 17α- methyltestosterone and isolation of MT-degrading bacterium from sediment of Nile tilapia masculinization pond. Water Science and Technology 59, 261–265.

Homklin, S., Ong, S.K., Limpiyakorn, T., 2012. Degradation of 17α-methyltestosterone by *Rhodococcus* sp. and *Nocardioides* sp. isolated from a masculinizing pond of Nile tilapia fry. Journal of Hazardous Materials 221–222, 35–44.

Kashindye, B.B., Nsinda, P., Kayanda, R., Ngupula, G.W., Mashafi, C.A., Ezekiel, C.N., 2015. Environmental impacts of cage culture in Lake Victoria: the case of Shirati Bay-Sota, Tanzania. SpringerPlus 4, 475. https://doi.org/10.1186/s40064-015-1241-y.

Lin, C.K., Yi, Y., 2003. Minimizing environmental impacts of freshwater aquaculture and reuse of pond effluents and mud. Aquaculture 226, 57–68.

Lin, C.K., Shrestha, M.K., Yi, Y., Diana, J.S., 2001. Management to minimize the environmental impacts of pond effluent: harvest draining techniques and effluent quality. Aquacultural Engineering 25, 125–135.

Ling, M.-P., Hsu, H.-T., Shie, R.-H., Wu, C.-C., Hong, Y.-S., 2009. Health risk of consuming heavy metals in farmed tilapia in central Taiwan. Bulletin of Environmental Contamination and Toxicology 83, 558–564.

Megbowon, I., Mojekwu, T.O., 2014. Tilapia sex reversal using methyl testosterone (MT) and its effect on fish, man and environment. Biotechnology 13, 213–216.

Mlalila, N., Mahika, C., Kalombo, L., Swai, H., Hilonga, A., 2015. Human food safety and environmental hazards associated with the use of methyltestosterone and other steroids in production of all-male tilapia. Environmental Science and Pollution Research 22, 4922–4931.

Njiru, J.M., Aura, C.M., Okechi, J.K., 2018. Cage fish culture in Lake Victoria: a boon or a disaster in waiting? Fisheries Management and Ecology 1–9. https://doi.org/10.1111/fme.12283.

Pandian, T., Kirankumar, S., 2003. Recent advances in hormonal induction of sex-reversal in fish. Journal of Applied Aquaculture 13, 205–230.

Rico, A., Oliveira, R., McDonough, S., Matser, A., Khatikarn, J., Satapornvanit, K., et al., 2014. Use, fate and ecological risks of antibiotics applied in tilapia cage farming in Thailand. Environmental Pollution 191, 8–16.

Santiago, A.E., 1994. The ecological impact of tilapia cage culture in Sampaloc Lake, Philippines. In: Chou, L.M., Munro, A.D., Lam, T.J., Chen, T.W., Cheong, L.K.K., Ding, J.K., et al. (Eds.), The Third Asian Fisheries Forum. Proceedings of the Third Asian Fisheries Forum, 26–30 October 1992, Singapore. Asian Fisheries Society, Manila, Philippines, pp. 413–416.

Santiago, A.E., Arcilla, R.P., 1993. Tilapia cage culture and the dissolved oxygen trends in Sampaloc Lake, the Philippines. Environmental Monitoring and Assessment 24, 243–255.

Troell, M., Berg, H., 1997. Cage fish farming in the tropical Lake Kariba, Zimbabwe: impact and biogeochemical changes in sediment. Aquaculture Research 28, 527–544.

White, P.G., Shipton, T.A., Bueno, P.B., Hasan, M.R., 2018. Better Management Practices for Feed Production and Management of Nile Tilapia and Milkfish in the Philippines. In: FAO Fisheries and Aquaculture Technical Paper No. 614. FAO, Rome, pp. 98.

WWF (World Wildlife Fund), 2011. Better Management Practices for Tilapia Aquaculture: A Tool to Assist with Compliance to the International Standards for Responsible Tilapia Aquaculture. World Wildlife Fund, Inc. Version 1, pp. 54.

Yap, C.K., Jusoh, A., Leong, W.J., Karami, A., Ong, G.H., 2015. Potential human health risk assessment of heavy metals via the consumption of tilapia *Oreochromis mossambicus* collected from contaminated and uncontaminated ponds. Environmental Monitoring and Assessment 187, 584.

Yi, Y., Lin, C.K., Diana, J.S., 2002. Recycling pond mud nutrients in integrated lotus-fish culture. Aquaculture 212, 213–226.

Index

'*Note:* Page numbers followed by "t" indicate tables and "f" indicate figures.'

C

M

N

O

P

R

S

9780128165096